THE UNIQUE HERBAL

NEW INSIGHTS INTO ANCIENT MEDICINES

VOLUME FIVE (S-Z)

ROBERT DALE ROGERS (RH) AHG

CONTENTS

ARBUTUS 189

BALMONY. 180

BEARBERRY. 189

BLUE DEVIL. 225

BROOKLIME 96

BUCKBRUSH 64

BUTTER AND EGGS. 166

CALLA LILY 231

CANKER ROOT. 118

CHAFFWEED 13

CHELONE 180

CORALBERRY. 64

COSTMARY 154

CULVER ROOT 96

FALSE CARAWAY. 261

FRINGE CUPS. 9

GAYWINGS 77

HOLY GRASS 149

INDIAN CURRANT 64

JERUSALEM ARTICHOKE 121

JUNE BERRY. 1

LADY'S SLIPPER 263

LEPTANDRA 96

MARSH ROSEMARY. 118

MILKWORT 77

PACIFIC MADRONE. 189

PARACRESS 110

SASKATOON 1

SAXIFRAGE 8

SCARLET PIMPERNEL 13

SEA BUCKTHORN 21

SEA LAVENDER 118

SELF HEAL. 32

SENECA SNAKEROOT 77

SHEPHERD'S PURSE. 43

SHINLEAF 245

SINGLE DELIGHT 245

SKELETON WEED 53

SKUNK CABBAGE 55

SNAKEROOT, BLACK 84

SNAPDRAGON 166

SNEEZEWEED 60

SNOOPY FLOWER 77

SNOWBERRY 64

SNOWDROP. 90

SOW THISTLE 69

SPEEDWELL. 96

SPILANTHES 110

STAR OF BETHLEHEM 115

STATICE 118

SUNFLOWER 121

SWEET CICELY 142

SWEETGRASS. 149

TANSY 154

TELESONIX 8

TOADFLAX 166

TOOTHACHE PLANT. 110

TULIP. 173

TUMBLEWEED 177

TURTLEHEAD 180

TWINFLOWER 187

VIOLET. 204

VIPER'S BUGLOSS 225

WATER ARUM 231

WATER CARPET 9

WATER PLANTAIN 234

iii

WILD RICE 239
WINTERGREEN 77
WOLFBERRY 64
WOOD NYMPH 245
WOOD SORREL 253
WOUNDWORT 32
YAMPA 261
ZINNIA 271

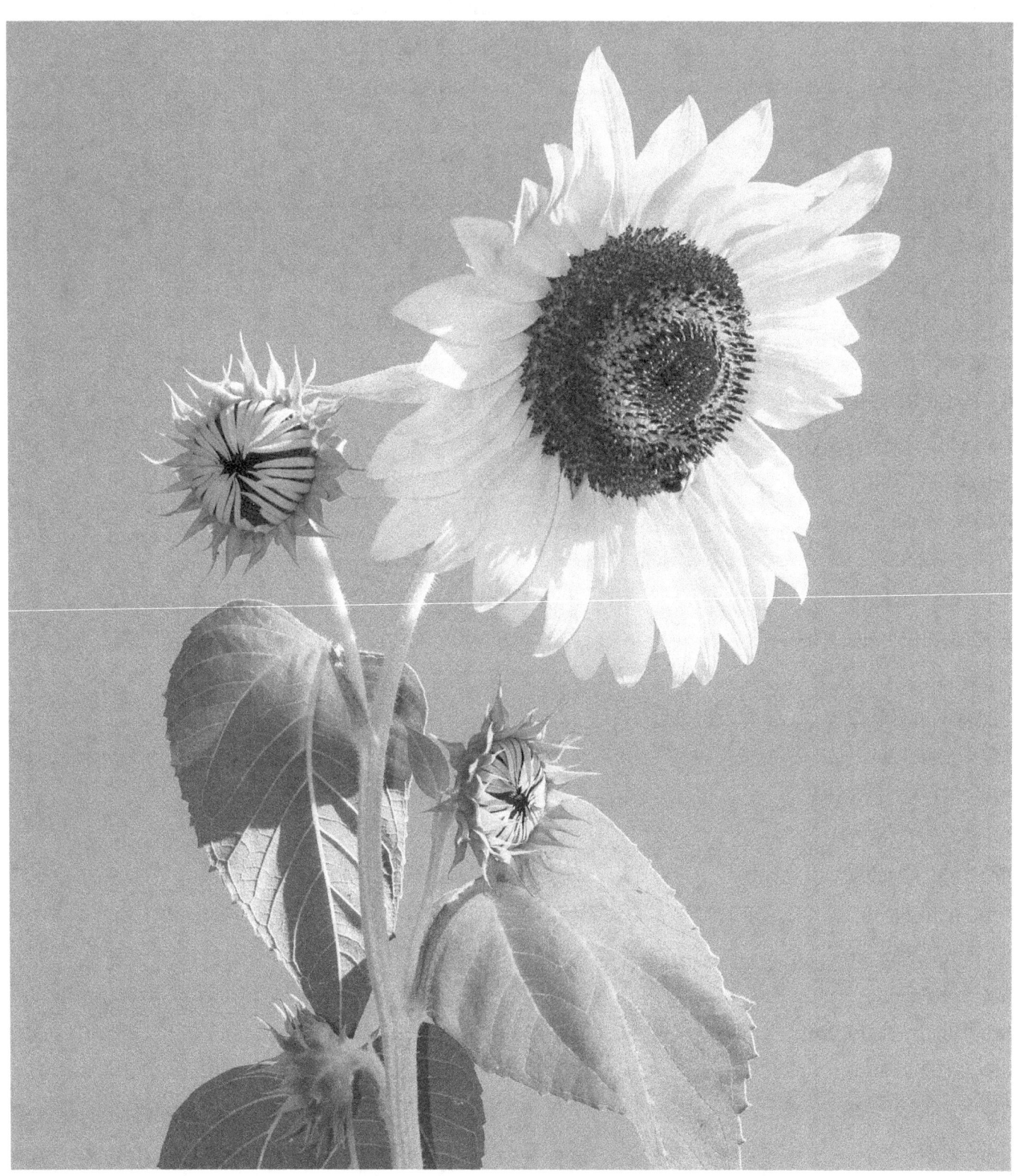

INTRODUCTION

Over the years,I have accumulated some information, a bit of knowledge and even a little wisdom about medicinal plants.

Many of the healing herbs in this volume set are relatively unknown; and some are little used in day-to-day clinical practice. Some are well known, but not utilized to their full extent of possibilities.

It is my hope that these pages may lead to a new and expanded materia medica, and a wider appreciation of many, often neglected, overlooked, and useful medicinal plants.

North American herbals tend to repeat, with increasingly useful additions, the same hundred or so plant medicines. The purpose of this book is to expand that awareness and hope that other herbalists will begin to look at the plants in their backyard and explore, observe and experience for themselves.

In turn, we could reconnect and continue the work begun in past centuries by the Eclectics and other plant people.

Like some of my previous publications, this book records indigenous use of medicinal herbs, garnered respectfully from the oral tradition, as well as work by various cultures around the world, the Eclectic physicians, modern herbalists, and recent scientific findings on various plant constituents.

It also includes homeopathic usage, essential oils, hydrosols, gemmotherapy, flower essences, personality traits, spiritual properties and astrological correspondences.

Please contact me if you wish to contribute;I am always learning.

Some Other Books by Robert Dale Rogers - www.amazon.com/author/robertdalerogers

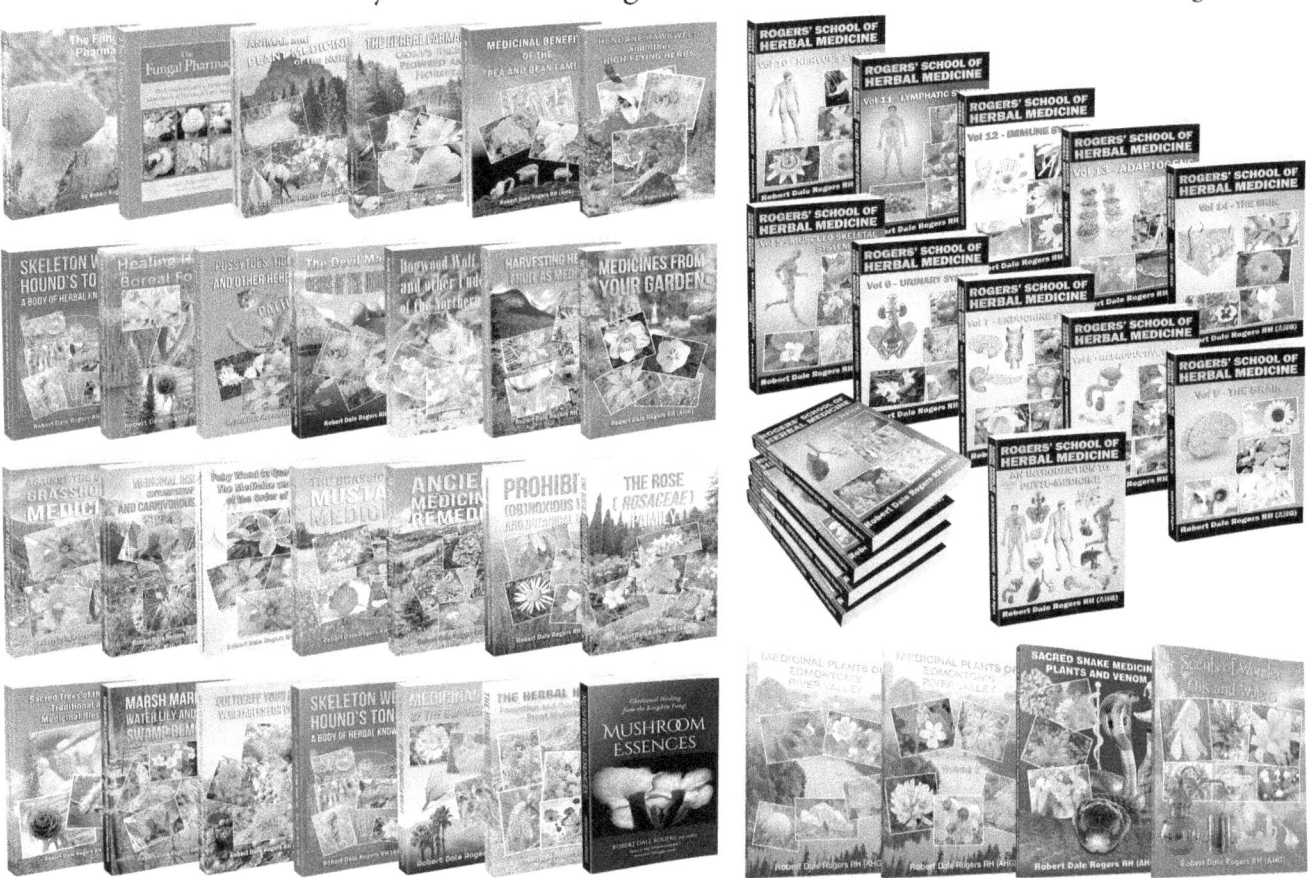

www.selfhealdistributing.com or www.scentsofwonder.ca - email: scents@telusplanet.net - Fax: 1 780-439-9540

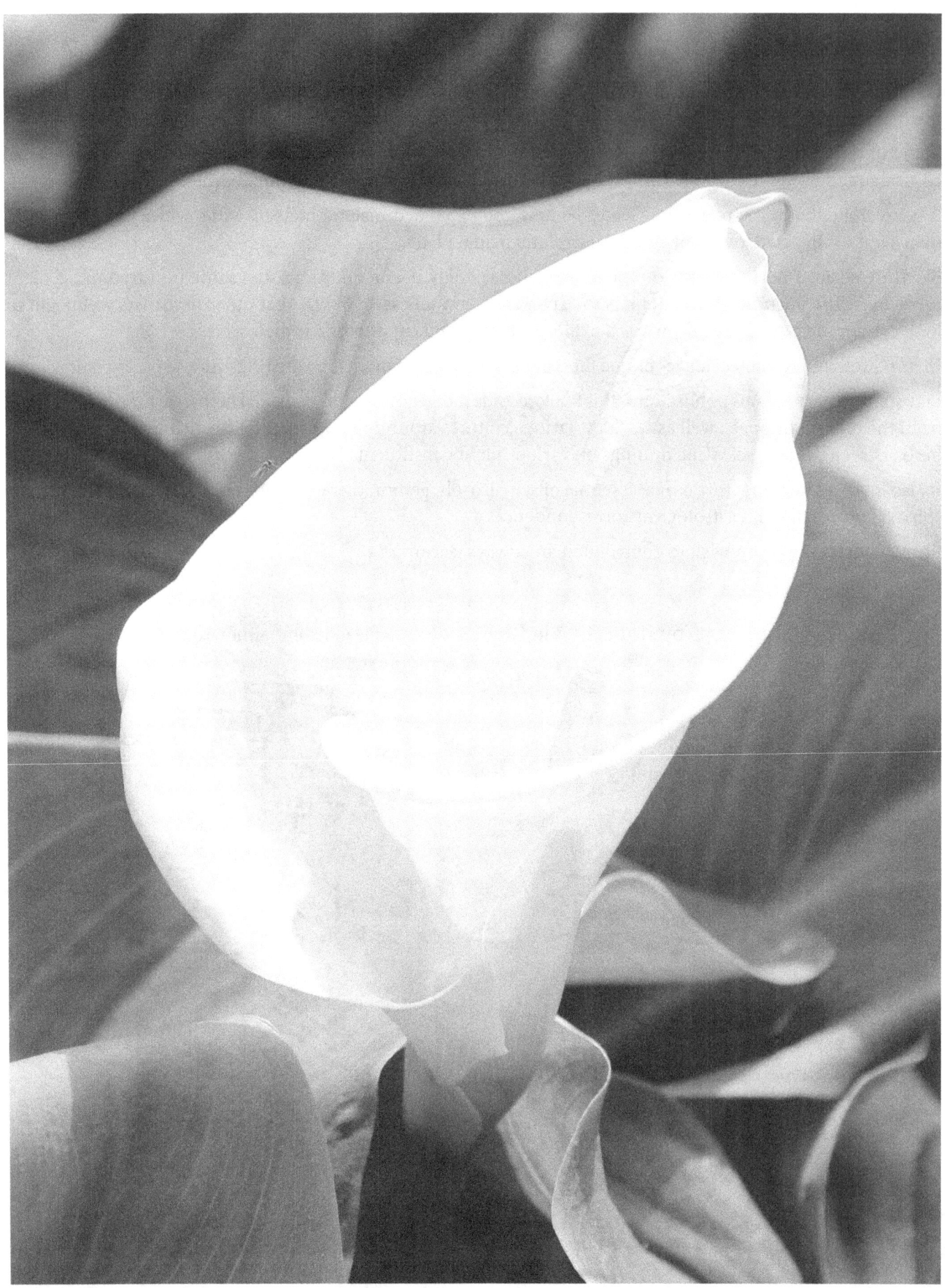

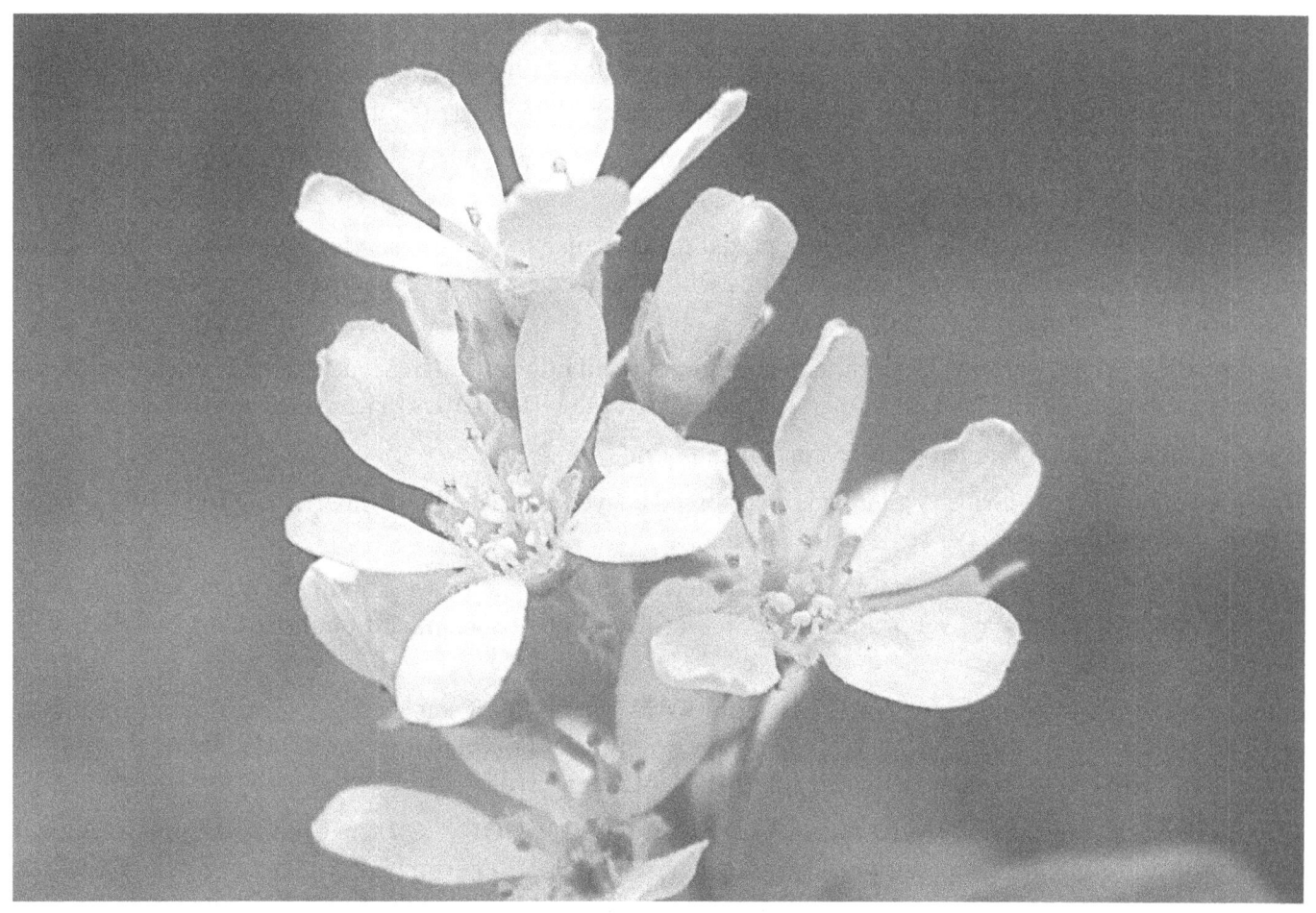

SASKATOON FLOWERS

SASKATOON
SERVICE BERRY
JUNE BERRY
(*Amelanchier alnifolia* [Nutt.] Nutt. ex M. Roem)
(*Aronia alnifolia* Nutt.) not accepted
CANADIAN SERVICE BERRY
(*A. canadensis* [L.] Medik)
PARTS USED- berry, flower, bark

Budding, the service tree, white
Almost as white beam, threw
From the under of leaf upright
Flecks like a showering show.

G. MEREDITH

Amelanchier is derived from local French name for related *A. ovalis* in region of Savoy. Alnifolia derives from Latin **ALNUS** for alder; and **FOLIUM** for leaf, presumably due to their similar appearance. Unfortunately they don't look similar.

Serviceberry originates from use of the snow-white flowers for Easter Sunday service by Puritans. It was traditionally called a service tree, a corruption of cerevisia, because a kind of ale was brewed from the berries. I believe there is a more likely origin. Early pioneer families had to wait until spring to bury their dead, and the early white blossoms were used to cover the grave, and this was the service they provided.

1

Another possibility is corruption of old botanical name Sorbus, formerly applied to the genus. Who knows for sure!

Saskatoon appears to originate from the Cree name **MIS-SASK-WA-TOOMIN**, or **SASKAHTÔMINA** meaning "tree of many branches or wood"; or "big berry". Early settlers then shortened it to the present name.

The beautiful city of Saskatoon derived its name from the profusion of berry producing trees in its river valley. The Chipewyan call the tree **KIN JIE.**

The berries, or pome fruit to be correct, are prized for their use in pies, preserves, ale and wine. The Native tribes of Alberta stored them for winter use, along with chokecherries, and blueberries. And of course, it is still a favorite winter browse of moose, deer and elk.

Traditionally, the fruit was sun-dried, either whole, or pounded into patties. In Montana, the Flathead powdered the leaves of bergamot and field mint, then sprinkled it over the fruit patties to keep flies away while drying.

These saskatoon loaves weighed up to ten or fifteen pounds.

The Gitksan of northern British Columbia often spread a layer of crushed bunchberries on top of the berries, **GYAM**, before rolling, to better stick them together.

The dried fruit was used in various ways. It was added to stews, or mixed with flour, sugar and water to make sweet puddings, after the arrival of Europeans. It was used in pemmican, and pounded into buffalo, elk or moose meat and fat.

Pemmican may be from the Cree **PIMII**, "fat", and **KAN** "prepared". It was usually prepared from wild meat dried and braised over a fire. The Blackfoot name for dripping fat or lard is similar, **POMIS**. The Cree word, in particular, is remarkably similar to the Greek **PIMELE** meaning lard or fat.

The Blackfoot call the shrub **OKO-NOK**, and the berry **OO-COO-NOO-KEN**. They made a sausage of animal fat and iron and copper-rich Saskatoon pomes. They were placed on a perforated skin, out of reach of children and animals. When dry, they were mixed with fat and stored in hide bags made of fetal deer or mountain sheep. The berries were combined with fat and stuffed into animal intestines tied at each end. This was then boiled and eaten like sausage.

They made a dye from the dark berry juice. The young Blackfoot girls played a game while gathering the berries. After some harvesting, they would sit together and hold their breath while another called out "tops, tops, tops" at a regular beat.

Each girl then put a berry in her bag for every call and the one who held her breath the longest, won all the other girl's berries.

The Blackfoot used Saskatoon blossoms to symbolize spring, when performing the tobacco planting ceremony. The berry juice was used for the relief of earaches.

Even the leaves were crushed and mixed with blood, dried and used to make richer broth for winter soups. The leaves were combined with dry chokecherry cambium as tea for nursing mothers with a colicky baby.

The neighboring Blackfeet from Montana used the leaf and twig tea for high blood sugar. Recent work has found potent intestinal alpha glucosidase inhibition, and delayed absorption of carbohydrates, similar to drug Acarbose. Zhang AJ et al, *J Ethnopharm* 2012 143(2): 481-7.

The Blood tribe cooked the fruit for stomach and liver trouble.

The hard, weighty, straight and flexible stems were prized for arrow shafts.

They were first soaked in warm water and bitten with teeth, to break the fibre and prevent warping. The stems were fire-hardened to preserve their shape and strength.

It was used for tipi stakes, closure pins, digging implements, spears, bows and canoe cross pieces.

The wood is hard, straight and tough, and by heating over a fire, can be bent and twisted while still hot. When the first voyageurs saw arrows made from Saskatoon wood they call the tree **BOIS DE FLECHE.**

Spring and summer bark can be made into cordage, possessing about the same strength as Wolf Willow.

When saskatoon branches were cut, the shoots next year were just right for basket rim hoops. Then, a couple of years later, the fruit quantity and quality related to this "pruning".

The Wood Cree of Saskatchewan used the root as an ingredient in decoctions for teething, chest pain, coughs, lung infections and to prevent miscarriage. Other tribes used the inner bark to control menstrual flow and as a strengthening tonic during and after childbirth. The roots and stems were decocted for treating tuberculosis, while the root was used for coughs, colds, and lung infections.

Muscle spasms and pinched nerves causing temporary back "paralysis", benefitted from root decoctions.

The buds were best boiled for diarrhea, while the branch bark was decocted for pleurisy and inflammatory diseases.

They combined snowberry and saskatoon stem bark in decoction to induce sweating and treat fevers.

As well, they immersed four to five pieces of barked stem sticks in boiled sturgeon oil for about ten minutes to help keep the oil fresh during storage. This natural preservative nature should be further explored.

The Dene boiled the berries and drank the liquid cool for whooping cough. The stems were decocted for urinary problems and "infection inside their waistline". The small buds were picked from the stem, crushed and boiled for headache, sore stomach and diarrhea, after it cooled down. I believe they called it **KIIACHII,** and used the stem tea when their sides were sore. The Dogrib call the tree **TCHE KI EH.**

Métis boiled the fruit of **LII POO-AIR** for eardrops. The strained water was cooled and inserted.

Other Natives place a grid of green Saskatoon sticks in the bottom of birch bark cooking baskets to prevent them from being burned through by hot rocks.

The Chippewa tribe made a decoction of the berries, bark and root for preventing miscarriage after a fall; to stop excessive menstrual bleeding; abdominal cramps; and to help smooth the menopausal transition.

The Cheyenne made a red beverage tea of the leaves, although the fruit pit and leaves contain cyanide compounds that give the benzaldehyde flavour of dried almonds. It is a pleasant and safe drink in small amounts. Sap from Manitoba maple trees was mixed in the tea when available.

The Cheyenne mashed the ripe berries and fed them to both young and old for loss of appetite, usually following an illness. The juice stimulates appetite, as well as providing valuable nourishment to the weak.

The Cheyenne name is **HE TAN I MINS** meaning male berry, and the Lakota call it **WIPANZUTKAN** in reference to something that cracks bones.

The equivalent of the month of June, called June Berry Moon, was called **WI PAZUKA WASTE WI.**

Both the Ponca and Omaha name means "gray wood", and the Winnebago call it red fruit. The Crow of southern Montana name is **BAACHUUAWUULEETE** meaning "berry without big seeds." The Navajo considered it one of the sacred Life Medicines.

Lewis and Clark reported on a type of bread made with combination of berries, pounded seeds of balsam root and lamb's quarter seeds.

The Thompson decocted dried bark to take warm internally and wash externally for ensuring the removal of afterbirth.

The dried bark was infused to stop menstruation after giving birth, and act as a form of birth control. The fresh bark is more of a tonic.

Other tribes used saskatoon and maple twig decoctions for the mother after childbirth. Decoctions of bitter cherry and saskatoon wood or stems were used for birth control.

The dried root or inner bark slows excessive menstruation, helps remove placenta, prevents miscarriage and serves as a contraceptive, suggesting multiple uses for "female" conditions.

The Okanagan considered serviceberries their most important type of berry. Nine varieties were recognized, even though botanists delineate only three varieties within Okanagan territory, according to renowned anthropologist Nancy Turner.

The Carrier of British Columbia used the bark and stems to make fish traps and baby baskets. The berries were mixed with a "flour" paste for dessert.

The Crow of Montana and Shoshone decocted the inner bark and berries as eye drops for treating snow blindness. The Iroquois planted their corn when the tree blossomed.

Mors Kochanski says that there are four plants and fungi native to Western Canada that help increase the production of endorphins. They are the diamond willow fungus, the tips of buffalo berry branches, bunchberry leaves, and saskatoon root.

He mentions that the root of the latter, when boiled, yields oil that was used in times of famine.

Cattle fed saskatoon twigs show signs of cyanide poisoning attributed to prunasin breakdown. On healthy rangeland this will not cause a problem, but only if there is nothing else to eat.

Saskatoon trees are an excellent bio-indicator of sulphur dioxide and ozone emissions. Krupa et al, in *Environmental Pollution* 2001 111:3.

Commercial saskatoon berry production on the prairies is about 3 million pounds annually. Yields of up to 10 tonnes/ha can be realized. The most popular varieties grown commercially are *Smoky, Northline* and *Thiessen*. The latter variety was discovered by Isaac Thiessen in 1902 and has large fruit, but blooms early, risking frost damage.

Recent work at Olds College by Bakowska-Barczak et al, *J Ag Food Chem* 2008 56:21 found the Nelson cultivar the highest in polyphenols and antioxidant activity.

Saskatoon Juniper rust is fungi best controlled by planting orchards at least a half-mile from any junipers.

MEDICINAL

CONSTITUENTS- berries- contain significantly higher amounts of protein, fat, fibre, calcium, magnesium, potassium, manganese, barium and aluminum; and lower contents of phosphorus and sulphur than blueberries. Main acid is malic, major sugars, fructose and glucose.
Specifically, protein 1.3 grams, vitamin C 16 mg, iron 0.96 mg, calcium 88 mg and potassium 244 mg per 100 grams.
Dry weight composition of the Smoky berry is 9.7% protein, 4.2% fat, 19% fibre, with significant amounts of iron, manganese, zinc and traces of the important molybdenum.
Energy value is also 70% higher than blueberries at 85 Ca vs. 51. Saskatoons supply nearly 34% of recommended daily allowance of manganese.
Anthocyandins, 86-125 mg/100 grams present in fresh berry, including cyanidin, pelargonidin and malvidin. Various flavanols are present including rutin, hyperoside, avicularin, quercetin. The flavonoids of the fruit comprise four glycosides, one aglycone and three caffeic acid esters. Cyanidin 3-galactoside accounts for about 61% of anthocyanins, and its 3-glycoside for another 21%. The berries contain 29 polyphenolic compounds, four anthocyanins, nine phenolic acids, nine flavonols, seven flavan-3-ols, three triperpenoids, seven carotenoids, five chlorophylls and four tocopherols. (-)-epicatechin is most abundant proanthocyanidin.
Seeds- up to 18.7% oil
Leaf- prunasin (HCN), quercitin 3-galactoside and 3-glucoside, (-)-epicatechin, chlorogenic acid.
Stem- flavanone and flavonol glycosides (55% of phenols), catechins (38%) and hydrobenzoic acid. The proanthocyanidin of stems and leaves is from 10-14%, compared to only 3% in berries. The dry stem contains from 2.2 to 6.5 mg/g of eriodictyol 7-glucoside.
A. canadensis fruit- 4.8 mg% carotenoids, 269.6 mg% ascorbic acid, 900 mg% phenol carboxylic acids, 1600 mg/kg bioflavonoids, 4% pectins, 80 mg/kg iron, 93 mg/kg manganese, 20 mg/kg zinc, 3 mg/kg copper.

Saskatoon berries (pomes), when still unripe, can be picked and used dried or fresh for diarrhea and watery stools. A decoction is made, as described below.

Of course, once the berries ripen, the fruit can be quite laxative in large quantities. The berries are high in iron and copper, both important minerals for proper red blood cell production and other metabolic functions.

When using the bark, root or berry decoctions remember to use the tea warm in the first trimester of pregnancy for preventing miscarriage. Use the tea cool to prevent hemorrhaging and menopausal symptom relief.

The cooled tea, well-strained is used for vaginal discharge due to yeast infections (*Candida albicans*), and endometriosis.

An infused tea of flowers and leaves helps alleviate nausea associated with stomach flu.

A tincture of the bark combines well with chokecherry bark in a cup of warm water every three to four hours for low energy associated with prolonged or heavy menses.

Anti-viral plant screening conducted at University of British Columbia by McCutcheon et al, showed saskatoon plant methanol extract very active against enteric bovine coronavirus. This is closely related to respiratory syncytial virus, as both are single strand RNA viruses that infect mucosal membranes. *J Ethnopharm* 1995 49 101-110.

Previous testing with water extracts of the leaves, indicated activity against gram- negative bacteria. The bark has analgesic properties, not fully understood.

The only European relative, Showy Mespilus (*A. ovalis/A. vulgaris*) has been shown in vitro to contain ACE inhibitors, or angiotensin converting enzymes. This should be further examined in our local species, as natural ACE inhibitors can be useful for lowering high blood pressure. Plant extracts of *A. ovalis* reveal anti-bacterial activity. *Phytotherapy Research* 2000 14:8.

Dr. David Kitts has studied the anti-oxidant activity of Saskatoon Berries, for the *Saskatchewan Agricultural Development Fund*, but this information is not easily available. Work by Hu et al, *Food Res Int* 2005 38 found the berries to be strong scavengers of free radicals.

The fruit flavonoids are potential inhibitors of hepatitis C protease and helicase proteins. Khan M et al, *Bioinformation* 2013 9(19): 978-82.

Fruit from the related *A. canadensis* and *A. arborea* inhibit COX-1 and COX-2, suggesting a moderation of inflammatory conditions.

Jarkko Hellstrom et al, *J Ag Food Chem* 2007 55:1 isolated procyanidin oligomers from the berries, and found they consist mainly of epicatechin units linked by B-type bonds.

Wang & Mazza found a concentrated extract inhibited nitric oxide production in macrophages, suggesting protection against inflammation and cardiovascular risk.

Work by Kraft et al, *J Ag Food Chem* 2008 56:3 found the non-polar parts of fruit inhibit aldose reductase, and moderate expression of IL-1beta, an anti-inflammatory marker.

The polar parts reduce inflammation and improve glucose uptake via insulin-like effect.

The high content of flavonoid antioxidants is responsible for the anti-inflammatory, anti-diabetic and chemo-protective effects of fruit. Jurikova T et al, *Molecules* 2013 18(10): 12571-86.

Orchard Mist Products, from Medicine Hat, will soon release Prairie Berry Ice Blast, which are frozen confections with saskatoon, black currant or blueberry juices. Antioxidants in a frozen form!

Saskatoon berry juice is very rich in proanthocyanidins, 1363mg/100 ml.

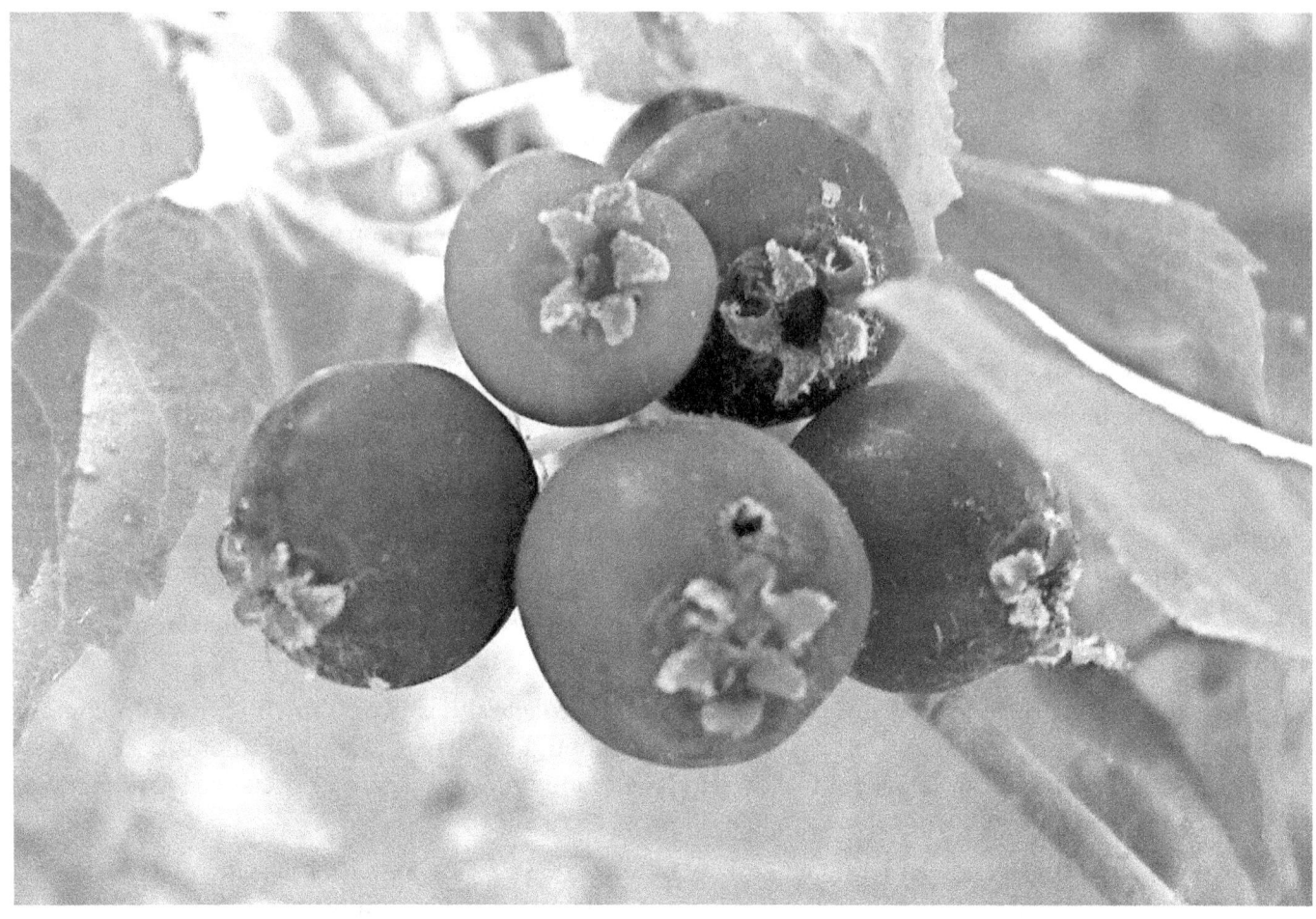

UNRIPE SASKATOON FRUIT

POME WAX

The pome is coated with an epicuticular wax, with two major components, nonacosane and nonacosan-10-ol making up half the total wax.

Other waxes include alkanes, long chain esters, primary and secondary alcohols and saturated fatty acids. Tetracosanol, hexacosanol and octacosanol decreased from young immature berry until red and then increased when purple. On the other hand, arachidyl alcohol increased in red pomes and then decreased when fruit turned purple.

SEED OIL

The seed oil varies with variety, ranging in yield from 9.4-18.7% for the cultivar Thiessen. The oil is rich in alpha tocopherol, and sterols up to 15.771 mg/gram. At least 13 triacylglycerols (TAGS) have been identified. Bakowska-Barczak et al, *J Ag Food Chem* 57:12.

HYDROSOL

A hydrosol can be prepared from Saskatoon bark and twigs. It is used for energy, especially when lost through heavy bleeding during menses. Take two drops in pint of water.

It can be used to wash infected wounds, and in larger doses internally for diarrhea.

FLOWER ESSENCES

Saskatoon flower essence is related to the soul qualities of giving thanks. It is difficult for many to think of prayer, as other than a religious ritual. Saskatoon essence can be taken to connect the inner self and the higher spirit, in a way that is free of dogma.   **PRAIRIE DEVA**

Saskatoon flower essence facilitates communication between all parts of the brain to support whole brain integration and functioning with ease.   **TREE FROG**

Saskatoon flower essence aids in co-ordinating interaction, and communication between all levels of the mind/brain.   **WILD ROSE**

LEAF ESSENCE

Snowy Mespilus (*A. canadensis*) essence can help treat infertility without discernable cause. Women should take it for up to six months. It is also useful for men in cases of low sperm count or poor motility over a similar time frame.   **FALLING LEAF**

PERSONALITY TRAITS

The Saskatoon tree is a late, but sure fruiter, bearing shining red berries as a harvest for the birds right through the winter. It means prudence.   **POWELL**

MYTHS AND LEGENDS

The Klamath natives trace their origin to this plant. In one myth, "Old Martin" caused the first people to be made from Saskatoon bushes. In the mythology of the Achomawi of northern California, Saskatoon wood and shaving were used to create humans.

Silver-Fox and Coyote lived together. Silver-Fox gathered some service-berry sticks, and whittled them down nicely, working all night. The shavings were to be made into common people; the finished sticks, into the best kind of people. About sunset the next day he was ready to make them alive. They turned into people; and Silver-Fox sent them away, some in one direction, some in another. Then he and Coyote had a big feast. Coyote wanted to imitate the deed, and so copied everything he had seen Silver-Fox do. Just as before, the sticks and shavings became people just about sunset. As soon as this happened, Coyote ran after some of the women, and after a chase caught them; but as soon as he touched them, they turned back into sticks and shavings.

RECIPES

ROOT, BERRY AND BARK DECOCTION- Take one tablespoon of berries, and two each of bark and root to two liters of boiling water. Reduce to simmer for thirty minutes.

Allow to cool.

TINCTURE- Take one part of 24 hour wilted bark to 5 parts of 40% alcohol and soak for two weeks, shaking daily. Dose is five to twenty drops as needed.

SASKATOON ALE- Place three cups of fresh saskatoons in a blender with one quart of water and puree. Slow boil with three more quarts of water for one hour, cool and strain through sieve. Add two pounds of malt extract and then add yeast at 70° F. Ferment.   **BUHNER**

PROPAGATION- In order to grow Saskatoon from seed, it is necessary to eliminate the germination inhibitors in the fruit. In nature, this is done via the digestive tract of squirrels and birds.

SAXIFRAGE AND RELATED SPECIES

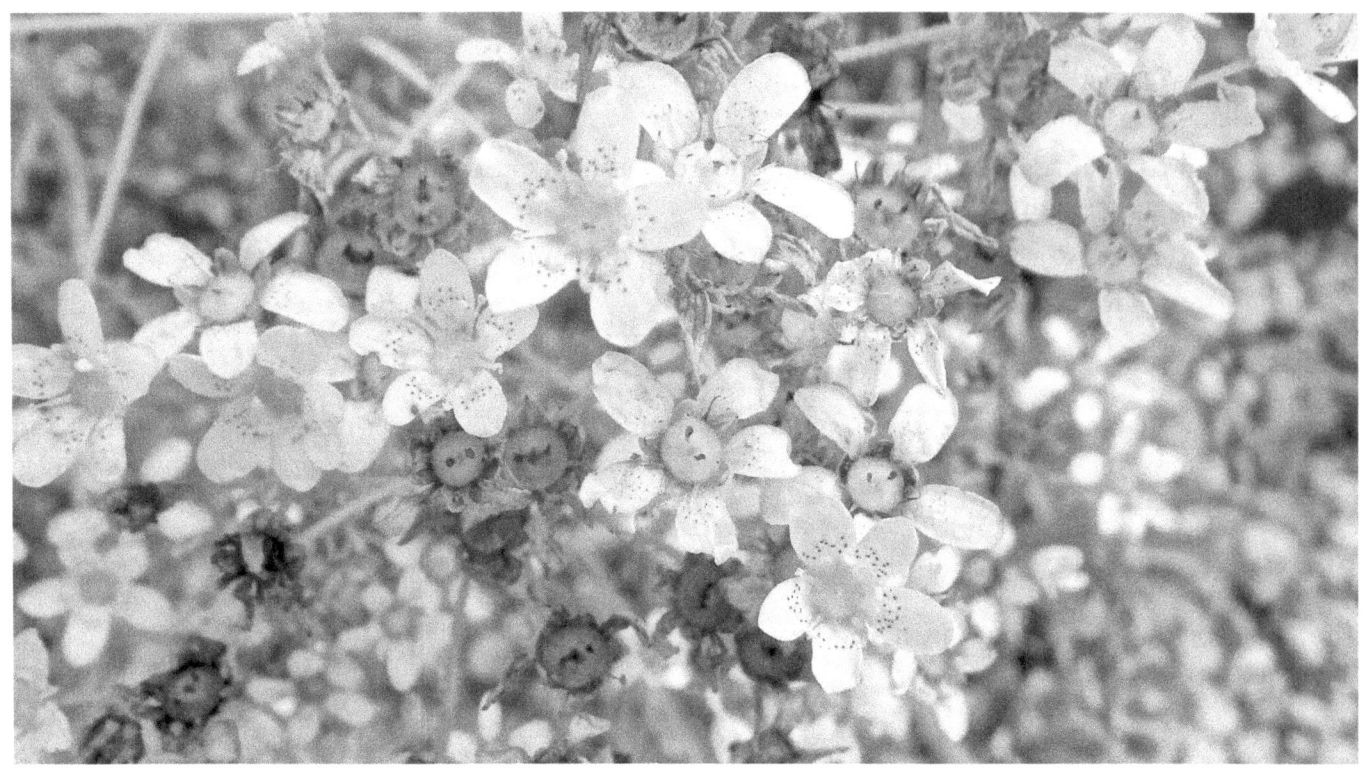

SAXIFRAGE HOSTII

STIFFSTEM SAXIFRAGE
(*Saxifraga hieraciifolia* Waldst. & Kit. ex Wild)
                                        not accepted
(*Micranthes hieracifolia* [Walkst. & Kit. ex Willd.] Haw.)
REFLEXED SAXIFRAGE
(*S. reflexa* Hook.) not accepted
(*M. reflexa* [Hook.] Small)
ALASKA SAXIFRAGE
RUSSET HAIR SAXIFRAGE
(*S. ferruginea* Graham) not accepted
(*M. ferruginea* [Graham] Brouillet & Gornall)
JENNY CAKE
(*S. arguta* auct. non D. Don) not accepted
(*M. odontoloma* [Piper] A. Heller)
HEART LEAF SAXIFRAGE
(*S. nelsoniana* D. Don) not accepted
(*M. nelsoniana* var. *nelsoniana* [D. Don] Small)
SPOTTED SAXIFRAGE
YELLOW DOT SAXIFRAGE
(*S. bronchialis* L.)
PRICKLY SAXIFRAGE
(*S. austromontana* Weigand) not accepted
(*S. bronchialis* ssp. *austromontana* [Weigand] Piper)

PURPLE SAXIFRAGE
(*S. oppositofolia* L.)
TRI-POINTED SAXIFRAGE
PRICKLY SAXIFRAGE
MOUNTAIN TOP GRASS
(*S. tricuspidata* Rottb.)
(*Leptasea tricuspidata* [Rottb.[Haw.)
STRAWBERRY BEGONIA
MOTHER OF THOUSANDS
CREEPING SAXIFRAGE
(*S. stolonifera* Meerb.)
(*S. sarmentosa* L.f.)
YELLOW MTN. SAXIFRAGE
(*S. aizoides* L.)
(*L. aizoides* [L.] Haw)
AIZOON SAXIFRAGE
(*S. aizoon* Jacq.)
(*S. paniculata* Mill.)
LEATHER LEAVED SAXIFRAGE
(*S. amplexifolia* Sternb.)
(*Leptarrhena pyrolifolia* [D. Don] R. Br. ex Ser.)
TELESONIX
HEUCHERA-LIKE BOYKINIA

8

ALUM ROOT BROOKFOAM
(*Boykinia heucheriformis* [Rybd.] Rosend.) not accepted
(*Telesonix heucheriformis* [Rybd.] Rybd.)
FRINGE CUPS
BIG FLOWER TELLIMA
(*Tellima grandiflora* [Pursh] Douglas ex Lindl.)
GREEN SAXIFRAGE
NORTHERN GOLDEN SAXIFRAGE

NORTHERN WATER CARPET
(*Chrysosplenium tetrandrum* Th. Fries)
(*C. alternifolium* var. *tetrandrum* [Th. Fr.]
                    N. Lund ex Malmgren)
GOLDEN SAXIFRAGE
(*C. iowense* Rydb.)
(*C. alternifolium* ssp. *iowense* [Rybd.] Hulten)
WATER CARPET
(*C. americanum* Schwein. ex Hook.)
PARTS USED- leaves, roots, flowers

Here's Golden Saxifrage, in vernal hours,
Springs up when water'd well by fertile showers:
It flourishes in bogs where waters beat,
The yellow flowers in clusters and complete.
Adorn'd with snowy white, in meadows low,
White Saxifrage displays a lucid show....

                                        JAMES CHAMBERS

Mary, Mary quite contrary
How does your garden grow?
With silver bells and cockleshells
And Pretty Maids, all in a row.

Saxifrage is from the Latin, **SAXUM**, meaning rock and **FRANGERE**, to break. This has two possible meanings. One is that the plant, which grows on rocks, is capable of breaking them down to soil. The other is in allusion to the medicinal benefits of the plants on kidney or gall bladder sand, gravel and stones.

Boykinia is named in honour of Samuel Boykin, an American physician and botanist who lived in Georgia in the early 19th century.

Tellima is an anagram of Mitella, its first genus designation. Grandiflora means large flowered. Bronchialis refers to its use for bronchitis.

Chrysosplenium is from the Greek **CHRYSOS** meaning gold, and **SPLENE**, for spleen, due to the spleen shaped flowers. Tetrandrum refers to the four lobed calyx and stamen. Iowense refers to Iowa, possibly the first site of discovery.

Pretty maids is another name for the European Meadow Saxifrage (*S. granulata*).

The plants leaves were believed to resemble the human spleen, and of course, good for diseases of that organ, according to the doctrine of signatures.

Saxifrage, like other wild plants, has sticky, hairy stems that discourage ants and other walking insects from robbing pollen and nectar.

Saxifrage was suggested by Hildegard de Bingen, for jaundice, the seed being ground into wine. "This extinguishes the jaundice which arises from an excess of gall, often producing in a person matter as hard as stone."

In Russia, infusions of Saxifrage root were used as a contraceptive, and in 16th century Europe, the plant was used to increase flow of breast milk.

Stiff stem Saxifrage was utilized by native people for baiting traps intended for martens; often boiled with Whitlow Grass (*Draba breweri*), and bog blueberry (*V. uliginosum*).

Reflexed Saxifrage was reserved for trapping fox, often combined with Small Blacktip Groundsel, and dried fish for this exact purpose.

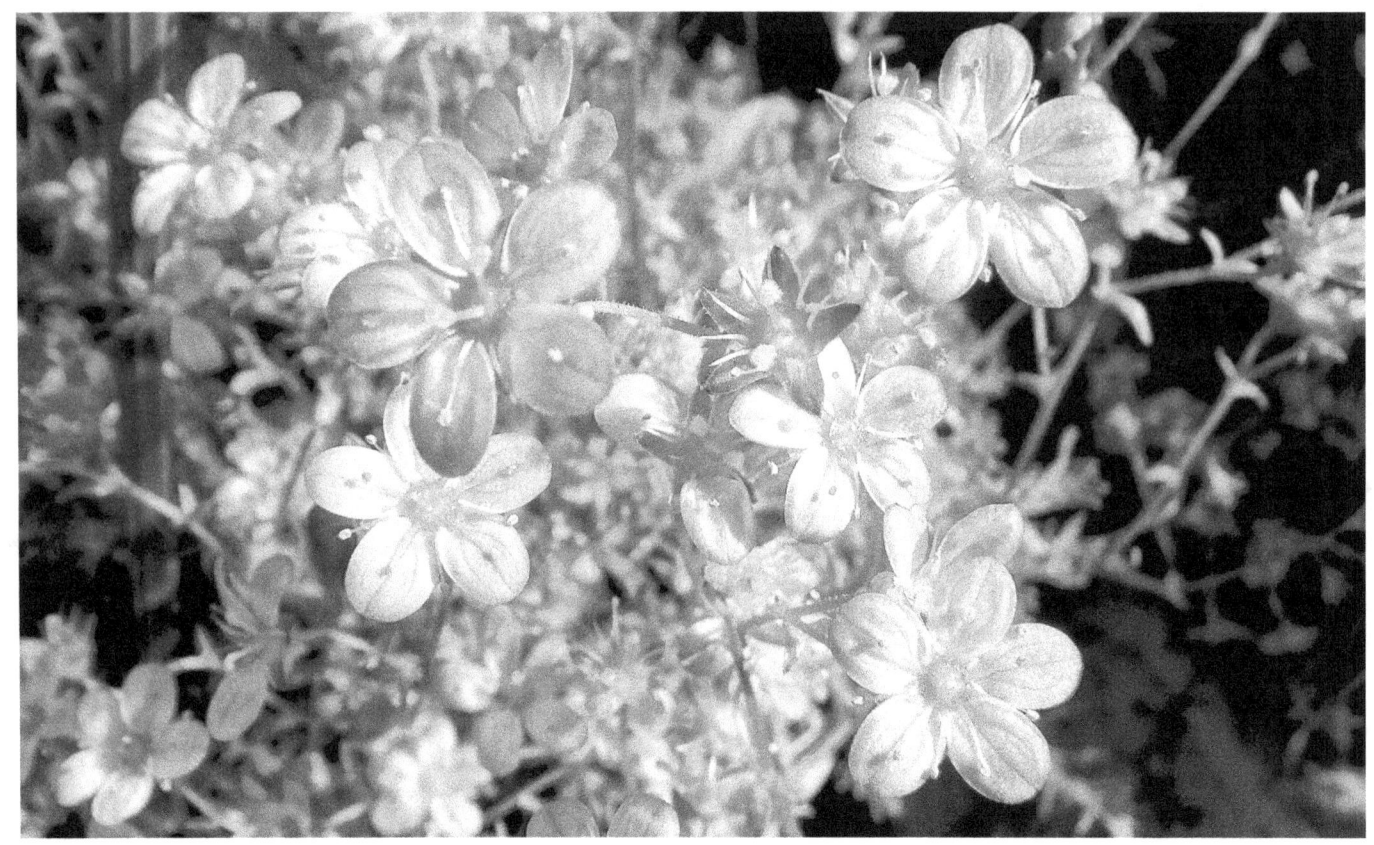

SAXIFRAGE

Alaska Saxifrage root and leaf decoctions were used by the Bella Coola to cure "strangulation of the bladder".

Purple Saxifrage is known to the Inuit of Baffin Island as **AUPILATTUNNGUAT**. Etymologically this means, "resembling something red". They are the first flower to come out in spring, which are considered quite tasty when combined with seal blubber. The leaves are used for tea. The flowers are eaten for general health, or for sickness.

The Dena'ina of Alaska call this plant **SHLUJEGA**, meaning my claw, due to the arrangement of small, opposite leaves close together in four rows.

Strawberry Begonia (*S. stolonifera*) is an introduced hardy, perennial from south-east Asia. In Japan, the leaves of Saxifrage species are made into tea, or into tempura fritters.

Various cosmetic products, produced by Revlon, contain this plant extracts, including Even Out Makeup Cream, Concealer, Makeup Natural Tan, and Foundation.

Aizoon Saxifrage is introduced into rock gardens from Europe. Also called Live Long Saxifrage, it comes in a variety of floral colours, and is hardy to zone 2-3.

Leather-leaved Saxifrage was used by the Aleuts, as a leaf infusion for influenza. The Thompson of British Columbia made a poultice of the freshly chewed leaves for wounds and sores.

It has bright purplish red flowers and stems that look attractive in a native garden or moist part of the yard. The perennial transplants well.

The Thompson call Prickly Saxifrage, **SK'IKENS A KOZAMAI'AT** meaning "companion of rock lichens", in reference to their preferred area of growth. Natives of present day Nunavut gathered the tops of **KAKILLARNAT** for summer food.

Telesonix is a perennial member of the Saxifrage family found in rocky outcrops and limestone slopes of the alpine.

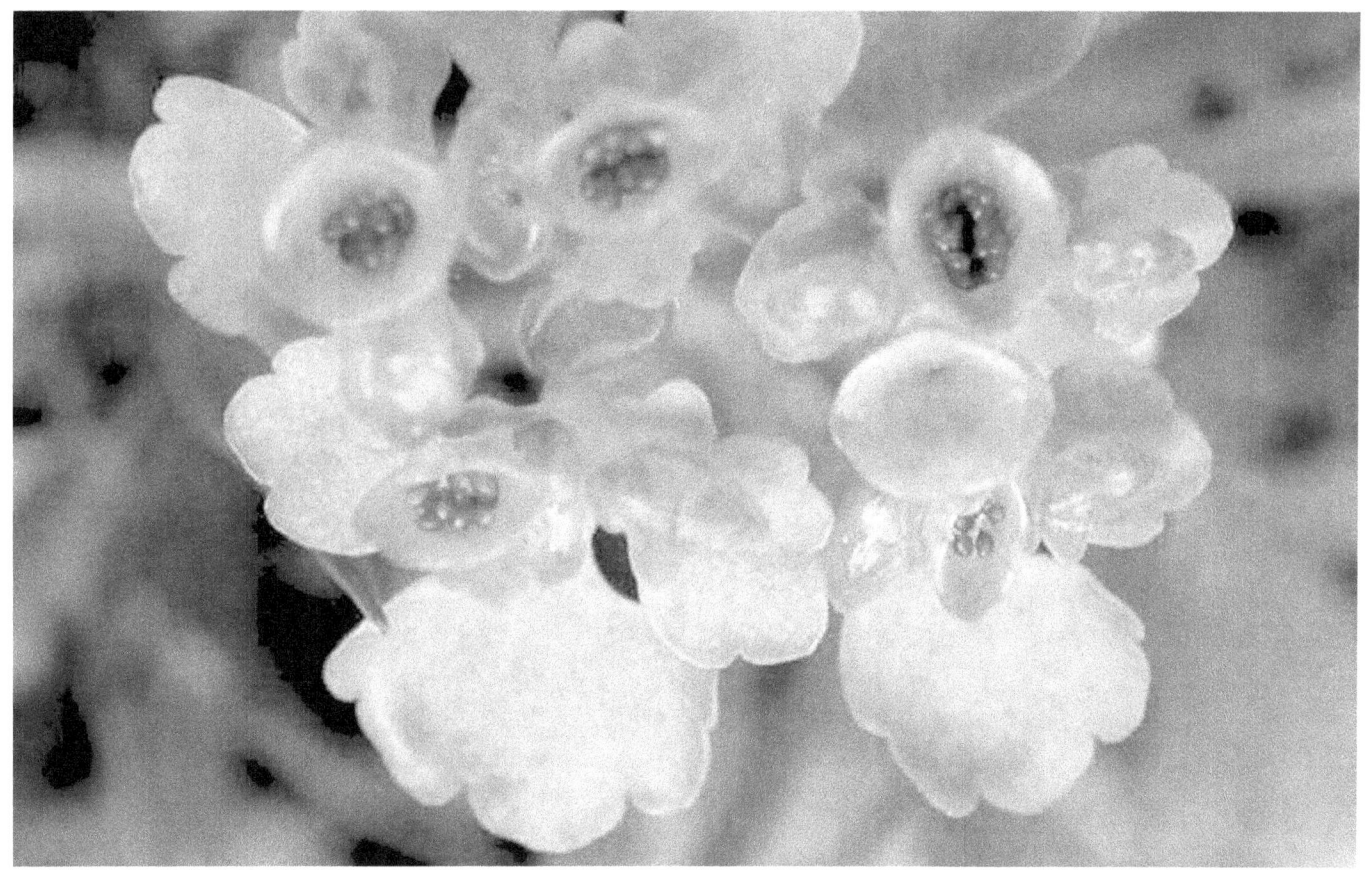

GREEN SAXIFRAGE

The Cheyenne used infusion of the dried plant, called red medicine, for treating hemorrhage of the lungs. The Quileute of British Columbia, used raw leaves of the closely related *Boykinia elata* to treat tuberculosis.

Various *Chrysosplenium* species were used, according to an 18th century Nottinghamshire doctor as an ointment for glassmakers. It was a well-kept secret for curing burns caused by hot metal.

Fringe Cups are restricted to the southwestern portion of Alberta. The Skagit made a decoction of the pounded plant to restore appetite, and for any general form of illness.

Green Saxifrage is common to the northern and boreal forest, as well as the montane and alpine regions of the Rockies. Golden Saxifrage prefers marshy regions throughout Alberta, central Saskatchewan and southwestern Manitoba. The latter is more commonly found in north and central Alberta.

The Slave call *S. tricuspidata*, Mountain Top Grass, **SI TAHKO TOH**.

The Inuit of Baffin Island refer to it as **KAKILLARNAT** meaning, "that which causes prickly feelings"; as well as **TIINNGUAT** meaning "tea substitute"; and even **A'SAAT**. The latter name might be onomatopoeia in reference to the sound a person may make when pricked "A'AA", or "ouch". The dried leaves taste like black tea, and the small white flowers are edible.

The prickly plant was gathered and used as a mattress for puppies to harden the pads on their paws, so that they were toughened for walking on sea ice as a sled dog.

The tea was put on cuts. The leaves are used for wound healing.

Water Carpet inhabits shallow, cool waters of Saskatchewan and Manitoba.

Pretty Maids are a double form of the European Meadow Saxifrage (*S. granulata*).

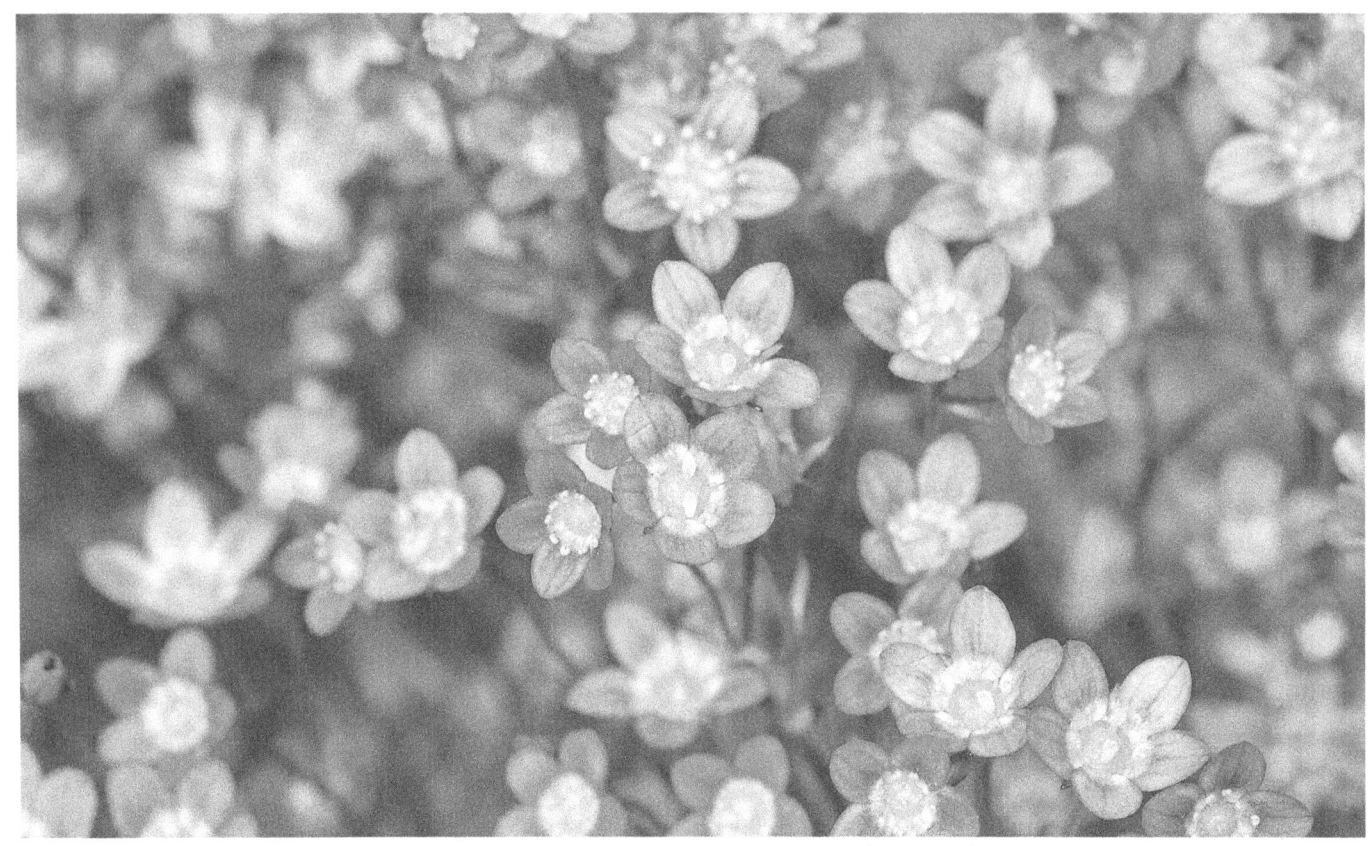

PURPLE SAXIFRAGE

MEDICINAL

CONSTITUENTS- potassium nitrate, potassium chloride, bergenin, arbutin, saxifragin (quercitin-5-glucoside), quercitrin (quercitin-3-rhamnoside).

Strawberry Begonia (*S. stolonifera*) is used in traditional Chinese Medicine. Its name **HU ERH TSAO**, means Tiger Ear Leaf, due to the ear shaped leaves. Other names include **FU ERH TS'AO**, Buddha's Ear Grass, **T'IEN HO HSIEH**, Heavenly water lily leaf, **SZU SZU TS'AO**, Thready Grass, and **HSIEH HO TS'AO** or Crab Shell Grass.

The leaves are considered mild, bitter, and pungent in flavour; cold in property.

The fresh juice of the plant is used to cure otitis media due to its bacteriostatic or bactericidal activity.

The herb removes heat, toxins, dissolves swelling, controls pain, cools the blood and controls bleeding.

This makes it an excellent choice for either acute or chronic otitis media, bleeding from external trauma, carbuncles, incised wound toxin, insect stings, or hemorrhoids.

A study of 42 patients compared herbal ointment with cortisone for treating chronic eczema, applied twice daily for four weeks. Similar benefits were noted for both groups. Xu et al, *Zhong Xi Yi Jie He Xue Bao* 2008 6:12.

Work by Chen et al, *Bioorg Med Chem* 2008 16:13 found quercitin, extracted from this plant, helped induce apoptosis in gastric carcinoma cell lines.

Water extracts exhibit anti-tumor effect on Lewis lung tumors. Liu D et al, *Bioorg Med Chem Lett* 2016 26(19): 4671-8.

Saxifrage species seeds contain alpha linolenic acid, and generally gamma tocopherol as the vitamin E component.

HYDROSOL

Saxifrage water causes piss and removes stone and gravel from the kidney and bladder, according to Brunschwig, in Book of Distillation 1530.

FLOWER ESSENCES

Purple Mountain Saxifrage (*S. oppositifolia*) flower essence is for grounding wisdom from the higher self, and helping one tune into and make practical use of information from celestial origins. **ALASKA**

Leather leaved Saxifrage (*L. pyrolifolia*) flower essence is for mental versatility, and acceptance of one's freedom and abundance. Finding a centered state so that one does not become sidetracked by the myriad variety and depth of the emotions. **CANADIAN FOREST**

Lyall's Saxifrage flower essence helps ease self-absorption and increases outer appreciation. **ROCKY MOUNTAIN**

SCARLET PIMPERNEL
(*Anagallis arvensis* L.)
FLAXLEAF PIMPERNEL
(*A. monelli* L.)
(*Lysimachia monelli* [L.] U. Manns & Anderb.)
FALSE PIMPERNEL
CHAFFWEED
(*A. minima* [L.] E.H.L. Krause)
(*Centunculus minimus* L.)
PARTS USED- flowering tops, leaves

Closed is the pink-eyed pimpernel,
'T will surely rain, I see, with sorrow,
Our jaunt must be put off to-morrow. **JENNER**

Anagallis was named by Linnaeus after the Greek **ANAGELAO**, to laugh aloud. It may come from **ANAGALLO**, to decorate; or **AGALLEIA**, to delight in, and **ANA**, again.

Both its Dutch and German common names, **GUICHELHEIL** and **GAUCHHEIL**, reinforce this idea. Guich or Gauch means fool or idiot, but also cuckoo, and Heil means to heal.

Or, it may simply derive from Latin **ANAGALLIS**, meaning unpretentious, without boasting, or adornment.

Scarlet Pimpernel is an introduced annual that has taken to the prairies, growing in waste fields and sandy roadsides. The flower is more pink or salmon colored than red.

It has been called the Poor Man's Weatherglass due to the habit of closing at the first sign of rain. As it is, the flowers, even on a bright, cloudless day, only open from 8 AM and close before 3 PM. Linnaeus, the father of botanical classification, noticed this one day on a walk, and began the concept of floral clocks. See below.

Scarlet Pimpernel, said to have appeared on the soil at Calvary when the drops of Christ's blood fell to the ground, was considered very efficacious in countering the spells of witches, especially their nasty trick of embedding splinters in one's flesh.

While Scarlet or Common Pimpernel introduced itself in grains; the Blue flowered Flax leaf Pimpernel is a native biennial or perennial of North Africa. It is a compact plant often grown in dry pockets of rock gardens, or found in hanging baskets.

Gerard wrote, "the pimpernel with the blue flowers helpeth the fundament that is fallen down". (This is probably *A. caerulea*- a different species).

The red form was often known as male pimpernel; the blue form, the female.

In the 16th century, Scarlet Pimpernel shows up in English Herbals as **BIPINELLA**, originally applied to the unrelated Salad Burnett.

The plant name was used, by Baroness Orczy, as the title of a novel about the French Revolution, called Scarlet Pimpernel, written in 1905.

It was used chiefly as a cosmetic, to dispel sadness, and as a universal panacea. "No heart can think, no tongue can tell the virtues of the Pimpernel".

Pliny says to use it in liver complaints, because it removes the depression that follows liver trouble.

The medieval physicians of Myddfai suggested the plant for fevers, abdominal complaints, festering swellings and excessive menstruation.

The Greeks used it for diseases of the eye, according to Grieve, and Culpepper says that "it helpth them that are dim-sighted"; the fresh juice mixed with honey and dropped into the eyes.

"The distilled water or juice is much celebrated by French Dames to cleanse the skin of any roughness, deformity, or discolourings thereof."

John Hill (1756) said that the whole plant dried and powdered is good against epilepsy... the flowers alone have been found useful, 20 grains dried being given four times a day.

The expressed juice has been given in dropsy, and obstructions of the liver and spleen. A tincture has been used for irritability of the urinary passages, having been found effective in cases of stone and gravel.

In Gerard's day, a preparation of the herb called **DIACORALLION** was given for gout.

The leaves can be eaten in salad in small amounts only.

In India, scarlet pimpernel is used for inflammation, sores, as well as liver and kidney pain. A leaf extract has been used in India to expel leeches from the nostrils of dogs.

The root contains cyclamin, a saponin toxic to fish.

In Taiwan, the plant is used to remove toxins, and to treat fish poisoning, brain disease, epilepsy, edema, swollen liver and spleen, and calculus.

In Ecuador, according to a 1945 report by Prieto, "a plaster is made by grinding this plant and one is placed on the forehead and a similar one on the back, and then an infusion is drunk; supposed to get rid of intestinal worms".

Another report in 1945 by Steyermark says Scarlet Pimpernel is "used as a worm medicine; mash up green plant, squeeze out the liquid and drink 3 spoonfuls when you have worms in the stomach (symptoms are itching of the nose), after drinking the worms are reputed to leave".

The Chumash of California may have used the introduced plant to treat wounds, using the boiled plant as a poultice. Modern day usage is as a wash for sores, eczema and ringworm.

The plant accumulates heavy metals such as lead, copper and zinc in the roots and may be used for bio-remediation.

Scarlet Pimpernel has been related to cattle and sheep poisonings in Uruguay and Australia.

Flax-leaved Pimpernel is a perennial from southern Europe that is planted as an annual on the prairies. It is prized for its clear, gentian blue flowers.

False Pimpernel (*A. minima*) is a small, hairless annual native usually found in moist soil and mud by ponds in southeastern Alberta and parts of the southern prairies.

The Mahuna used Chaffweed, as it is known, as an infusion to treat gonorrhea, when the bladder and urinary tract began to fail.

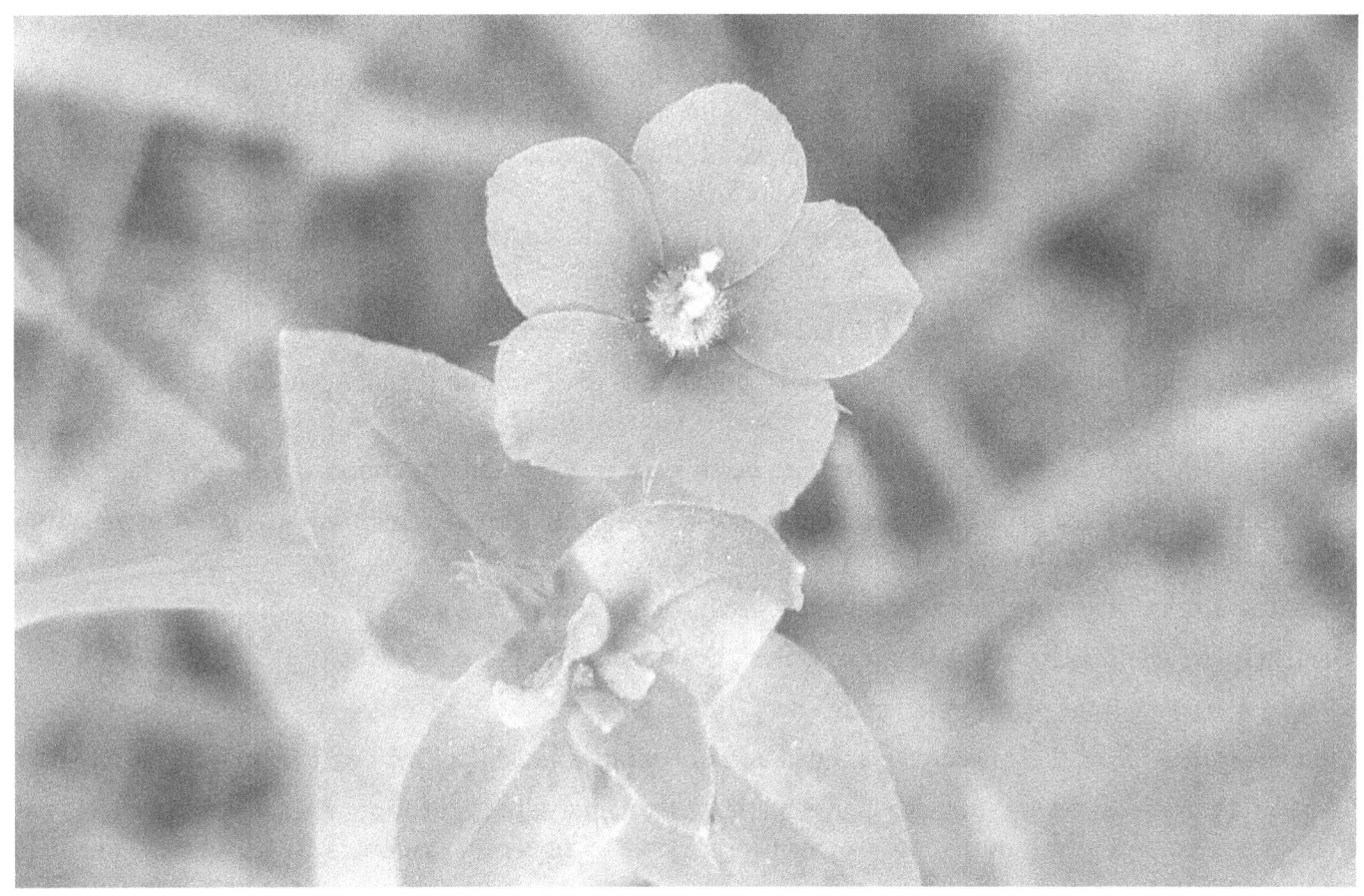

SCARLET PIMPERNEL

MEDICINAL

CONSTITUENTS- *A. arvensis-* triterpene saponins, including anagalline, anagallosides and desglucoangallosides; various oleanane glycosides called anagallosaponins; and cucurbitacin glucosides; including cyclamin. Chief sapogenine is 13,28-epoxy-16-oxooleanan; while another saponin, 23-hydroxyproto-primulagenin is also found. Various flavonoids and caffeic acid derivatives also present; as well as a pepsin-like ferment.
root- cyclamin
A. monelli- aerial parts0 anamighrinal, 3-(O)-alpha-L-rhamnosyl)quercitin: 2,5-dihydroxy-benzoic acid 3'-formly-5'-hydroxy-phenyl ester.

Scarlet Pimpernel is used in nephrotic syndromes, ascites, bronchorrhea, and for digestive, respiratory and cutaneous fungal infections. It is also a mild cardiac stimulant, used for right-sided cardiac insufficiency and depression.

The herb has also been used for rhinitis, allergic asthma, and hepatic insufficiency.

Work by Puri et al, *J of the Nepal Medical Association* 1997 36:123 reported on the use of Scarlet Pimpernel to lower serum cholesterol, glucose and triglyceride levels; as well as exhibiting anti-atherosclerotic activity.

Triterpene saponins were shown as effective as anti-viral drugs treating herpetic keratitis in laboratory studies.

The same saponins were found effective against the herpes simplex (cold sores), adenovirus II and polio virus, type II. Amoros et al, *Antiviral Research* 1987 8.

The cucurbitacins and saponins in full amounts tend to create anal itching, burning, and bloody stools in some individuals.

Scarlet pimpernel water extracts exhibit anti-fungal activity.

Triterpenoglycoside, anagalloside and aglycon anagalligenones isolated from the plant, display inhibitory results against a number of microorganisms.

Cyclamin, a triterpene saponin, is found in root and aerial parts. It synergistically enhanced the inhibitory effect on Bel-7402 liver cancer cells by 41-64% with 5-fluorouracil, by 57-79% with cisplatin and by 62-74% with epirubicin. Li Q et al, *Planta Medica* 2014 80(5): 409-14.

Ali-Shtayeh et al, *Mycoses* 1999 42 found water extracts of the herb significantly anti-fungal against *Microsporum canis, C. albicans, Trichophyton violaceum,* and *T. mentagrophytes.*

In China, the plant known as **CHIEN FENG HUNG**. It has a sour and astringent flavour.

The herb stimulates the flow of bile. If too much bilirubin is released into the blood stream it tends to cause increased skin itching.

Michael Moore suggests it is a simple short term laxative for cases of water retention and poor fat digestion.

A recent study found the plant exhibits moderate hormone-sensitive lipase inhibition, suggestive of benefit in insulin resistance. Bustanji et al, *J Med Plant Res* 2011 5:18.

Water extracts show uterine contracting activity in human uterine tissue.

The triterpene saponins have demonstrated activity against human sperm.

Methanol extracts of the plant demonstrate estrogenic activity in the Allen Doisy test.

Saponins isolated from the powdered plant with alcohol demonstrated hemolytic activity in human blood.

This is to be expected. Many years ago a presentation to students at the U of Alberta, Faculty of Medicine led to the assertion by a professor that I was being irresponsible by suggesting saponins are useful parts of plants for human health.

The hemolytic concept was brought up, suggesting that a hypothermic syringe of saponins injected into human blood vessels would kill red blood cells.

To which I responded, "What idiot would do that?" This brought on much laughter and chagrin. Ironically, I am now an assistant clinical professor in family medicine at this university.

Acetyl saponins isolated from the plant kill parasites. This would appear to support the traditional belief that the plant protected sheep from cranial tapeworms, or gid, as in giddy, delirious or insane. The herb was brewed and given to enraged, hysterical farm animals, and a folk cure for rabid animal bites, used both externally and internally.

Dr. Mitchell suggests adding a vitamin B complex and 50 mg B6, with a daily cup of tea, for melancholy.

In Germany, the herb is used to treat depression, disorders of the mucous membranes, hemorrhoids, herpes, painful kidney disorders, liver disorders, poorly healing wounds and pruritis.

Rudolf Steiner's early work has led to a medicine produced from *Kalium sulfuricum* (potassium sulphate) modeled on the Anagallis herb.

For skin rashes and irritation, apply the tincture diluted in water to affected area.

The herb is used as adjunct therapy for a number of various carcinomas, and is used both internally and externally to treat pain of the joints.

The herb extract strongly inhibits *Candida albicans*. Methanol extracts show inhibition of COX 1 and 2, while water extracts exhibit anti-oxidant activity. Lopez et al, *J Ethnopharm* 2011 134(3):1014-7.

Work by Hilal et al, *Egyptian Journal of Bilharziasis* 1988 10:1 examined ethanol extracts and purified saponins of *A. arvensis*.

Molluscicial and cercaricidal properties were observed, especially from the isolated saponins.

HOMEOPATHY

Scarlet Pimpernel (Anagallis) has a marked action on the skin, characterized by great itching and tingling everywhere, especially the hands, fingers, and palms. Ulcers and swelling of the joints are also common, as well as rheumatic and gouty pains, with cramping in the ball of the thumb.

It possesses the power of softening flesh and destroying warts. It helps, like silicia, to expulse splinters from deep in the skin.

Skin rough and dry, dry bran-like tetter in rings, groups of small vesicles.

The urethra may be irritated, that is sometimes relieved by sex. There may be burning pain on urination, with the stream separating into several streams, with an urgency to press before it passes.

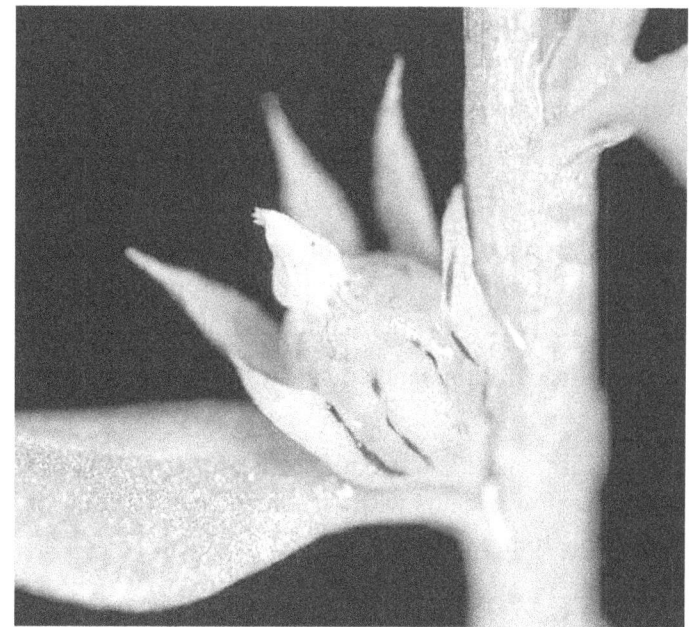

CHAFFWEED (Courtesy of southeasternflora.com)

There may be headaches over the supra-orbital ridges, a sick headache, made better from coffee. There may also be a great hilarity emotionally.

Lively, more gay than usual, with great joy. In high spirits, takes pleasure in everything, very joyful feelings, without thinking of anything in particular.

DOSAGE- First to 3rd potency. If not exact symptoms compare with primrose or buckwheat. The mother tincture is prepared from the fresh flowers, and has a slight olive colour, a sweet, somewhat nauseous herbaceous odour, and a nutty, slightly astringent taste. Self experiment by Schreter in 1846. Summary of symptoms by Fitz published in 1891, may include proving by Gunther and his son with tincture in 1854.

FLOWER OIL

Scarlet Pimpernel makes an excellent sun infused oil for a variety of skin complaints of viral and fungal origin. Take one part fresh flowers to five parts canola oil and sun infuse for 10-14 days. Use low temperature crockpot in cooler climates.

ESSENTIAL OIL

An essential oil, from the dry plant has been obtained and has a specific gravity of 0.980. It has a harsh, pungent taste and pronounced odour.

HYDROSOL

The distilled water is much esteemed by French dames to cleanse the skin from any roughness and deformity, or discolouring thereof. The distilled water is no less effectual to be applied to all wounds that are fresh and green, or old, filthy, fretting and running ulcers.   **CULPEPPER**

FLOWER ESSENCES

Scarlet Pimpernel flower essence stimulates the crown, heart and pituitary chakras. It helps re-awaken and re-affirm love.   **RUNNING FOX FARM**

Scarlet Pimpernel flower essence assists people who have trouble with their father image, men who have trouble relating to women, and people who have trouble developing a loving nature.

Weakness in the pituitary gland and chakra cause a weakened sense of personal identity and even, a fear of society.

When the awakened kundalini travels up the spin, pimpernel helps it penetrate and activate each main chakra.

GURUDAS

Scarlet Pimpernel is a powerful catalyst, and for this reason, it should be used with caution. (It) is helpful for those who have done some inner work but are somewhat frustrated by a lull in the process. It is as if there is something there to work on but it is not entirely within reach.

DALTON

Scarlet Pimpernel essence helps hidden issues come to the surface into consciousness so they can be healed.

BRYNAHERB

Scarlet Pimpernel is a useful essence for someone emotionally entangled with another person. There are two states the flower deals with—either being obsessed or being "possessed" by someone else. In either case they are unable to break free.

BAILEY

SPIRITUAL PROPERTIES

Pimpernel has an upward motion through it. Its circulation and strength are derived from this motion, which can be observed by those who work with this signature on the etheric levels. Because of this upward motion, energy associated with an area in which there is a blockage or a particularly strong expression in life is spiritualized.

It changes your point of view. This is not the same as raising energy through kundalini yoga. It is a way to spiritually understand God's purpose. God's way of expression and an understanding of how these things are beneficial for you in your relationship with God are brought more closely into focus.

There is some concentration of psychic energy as a result of this motion. Whichever chakra has blocked energy or a strong amount of energy associated with it, can have its energy released and raised to the next chakra.

Individuals developing the abilities of self-expression may find psychic gifts such as clairvoyance, telepathy, and deeper understanding of the self associated with the third eye, becoming stronger and more focused.

Deeper states of healing may result as individuals who work with love use this herb.

In Lemuria, pimpernel was used extensively in dance. The devic spirits associated with this plant were quite clear and easy to work with, and indeed, they even helped to choreograph some of the dances.

Joyousness, motion, and strength were imparted as a result of this dance. The devic spirits have continued to maintain this energy. Today, mankind is not able to dance in such a fashion; however, there is karmic purpose to wait and allow this when mankind is ready.

The emotional and etheric bodies are cleansed, and the tubercular and cancer miasms are eased.

GURUDAS

PERSONALITY TRAITS

One of my favorite plants for helping with Fire imbalance is scarlet pimpernel, Anagallis arvensis.

My dream journey to the spirit of this plant took me through long stretches of cold dark space until I arrived at a small distant planet. The sphere seemed deserted until I got to the remotest part, where I saw a gruff unshaven man dressed in a tight t-shirt and black pants.

"Are you the spirit of scarlet pimpernel?" I asked.

"What's it to ya?"

"Well, I..."

"Listen buddy, why don't you just take off to the next solar system. There's some nice flowers over there. Scram."

This had to be the spirit of Scarlet Pimpernel! He was showing the same bitterness and the same over-protectiveness in the dream as he did in waking reality. I remembered that the warmth of the sun would get him to open up and share his beauty.

"I love your flowers!" I said. "They have the wildest color combination! It makes me happy to look at them! You must be a beautiful guy behind that gruff front!"

He cracked a little smile and blushed. I went on, "What are you doing here all alone on this frigid little planet?"

A tear trickled down the tough guy's cheek. "People are so cold, so heartless!" he said. "They can hurt you if you let your guard down. I take everything to heart-I'm too vulnerable, I guess".

He didn't need to say any more to let me know he had medicine for the heart protector. When he saw I understood his act, he threw back his head and laughed uninhibitedly.

"May I use you?" I asked. "Will you share your medicine with others?" In reply he took my hands and we danced in a circle, abandoning ourselves to joy.   **COWAN**

Such mental pathology is most frequently encountered in younger people who are engaged in intensive spiritual practices and who, at a certain point, feel that they have attained a super-conscious state. While it is clearly apparent to the observer that the affected individual looks full of joy, the state is an unhealthy one, leading to irresponsible behaviour. The insanity is not overt; it is not readily apparent that the patient's mental state is unbalanced. Usually the person claims that he has a high spiritual consciousness and has, therefore, transcended the necessity of attending to earthy, practical matters; he feel he need do nothing mundane at all. He is quite willing to discuss his inner spiritual state with anyone who comes along…The Anagallis state is one which can be seen in those taking drugs, such as amphetamines or cocaine, which exert an exactly similar effect: the speeding up of mental processes.   **GEORGE VITHOULKAS**

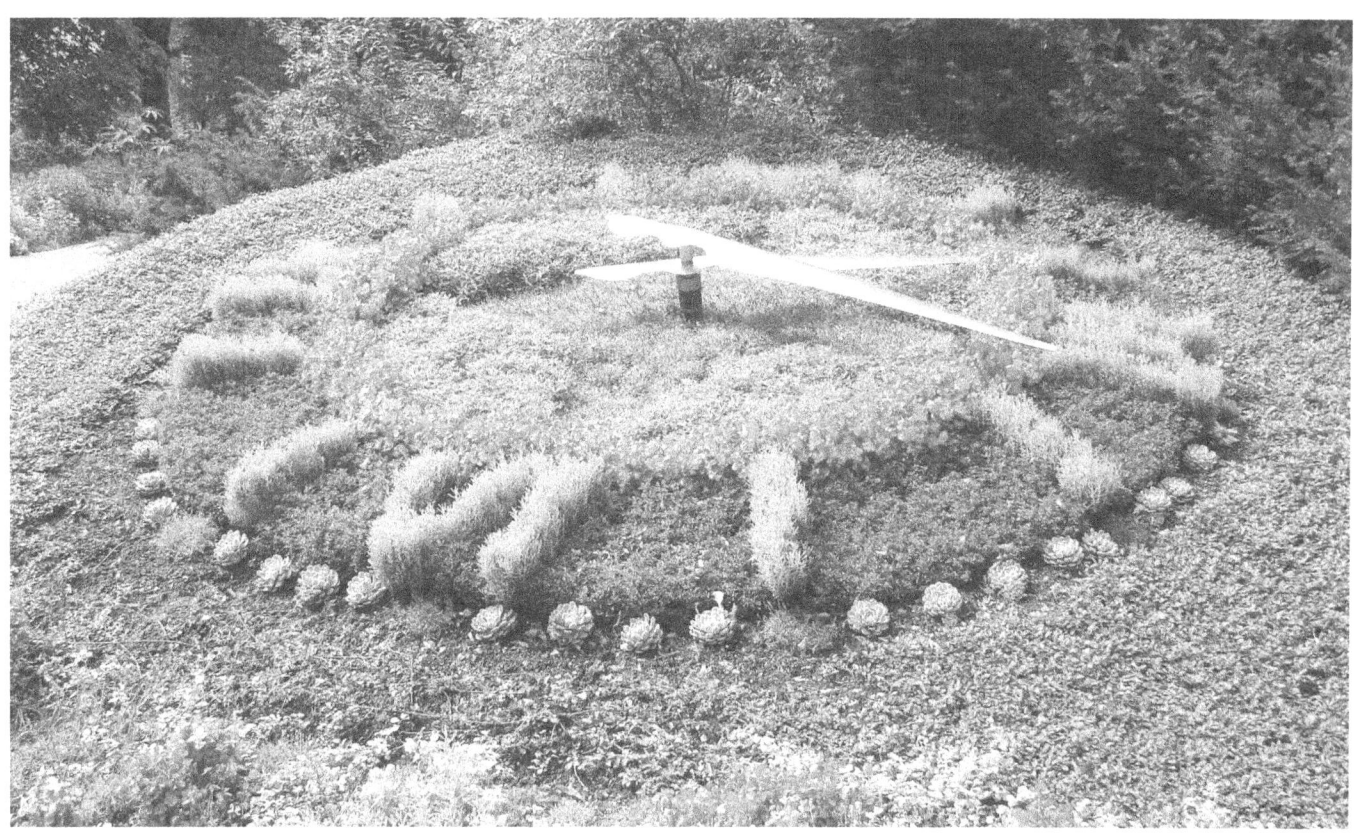

FLORAL CLOCK

19

There are a number of issues that involve when, and if, a flower opens. Light is an obvious one, although bindweed and other night blooming flowers are the exception to this rule.

Mainly, the flowers open to maximize cross pollination, and when nectar will attract the most pollinators. Here are some of the flowers you may include in a northern floral clock.

2-8 a.m.-	Bindweed (*Calystegia sepium*)
3-5 a.m.-	Goat's Beard (*Tragopogon* sp.) close at noon
4-5 a.m.-	Corn Poppy (*Papaver rhoeas*) Chicory (*Cichorium intybus*)
5-6 a.m.-	Dandelion (*Taraxacum spp.*) Nipplewort (*Lapsana communis*) Iceland Poppy (*P. nudicaule*) Day Lily (*Hemerocallis fulva*) Sow Thistle (*Sonchus* spp.)
7-8 a.m.-	Common Lettuce (*Lactuca sativa*) Scarlet Pimpernel Calendula (*Calendula officinalis*) Water Lily (*Nymphaea* spp) Chicory (*Chicorium intybus*)
8-9 a.m.-	Hawkweed (*Hieracium* spp) Pinks (*Dianthus* spp) Yellow Water Lily (*Nuphar lutea*)
9-10 a.m.-	Mullein (*Verbascum* spp.) Sandwort (*Arenaria* spp.) Purslane (*Portulaca* spp.) Chickweed (*Stellaria media*)
11-noon-	Star of Bethlehem (*Ornithogalum umbellatum*)
Noon-	Ice Plant (*Mesembryanthemum* spp)
1 p.m.-	Carnation (Dianthus sp.)
2 p.m.-	Thistle (*Carlina* spp)
4 p.m.-	Lance leaved Plantain (*Plantago lanceolata*) Four O'Clocks (*Mirabilis* spp)
6-8 p.m.-	Evening Primrose (*Oenothera* spp) Flowering Tobacco (*Nicotiana alata*) Annual Stock (*Matthiola incana*)

RECIPES

TINCTURE- 30-45 drops as a total daily dose. The fresh plant tincture is made at 1:2 and 50% alcohol.

POWDER- 1.8 grams four times daily.

INFUSION- One half teaspoon of dried herb to each cup of boiling water. Infuse ten minutes. Take three times daily, or hourly for edema and water retention. The fresh leaf infusion is superior.

CAUTION- Scarlet Pimpernel should not be used medicinally for longer than 2-3 weeks.

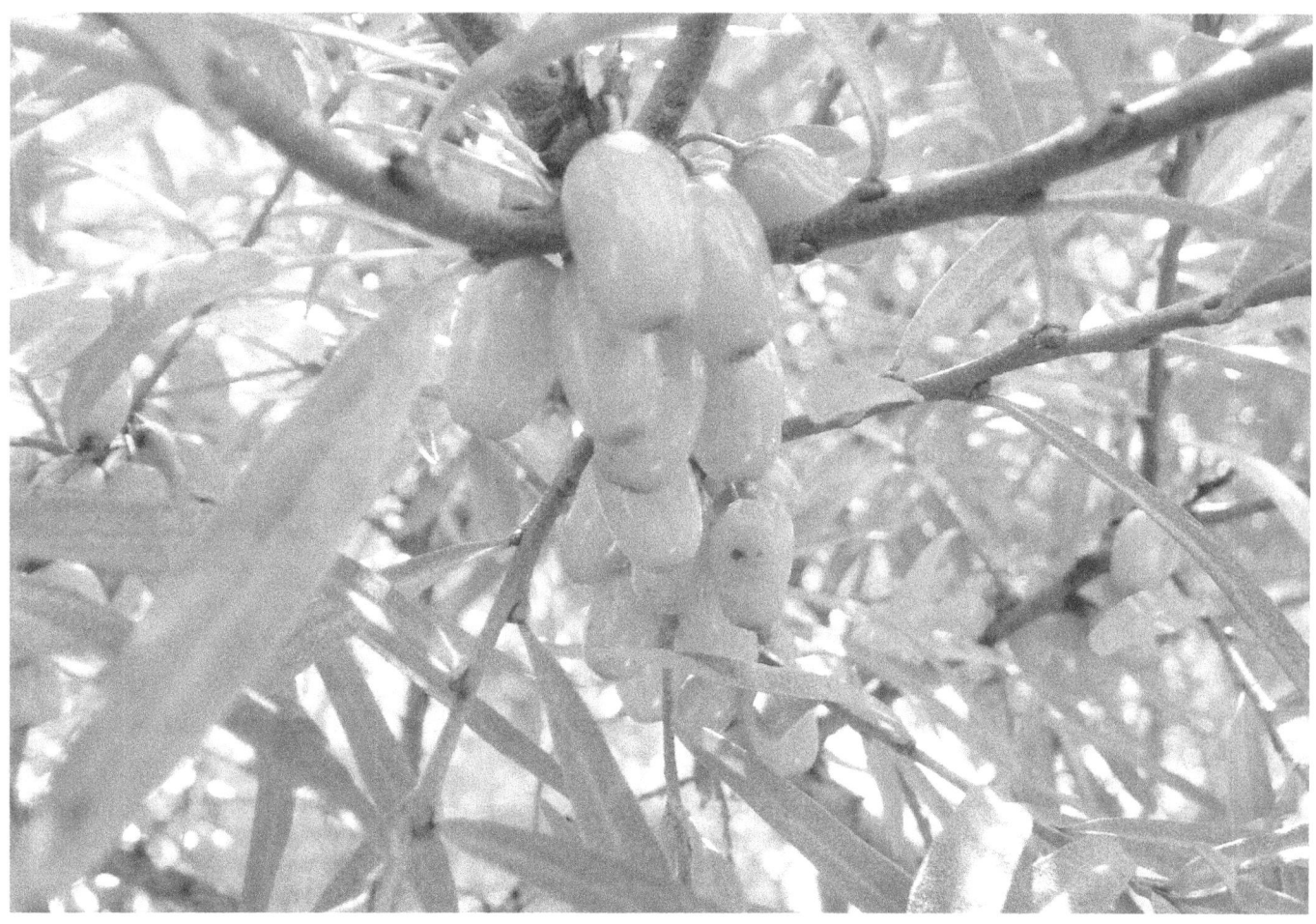

SEA BUCKTHORN BERRIES

SEA BUCKTHORN
(*Hippophae rhamnoides* L.)
PARTS USED- berries, flowers, leaves

Look around you, Gabrielle. Lush Prairie. And those bushes with orange berries? See them, on those dunes?

Sea Buckthorn! It grows wild here, and the oil works wonders on horses.   **XENA, PRINCESS WARRIOR**

Hippophae means "giving light or sight to a horse" based on curing equine blindness, or "shining underneath", alluding to the silvery underside of leaf. In Greek, **HIPPOPHAES** means, a shiny plant.

HIPPOS is Greek for horse, and **PHAEITHON**, "shining", **PHAINO** meaning "light". The berries were said to be a favourite food of Pegasus, the Greek flying horse and constellation.

Rhamnoides is from Greek **RHAMNOS** due to resemblance of spines from Rhamnus or Buckthorn species, or from Celtic **RHAM**, a tuft of branches.

Originally a native of Europe and Asia, sea buckthorn was imported for its ornamental value, as well as drought and salt tolerant qualities to the Canadian prairies. It is closely related to wolf willow and russian olive.

In fact, since 1982, over one million seedlings have been distributed through a federal shelterbelt program of PFRA.

The plants are extremely winter hardy and bear annual fruit in their second year. Male and female plants are both required for fruit production.

21

The variety of male plant chosen appears significant, with hybrid pollens increasing oil content from 8-33%, and vitamin C content by 17-137% in Russian experiments.

Cultivars in Russia are now thorn-less, and yielding up to 12 tons per hectare; compared to 0.3 tons for natural wild stands.

Work by researchers at Indian Head, Saskatchewan, has developed two cultivars with few thorns, and fruit good for processing and mechanical harvest. Orange September and Harvest Moon were released in 2005 and are hardy to zone 2a on the prairies.

The trees can withstand winter temperatures down to minus 43 degrees C. Like alder, the roots of Sea Buckthorn have established a relationship with *Frankia* bacterium, that helps convert atmospheric nitrogen into a usable form.

Mature, seven year-old plants will produce from 5-12 kilos or more of fruit per year.

The seeds contain 30% protein, an after oil production, as a valuable high-protein supplement in food manufacture.

The berries were traditionally eaten with milk and cheese by the Tartars and Siberians, made into a jelly, or cooked in meat or fish sauce.

The seeds are quite sour, with a pineapple-like scent, and a passion fruit-type flavour.

The plant is widely used for medicinal properties throughout the world. In Tibet, the orange fruit is given to those with stomach sluggishness and lazy digestion.

Several Tibetan medical texts, including the Shel-Ireng describe the uses of sea buckthorn, known as **DHAR-BHO**, or **TAIRUA**.

Sibu Yidian, the 8th century Tibetan medical book, contains 30 chapters on its benefits. In 1977, it was listed for the first time in the *Chinese Pharmacopoeia*.

The leaves, stems, and roots produce a yellow dye. Decoctions of the berries have been used on various skin eruptions.

In Nepal, women use the orange-red fruit juice to decorate their lips and forehead. The berries are boiled with silver jewelry to take off the tarnish.

The berries and leaf tissue contain an ice-nucleating compound with a number of potential industrial applications.

This compound occurs frequently in nature, as the temperature drops in fall, certain types of bacteria that grow on leaves produce elevated amounts. When the organisms freeze at several degrees above zero, the resulting ice crystals sustain the damage that causes the leaves to discolor and fall. Species of ice-nucleating bacteria are the key to commercial "snow-making" at ski resorts, and application in frozen foods.

A patent was issued in June of 1997 to a European group, and is the first patent on ice-nucleating compounds from a plant.

The frozen berries make an excellent ice-wine. Jack Winniski from Pearl Creek Farms near Melville, Saskatchewan has over a thousand trees, and sells root cuttings across Canada.

He says, "the leftover pulp makes excellent feed for horses. It gives them a sleek coat. It is said that Alexander the Great always camped near Sea buckthorn groves, so his horse, Bucephalus, could get a good nutritional feed every night". Xena would agree!

The fall berries are firm enough to pick with a coarse comb, but later the flesh becomes so liquid they burst at the least touch. Mears and Hillman report in Wild Foods, "by this stage the best way of harvesting them is to grip the base of a fruit covered branch and slide your hand up the stem, crushing the berries from bottom to top and letting the juice drip into a receptacle held immediately below."

Betty Forbes, president and CEO of Nvigorate produces berry products, including a tart, orange-colored sorbet that is so refreshing. Visit www.nvigorate.ca .

Birds enjoy the fermented berries, and like mountain ash berries, they cause drunkenness and dangerous acrobatics in our feathered friends.

The juice can be strongly purgative in some people so caution is advised.

Work in China, *Journal of Jilin Agricultural University* 1999 21:2 looked at solving the problem of separating seed kernel and shell. The method includes cleaning, shelling, sieving, separating, and processing the seed kernel and processing the seed shell. The optimum separation floating velocity is 4.1 metres per second for seed kernels and shells on the first sieve, with a loss rate of 7.5% for kernels and 12% shell rate in kernels.

Some 200 hundred finished products in eight different categories such as soft drink, food, wine, medicine, health protection, forage and additives are produced at 150 processing plants in China. One hectare of trees can yield up to 15 tons of juice.

Fruit leather is a great product, combining well with apple.

The fruit may be supplemented into broiler chicken feed at 0.05%, improving feed intake, average daily gain and final body weight at 42 days. Ma JS et al, *Poult Sci* 2015 94(11): 2641-9.

Seed germination is best achieved with a 48 hour soak in 20 degrees Celsius water.

The *Prairie Agricultural Machinery Institute* in Portage la Prairie, Manitoba has developed a berry harvester that does not damage trees.

A fast analysis of sugars, fruit acids and vitamin C in different varieties has been developed in Finland. Tiitinen K et al, *J Ag Food Chem* 2006 54:2508-13.

MEDICINAL

CONSTITUENTS- berries- vitamin C (600 mg per 100 grams). Total sugars range up to 6.6%, composed mainly of glucose, fructose, saccharose and arabinose.
Water-soluble polysaccharides (2-3%) include xylose, D-galacturonic acid, L-arabinose, D-glucose, L-rhamnose. The fresh fruit contains 19 carotenoids, with a yield of 165 ppm. The most abundant in one study conducted in Kiev, Ukraine in 1989, was beta-cryptoxanthin (18.4%), beta-carotene (15.8%), lutein (14.2%), and taraxanthin (12.4). The carotenoids with provitamin A activity was 48% of the total.
Smaller quantities of various vitamins B, E, K and P; sugars (glucose, fructose), pectins, wax, essential oils, phospholipids, amino acids and sterols. The fruit is quite acidic (pH 2.9), but pleasant. Phylloquinone content of the fruit is up to 1.3mg/ per 100 grams.
Flavonoids include isorhamnetin (the major one), catechin, leucocyanidin, flavonol, narcissin, myricetol, caffeic acid, rutin, quercitin, and delphinidin; as well as abscisic acid. Fruit contains chiefly malic acid, with some acetic, citric, tartaric, ursolic and quinic acids; as well as sugar alcohols like mannitol and quebrachit.
It also contains serotonin, and 35 mg of S-methylcysteine per gram of fresh fruit, as well as betaine. The fruit is significantly higher in cobalt than other fruit, with copper levels twice that of apricots and red currants. Also present in leaves, shoots, buds and berries is plastochromanol-8.
Seeds- proanthocyanidins, flavonoids, fatty acids (see below), hippophins C-F, K-M (flavonol glycosides).
Leaves contain up to 3068 mg/100 grams of flavonoids including isorhamnetin, kaempferol and quercitin, gallic and ellagic acid, four C-glycosidic ellagitannins, six hydrolysable tannins comprising 12%, 2.6% free carbohydrates (glucose, fructose and saccharose), carotenes, Vit C 259 mg%, and E, and B complex, especially B6, and B12. Manganese is 55 mg/kg and iron content is 77.5 mg/kg.
twigs, leaves- harmalol, Beta amyrin oleyl alcohol acid.
flowers- 1.2% free carbohydrates
bark- serotonin, 5-hydroxytryptamine (0.3-0.3%), harmol
root-harmol

The bright orange fruit is gathered when ripe, but not yet soft. They are pressed into juice used in syrups and preserves; and highly valued for their nutritive properties. The juice should be produced without contact to any metal substances except stainless steel.

It combines well with blueberry for improving eyesight, night blindness and vision. This may be due, in part, to the presence of zeaxanthin dipalmitate, which has been shown useful in prevention of macular degeneration.

A study of 31 type 1 diabetic children, given a supplement of blueberry and sea buckthorn fruit for two months, noted significant decreases in glycosylated hemoglobin. Nemes-Nagy et al, *Acta Physiol Hung* 2008 95:4.

It is very useful in prolonged illness, to fight general weakness and fatigue. It helps those prone to bleeding gums and mucous membranes.

It offers protection from colds and flu, especially in later winter and early spring.

The unripe fruit can be used to treat diarrhea, dysentery and staunch bleeding.

The juice has been found to block the endogenous formation of nitrosamine compounds and thereby prevent tumour production.

In 1989, Peizhen et al reported that concentrated sea buckthorn juice significantly inhibits the growth of sarcoma, lymphocytic leukemia, and human gastric cancer cells.

Work by Suleyman et al, *Phyto Res* 15:7 found hexane extracts possess anti-ulcer activity.

Cold pressed juices constitute an emulsion containing an oil phase, a liquid phase and particles of the flesh. It is important to process the juice properly to obtain maximum benefit.

Eighty overweight women were enrolled in a randomized crossover study looking at sea buckthorn fruit and oil. Sea buckthorn effects were mainly on serum triglycerides and very low density lipoprotein (VLDL). Larmos PS et al, *Am J Clin Nutr* 2013 98(4): 941-51.

In the *Journal of Chinese Materia Medica* of June 1994, sea buckthorn seed oil showed liver protective action. It inhibited the rise of MDA in rat and mice liver, and markedly checked the depletion of GSH (glutathione).

Mizina et al in 1999 found rats exposed to X-ray irradiation, and taking sea buckthorn juice had increased lifespan, normalization of basal activity, and response to ACTH. Work by Goel et al, *Phytother Res* 2003 17:3 found alcohol extract of the berries protected mice against lethal gamma radiation.

An *Acta Pharmacologica Sinica* July 1994 study showed flavones from sea buckthorn prevented heart arrhythmia in guinea pig experiments.

Cheng et al, *Life Science* 2003 72:20 found the total flavones from sea buckthorn fruit prevented *in vivo* thrombosis, and *in vitro* inhibition of platelet aggregation.

The flavones stimulate IL-6 and TNFalpha secretion, suggestive of immune support. Mishra et al, *Phytother Res* 27:11.

The fruit reduced C-reactive protein, a marker of inflammation and cardiovascular. Larmo et al, *Eur J Clin Nutr* 2008 62:9.

Work by Koyama et al, *Clin Hem Microcirc* 2009 41:1 found fruit reduces hypertension stress on ventricular micro-vessels. The fruit possesses anti-platelet activity. Olas B et al, *Oxid Med Cell Longev* 2016:4692486.

The fruit pulp has been studied for its anti-inflammatory properties by Sabynich et al, *Rastitel'nye-Resuray* 1994 30:3.

The thick fruit pulp suppressed carragenan-induced edema, UV-induced erythema and exudative peritonitis. It increased capillary resistance, retarded the rate of tissue damage during acute inflammation and delayed the development of granulating fibrous tissues.

The marc from pressed berries contains isorhamnetin that is anti-oxidant and could be used in various preparations. Pengfei et al, *Plant Foods for Human Nutrition* 64:2.

The berries contain up to 0.36% betaine, a substance found in beets, and associated with curing ulcers and reducing arteriosclerosis risk.

The fruit phenolics show inhibition of blood platelet adhesion, suggestive of benefit in prevention of cardiovascular disease. Olas B et al, *J Physiol Pharmacol* 2017 68(2): 223-9.

A very interesting study on children with functional dyspepsia, found the fruit increased levels of appetite factors, leptin and neuropeptide Y, increased gastric emptying, digestive function, children's growth and development. The control drug domperidone was much less effective. Xiao M et al, *Hell J Nucl Med* 2013 16(1): 38-43.

Jagetia et al, *J Clin Biochem Nutr* 2007 40:2 confirm radiation protective mechanisms. The compound quassin is believed involved.

In fruit pomace extract, the oligomeric proanthocyanidins account for 75% of antioxidant activity. Rosch et al, 2004.

Work by Geetha et al, *J of Ethnopharm* 2002 79:3 found seabuckthorn fruit and leaves possess anti-oxidant and immune modulating activity.

Ethanol extracts of fruit show activity against *Bacillus cereus, E. coli, S. aureus* and *Pseudomonas aeruginosa*. Kokoska et al, *J Ethnopharm* 2002 82 51-3.

After oil has been removed from the seeds, their flavonoids induce apoptosis in liver cancer cell lines. Sun et al, *Zhong Yao Cai* 2003 26:12.

A water extract of the seeds is highly anti-oxidant and found active against *Listeria monocytogens* and *Yersinia* species. Chauhan et al, *Fitoterapia* 2007 78 7:8.

When fed to Zucker diabetic rats, water extracts of seed residue, after pressing, reduced body weight, serum glucose, and total cholesterol suggesting use for metabolic syndrome. Zhang et al, *J Food Biochem* 34:4. Similar results were found from seed protein. Yuan H et al, *Food Funct* 2016 7(3): 1610-5.

The seeds contain proanthocyanidins that give protection against visible light-induced retinal degeneration, *in vivo*. Wang Y et al, *Nutrients* 2016 8(5).

Procyanidins from seeds induce apoptosis of MDA-MB-231 breast cancer cells by inhibiting fatty acid synthase. This compound is over-expressed in many human cancers. Wang Y et al, *Tumour Biol* 2014 35(10): 9563-9.

Ursolic acid, found in other medicinal herbs, has function similar to adrenocorticol hormone.

Water extracts of the fruit act as an anxiolytic agent, suggestive of nervous system benefit. Batool et al, *Pak J Botany* 2010 41:6.

The fruit extracts and their various compounds are not adversely affected by treatment with heat. Ursache FM et al, *Food Chem* 2017 233: 442-9.

Some of the commercial products available with Sea-buckthorn constituents include:

From Russia-	Vicalin (for ulcers)
	Oblepicha oil (for skin)
Austria-	Biodoat (with honey)
Switzerland-	Exsativa (sexual enhancer)
China-	Xianshai Beer (Medicinal Beer)
	Natural Shai Drink (Fruit Juice)

During the 1988 Olympic games in Korea, two sea buckthorn sports drinks "Shawikang" and "Jianibao", were official beverages.

Sea Buckthorn International in Summerland, British Columbia has been a long time proponent of this medicinal plant. Soy sauce and vinegars containing sea buckthorn berry have recently appeared on the market. The organic juice is widely available.

Sea Buckthorn juice was supplied to Russian cosmonauts, to enhance resistance to stress. Work by Eccleston et al, *J Nutr Biochem* 2002:13 showed the antioxidant rich juice moderately decreased LDL levels to oxidation.

The fruit protects against haloperidol-induced orofacial dyskinesia. Batool et al, *Med Sci Monit* 2010 16:8.

Both fruit and leaf extracts show activity against MRSA (methicillin-resistant *Staphylococcus aureus*). Qadir MI et al, *Pak J Pharm Sci* 2016 29(5): 1711-13.

Extracts were found against methicillin-resistant *S. epidermis*, equal to and synergistic with gentamycin and ofloxacin. Abidi SH et al, *J Infect Dev Ctries* 2015 9(9): 925-9.

An animal study found pre-treatment with the leaf extract protects the brain and neurotransmitters from radiation damage. Bala M et al, *Pharm Biol* 2017 55(1): 1833-42.

The leaves contain an analog of sea buckthorn fruit, and some of the pharmacological action. Hydrocarbons, triacylglycerols, free fatty acids, carotenoids, aldehydes, and triterpene acids are all present. Beta-amyrin derivatives help dilate blood vessels and lower blood pressure. Ge Xiaoyan et al, *J Chinese Herbs* 1986 17.

The flavonoids (isorhamnetin and quercitin) are efficacious in hypertension and coronary heart disease.

Work by Zhang et al, *J Chin Cardiovas Dis* 1987 15:2 in a double-blind randomized trial, found remission of angina and improved ECG readings, superior to the drug isosorbide dinitrate.

Leaf flavonoids change the dynamics of heart contraction, including diastolic pressure of left ventricle, cardiac output, heart stroke index and myocardium improvement.

Heart arrhythmia, due to ventricular fibrillation, or atrium function was corrected with flavonoids. Liu Feng Ming et al, *J Chin Pharmacology* 1989 5:1.

Isorhamnetin has been shown to protect against cardiac hypertrophy by blocking P13K-AKT pathway. Gao L et al, *Mol Cell Biochem* 2017 429(1-2): 167-77.

It also suppresses proliferation of colon cancer cells. Li C et al, *Mol Med Rep* 2014 9(3): 935-40.

Isorhamnetin may be therapeutic in treatment of endotoxin-induced sepsis. Jayashankar B et al, *Int Immunopharmacol* 2014 20(1): 89-94.

Isorhamnetin, kaempferol and quercitin oral bioavailability is enhanced by taking IP6(phytic acid) at the same time. Xie Y et al, *Fitoterapia* 2014 93: 216-25.

The leaf ethanol extracts show activity against mycobacterium. Hydrogels containing leaf extracts enhance wound healing in a rat model. Kim J et al, *Int J Biol Macromol* 2017 99: 586-93.

The leaves are anti-bacterial and show activity against *E. coli. Salmonella typhi, Shigella dysenteriae, Streptococcus pneumoniae* and *Staphylococcus aureus*. Yogendra Kumar MS et al, *Food Chem* 2013 141(4): 3443-50.

They contain salicylates and can be helpful as a tea for inflammation and insomnia.

Significant amounts of B12 were detected in plant (37μg/100g dry weight. Other interesting findings are couchgrass (26μg/100g) and elecampane (11μg/100grams). Nakos M et al, *Food Chemistry* 2017 216:301-8.

Work by Goetha et al, found leaf extracts protective of animals subjected to chromium-induced oxidation. *J Ethnopharm* 2003 87:2.

Saggu et al, *J Pharm Pharmacol* 2007 59:12 found leaf extracts prevent oxidative stress in liver cells. Neuronal cells were protected from oxidative stress. Cho CH et al, *J Microbiol Biotechnol* 2017 May 24.

Ethanol leaf extracts show activity against *Helicobacter pylori*, implicated in gastric and duodenal ulcers. Li et al, *J Ethnopharm* 98 329-33.

Leaf tinctures help down-regulate adipogenic and lipogenic gene expression, suggesting a possible benefit in obesity and related blood glucose and lipid disorders. Pichiah PB et al, *Nutr Res* 2012 32(11): 856-64.

Leaf extracts show potential to delay onset and/or progression of cataracts. Dubey S et al, *Vet Ophthalmol* 2016 19(2): 144-8

Saggu et al, *Food Chem Tox* 45:4 suggests the leaf extract is a potent adaptogen, with further study needed. A follow-up study by the author in *Phytother Res* 22:9 found a 70% extract of the dry leaf enhanced physical performance.

The leaf shows anti-Dengue virus activity in work by Jain et al, *Phytomed* 2008 15:10.

Leaf extracts exhibit immune-modulating effect, either enhancing or reducing its capacity to required levels. This suggests benefit in inflammatory conditions, including auto-immune responses. Tanwar H et al, *Inflammopharmacology* 2017 April 13.

A 70% ethanol extract of the branches show *in vivo* anti-tumor and anti-inflammatory activity. Yasukawa et al, *Fitoterapia* 80:3.

Leaf extracts inhibit acetylcholinesterase, suggestive of possible benefit in cognitive disorders. Attrey DP et al, *Indian J Exp Biol* 2012 50(10): 690-5.

Aerial part tinctures show activity against acute myeloid leukemia cells, and enhanced by vitamin D_3. Zhamanbayeva GT et al, *Biomed Pharmacother* 2016 82:80-9.

Leaf and twig extracts show significant anti-*Candida albicans* activity, and enhanced activity of fluconazole and caspofungin; decreasing biofilm formation by 80%. Sadowska B et al, *Microb Pathog* 2017 107: 372-379.

Leaf extract inhibits the rapid proliferation of C6 glioma cells, via apoptosis. Kim SJ et al, *Appl Biochem Biotechnol* 2017 Feb 8.

Tincture extracts at 350 mg twice daily were given to 28 patients in a DB, PC trial for idiopathic nephrotic syndrome. The other 28 patients received standard treatment of dietic advise. After three months the sea buckthorn group show improvement in symptoms of edema, anorexia and oliguria. Urinary protein and cytokines showed a significant decrease, and albumin levels were elevated. Singh RG et al, *J Assoc Physicians India* 2013 61(6): 397-9.

Sea Buckthorn pollen is an effective medicinal remedy for skin, severe burns, eczema and allergies. Research in Russia, by Panteev et al, has resulted in suitable cultivars for pollen production.

Work by Podder B et al, *Mol Med Rep* 2013 8(6): 1852-60 suggests sea buckthorn extracts may be useful for various oxidative stress-related diseases.

Russian research found hippophan (5-hydroxytryptamine) isolated from the bark, inhibited tumour growth. Sokoloff et al, 1961.

This compound, 5HT, found in fruit stems and peel, is a neurotransmitter and regulator of blood pressure, body temperature and hormone levels. In fact serotonin is widely found in plants, fungi, insects—throughout nature, acting as a hormone that helps all living creatures adapt to their environment.

GEMMOTHERAPY

The young leaf sprouts of sea buckthorn are useful for colitis and other inflamed conditions of the gastrointestinal tract.

DOSE- 20-40 drops of 1D glycerine macerate up to 3 times daily. Produced and proved by author.

Bud extracts show activity against influenza A H1N1 virus. Torelli A et al, *J Prev Med Hyg* 2015 56(2):51-6.

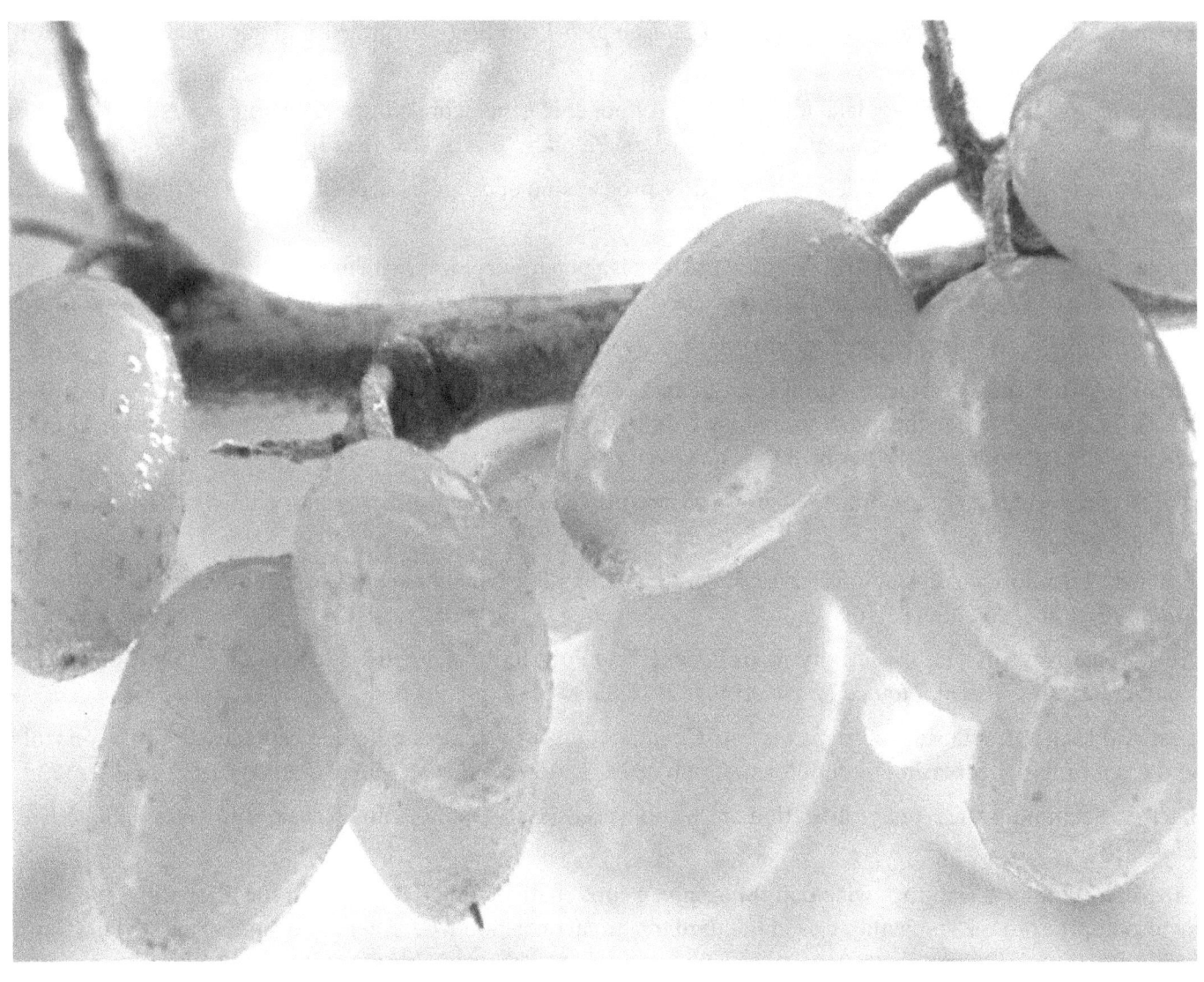

SEA BUCKTHORN FRUIT

FRUIT AND SEED OILS

Fixed or fatty acid oils from sea buckthorn fruit and seeds contain mainly unsaturated linoleic acid (C18), and saturated palmitoleic (C16) acids. The waxy constituent is mainly nonacosane. The oil content can be up to 34% in dried fruit.

Specifically, the fruit contains just over 5% fatty acids, and the seed over 9%. The fruit coat oils are mainly saturated over 75% oleic acids, as well as rich in palmitic and palmitoleic acid (omega-7).

The seed oil is predominately unsaturated fatty acids with 33- 40% linoleic, 15-22% alpha linolenic, and 17% oleic acids.

A cycloartane terpenoid, 24-methylenecycloartane; and 24-Z-ethyliden-ecycloartanol, were isolated from the unsaponifiable part of the oil by Glazunova et al in 1994. Present in sterol fraction of the unsaponifiable portion are triterpene alcohols, higher fatty alcohols, beta sitosterol, citrostadienol, uvaol, alpha and beta amyrins, 24-ethylcholest-7-en-3beta-ol and erythrodiol.

Among the carotenes are alpha and beta-carotenes, lycopene, cryptoxanthin, zeaxanthin, taraxanthin and phytofluin. Alpha, beta, delta and gamma tocopherols constitute 93-98% of seed tocopherols and tocotrienols; whereas the fruit is 76-89% alpha tocopherols.

Phytosterols are beta-sitosterol (the major one), b-amirol and erithrodiol.

Sea buckthorn oil reduces inflammation, is anti-bacterial, relieves pain, and promotes regeneration of skin. It can be used in skin grafts, and the treatment of corneal wounds.

A study in China on 350 patients treated with a beauty cream containing sea buckthorn oil, found positive effect on xanthopsis, melanosis, senile wrinkles and freckles.

Veterinarians have successfully controlled foot rot in sheep with applications of the oil and paste from sea buckthorn. Studies in Romania indicate significant wound healing properties attributed to sea buckthorn oil extract.

Sea buckthorn oil, rose oil, and plantain seed oil all produced therapeutic action on chemical burns of laboratory rabbit eyes. *Russian Clinical Pharmacology Journal* 1992.

The fruit oil, rich in omega-7 given orally, restored tear secretion in dry eye models. Kimura Y et al, *Nutrients* 2017 9(4).

In Germany, the fruit and seed oils are used externally for radiation damage, including x-ray and sunburn.

A study conducted in Russia in 1987 followed the treatment of gastric and duodenal ulcers using sea buckthorn oil.

The group of 30 men and 23 women had suffered from six months to fifteen years. After giving one dessertspoonful three to four times daily for three to four weeks, there was an absence of pain and dyspepsia in 86 % of patients.

There was healing of ulcer tissue, and improvement in the defense factors and regenerative processes of gastric mucous and blood flow to the stomach wall. T and B lymphocytes, and immunoglobulin production improved as well.

A double-blind, randomized, crossover study of sea buckthorn oil given to hemodialysis patients showed not improvement in all health parameters. Rodhe Y et al, *J Ren Nutr* 2013 23(3): 172-9.

Sea buckthorn and olive oil show healing benefit on full-thickness burn wounds, superior to silver sulfadiazine. Edraki M et al, *Adv Skin Wound Care* 2014 27(7): 317-23.

A comparative study, in the *Chinese Journal of Vet Medicine* 1997 23:6 on the effects of seed vs. fruit oil on immune systems of mice, found both worked well at high dosage but the seed oil effect was better.

Palmitoleic acid is a relatively rare fatty acid, and a component of skin fat, explaining in part, its support of cell tissue and wound healing.

The oil is useful in post-operative wounds of tonsillitis, and traumatic perforation of tympanic membrane. In 56 cases, it was found the oil helped reunite the valvulae of perforated edges, facilitated exudation and hematopedesis of tissue fluid of the wound and reunion of tympanic membrane. Fan Yulin et al, *Sea Buckthorn* 1991 4:2.

The fruit oil helped restore balance to hyperthyroid conditions. Chen et al, *Hippophae* 1998 1:4.

It also alleviates insulin resistance through the P13K/AKT pathway in type 2 diabetes mellitus cells, and diabetic rats. Gao S et al, *J Agric Food Chem* 2017 65(7): 1328-36.

Aubrey Organics, a manufacturer of quality cosmetics out of Tampa, Florida markets a skin care line with sea buckthorn pulp oil. The Body Shop uses the oil in several of its sunscreen products.

The Russian cosmonauts have used the oil to protect them from cosmic radiation for decades. Work by Gao et al, *World J Gastroenter* 2003:9 reported the fruit useful for prevention and treatment of liver fibrosis.

A combination of sea buckthorn and Saint John's wort oils may be useful in the treatment of endometriosis. Ilhan M et al, Taiwan *J Obstet Gynecol* 2016 55(6): 786-90.

Sea buckthorn oil, taken orally at three grams daily, shows benefit on vaginal atrophy in postmenopausal women. Larmo PS et al, *Maturitas* 2014 79(3): 316-21.

Work by Cao et al, *Zhong Yao Cai* 2003 26:10 found flavonoids from the seed and fruit residue reduced serum glucose, cholesterol and triglyceride levels.

Carbon dioxide extracts show inhibition of platelet aggregation. Work by Cheng et al, *Life Sci* 2003:72 reported a total flavone extract exhibits inhibitory effect similar to aspirin on platelet aggregation. This suggests possible use in preventing cardiac and cerebral thrombosis.

The seed oil, taken internally, appears to significantly reduce plasma cholesterol, LDL, atherogenic index and LDL/HDL ration. Basu et al, *Journal of Phytomedicine* 14:6.

It appears to restore natural killer cell activity. Ren Lisa et al, *Hippophae* 1992 5:4. The oil increased IL-2 function that helps strengthen the immune system.

Sea buckthorn oil increases NK cell cytotoxicity in chronic stress, by suppressing ACTH, cortisol, IL-1beta and TNF-alpha levels, and increasing 5-HT and IFNgamma levels. It up-regulates the expression of perforin and granzyme B. Diandong H et al, *Int J Immunopathol Pharmacol* 2016 29(1): 76-83.

Seed oil may be useful in treatment of depression. A preliminary study in chronic, unpredictable mild stress in rats found increased levels of pimelic and palmitic acid in urine, and lower levels of suberic acid, citrate, phthalic acid, cinnamic acid and Sumiki's acid. Tian JS et al, *Food Funct* 2015 6(11): 3585-92.

The oil reduces lipid oxidation due to content of SOD or superoxide dismutase, also found in the leaves. Animal studies have shown the oil postpones senility and prevents lipid peroxidation. Rui Livin et al, *Proceedings of Int Symposium Seabuckthorn* 1989.

Sarcoma 180, lymphatic leukemia, and B16 cancer cell formation have been inhibited by oral administration of seed oil. Zhang et al, *Hippophae* 1989 2:3.

Human leukemia cells and Ellis ascites carcinoma are inhibited by oil obtained from fruit pressings. Yang Jian Ping et al, *Int Symposium Seabuckthorn*, Xi'an China 1989.

Sea buckthorn oil has close to 200 properties, including blood circulation, oxygenation of skin, and removing excess toxins from the body. It easily penetrates the epidermis, and protects against infection, prevents allergies, reduces inflammation and inhibits the aging process. Zielinska A & I Nowak. *Lipids Health Dis* 2017 16(1): 95.

The seed residue, leftover from oil extraction, blocks angiotensin signals and improves insulin sensitivity, suggesting use in cardiovascular and diabetic conditions. Pang et al, *J Ethnopharm* 117:2.

Flavonoids derived from seeds reduced obesity, triglyerides and suppression of adipose tissue inflammation via PPARgamma and PPARalpha gene expression. Yang X et al, *Pharm Biol* 2017 55(1): 1207-14.

To encourage the industry in Western Canada, a processing plant is necessary. Although published in Russian, an article by Varlamov in *Traktory-i-Sel'skokhozy-aistvennye-Mashiny* 1998 10 contains plans for a factory, including diagrams of the process stages and suggested layout of equipment, such as choppers, crushers, pumps, centrifuges, filter presses, etc.

To make your own fruit oil, see recipes.

LEAF OIL

The unsaponifiable part of an ethereal extract of sea buckthorn leaves yields lipids with medicinal use.

It is similar in composition to the pericarps, with high aliphatic esters, and cyclic acid of triterpene nature present. The intracellular lipids are mainly esters of various alcohols with higher fatty acids, as well as triaclyglycerols, carotenoids, aldehydes, and phytol, campesterol nortriterpene alcohols and polyprenols.

Leaf extracts using sunflower oil have shown effect on repair processes like the rest of the plant. The surprising amount of carotenoids, up to 600mg/% from the leaves is worthy of further investigation.

The main fatty acids in leaf extracts were palmitic and linolenic.

CO_2 extractions augment immunity in response to tetanus and diphtheria toxoids, and may hold promise for balanced Th1 and Th2 directed adjuvant for veterinary and human vaccines. Jayashankar B et al, *Int Immunopharmacol* 2017 44: 123-36.

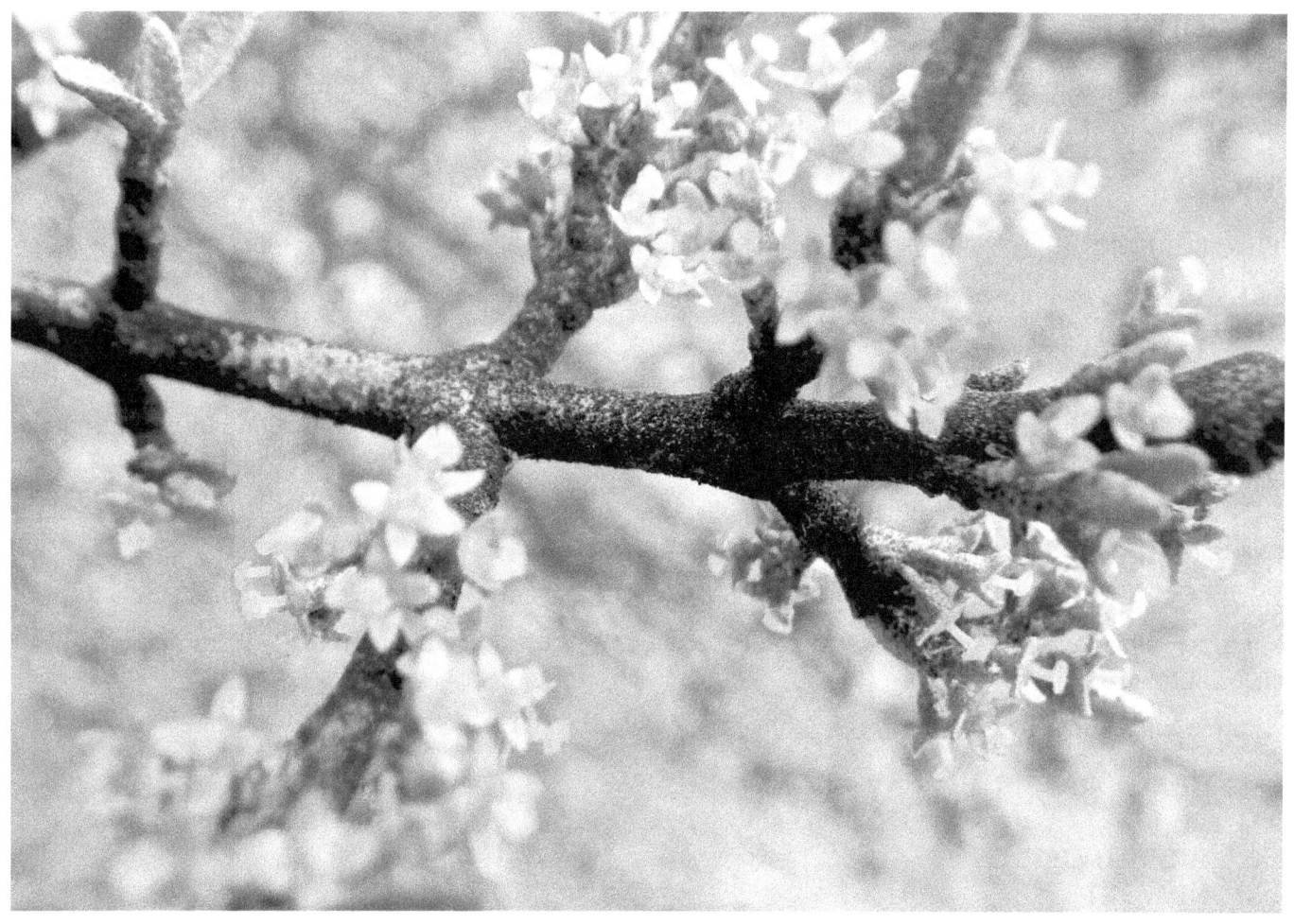

SEA BUCKTHORN FLOWERS

ESSENTIAL OILS

CONSTITUENTS- fruit- over sixty components, including ethyl hexanoate, 3-methylbutyl benzoate, 3-methylbutyl octanoate; various aliphatic esters. Terpenes and aromatic compounds are extremely low. Carotenoids are present in 1900 IU of provitamin A per gram. Yield is 36 mg/kg.

Carbon dioxide extractions of fruit appear to be the most useful form for cosmetic and external application.

The fatty acids, essential oils and waxes are retained in a relatively stable and easy to use form. The oil is added, at no more than 5% dilution, as anti-wrinkle, skin softener, wound healing and increased skin granulation. It has good application in various ointments, suppositories, balsams, aerosols and cosmetic creams.

FLOWER ESSENCES

Sea buckthorn flower essence is best suited to individuals truly weighed down with poverty consciousness. Because the pattern of scarcity is so well entrenched, it is difficult for any movement to be made with regards to prosperity. Sea buckthorn flower essence helps shift mental and emotional focus, so that other possibilities can take root.

Sexuality and abundance are so inter-related on a spiritual plane, that distortions of one with affect the other directly. **PRAIRIE DEVA**

Sea Buckthorn essence helps give fresh perspectives; un-involvement; protection from harmful influences; understanding emotions. **GREEN MAN**

PERSONALITY TRAITS

She forms a bridge between sea and land. Where the sturdy sand grasses are sculpting dunes, she feels at home. She's the queen of poor, sandy soil, vanishing as soon as humus forms and the soil becomes richer.   **LEAF**

RECIPES

TINCTURE- 1-2 ml daily. A tincture is made from the leaf at 1:4 ratio with 60% alcohol.

FRESH JUICE- 2-4 ounces daily. The compound pheophytin may be useful as a marker of berry ripeness. Andersson et al, *J Ag Food Chem* 2009 57:1.

Preserving fresh juice in ice cubes has many advantages.

LEAF INFUSION- One part dried leaf to 32 parts boiling water. Steep for one hour. Combine with Boneset, in equal parts for Dengue fever.

VINEGAR- Equal parts of fresh berries and apple cider vinegar. Leave for two weeks, shaken daily. Great for salads and skin.

FRUIT OIL- Cover fresh berries with olive oil for 6-8 weeks in container that breathes. Mash thoroughly and strain.

For more information on sea buckthorn products, contact Seabuckthorn International in Summerland, BC or check out their website.

Another interesting site is www.icrts.org/china.htm

SELF HEAL
ALL HEAL
HEART OF THE EARTH
WOUNDWORT
(***Prunella vulgaris*** L.)
PARTS USED- leaves and flowers

My garden grew Self-heal and Balm,
And Speedwell that's blue for an hour,
Then blossoms again, O, grievous my pain,
I'm plundered of each flower. **DEVONSHIRE SONG**
"No one wants a surgeon, who keeps prunelle."   **FRENCH PROVERB**

Prunella is believed derived from the Old German **BRUNELLA** quinsy or diphtheria, an inflammation of the mouth, from **BRAUNE**, a sore throat with brown tongue, or less likely, from **BRAUN**, for the brown seed heads. Others believe it has roots in the Latin **PRUNUM**, or purple, for the colour of the flowers. In the doctrine of signatures, the flower has an obvious throat and mouth. One author believes it stems from the French **BRUNELLE** meaning little plum, or the Latin **PRUNELLA** for little prune.

Self Heal is a naturalized, circumpolar and common perennial often overlooked for several reasons. That it is low growing is obvious. But because it is perceived as "wound healing" and has an All Heal reputation, science-oriented herbalists tend to dismiss it. Which is really unfortunate, as you will see.

My wife and I once operated a store and clinic called *Self Heal Herbal Centre*. I always loved the plant and we now have a company specializing in flower essences and essential oils, the latter aromatherapy line called *Scents of Wonder*.

Many years ago (25?) we attended Expo West in Anaheim and I took along freshly printed business cards with a line drawing of self heal with its latin binomial printed below. Much to my surprise I received several months later, a letter address to Dear Prunella. Ha Ha.

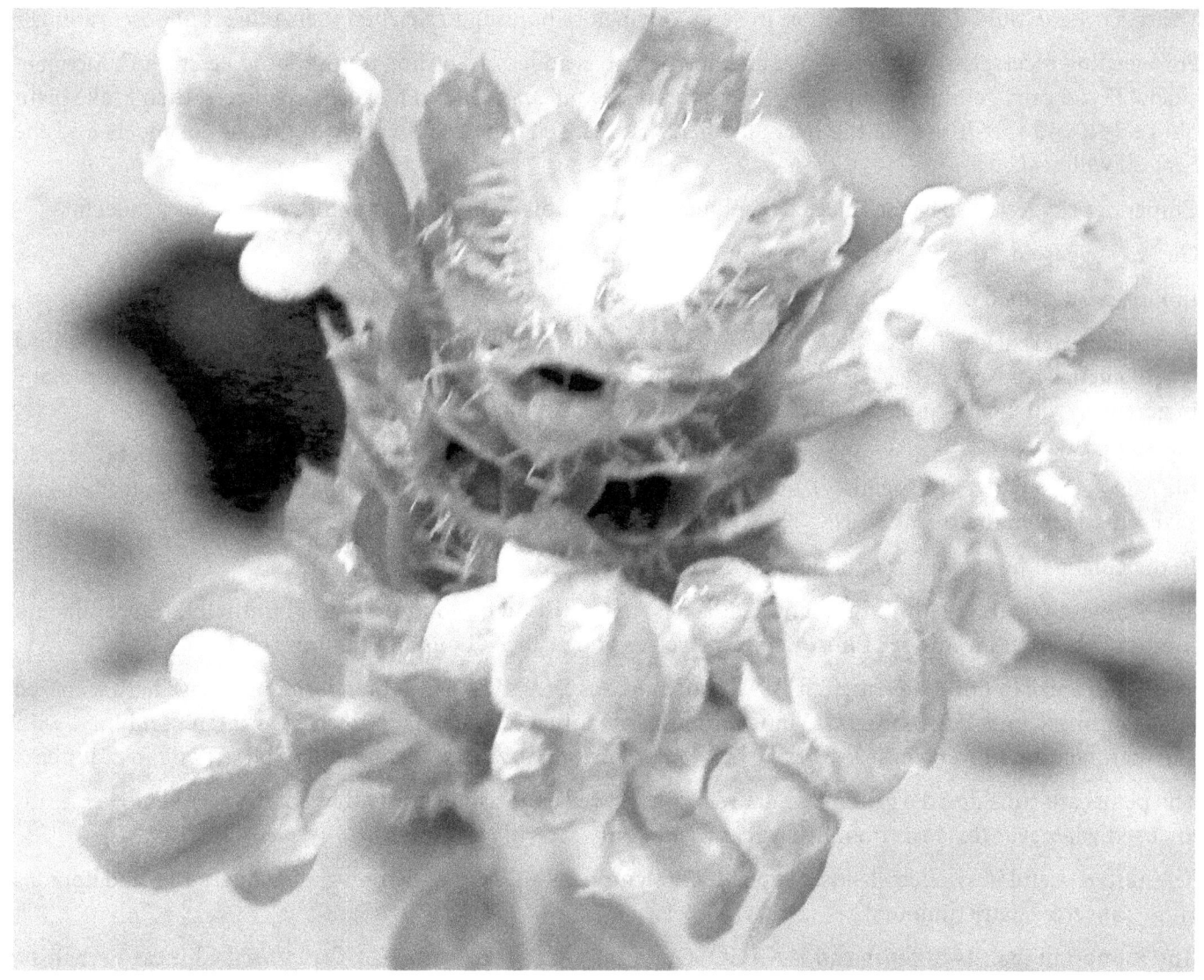

SELF HEAL

The aerial parts are cold, bitter and somewhat acrid.

The Blackfoot used the plant decoctions for cleansing wounds, and for healing saddle sores on their horses. The Natives of BC soaked the plant in cool water to make a tonic beverage, or to treat gas and other stomach problems.

The Cree chewed the leaves or used infusions as a gargle for sore and inflamed throats. The Iroquois gave it to babies that cried too much, and to relieve sickness caused by prolonged grieving over the loss of a loved one.

Chippewa people named the introduced plant, **NAME' WUSKONS'**, using the root along with catnip in decoction as a physic, or strong laxative.

Further south, the Cherokee call it **DI DO DI**, or spoon, using it as special female medicine, a carminative and for treating hemorrhage. Other sources suggest the Cherokee call it **GA NI QUI LI SKI**, and use it to wash wounds.

The Quileute of Washington state put the plant juice on boils. The neighboring Chehalis don't use the flower, but say that when not quite open it has a face like a person. This is true!

The Karuk also pick off the flowers and use the aerial parts for convulsions, bleeding gums, in salves for ulcerated sores and in cough formulations with chokecherry bark and yerba santa.

Various tribes would drink the root tea in ceremony before hunting to sharpen their powers of observation.

For bleeding ulcers, a tea is made to which knox gelatin is added, according to Josephine Peters, a Californian elder. "If you can't get the gel out of the Solomon seal (*Smilacina stellata*) for bleeding ulcers, then I take plain old gelatin and mix it in with the heal-all when you drink it. The gelatin seals the tissue for ulcers and the heal-all will heal.

Culpepper suggested the fresh juice be combined with rose oil and rubbed into the temples for headache.

Gerard suggested, "there is not a better wounde herb in the world."

In Europe, it gained prominence for contagious fevers amongst German armies in 1547 and 1566.

Parkinson's Herbal (1640) records. "This is generally called prunella and brunella from the Germans who called it brunellen, because it cures that disease which they call die brun, common to soldiers in camp, but especially in garrison, which is an inflammation of the mouth, throat and tongue."

The tender, young leaves make an acceptable potherb or salad addition. In China, its use for food dates back to the Ming dynasty (late 16th century), or earlier. In Hunan province, it is eaten as part of glutinous steamed rice cakes, made from the spring buds.

In the Guangdong region, a tasty soup or cool tea is preferred.

The Chinese use the seeds for anxiety, headaches, hepatitis, high blood pressure, ophthalmia, scrofula and tinnitus. The leaves were used for the above as well as gout, cancer, boils and tumours.

The flower spike or flowers are used in TCM, and known as **XIA KU CAO** in Mandarin, meaning "herb withered after summer" and **HA BU CHOU** in Cantonese; meaning Summer Dry Herb. It is often combined with Chrysanthemum flowers for fever, headaches, hypertension, dizziness, vertigo and hyperactivity in children.

The plants are considered a cardiovascular relaxant, as well as a vasodilator and hypotensive. The flower heads are used whenever toxicosis from heavy metals, or gouty arthritis is present.

The herb is useful in swollen glands, lymphadentis, lymphangitis, cervical lymph gland congestion, and lipomas (non-cancerous fatty tumours).

The Kampo herbalists of Japan call it **KAGOSO**, and use it in the manner of Traditional Chinese herbalists. In Korea, it is known as **HAGOCHO**.

The first record of use is found in the early monograph *Sehn nong ben cao jing*.

Among the Amchies of the Himalayas, Self Heal leaves and flowers are used in cerebral and brain disorders, as well as colds, headaches and gastric disturbances.

In Ireland, the herb was used as a heart remedy and sudden stroke as well as de-worming children, piles, eczema, renal colic and "weak blood".

In fact, it is one of the seven herbs that nothing natural or supernatural can harm. The other plants are vervain, speedwell, eyebright, mallow, yarrow and St. John's wort.

Self Heal represents the 22nd Nordic Rune, Ing.

In a study on nectar secretion of members of the Lamiaceae family, it was found that Self Heal was the highest producer per flower/per day.

It companion plants well with Betony and Violets.

Work by Colin Kingshott with *Plant Bio Signatures* or Florachology has found that Self Heal emits its strongest vibratory patterns at 12 am. This suggests that each plant emits energetic fields at different times, and flower essence preparations are optimized, by measuring these fields.

MEDICINAL

CONSTITUENTS- triterpenoids (64) including ursolic, betulinic, gluconic and oleanolic acids, hyperoside, beta amyrin, euscaphicacid, rosmarinic acid (up to 6.1%), caffeic acid, prunellin, two steroidal triterpenoids; rutin, tannins, bitters, resin, aucubin, and coumarins including umbelliferone, scopoletin, and esculetin.
Also includes danshensu (salvianic acid A), butyl rosmarinate, salviaflaside, tanshinon, rhein and autantiamide acetate, as well as lupeol, betulic acid, uvaol, ethyl coffeate, and beta amyrenone.
Flavonoids include delphinidin, cyanidin, luteolin, isoorientin, and cinaroside.
Sterol glycosides include beta-sitosterol, stigmasterol, stigmast-7-en-3-betal-ol, spinasterol. Monoterpenes include d-camphor and d-fenchone.
Contains up to 68% potassium chloride of the soluble salts; as well as vitamins A, B1, C, K, and trace minerals including zinc, copper and high amounts 4.5% of magnesium.
root- 1.4% calcium, betulinic acid, endophytic fungi (XKC-S03).
A thorough review of the phytochemistry and pharmacological activities by Bai Yubing et al, *Food Chemistry* 2016 204:483-96 has great detail into constituents for those interested.

Self Heal, like fleabane and shepherd's purse, has a well-deserved reputation as a vulnerary or wound healer. It behaves like them as a true hemostat in both active and passive bleeding.

Cool, dry and astringent infusions help reduce inflammation of the mouth, gums, throat and ears. External washes help relieve sore eyes, blepharitis, conjunctivitis, and other redness and inflammation of the eyes from tiredness and strain. As well, *Prunella vulgaris* extracts, in the form of eye drops, showed good success in clinical cases of herpes keratitis; 38 patients treated with prunella eye drops were cured, 37 others improved and only three did not benefit, out of 78 patients.

Prunella could be considered in helping reduce the intra-ocular pressure associated with glaucoma.

It combines well with water plantain that improves fluid drainage, and apigenin rich herbs such as parsley, chamomile, feverfew and chrysanthemum.

At one time, Self Heal was exported from England all over the world and used by opera singers for throat and bronchial afflictions. One of its greatest abilities is clearing heat from the body, particularly an overactive liver.

Research from China indicates that it plays a role in blood pressure reduction, due to this cool and soothing quality, reducing hyperactivity of the liver. In TCM, the flower spikes are combined with puncture vine (*Tribulus terrestris*) fruit, white peony root, water plantain rhizome and chrysanthemum flowers for liver fire and liver yang conditions.

As well, its mild diuretic properties reduce swelling and edema.

In one study of 42 hypertensive patients, the herb showed good results. *Fujian Jian Zhong Yi Yao* 1959 4:41. In some cases of hypertension, unresolved or suppressed anger can be problematic.

Decoctions of the herb and pulsatilla root have been shown effective in the treatment of tuberculosis of the cervical lymph nodes; the enlarged glands gradually subsiding or shrunk significantly in two to four weeks. Inflamed lymph nodes, swollen, enlarged and hard will respond.

Nodules in the inguinal canal also respond.

Self Heal combines well with red root and figwort in the treatment of lipomas, those fatty accumulations under the skin that move when touched. Cystic breast disease and hemorrhoids respond well to the combination, adding dandelion leaf and rhaponticum (maral root).

It combines well with hop flowers. Out of 21 cases of pulmonary tuberculosis, 17 benefited, and it was markedly effective in reducing cough, fever and chest pain, and increasing appetite.

The plant makes a useful addition to wound, burn and skin salves.

Fresh plant poultices or the juice can be applied to insect bites, boils, carbuncles, sties, gum or canker sores; as well as cracked nipples. David Winston says that a native elder told him compresses are very effective for removing splinters of wood, metal or glass.

A 5% ethanol tincture was administered to mice suffering intestinal inflammation, with greatly reduced severity of mucosal inflammation, suggesting a trial in colitis. Haarberg KM et al, *World J Gastrointest Pharmacol Ther* 2015 6(4): 223-37.

Self Heal helps moderate and regulate menstrual bleeding both internally and with douching. It relieves hot and irritated in-between period bleeding, especially when due to liver congestion.

Diarrhea and hemorrhoids are likewise relieved with cool infusions orally and/or retention enemas.

Self Heal contains high levels of rosmarinic acid, (6.1%), a phenolic type anti-oxidant that shows great promise as a cancer preventative. Rosmarinic acid, according to James Duke, helps suppress thyroid hormone production in both over-active thyroid conditions such as Grave's Disease, and raises them in hypoactive thyroid. For these purposes it combines well with Bugleweed, Vervain, Motherwort or Radish, according to whole picture pattern.

The fresh plant juice helps increase production of adrenocortical hormones, helping restore and support adrenal function that is hypoactive.

Work in China has shown the plant to be leukocytogenic.

Ursolic acid is a constituent considered both antibiotic and anti-tumour. Work by Achina et al, *Oncol Rep* 14:2 has found ursolic acid active against endometrial cancer cells.

Ryu et al, *Planta Medica* 2000 66 found ursolic acid to be the most important anti-inflammatory compound in the plant.

Work by Xiong et al, *Zhong Yao Cai* 2003 26:8 found ursolic acid promotes bile secretion, and significantly protects the liver from toxic chemicals.

Ursolic acid also appears to modulate human dendritic cells in a manner favouring Th1 via considerable activation of interferon gamma. Jung TY et al, *Eur J Pharm* 2010 643:2-3, suggests its use as an adjuvant for vaccine cancer immunotherapy.

Modern research has found the herb inhibits *Bacillus dysenteriae* and *Mycobacterium tuberculosis*.

In a small study of 18 cases of pulmonary tuberculosis, a success rate of 78.5% was found after a period of time taking a herb decoction only. *Zhong yi Za Zhi* 1961 11:147.

Older *in vitro* work shows inhibition against *Shigella spp, Salmonella typhi, E. coli, Pseudomonas aeruginosa*, and *Streptococcus species*.

A lectin, isolated from aerial parts shows activity against *S. typhi, E. coli*, and *Klebsiella pneumoniae*. Mustafa et al, *J Pharm Res* 2011 4:10.

Drug-resistant *Mycobacterium tuberculosis* induced in rats was significantly reduced with self heal. Enhanced cell-mediated immunity was due to up-regulating levels of genetic transcription. Lu J et al, *Mol Med Rep* 2013 May 27.

Four organic acids, including betulinic acid, were found to have strong inhibitory activity against allergenic tests.

Research from China has shown Self Heal to contain prunellin (possibly a sulphated polysaccharide) that inhibits HIV-1 replication in hot water extractions at a dosage of 16 mcg/ml. Chang 1988; and Zhang 1990.

Yao et al, in March 1992 issue of *Virology* showed that prunella extracts block cell to cell transmission of the virus and interfere with the virus's ability to bind with T cells.

In fact, prunellin is more effective than retrovir (AZT) in inhibiting reverse transcriptase activity.

This work by Canadian researchers followed the identification of prunellin, a complex sugar, by Tabba and other scientists at the University of California at Davis.

Work by An et al, *Life Science* 2001 68: 14 removed polyphenols from self heal, and found the herb exhibited moderate anti-HIV activity.

In November of 1999, a research team at Dalhousie University in my hometown of Halifax, Nova Scotia, isolated a polysaccharide from *P. vulgaris* with specific activity against *Herpes simplex* virus. Its mode of action appears to be different that from other anionic carbohydrates such as heparin. It stops the virus from growing within cells, and prevents it from binding to cells.

Water extracts (infusions) seem to work best with post infection and simultaneous infections, while the ethanol extract (tincture) works best at pre-infection stage.

An 80% ethanol extract was found to reduce inflammation of *herpes labialis*. Reichling et al, *Forsch Komplement* 2008 15:6.

In one study of 78 cases of herpetic keratitis, causing by the virus, 38 treated with prunella eye drops were cured and 37 improved. Only 3 patients did not benefit.

Dextrin sulphate is another anti-HIV substance found in Self Heal. The related Dextran sulphate is present in the Chinese Violet (*V. yedoensis*), and appears to inhibit viral binding and replication. Rosmarinic acid inhibits multiple enzymes of HIV including DNA polymerase, RNase H and Integrase activity.

Water extracts inhibit HIV-1. Oh C et al, *Virol Journal* 2011 8:188.

Zhang et al, *Antiviral Res* 2007 75:3 found a lignin polysaccharide complex inhibits viral binding in HSV 1 and 2 and penetrates host cell walls.

Recent work suggests self heal exhibits potent anti-Ebola viral activity. Yang Y et al, *J Med Virol* 2017 89(5): 908-16. This follows up work by Zhang X et al, *Antiviral Res* 2016 127:20-31 that found water extracts exhibit anti-Ebola virus activity. Their research suggests the extract directly binds, and blocks early viral event, and enhanced the activity of monoclonal antibody MAb 2G4.

Ethanol extracts significantly improved cellular immune function of mice infected with multi-drug-resistant *Mycobacterium tuberculosis*. Lu J et al, *Journal of Medical Colleges of PLA* 2011 26(4): 230-7.

Studies by Lee et al (1988) showed self heal extracts exhibit moderate anti-mutagenic activity in lab studies. The flower petals show activity against sarcoma 180, cervix cancer-14, as well as thyroid, esophagus and breast cancer, and hepatoma of the liver.

Prunella exerts anti-cancer activity on human breast carcinoma-associated fibroblasts, by inhibiting basic fibroblast growth factor, thus inhibiting breast cancer SKBr-3 cells indirectly. Hao J et al, *Chin J Integr Med* 2016 Sept 1.

Zhang et al, *Zhong Yao Cai* 2009 32:6 found *Prunella* significantly inhibits Jurket cells and exhibits anti-tumor effect.

The herb appears to reduce proliferation, induce apoptosis and stop migration of cancers on endothelial cells. Xiong-Zhi et al, *J Med Plant Res* 2011 5:17.

Rosmarinic acid from this herb inhibits metastasis of breast cancer cells to bone tissue. Xu Yichun et al, *Planta Medica* 76:10.

Oleanolic acid from the herb induced apoptosis in lung adencarcinoma cell lines via down regulation of Bcl-2 expression and upregulation of Bax and Bad expression. Feng et al, *Asia Pac J Cancer Prev* 2011 12:2.

Polysaccharides show activity against adenocarcinoma associated with lung cancers as well as immune modulation and increased thymus and spleen function. Feng et al, *Molecules* 2010 15:8.

The herb contains more rosmarinic acid, than the herb rosemary.

Work by Won et al, *Eur J Immunol* 2003 33:4 found rosmarinic acid inhibits TCR signaling and subsequent T cell proliferation.

Self heal, marijuana and ashwaghanda all exhibit anti-inflammatory, anti-arthritic and anti-rheumatic properties. All three may be useful in treating auto-immune conditions such as rheumatoid arthritis. Zaka M et al, *J Mol Graph Model* 2017 74: 296-304.

This rosmarinic acid content is helpful in Grave's Disease, or in suppressing any hyperactive thyroid condition, as mentioned above.

This is interesting, as Prunella flowers are considered a specific for eyeball pain in the afternoon or evening. One symptom associated with hyperthyroidism is eyeball bulge, and increased hypertension.

Work by Yang et al, *Zhongguo Zhong Xi Yi Jie* 2007 27:1 looked at the benefit of this herb on 56 cases of hyperthyroidism, 24 cases of hypothyroidism and 18 cases of goiter. Treatment was found superior to western orthodox medical approaches in terms of gland size and other parameters after one month.

Rosmarinic acid is useful in various autoimmune inflammatory conditions, and helps prevent tissue rejection in human skin grafts. It protects the lungs in chronic disease and prevents arterial blocking from lipid deposits.

Rosmarinic acid is anti-oxidant, anti-inflammatory, and helps reduce histamine release from mast cells. Sanbongi et al, *Free Rad Biol Med* 2003:34 found it inhibits lung injury from diesel exhaust particles, by reducing the expression of the macrophage inflammatory protein-1alpha.

Ursolic acid is also present in the herb in decent amounts. A mouse study found that ethanol extracts of self heal flowers, containing ursolic acid, enhanced sleep duration through GABA A receptors, suggesting benefit for insomnia. Jeon SJ et al, *Eur J Pharmacol* 2015 762: 443-8.

The herb inhibits mast cell derived allergies and cytokine cascade in water extract experiments by Kim et al, *Exp Bio Med* 232:7.

Beta amyrin and euscaphic acid suppress release of histamine, helping contribute to anti-allergic inflammatory effect. Choia HG et al, *Nat Prod Commun* 2016 11(1): 31-2.

Both the herb and rosmarinic acid significantly eliminate reactive oxidative stress and diminish IL-6 release preventing damage to UVB exposed skin. Vostalova et al, *Arch Dermatol Res* 2009 Oct 28.

Toshiaki et al, *Nephrol Dial Transplant* 2000:15 found rosmarinic acid inhibits cytokine-induced mesangial cell proliferation and suppresses platelet-derived growth factor.

Rosmarinic acid is useful in kidney disease, including suppressing proteinuria, suppressed mesangial IgA deposition and significantly suppressed serum IgA levels in HIGA mice. Makino et al, *Nephr Dialysis Transplant* 2003 18.

Water extracts suppress renal inflammation and fibrosis, and targets glomerulonephritis and glomerulosclerosis associated with diabetic nephropathy. Namgung S et al, *Am J Chin Med* 2017 45(3): 475-95.

It may also ameliorate type 1 diabetic complications, due in part to a rich fraction of caffeic acid. Raafat K et al, *Biomed Pharmacother* 2016 84: 1008-18.

Decoctions inhibit alpha-amylase, alpha-glucosidase and alpha-maltase, reducing post-prandial hyperglycemia. Wu HP et al, *Journal of Nanjing University of Traditional Chinese Medicine* 2009 25(5): 361-3.

Water extracts inhibit diabetic atherosclerosis in type two diabetic mice, increase creatinine clearance and reduce total cholesterol, triglycerides and LDL. Hwang SM et al, *The American Journal of Chinese Medicine* 2012 40(5): 937-51.

William LeSassier believed the plant strengthened and pumped the kidneys especially in combinations involving dental decay.

Work by Psotova et al, found rosmarinic and caffeic acids work better together than separately in anti-viral, anti-microbial and anti-oxidant activity. *Phytotherapy Research* 17:9.

Plant tinctures may enhance cognitive function, in part by up-regulation of adult hippocampal neurogenesis, associated with neuronal plasticity. Park SJ et al, *Phytother Res* 2015 29(11): 1814-21.

Plant tinctures appear to reduce neuro-inflammation, suggesting benefit in anti-dementia dietary supplementation. Qu Z et al, *J Agric Food Chem* 2017 65(2): 291-300.

The same author found the whole herb and rosmarinic acid gave improved protection to cardiomyoctes subjected to doxorubicin induced oxidative stress. *Fitoterapia* 76:6.

The herb is protectant to liver cells by increasing expression of heme oxygenase-inducing activity. This is especially true of one of the constituents, 23 hydroxy-ursolic acid. Jeong et al, *Biol Pharm Bull* 2008 31:3.

Harput et al, *Phytother Res* 20:2 found the plant increased proliferation of lymphocytes, while suppressing nitric oxide production. It stimulated macrophage activity without cytotoxicity.

Recent work by Han et al, *Food Chem Tox* Oct 2008 found water extracts stimulate macrophage activity via NFkappaB transactivation and mitogen activated protein kinase activation. Zhang et al, *Zhong Yao Cai* 2006 29:11 found *Prunella* to suppress proliferation of Raji cells, probably by inducing apoptosis; suggesting another lymphoma treating herbal tool.

Work by Il Kyun Lee et al, *Arch Pharm Res* 2008 31:12 found ursolic acid extracted from the flower head active against various cancer cell lines including A549, SK-OV-3, SK-MEL-2 and HCT15.

The herb may have application in periodontitis, based on work by Zdarilova et al, *Toxicol in Vitro* 2008 Dec 30.

The herb shows anti-estrogenic activity and may have application in treatment of endometriosis and hormone sensitive cancers. Collins, *Biol Reprod* 2009 80:2.

Ethanol extracts may be helpful in treating cognitive impairment via NMDA receptor signal pathways. Park et al, *Food Chem Toxicol* 2010 48:6.

Methanol extracts significantly inhibit lipase activity. Cheng-Dong Zheng et al, *J Chin Med Assoc* 2010 73:6.

Self Heal combines well with Hawthorn berries in the treatment of hyperactivity in children. Even the roots can be used, as a vermifuge.

An endophyte from root suppresses activity of gastric cancer, *in vitro* and *in vivo*. Tan J et al, *Oncol Lett* 2015 9(2): 945-9. The root also contains betulinic acid, a known anti-cancer, anti-viral compound.

HOMEOPATHY

Prunella is for the treatment of colitis and dysentery.

DOSE- Tincture to sixth potency.

CELL SALTS

Kali Mur (potassium chloride) molecules build fibrin, a building block for skin and connective tissue. In venous blood, fibrin amounts to 0.3% parts and when levels fall lower the blood fibrin thickens, causing pneumonia, pleurisy, and mucus congestion.

If the body cannot throw out the thickened fibrin, it clogs up the arteries as well as auricles and ventricles of the heart.

Earaches with swelling of Eustachian tubes, or swollen glands around ears with noises, snapping and cracking are indicated.

Symptoms worse from cold drinks, open air, dampness, motion, and fatty meals. Better from rubbing and letting hair down. Conditions that can be treated are Eustachian tube blockages, sinus problems, acne rosacea, varicose veins, white discharges, tonsillitis and difficulty digesting fats. **CARD**

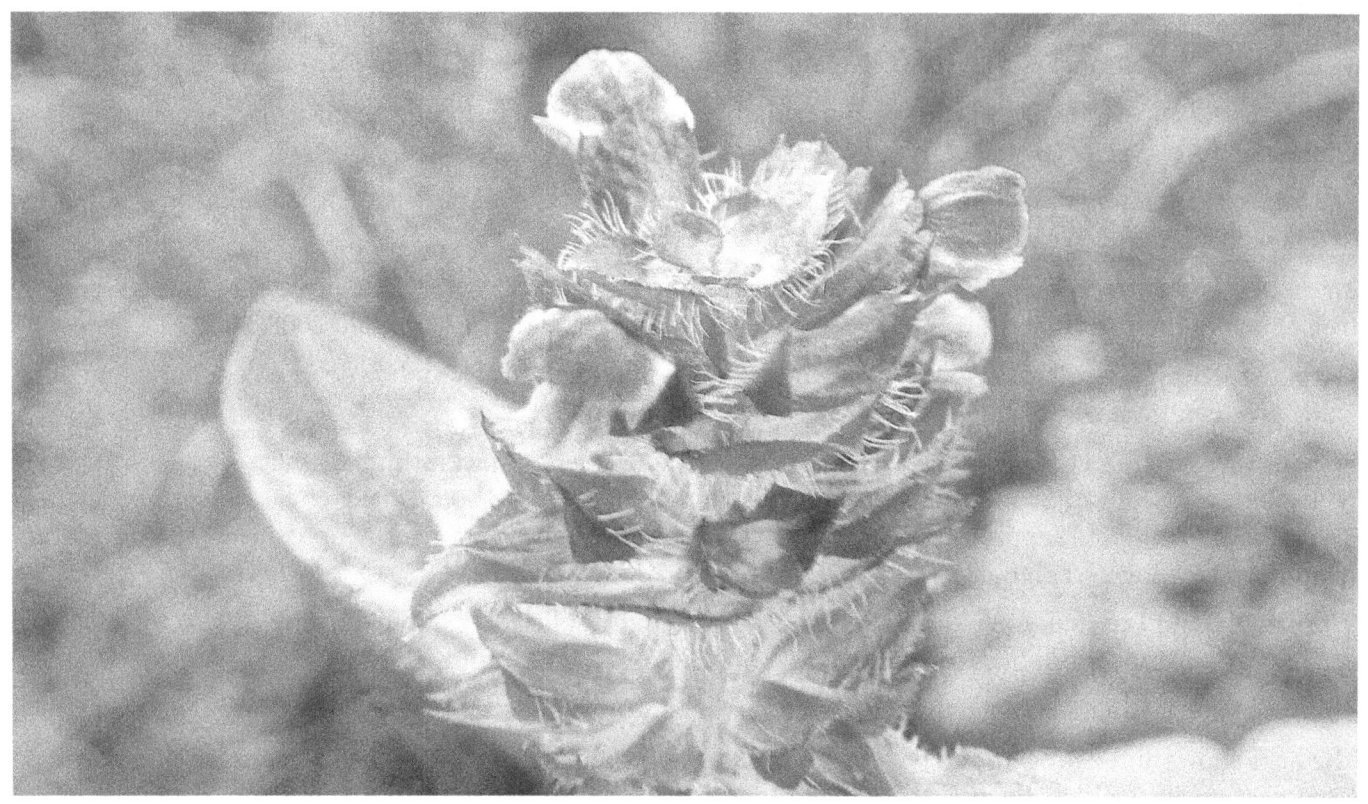

SELF HEAL FLOWER HEAD

ESSENTIAL OIL

CONSTITUENTS- fourteen chemical components including selin-11-en-4-alpha-ol 15%, cis-eudesma-6, 11-diene 9.4%, 1,10-di-epi-cubenol 8%, spathulenol 5.8%, germacrene D 5.1%, d- camphor, d-fenchone, hexadecanoic acid, flavonoids (0.14-0.19%), coumarins (0.26-0.40%), sesquiterpene lactones, isoquercitin. The yield is about 0.16% from the fruiting spikes.
A study in Ukraine identified mainly alpha-camphor, germacrene D, alpha pinene, beta-elemene and beta caryophyllene.

Although not a commercial commodity, self heal contains two and four cell essential oil glands. See hydrosols below.

HYDROSOLS

The distilled water of self heal is an excellent medicine for all injuries of the mouth, particularly quinsy and scurvy of the mouth, provided one gargles with it often.

Or, prepare the following gargle: Mix together three ounces of self heal water and plantain water...a small piece of cloth dipped in self heal water and repeatedly laid warm upon the affected place until it dries will prove exceedingly beneficial against all inflammations of the privates in both men and women.

Those who do not have the distilled water of self heal, or cannot get it, just use the freshly squeezed juice during the summer, or in the winter boil the dried leaves in water and use this instead.   **SAUER**

Prunella Dew (Xia ku cao lu) is the aromatic distillate of the fresh spikes, with properties similar to the herb. It is a popular beverage for summertime heat, and given to children for rashes and irritation. It can also be used for those with scrofula or thyroid conditions. The herb is cold and bitter, but prunella dew's effect is moderating, and it can be taken over a long period of time.

Prunella water is distilled in September for bloody diarrhea and dysentery. It causes women's soft breasts to become hard, according to Brunschwig in his 1530 Book of Distillation.

FLOWER ESSENCES

Self Heal flower essence, taken during fasting, helps the body assimilate minerals necessary for a good state of health. Surrounding the physical body is the thermal, a combination of the etheric and body's heat. Self Heal strengthens this region, helping you gain mastery over your skin temperature.

The thermal body acts as a breeding ground- hostile to harmful microbes and cultivating the needed. White corpuscles become more enzyme-like in property; with the spleen and colon becoming a point of concentration for re-assimilation.

The flower essence helps to ease doubts and confusion. Externally, it may be applied to athlete's foot. It also helps to cleanse quartz- just add two drops to pure water and immerse for ten minutes. Use when the sun is in Pisces.

DOSE- When fasting add 3-7 drops to water. **GURUDAS**

Self Heal flower essence is for those with the inability to take inner responsibility for one's healing, or those lacking the spiritual motivation for wellness, and are over-dependent on external help. The essence helps give self-confidence and self-acceptance. **FLOWER ESSENCE SOCIETY**

Self Heal flower essence is good for concentration during prayer or meditation, bringing one closer to ancient roots. It reduces spiritual skepticism, and aids in spiritual survival during intense emotional times. **MT. JULIUS**

Self Heal flower essence is for negative feelings of isolation; where one wishes to be alone and build a shell. Energy is diverted to work in an attempt to run from the inner self. The aloneness turns into loneliness; with a deliberate deadening of the senses.

Failure of a relationship, with all its pain, leads to defensiveness and a burial of the pain at a deeper level. It helps one enjoy their own company, and to communicate and interact in social groups. **NEW ZEALAND**

SPIRITUAL PROPERTIES

Self Heal, on the herbal and physical level, works with the body's ability to transfer medicinal properties. Spiritually, there occurs a powerful energy that leads to deeper absorption and ease of expression.

Used properly, this energy accelerates all spiritual processes. The herb and flower essence combine well for those individuals having trouble assimilating food, or making the switch to vegetarian diet.

Expressive abilities are made clear, as the etheric esophagus is activated.

This self-healing energy is useful for healing past hurts associated with traditional religious institutions and their expressions of God. There is greater understanding of vibrations associated with food, and extra energy is released from the throat chakra **GURUDAS**

This herb was once called a gift from God because of all its uses. If you're feeling anxious and stressed, add All Heal tea to your bathwater for relaxation and to release all of your worries.

Adding the flowers to a salad served to your beloved will improve your relationship and dispel any misunderstandings. **S. GREGG**

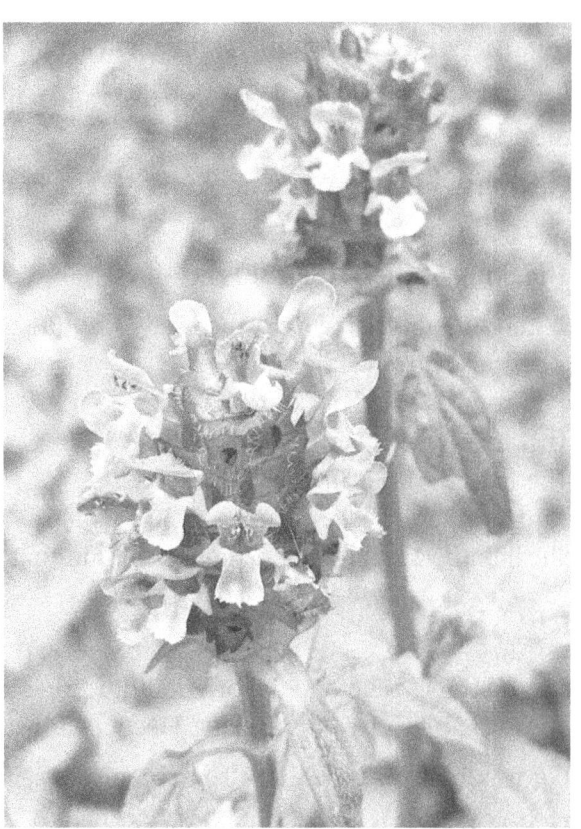

SELF HEAL BLOSSOMS

Self-heal waves her delicate purple wand and beckons us to come closer. She is a common herb or the common people. Never underestimate the common people as a force of transformation. It is through our commonality, our sharing and belonging to the community as a whole, that social change is born…The power of self-heal is the power of the people to heal on all levels…We now have and always will have the ability to heal ourselves. This knowledge is returning to us now, and knowledge is power.

Self-heal reminds us that we are always being supported and we always have everything we need in order to heal. **THEA SUMMER DEER**

MYTHS AND LEGENDS

The mother of a mayor suffered from scrofula with a swollen neck. All the doctors said there was no cure. One day, a herbalist came along who told the mayor he knew a herb to cure the disease. He climbed a nearby mountain, and came back with the herb that cured her.

Before he left, the herbalist told the mayor the herb only grew in summer.

The following winter, the governor came down with the same scrofula and swollen neck. The mayor, eager to help, told of the herb that had cured his mother. He climbed the mountain, but could not find the plant. Naturally, the governor was disappointed and the mayor embarrassed.

When the herbalist returned in the summer, the mayor blamed him.

"I made a point to tell you before I left that this herb cannot be found after the summer is over," said the herbalist. And so, the herb was named "see me not after summer". **HENRY LU**

PERSONALITY TRAITS

The eyeball is linked to terminal yin [liver]; if it worsens at night or on contact with cold herbs, this is constraint of yin fire in the terminal yin, unable to disperse. Naturally, one should not attempt to directly break it up with cold [because cold contracts]- this will just make it worse!

Prunella can dredge and unblock liver and gallbladder qi: "if wood is constrained, allow it to reach out" [says the adage].

Furthermore, because it contains pure yang qi it can disperse clumped stagnant heat in the midst of yin. **ZHANG SHAN-LEI**

The Song of the Self Heal Faery

When little Elves have cut themselves,
Or Mouse has hurt her tail,
Or Froggies arm has come to harm,
This herb will never fail.
The Faeries skill can cure each ill
And soothe the sorest pain;
She'll bathe and bind, and soon she'll find that they are well again. **CICELY MARY BARKER**

RECIPES

INFUSION- Take one tsp of dried flowerheads to one cup of boiling water and steep twenty minutes. Drink one cup up to three times daily. Decoct with same ratio for nine minutes for mouth gargles.

For tuberculosis combine 30 grams each of self heal and hop flowers to one litre of water. Drink 3-4 cups daily.

COLD INFUSION- as above, but cool water and let steep overnight.

TINCTURE- 10-20 drops as needed. The fresh plant tincture is superior. It is prepared at 1:3 and 70% alcohol from mainly flower heads and some leaves.

CAUTION- Do not use self heal in cases of diarrhea, stomachache, vomiting or nausea associated with digestive deficiency. Not recommended during pregnancy. Self Heal has some possibility of interfering with blood thinners.

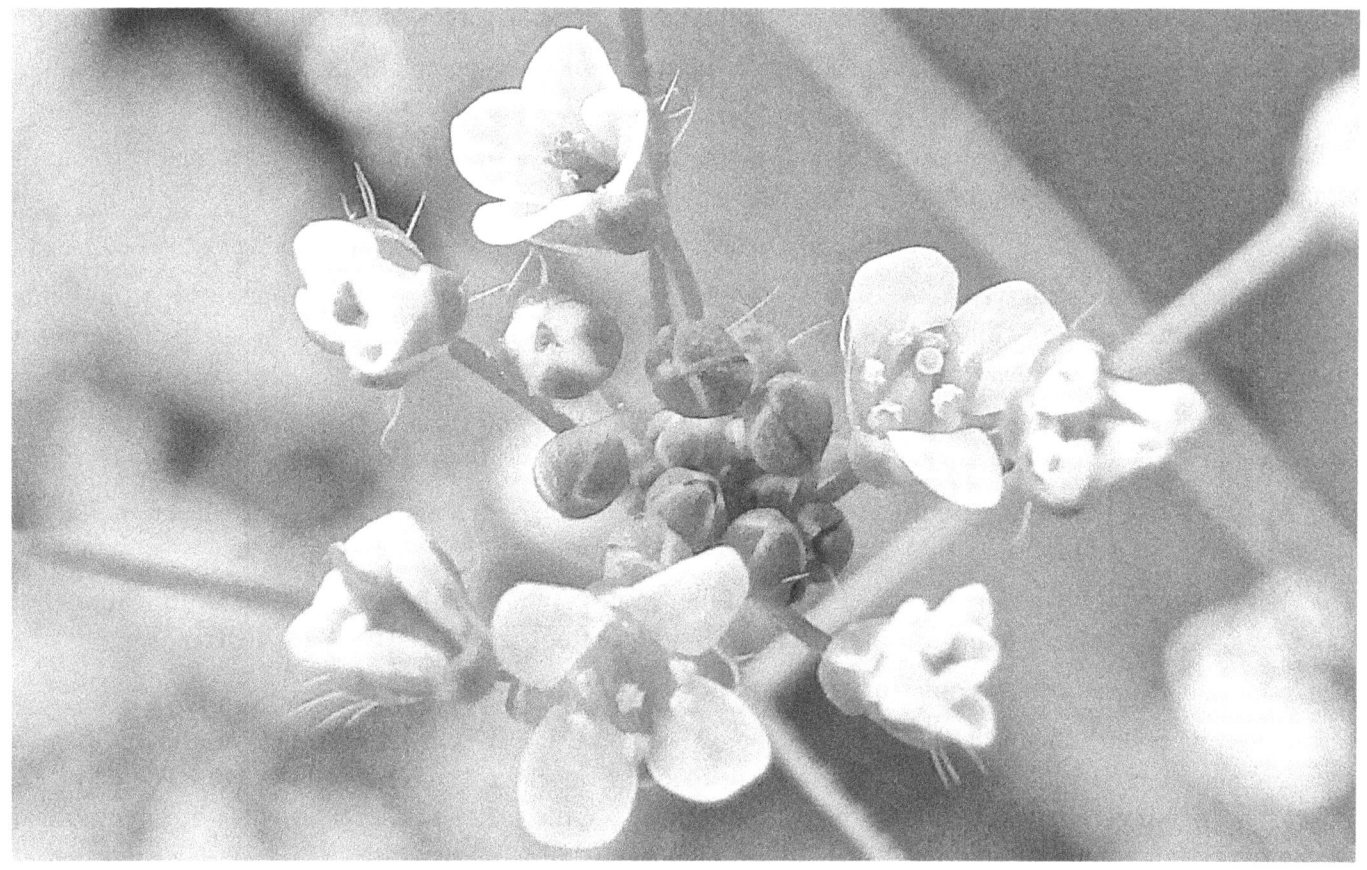

SHEPHERD'S PURSE

SHEPHERD'S PURSE
(***Capsella bursa-pastoris*** [L.] Medic.)
(***Thlaspi bursa-pastoris***) not accepted
PART USED- root, seeds, flower, leaves

Rocks covered with stonecrop, shepherd's purse, blue forget-me-not and little white sticky-stem are exquisite patchwork no earthly substance or human hand could produce.   **EMILY CARR**

The plant takes its common name from the purse or heart-shaped seedpod. **BURSA** is Latin for bag; **CAPSULA** means "small box or capsule" and **PASTORIS**, a shepherd. Traditionally, a shepherd's purse was made from the scrotum of a goat.

Thalaspi means cress of corruption.

This introduced annual was nicknamed salt and pepper in medieval England, where the seeds were used as a seasoning. See recipes below for a salt substitute made with wilderness plants.

The root is dried and substituted for ginger root.

In Yorkshire, a popular superstition involving Shepherd's Purse was opening the seed vessel. If the seed were yellow, you would be rich, but if green you would remain poor.

The tender new young leaves make a suitable potherb and in China they are sold commercially in the market. Herbalists call it **HU SHENG CAO** or "Life Preserving Grass", and consider it of benefit to the liver and stomach.

Other names are **JI CAI**, **DI CAI**, meaning earth vegetable, **JI YI CAI**, hen's wing vegetable, and **JAIO ZI CAI**, meaning upper-self vegetable.

The Japanese consider it an essential condiment in their barley-rice gruel, a ceremonial dish eaten on January 7th.

It does attract fungi, including *Cystopus* or *Albugo candidus,* and *Peronospora parasitica* that can be transmitted to other members of the mustard family.

The seedpods can be crushed after drying, and made into a flour or breakfast cereal. Combined with lamb's quarter, and plantain seed, it is often found in birdseed mixtures.

The seeds are extremely hardy, and can remain dormant for thirty years with one plant producing up to 64,000 seeds.

The heart-shaped seedpods were used in earlier times as part of a childhood teasing. Young boys would hide a mouthful of the hearts and then tell the girls that they can chew grass and spit out hearts. To their squeals of delight, it worked every time.

The Greeks and Romans considered the seeds an effective laxative, giving both a restorative and slightly stimulating effect.

According to Pliny, the seeds were used to warm, dissolve, and purify the bile, promote menstruation, kill the fetus, remove internal ulceration and abscesses and cure sciatica.

The Chippewa and other tribes made decoctions of the whole plant, including the root, for treating diarrhea, dysentery and unspecified stomach pain. It was known as Fire Root, or **I'CKODE'WADJI'BIK**.

The Menominee used infusions on skin exposed to poison ivy.

The Cheyenne refer to the plant as "Blue Medicine" **OTA?TAVE-HESEEO?OTSE**. The stems and leaves were powdered and put into cold water, and drunk for headaches. The Cherokee call it **DE GA LO DI, YV WI YA HI**, meaning Indian bag, in reference to the purse-like shape of the seed pods. It was used alone or combined with alumroot or wild geranium to stop bleeding of a menstrual or urinary nature.

The Karuk name **CHANTINNIHIICH** means "imitation ticks". The top of the plant, including flowers in bloom and seedpods were steeped. Once the tea turns cold it turns to a cold, white slime or gel. It was used for bleeding ulcers, diarrhea and childbirth hemorrhages.

The tiny seeds were gathered, roasted and eaten as a pinolé or bread by the Cahuilla, Mendocino and Apache.

Traditionally, the plant has been added to the regular diet in Northern Europe to inhibit the estrus cycle; hot infusions have been used as an emmenagogue.

Culpepper said that "the juice.... being dropped into the ear, heals the pains, noise and muttering."

It was once used as a substitute for quinine in malaria, and other protozoal fevers; as well as preventing epidemic encephalitis.

Dodoens in 1578 recommended it to staunch nose bleeding, spitting blood, blood to stop, toothache, urine flux, earache, ulcers of ear, ears running, straightness of breath, stranguary, venomous bitings, fevers, creeping and running sores, fistulas, erysipelas, swellings, indurations, shingles, new wounds, and rheumatic affections.

Count Mattei of Bologna, Italy created seven "marvelous medicines" based on certain vegetable electricity's found in this plant as well as Knotgrass, Water Betony, Cabbage, Stonecrop, Houseleek, Feverfew and Watercress. This herb furnished the so-called blue electricity for controlling hemorrhage. Which it does, very well.

In Japan, the plant extract was patented for use as a high calcium juice source and coagulating agent for flavoring tofu.

One 10th century Chinese herbal wrote the seed, "brightens vision, clears nebula, and detoxifies. Long term ingestion makes one see objects clearly".

In India, the plant is a remedy for atrophy of the limbs, by rubbing the affected areas with an alcoholic extract.

In Portugal, hot infusions are given as a diaphoretic while in Germany it is sometimes included in herbal combinations for treating late onset diabetes, probably due to it's organic chromium content.

The herb is used in Bolivia to stimulate uterine contractions at birth.

Dr. Cook, one of the great Eclectic physicians noted, "it is somewhat of a stimulating expectorant". He suggested combining with agrimony and cornsilk for kidney problems, and with partridge berry and crampbark for female weakness.

The plant seed is a closet carnivore that unlike the obvious sundew, indulges secretly. The young seeds, under cover of soil, snare whatever protein rich prey is available, by secreting a sweet, sticky substance. They then absorb the nutrients to gain strength to produce a new plant. The ability to produce protease and absorb amino acid suggests a unique carnivorous seed.

Scientists at the University of Tulane have discovered the seed, when placed in water, releases a mosquito attractant and gummy substance that binds the mouth of the larvae to the seed. The seed then releases another substance that destroys three quarters of the larvae in three days. Just one pound of seed has the power to destroy one million mosquito larvae, with not side effects. More research is surely warranted.

The dried plant can be placed under carpets and mats to discourage lice, fleas and other small vermin. The herb has some potential as a bio-monitor of heavy metals such as lead, cadmium, zinc and copper.

MEDICINAL

CONSTITUENTS- acetylcholine, amino phenols, histamine, sinigrin, choline (0.2%), inositol, 22 amino acids including proline, tyramine, diosmin, bursine, potassium+ bursilate, choline, essential oils, sinigrin and other mustard glycosides, fumaric, malic, tartaric, oxalic, citric, pyruvic, glutamic and bursic acids, garbanzol, saponins, vitamins A, K and C (0.5%), chromium (8.8 ppm), iron, calcium, coumarins, alkaloids yohimbine, ergocristine, and various flavonoids and their glycosides like sitosterol, diosmin, hesperidin, robinetin, rutin , and flavonoids such as luteolin-7-rutinoside and gossypetin hexamethyl ether, luteolin 7-galactoside quercitin 7-rutinoside and luteolin 7-rutinoside.
Polypeptides of an undetermined structure present; as well as chymosin, a digestive enzyme.
Only the seeds contain cardio-active steroids, and protease.
It was found that in healthy plants during flowering the coumarin derivatives were from 0.03-0.05%, but in fungus infected plants this rose to 0.58-0.75% (15-20 x increase).
Roots- shepherin peptides

Work by Tiberiu, Romania 1983 found the herb contains much higher content of free amino acids than many plants. It is especially high in histidine, arginine and lysine as well as other protein bound amino acids. The herb is cool and drying.

The vitamin K content is considered only a part of the blood clotting abilities of shepherd's purse. It covered with *Cystopus candidus, Albugo candida* or *Peronospora parasitica,* fungi that may well hold the key to some of its anti-hemorrhage effect.

It is well known to herbalists that only fresh plant tinctures have any significant anti-hemorrhagic effect.

Bursic acid possesses hemostatic properties, but only in increased amounts.

Earlier work by Kuroda & Takagi, *Nature* 1968 220 attempted to articulate the physiologically active substances in the herb, but more is yet to be found. Other work by the lead author dismissed hypotensive effects being due to presence of cholinergic compounds.

Some authors believe the hemostatic action is due to high levels of oxalic and dicarboxylic acids, others to an unidentified peptide.

Vermathen et al, *Planta Med* 1993 59 found both water and 50% methanol extracts shortened re-calcification time of human citrated plasma by 50-60%, indicative of blood clotting.

Work by Jurisson et al, *Farmatsiya* 1973:22 found flavonoids reduced blood vessel permeability in mice.

Other authors, including Bisset Wichtl of Germany, believe the maximum activity is reached three months after preparation.

That is, the actives may form after preparation, and then slowly lose effect after long storage, under less than ideal conditions.

Shepherd's Purse is very useful in all types of excessive bleeding from menstruation, to nosebleeds, to internal hemorrhage. For nosebleeds soak a cotton ball in fresh infusion and insert. It can also be used liberally on deep external wounds that refuse to stop bleeding.

During World War I, when other standard herbal medicines for staunching wounds were not available, they turned to this herb.

Midwives revere the herb for its ability to stop severe postpartum hemorrhage. Ironically, it is a smooth muscle contractor, and therefore a uterine stimulant, promoting and enhancing labor, if given before hand.

However, in one case I know of, the fresh tincture was given during labor to prevent bleeding, and this only encouraged the formation of huge blood clots that were not only painful to pass, but preventing the uterus from "clamping down", and returning tone to the organ.

A single-blinded, randomized clinical trial of 100 women with vaginal birth confirmed its efficacy. Ten drops of a water/alcohol tincture was given to 50 women sublingually, and control group placebo. The amount of postpartum bleeding was access, and the mean decrease in amount of bleeding was significantly higher in herb group.

A water soluble substance, yet identified, contracted uterine tissue in an oxytocin-like manner in animal studies conducted by Kuroda et al, *Nature* 1968 220.

Maria Treben mentions its use in poor muscle tone of the uterus. In fact, this is a superb remedy for women with uterine atony, fibroids, excessive bleeding and dark clotted blood. It helps to tone and lift the uterus in both pre-menopausal and menopausal women.

In my own clinic practice, a 54 year old suffering huge dark blood clots and bleeding for nearly two weeks each month, had significant benefit within the first week. The bleeding was quickly confined to a five to six day cycle and was less painful and clotty by next period.

Ironically, large doses will often bring on delayed menses as in amenorrhea.

Matthew Wood correctly classifies this herb as a stimulating anti-hemorrhagic, as it acts best in situations where the blood is dark and oozing. This is in contrast to the cooling hemostat, yarrow, indicated with excited, red hemorrhage.

Two unidentified alkaloids have been found to elicit physiological activity on the uterus.

Induced uterine activity in the rat, equivalent to the effect of oxytocin 0.1 i.u., was unaffected by atropine, but inhibited by competitive inhibitors of oxytocin. Tyramine is a well-known uterine stimulant.

As it helps contract smooth muscles it can be useful in atonic conditions affecting the small intestine, lungs, tracheal, aorta and bladder. Work by Jurisson, *Tartu Riiliku Ulik Toim* 1971 270 indicates unidentified components cause smooth muscle contraction and sedative effect. The effects on smooth muscle were not due to acetylcholine or histamine activity. This agrees with its use in chronic diarrhea associated with poorly toned or relaxed intestinal tissue.

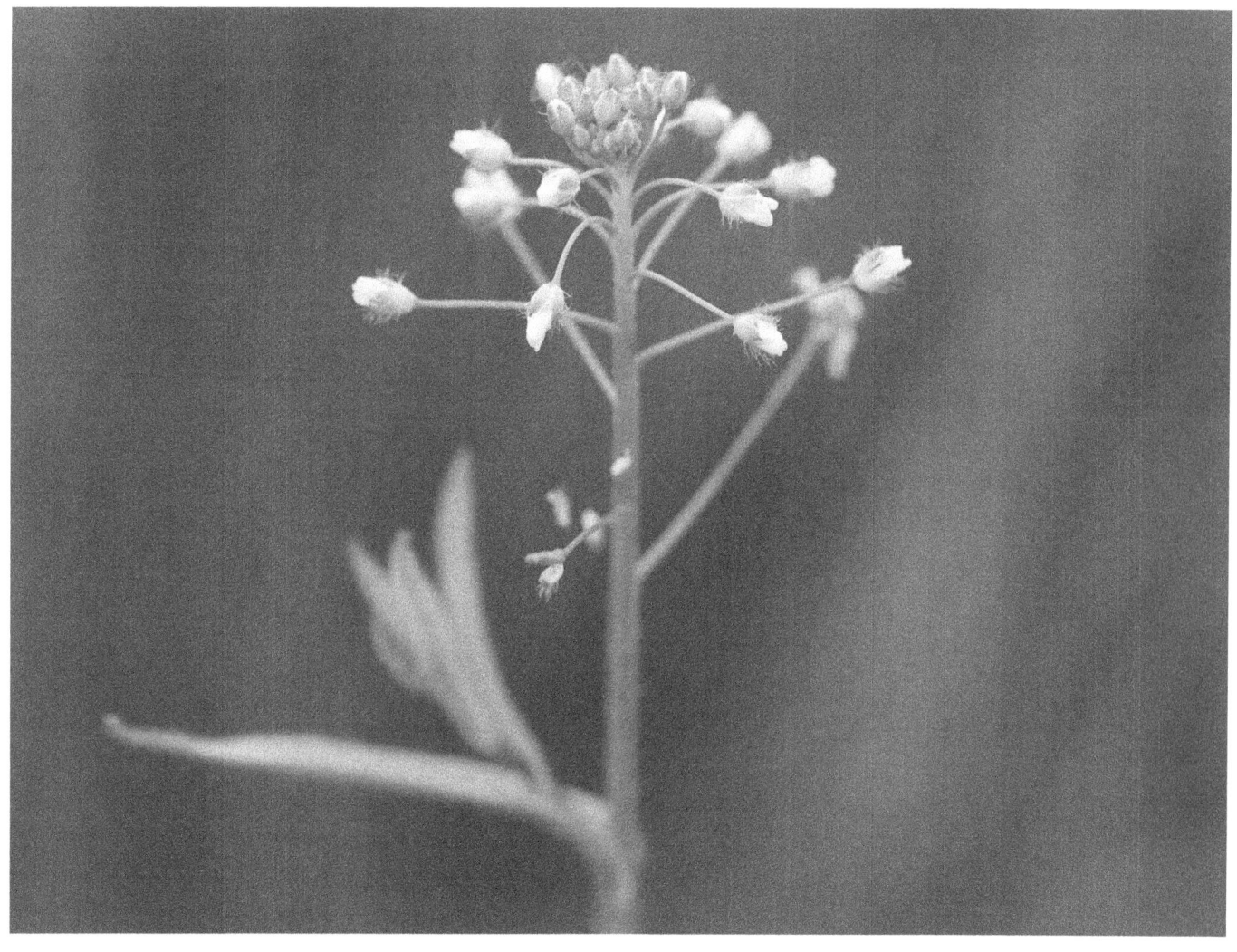

SHEPHERD'S PURSE FLOWERS

It helps remove sand and other sediment from kidney tubules, thus relieving blood from urine but also treating the irritation and congestion.

In fact, blood or mucous in the urine, painful urination, bladder ulceration, hot, burning cystitis, kidney stones or gravel, and edema are all helped by this rather malodorous tincture. It appears most useful in UTIs with Gram positive bacteria.

It works best in alkaline urine, suggesting addition of small amount of sodium bicarbonate to tea of tincture in water.

Shepherd's Purse helps the kidneys to excrete waste products, such as uric acid and phosphate type stones more efficiently. Both gout and pseudo-gout can be helped as the herb stimulates better phosphate recycling by the kidneys. It is a milder diuretic than parsley, but is less irritating to sensitive or inflamed kidney tissue, especially when bleeding is present.

Ethanol extracts show increased urine volume and glomerular filtration rates in mice studies. Kuroda et al, *Arch Int Pharmacodyn* 1969 178.

The herb may be helpful in non-specific atonic bladder, or where scar tissue may be affecting urinary flow. It helps relieve seminal vesicle irritation in men, sometimes related to sexual activity.

Vitamin K affects other proteins besides those involved in blood clotting. It adds a carboxyl group to glutamic acid in preformed proteins, thus activating them. Kidney protein is a vitamin K dependent protein formed in the kidneys. It functions by latching onto calcium and preventing its precipitation and deposition as calcium oxalate stones.

Another vitamin K dependent protein of relevance to the treatment of bone fractures and osteoporosis is osteocalcin. This protein only functions when activated by vitamin K, by binding calcium in bones.

It is worth noting that in patients with osteoporosis, tissue levels of osteocalcin are often only one third of normal. Since may seniors take aspirin for arthritis, and as a preventative for platelet aggregation; and since aspirin blocks vitamin K1 activity in the liver it may be contributing to the progression of osteoporosis.

It should be remembered for treating endometriosis originating from the heat of blood stagnation, and uterine fibroids causing excessive menstrual bleeding.

The herb has a soothing and regenerating effect on varicose veins, and hemorrhoids, combining well with horse chestnut. Various amines and flavonoids help strengthen capillaries, which in turn reduces their permeability. Jurisson et al, *Farmatsiya* 1973 22.

For women with liver complaints, or alcoholics, the herb can be helpful in repairing stomach ulcers, in combination with other herbs.

The fresh plant tincture has been shown in laboratory tests to suppress the growth of tumors, and prevent the induction of hematomas. Cytotoxic compounds were found in Lithuania in 1989.

Work by same author, reported in *Gann* 1981 72, found activity against cultured Ehrlich, MH134 and L1210 tumor cells.

Recent studies have shown that water and ethanol extracts increase the activity of membrane oxidase necessary for the defensive function of granulocytes. In fact, a 1977 patent in Japan was granted for neoplasm inhibition.

A study conducted at the University of Cairo in 1990, by El-Abyad et al, showed extracts of *Capsella bursa-pastoris* were effective against various fungi, including *Candida albicans*. Moskalenko, *J Ethnopharm* 1986 15 found weak anti-bacterial activity against Gram positive organisms.

Blood pressure is moderated; initially increasing because it is a sympathetic stimulant, and then decreasing to normalize. This muscarine-like effect is dose dependant as well. Both choline and acetylcholine stimulate cholinergic aspects of the autonomic nervous system, helping normalize neuromuscular function.

Duke suggests it may have application in glaucoma, but the author has not used it clinically for this purpose, and probably would not risk it.

It is helpful in congested veins and hemorrhoids with its astringent and decongesting properties; and stimulating effect on bowel movements.

The whole fresh plant is eaten or taken orally as an infusion for the prostate in northern Peru. Bussmann et al, *J Ethnobio & Ethnomed* 2010 6:30.

Externally, it is a good bath herb for wounds, and eczema, and for leucorrhea that is yellow and odorous. It combines well with White Deadnettle in the treatment of leucorrhea.

A fresh plant poultice will stop bleeding wounds, or as a weak substitute for mustard plasters in bronchitis and other respiratory conditions.

The fresh greens are used in Korea, as a potherb, tea or soup for their hypoglycemic effect. Studies conducted in 1992, using laboratory rats, confirm this effect, and suggest the plant shows potential for preventative and therapeutic approaches to alleviating the high blood sugar state in diabetes mellitus.

This could also be due, in part, to the high chromium level or another factor.

Research conducted over thirty years ago showed that fumaric acid in shepherd's purse inhibited the growth of Ehrlich tumor cells inoculated into mice (50-80%).

Fumaric acid has been found to prevent the development of hepatic neoplasm. Kuroda et al, *Japan Kokai* 1977 41.

Around that time, a patent for a neoplasm inhibitor was filed in the same country. As far back as 1969, Kuroda and Takagi were looking at the anti-inflammatory, anti-ulcer and diuretic effects of the herb. *Arch Int Pharm Therapie* 178.

Various phenolic glycosides in the aerial parts exhibit moderate inhibitory effect on nitric oxide production in LPS-activated BV-2 cells, suggesting anti-inflammatory activity. Cha JM et al, *Molecules* 2017 22(6).

Other research conducted by the same group showed extracts of the herb prevented the induction of hepatomas in mice fed azobenzene (hepato-carcinogen).

The herb reduced markedly, the development of cholangio-fibrosis, bile duct cell proliferation and hepatic cell degeneration.

Extracts show anti-thrombin and anti-cancer activity. Goun EA et al, *J Ethnopharm* 2002 81 337-342. Early work found extracts of the herb inhibit Ehrlich tumors in mice. Kuroda K et al, *Cancer Res* 1976 36(6): 1900-3.

Alcohol extracts inhibit growth and induce apoptosis of HSC-2 human oral cancer cells, via the Sp 1 protein. Lee KE et al, *Exp Ther Med* 2013 5(3): 789-92.

Fresh plants are covered in not only fungi, but also *Bacillus* bacterium. Of the twenty-five bacilli, eleven show resistance to antibiotics, and five are multi-drug resistant. Lee WJ et al, *J Food Sci* 2016 81:3: M684-91.

The herb is synergistic with *Tribulus terrestris* and licorice root against *Streptococcus mutans, S. sanguis, Actinomyces viscosus, Enterococcus faecalis, Staphylococcus aureus* and *E. coli*. Soleimanpour S et al, *Avicenna J Phytomed* 2015 5(3): 210-7.

Like other members of the Mustard family, the herb contains the isothiocyanante compound sulforaphane. This compound has significant anti-inflammatory activity and derived from this herb inhibits vancomycin-resistant *Enterococci* and Bacillus *anthracis* (anthrax). Choi WJ et al, *Korean J Physiol Pharmacol* 2014 18(1): 33-9.

Shepherd's purse helps calm the hyper-excitability of repletion heat in the Lungs that causes epistaxis, hemoptysis and epileptic seizures; especially in Water and Fire Yang constitutions. In Chinese medicine, the herb is most used for dysentery and eye problems, as well as internal bleeding, and post partum uterine bleeding.

The seed is used in TCM, for its normalizing effect and help in treating eye problems such as poor vision, eye pain, glaucoma, and nebula, or cloudy cornea.

Shepherd's purse root is juiced, and the resultant water used for treating blood shot eyes as an eye drop. Two glycine and histidine-rich peptides have been isolated from the roots. Park et al, *Plant Mol Biol* 2000 44:2 found the peptides, named shepherin I and II show activity against gram negative bacteria and fungi.

The flowers only, as an infusion, can be used to treat dysentery and uterine bleeding.

The herb has been found quite effective in preventing or treating measles in children. A 1970 report from eastern China found that a heavy decoction of one kilo of fresh herb and equal amounts of water is boiled down to 500 grams. When 150 children drank the decoction, only seven contracted measles. In the control group of 130 children who did not receive the decoction, 56 got the measles. It is often combined with equal parts Woolly Grass root for treatment of measles.

Recent pharmaceutical books on herbs, cite the presence of an unknown peptide with hemostatic, oxytocin-like activity. It appears that fungi-affected activity is not scientific enough!

The presence of the alkaloid yohimbine is interesting. PubMed cites over twenty-four thousands studies on this interesting compound.

HOMEOPATHY

This valuable medicine is anti-hemorrhagic and removes uric acid. It is very reliable for hemorrhage with uterine fibroids, nasal bleeding, and copious menstrual flow. Use it whenever each alternating period is heavy, or when one has barely recovered from one period and the other begins. Gums are full of blisters.

Chronic neuralgia, as well as kidney stones and sand and urinary frequency are indications for using this herb.

Hemorrhoids that bleed, chronic cystitis, and gouty diathesis are likewise resolved.

Other symptoms that appeared during the proving include: restless sleep, confused and unpleasant dreams, vertigo as if intoxicated, pressing frontal headache, sensation of dust in the eyes in morning, buzzing noise in ears after exertion, scurfy eruptions behind ears.

Milk from right nipple, with shooting pain in breast but was never pregnant.

Irritable and angry, after rising from bed. Very nervous, cross, and feels like fighting. Adversion to potatoes, and nausea after savoy cabbage. Craving for buttermilk and juicy fruit.

DOSE- Tincture to sixth potency. The mother tincture is prepared from the whole fresh plant in flower. First proving by Fincke with five females and ten males with tincture, 6c, 15c, 30c, and 1M between 1851-71. Proving was done by Malcolm Macfarlan at 9M in 1893.

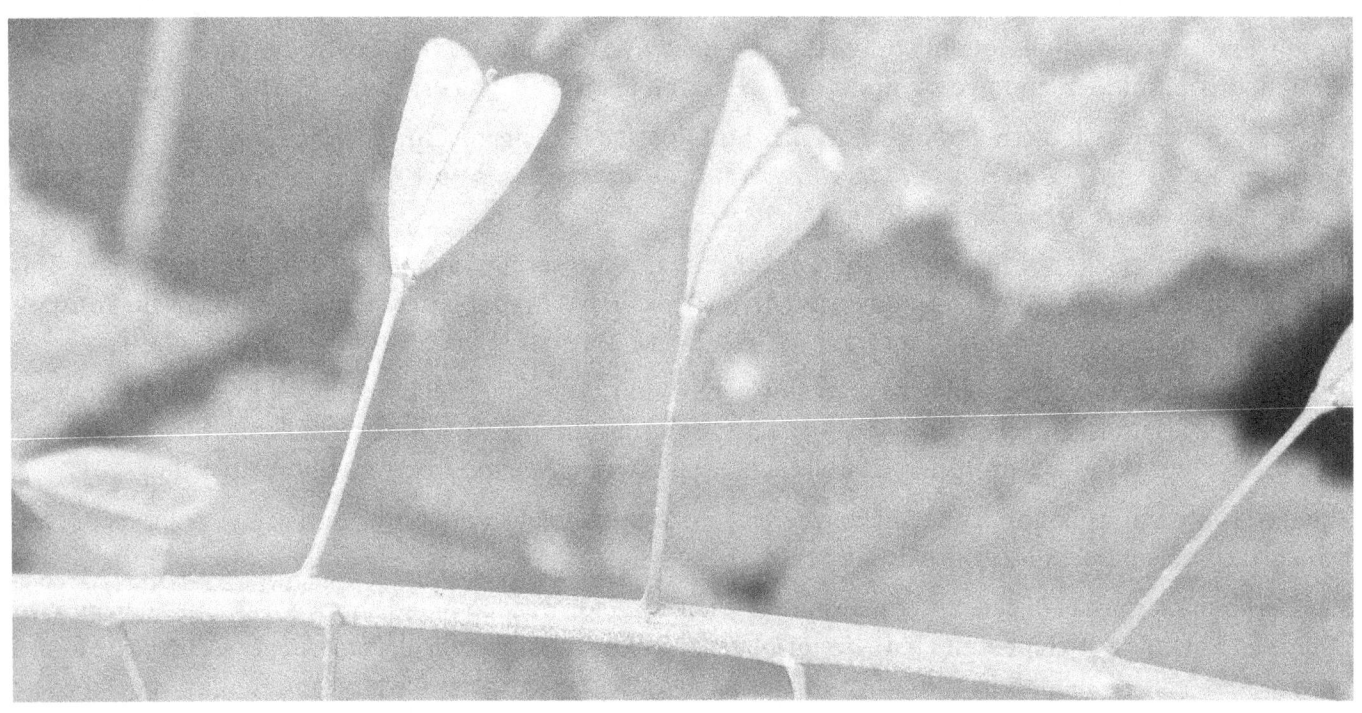

DISTINCT HEART-SHAPED LEAF

ESSENTIAL OIL

CONSTITUENTS leaf- camphor 0.02%, phellandrene, cis-3-hexen-1-ol, 3-Octanol, camphene, b- pinene, limonene, and 70 other constituents, with a yield of 0.02%
root- n-decane, n-dodecane, and minor constituents like geraniol, thymol, and carvacrol, with a yield of 0.03%.

Work by Nagai et al, *Chem Abstr* 1961 55 found the essential oil decreases blood pressure in lab animals.

The essential oil is not available available at the present time. It would probably be of little interest to the perfume industry, but possibly a useful counter-irritant in rheumatic afflictions.

SEED OIL

From the seed can be expressed an oil that yields 35%; with an iodine value of 128 and saponification value of 162.

HYDROSOL

The distilled water is made from the herb, roots and stalks and is good for all floods of blood of the belly, as well as dysentery, diarrhea or bloody urine. It heals bleeding wounds, stops menstrual bleeding, and stone in the bladder and kidney, according to Brunschwig, *Book of Distillation* published in 1530.

FLOWER ESSENCES

Shepherd's purse flower essence is related to the soul quality of fertility and feminine energy. It is useful for soothing the fear and negative emotions associated with various phases of the menstrual cycle. This essence is very useful for helping ease a young woman's fear of puberty, relating to issues such as breast growth, or the pain and shock associated with the onset of menstruation. It may help ease a woman's fear of a missed period, and the worry of pregnancy; or to soothe the emotional roller coaster of angst and guilt associated with a miscarriage or planned abortion.

Shepherd's Purse flower essence may help restore menstrual cycles in very athletic women producing excessive testosterone. Fertility issues associate with polycystic ovary syndrome (PCOS), for example, may also be helped. Shepherd's Purse combines well with Black Currant flower essence for issues of fertility. The flower essence may also be helpful in women with excess estrogen production, due to issues involving the pituitary; or estrogen/progesterone imbalance.

It may also help individuals who have a fear or history of repeated miscarriages, by relieving mental and emotional anxiety. For issues surrounding fertility consider combining this essence with She Oak from the Australian Flower Essences developed by Ian White, and/or fairy ring mushroom essence. Rogers (2016). And, of course, those suffering in-between-period bleeding, or heavy, and painful menstruation that is associated with feelings of guilt, childhood abuse, or anorexic/bulimic patterns of imbalance, may find it helpful.

Shepherd's Purse flower essence, taken together with fairy ring mushroom essence, may be useful in relaxing first time mothers-to-be, when taken at beginning of labour pains. It may help assist cervical opening and shorten transit time to delivery. Women moving into the pre-menopausal cycle of life, as well as the menopausal transition, will find Shepherd's Purse flower essence relieves fear and anxiety associated with moving into the unknown. The action of this essence is subtle and slow but deep acting. **PRAIRIE DEVA**

Shepherd's Purse essence helps one understand the right meaning of timing, and prevent unnecessary stress and too much pressure. **MARIANA**

SPIRITUAL PROPERTIES

When using Shepherd's Purse, there is an acceleration of life force. There is, as well, an enhancement of the essential instincts for survival. When the sun is directly overhead, an etheric flash of energy takes place. This is quite noticeable to those who are sensitive. Shepherd's Purse has the ability to absorb that energy and hold it within.

Individuals working the yoga and various meditative techniques will notice improvement with the use of this plant.

The devic order associated with it was given the task of allowing the sun's energies to be utilized by man. The third chakra is energized, the crown chakra is opened, and the root chakra more relaxed in the process of opening to life force. When the Sun repeatedly causes difficulty in certain astrological signs, there is great benefit in taking this herb. **GURUDAS**

BOTANICA POETICA

If you cut yourself in the wood
Shepherd's Purse is very good
A hemostat that will stop a bleed
It's a common, pretty weed
An astringent and diuretic
A urinary antiseptic
Use the parts that are aerial
You'll have a tea quite valuable
When you suffer from nosebleed
Capsella Bursa-Pastoris is what you need
Apply it on externally
Or drink it up internally
Stomach, lungs and uterus too
The entire herb is good to use
Excessive menstruation you can curb
When you take this friendly herb
Named for the shape of its seed pod
Think Shepherd's Purse to stop the bleed.

SYLVIA CHATROUX

RECIPES

INFUSION- Take one small handful of fresh plant to one pint of water. Steep for twenty minutes. Take 2-4 ounces every five minutes for serious bleeding.

DECOCTION- One ounce of fresh herb to one pint of water. Simmer slowly.

TINCTURE- fresh plant when in seed, pod including root is best- One tsp in water every five minutes until bleeding stops. 20-60 drops 3 times daily for kidney issues. Fresh plant tincture is made at 1:2 and 45% alcohol.

The mother tincture is made from the fresh plant including the root.

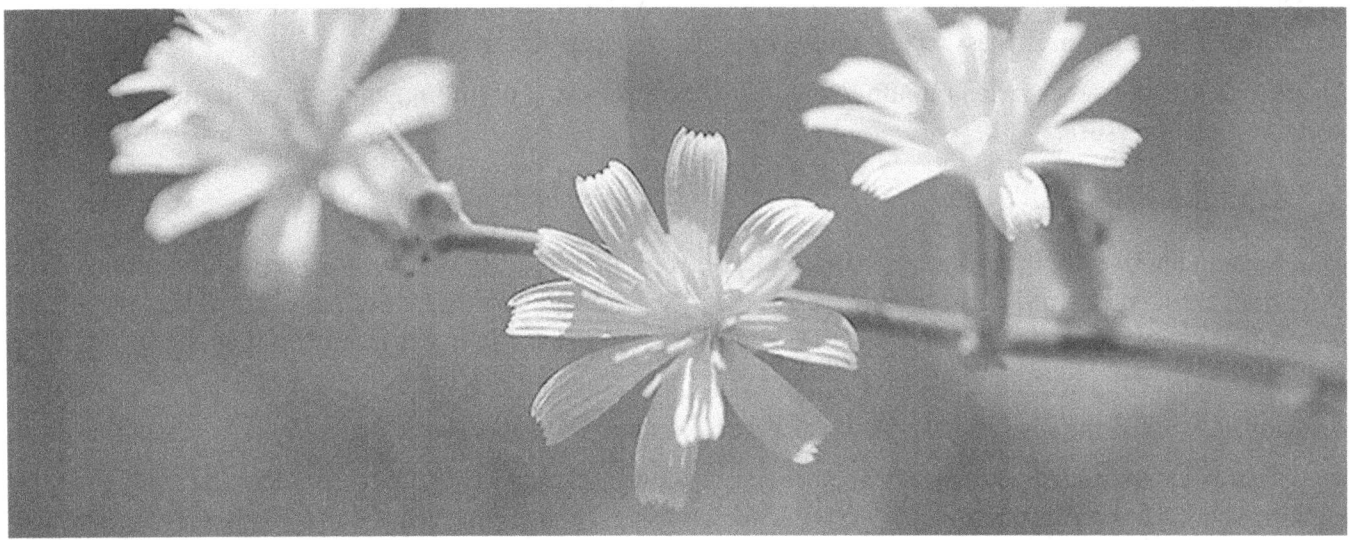

RUSH SKELETON WEED (Courtesy of Jose Ramon Vaquero Hedrosa)

EARACHE- In emergency, crush the fresh plant and squeeze several drops in ear. For nosebleed, chew into a moist pulp and insert into nostril.

BATH- Make decoction of leaves and seeds; add to bath for hemorrhoids or kidney pain.

SALT SUBSTITUTE- Take Shepherd's Purse leaves and seeds, wild mint, young Tansy leaves, peppergrass leaves and seeds, nettle leaves, lamb's quarter seeds, goldenrod leaves, yellow dock seeds, juniper berries, and wild carrot leaves, all dried. Blend in a food processor, or clean coffee grinder, and then sift through cheesecloth.

CAUTION- Shepherd's Purse taken over an extended time at high dosage may affect hypothyroid due to the iso-thiocyanates; is contraindicated in hypertension and may interfere with blood pressure medication. It may interfere with blood thinners.

The herb may aggravate those patients with known kidney stones; and those suffering thrombosis or phlebitis, or exaggerate the effects of sedative herbs or medications. Avoid during pregnancy and breastfeeding. Glucosinolates can taint milk.

RUSH SKELETON WEED
PRAIRIE PINK
HOGBITE
(*Lygodesmia juncea* [Pursh] D. Don ex Hook.)
(*Chondrilla juncea* L.)
ANNUAL SKELETON WEED
WILD ASPARAGUS
(*L. rostrata* [A. Gray] A. Gray)
(*Shinneroseris rostrata* [A. Gray] S. Tomb)
PARTS USED- stems, galls, latex

Lygodesmia is from the Greek **LYGOS**, meaning plant twig, and **DESME**, a bundle; both referring to its appearance. It may refer to Lygodesma, bound with twigs and sexually thwarted, by Artemis in Sparta. Chondrilla is an ancient Greek name, derived from the word for "lump", in allusion to the stem exudates.

Juncea means rush-like, referring to the look of the plant. Shinneroseris is named in honor of Lloyd Herbert Shinners, a 20th century Canadian born botanist, who specializes in Texas flora. Rostrata is from the Latin meaning, beaked, curved or hooked.

Skeleton Weed is a most unusual looking apomictic perennial, with stiff green stems, very few and tiny leaves, and small pink flowers. The plant is often covered in round insect galls, and found on dry, gravely soil. Its annual cousin is even more rare, and found in southeastern and east- central Alberta. It is invasive to North and South America, as well as Australia.

In fact, it is considered a prohibited, noxious weed in my province of Alberta.

Skeleton Weed (*L. juncea*) is known to the Blackfoot as Blue Sticks, or **OOT-SQUEEKS-SEE**. If you take the stems and boil them, the water does eventually turn blue.

The Blackfoot infused the stems to treat sore eyes, burning cough, while leaf tea was taken by nursing mothers to increase their milk flow.

They let the broken stem juice harden and gathered it for chewing gum. The stems most invaded by insects are said to be richest in medicinal value. The latex combines with saliva enzymes to produce a blue stain.

The whole plant was decocted for pregnant women of both the Blackfoot and Cree suffering from heartburn, vomiting and morning sickness common in the first trimester, or for relief of period pains.

The Cree call it **A KA KA NE PE WIK**.

The Cheyenne, Hopi, Blackfoot and other native women drank the stem tea to increase their breast milk flow.

The Cheyenne call it Milk Wood or Medicine, **MATANAA-HESEEO?OTSE** or **TATAWISSE'HEYO**, Blue Medicine.

The tea supposedly imparts a feeling of contentment to the mother and has an "inner power." The child that received this became healthy. It was often combined with Red Baneberry root for increasing breast milk production.

Decoctions of the juice were used to relieve heartburn, and infusions of the whole plant were an eye-wash.

It was brewed as a general tonic for children, and kidney trouble.

The related *L. spinosa* is called Big Medicine, and was an extremely important plant. The Cheyenne of Montana used it in nearly every medicine. For colds and mumps, the root was broken and boiled and taken internally and used for steaming. Work by Hart found others used it for tuberculosis.

The Stony used the plant to relieve fevers.

The galls of the plant were pulverized in a soft hide bag and the powder used as a diuretic tea.

The stem was infused and drank cool for a burning cough, or used to treat sore eyes.

The Blackfoot valued Skeleton Weed for treating the saddle sores and leg wounds of their horses. For this they rubbed infusions on the irritated surface, and drank internally to quell coughs. The horse was held down to the count of ten stones, after administration and then set free.

The stems, rich in resins and yellow-orange latex, were crushed, put into a storage bag and later used as footpads for moccasins. Newly tanned buffalo hides were made ochre red with a mixture of the stem juice and ochre to waterproof the hide.

Combined with lard, an infusion of the plant was applied as a hair tonic, to make it long and thick.

The Lakota chewed the plant resins, like gum, or made a tea of the whole plant to cure childhood diarrhea. They call it **MAKA' CANS'INHU**, meaning either Earth Sappy Wood Stem, or Skunk Resin Plant.

The plant galls, although yellow, produce a bright blue spit, and dye.

The aerial parts show strong inhibition of xanthine oxidase, at a level much higher than Labrador Tea (*Rhododendron groenlandicum*). This suggest possible use as an infusion for hyperuricaemia and gout. Pieroni A et al, *Phytother Res* 2002 16(5): 467-73.

The dry plant has a polyphenol content of 7.6% and oil content of 4.8%. Be careful of where the plant is picked, as it is a nitrate accumulator, like Horsetail.

Skeleton weed contains a high percentage of alpha linoleic acid, a precursor to omega 3 at over 56% of fat content. Morales P et al, *Food Sci Technol Int* 2012 18(3): 281-90.

Annual Skeleton Weed was smoked as a sedative by the Navaho.

FLOWER ESSENCE

Skeleton Weed flower essence is useful to those individuals who find themselves reactionary to authority figures. Usually stemming from past life experiences or from childhood, there is a fear/anger duality associated with those in uniforms, or positions of power.

Skeleton Weed flower essence helps one to see the Emperor with no clothes, and understand that these individuals are simply assuming their professional role, and you have choice regarding how you respond to their role-playing.

Slowly, over time, Skeleton Weed helps one find their true sense of self, and separate dogma from truth.
PRAIRIE DEVA

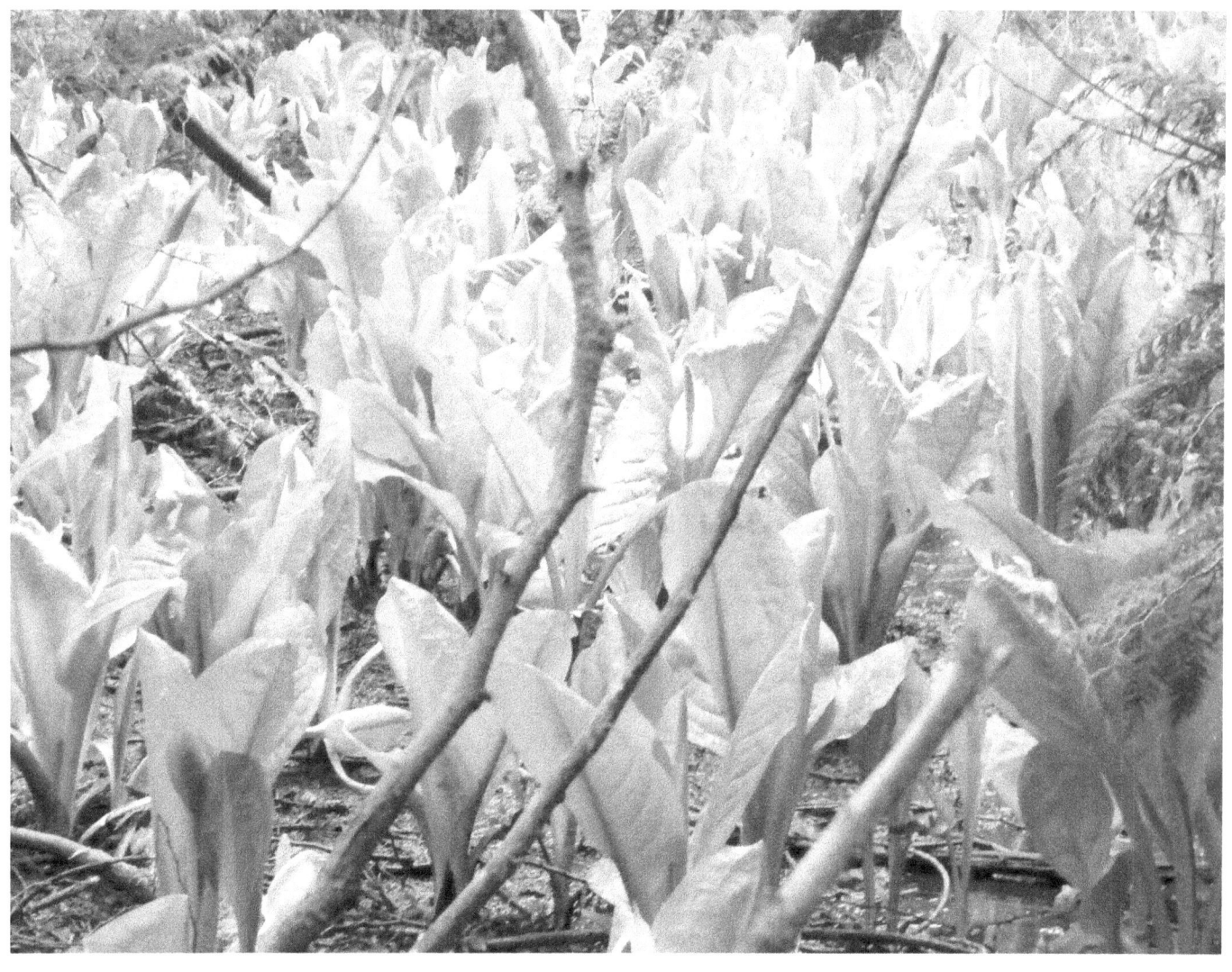

SKUNK CABBAGE PATCH

SKUNK CABBAGE
WESTERN SKUNK CABBAGE
SWAMP CABBAGE
SWAMP LANTERN
(*Lysichiton americanus* Hultén & H. St. John)
(*Lysichitum americanum* [L.] Schott, orth. var.) not accepted
EASTERN SKUNK CABBAGE
BEAR'S FOOT
(*Symphlocarpus foetidus* [L.] Salisb. ex W. P. C. Barton)
PARTS USED- leaves, root

In the swampy places and ditches of Greenville skunk cabbage grew- gold and brimming with rank smell-hypocrites of loveliness peeping from the lush green of their great leaves. The smell of them was sickening.
EMILY CARR

Skunk cabbage comes from its ill-smelling leaves, when first crushed. Lysichiton is from the Greek **LUSI**, or **LYSIS** and **KHITON**, meaning unfastened or loosened frock or tunic, in reference to how the spathe wraps around the central flower spike. Americanum means from America. In some texts, it is referred to as Swamp Lantern, or Yellow Arum.

Skunk Cabbage derives its name from the odour of the flowering plant that attracts flies for pollination. The scent is more of decay and rotting than skunk-like, but it surely does attract flies, bees and other insects. Foetidus means fetid, ill-smelling. Symplocarpus refers to the ovary, or fused fruit.

When bruised or cut, the leaves are skunk-like, the cut stems are more mustard or rotten, raw onion smell, and the flowers carrion-like. The overall impression is unpleasant at best. Bear and elk are fond of the roots and will plow up swamps to get them.

The flowers are pollinated by staphylinid beetle, *Pelecomalius testaceum*.

Western Skunk Cabbage grows in bogs and swamps of the temperate forests. It is closely related to Water Arum, or Wild Calla (*Calla palustris*), as can be seen by their similar appearance. Eastern Skunk Cabbage looks similar, but is in different genus.

Western Skunk Cabbage is related to Taro, a Polynesian relative, and important starch tuber. Skunk Cabbage is huge, reminding one of the pre-historic swamps full of dinosaurs and other massive creatures. It is not unusual to see leaves of five feet in length and several feet across. Under the right conditions, they can live more than 200 years.

It has adapted itself to cold climates. The skunk cabbage flowers push up through the damp mud, while leaves are still small. Like a warm-blooded animal, the clump of eastern skunk cabbage (*S. foetidus*) blossoms can raise its internal temperature, through thermogenesis, as much as 63 degrees Fahrenheit above air temperature. Its plant signature involves growing in cold, swampy areas, and treating cold, moist conditions. That is, the herb is warming and drying in nature.

Natives used the waxy leaves for storage, wrapping food and clothing in this ancient waterproof pouch. They can be folded into cones, useful for berry picking, or used like sheets of wax paper for storing fruits and vegetables while camping. The leaves are ideal for lining of steaming pits, a favourite cooking method of many Native tribes.

Various tribes roasted or dried the root, from which they prepared flour.

The leaves, at least when young, can be eaten after repeated boiling, and changing of water. Like Marsh Marigold, it contains calcium oxalate that can be very harsh to the mouth and body if not removed by cooking. The Lillooet of British Columbia recognized this, and their name for the plant means hot.

The Haida call it **HLGUN** meaning leaf. The leaves were used to carry salmon berries, line baskets, used in pit cooking and preservation of foods for winter storage. The central vein was heated to soften so that airtight packets can be completely formed and stored for long time. Skunk cabbage roots were used as bait on halibut hooks carved from yew trees, and looked like octopi underwater.

The Cree probably traded for the plant leaves, which they used on infected sores after softening the dried leaves in warm water. The plant was known as **PISKETE-PUKWA**, which means literally, in Cree, "individual leafed" plant.

There is not much record of medicinal use by Western Native tribes. The Cree of northern Alberta know the plant as **YOSKIHTEPAKWA**.

The Lower Stl'atl'imx ate the long white rhizomes, after cooking. They can be up to ten inches long, and were either baked or boiled.

Roasting destroys the calcium oxalate, as well as drying.

The raw, dry roots can be ground into a powder, for medicine as described below, or to blend with other flours for breads and stew thickeners.

Various tribes used the leaves as poultices for cuts, swellings, headaches, chest pains, and fevers. The Karuk infused the leaves for treating tuberculosis, helping relieve pain of terminally ill patients, and helping to ease them out emotionally, according to elder Josephine Peters.

The root is both a stimulant and anti-spasmodic, used in cough medicine, bronchial irritations, whooping cough, asthma, urinary obstructions and venereal disease.

The root was used for abortion, contraception and to facilitate childbirth. The root or root hairs were used like a styptic pencil to stop external bleeding.

The flowers were used by the Cowlitz, who heated and applied them to rheumatic joints.

The yellow bracts around the flowers were used by Molalla as yellow face powder.

Chilliwack placed the leaves under a pillow to help induce "power dreams".

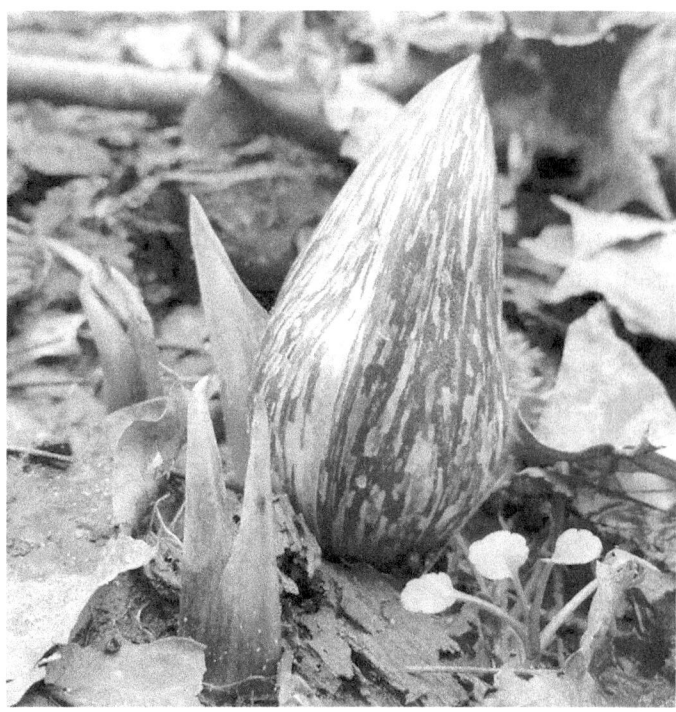
EASTERN SKUNK CABBAGE

The Mi'kmaq inhaled the odour of the crushed leaves of Eastern Skunk Cabbage (*Symplocarpus foetidus*) for headaches.

The Menominee mixed skunk cabbage root powder with other plant pigments, and after moistening, inserted it into the skin with a sharp fish tooth. This "tattoo" on the sick was not for decoration but to prevent illness from returning.

The fresh or dried fleshy fruits, without seeds, were mashed with Indian meal as a poultice for caking breasts, dissipating the hardness and congestion.

In some native traditions, a small piece of skunk cabbage helps bring good fortune in court cases. The color yellow, relates to Royal Canadian Mounted Police and the vertical yellow stripe on their pants.

Friends of mine falsely accused of growing marijuana some forty years ago, were given yellow ribbons to carry, by an indigenous healer at their court case. They were acquitted.

MEDICINAL

CONSTITUENTS- root- calcium oxalate, some unidentified aromatics, 5-hydroxytryptamine (5 HTP).
leaf- calcium oxalate, anthocyanins, kaempferol. The Eastern Skunk Cabbage (*Symplocarpus foetidus*) leaves are said to contain 5-hydroxytryptamine.
spathe/flower- skatole, cadaverine.

Western Skunk Cabbage root is most valued for medicinal purposes, but deteriorates very quickly in the dried form. As fresh root tincture, it is an excellent antispasmodic for painful cramps aggravated by stress and fear, according to Michael Moore.

It is a strong expectorant and bronchial anti-spasmodic, ideal for moist asthma that is suffered occasionally due to stress. It helps relieve the sense of panic and pain in the chest that accompanies shortness of breath, and labored, gasping gulping of air.

The root combines well with lobelia, or pleurisy root, keeping in mind that all have emetic properties in large doses.

Tremors and seizures will sometimes respond to the root's relaxing properties.

The root tincture is used for bouts of coughing that lead to vomiting, spasms and stomach pains, combining well with moose berry bark in such cases.

For asthmatics, vomiting of excess mucous can be a useful thing. For children, a cough and anti-spasmodic syrup can be made with honey.

It is more drying than gumweed, and most similar to expectorant and anti-spasmodic action of sweet coltsfoot (*Petasites*) root.

Taken in excess, western skunk cabbage root will cause nausea, as well as moderate gastric irritation, including diarrhea.

An ointment prepared from the roots can be used effectively on skin tumours and ulcerative, and indolent sores. It is an anodyne, or pain relieving ointment, that promotes healing of skin tissue.

Janice Schofield, in her excellent *Discovering Wild Plants*, has a recipe for Smoker's Tea.

An old patent medicine Skookum used Skunk Cabbage as the main ingredient.

Eastern Skunk Cabbage (*Symplocarpus foetidus*) also contains 5HTP; a tryptophan and serotonin and melatonin precursor.

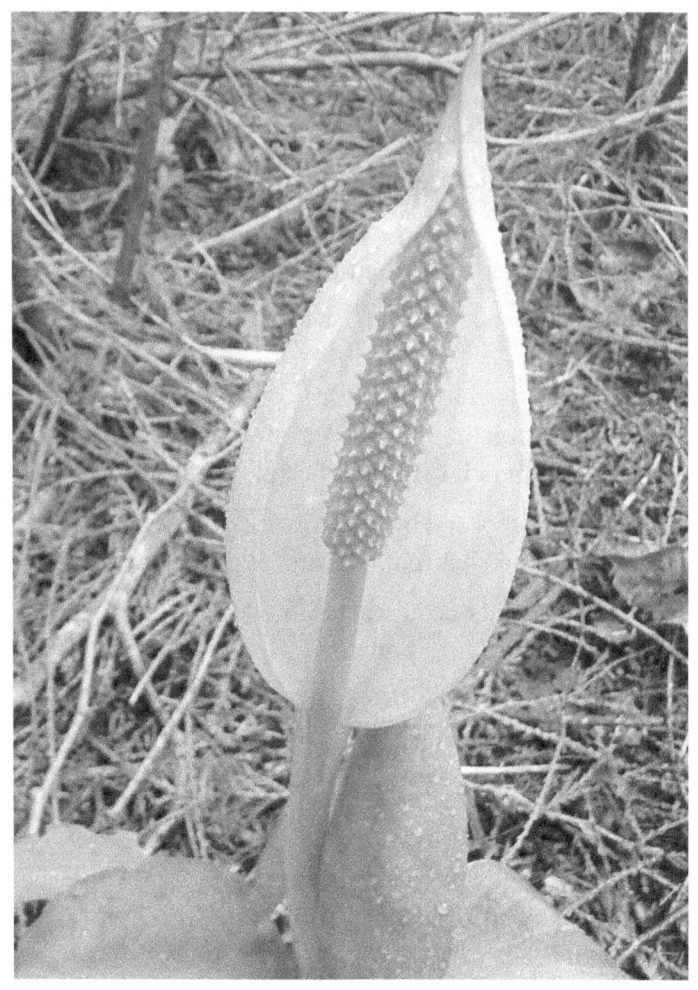

WESTERN SKUNK CABBAGE SPATHE

Our western version has been tested for its presence in the root. It may help explain its traditional use as a night-time tea for insomnia.

Work by McCutcheon et al, at the U of British Columbia 1995, found that extracts of western skunk cabbage exhibit anti-viral activity against bovine herpes virus type 1.

The plant is cytotoxic towards both sensitive and multi-drug resistant tumor cell lines. Karadeniz A et al, *Journal of Ethnopharmacology* 2015 168: 191-200.

ESSENTIAL OIL

The aerial parts of Eastern Skunk Cabbage have been both hydrodistilled and solvent extracted. The main components of former are p-vinyl-guaiacol (15%), 2-pentyl-furan (13.4%), and (Z)-ligustilide (9.5%). The main components from solvent method are 2-butoxy-ethanol (49.6%), ethyl-pentanoate (4.5%) and mesitylene (4%). Miyazawa M et al, *J Oleo Sci* 2015 64(12): 1329-36.

ROOT OIL

Take one part of dried rootstock finely ground to five parts of olive or canola oil by weight. Sun infuse for 10-14 days, or if weather is cold, you can slow simmer the dried root, cut into small chunks, in a low oven or crockpot overnight. Strain and preserve. Use as needed. For ointments, you can add beeswax, or use coconut oil from the start.

FLOWER ESSENCE

Skunk Cabbage flower essence when you feel stuck, stagnant or constipated in your life. This may express physically as large intestine/colon problems, deep skin issues- such as eczema, shingles or cancer, as thyroid imbalances or being overweight.

TREE FROG

MYTHS AND LEGENDS

The Kathlamet Indians of Western Washington tell a story about the Yellow Skunk Cabbage: "In the ancient days, they say, there were no salmon. The Indians has nothing to eat save roots and leaves. Principal among these was the skunk cabbage. Finally the spring salmon came for the first time. As they passed up the river a person stood upon the shore and shouted: 'Here come our relatives whose bodies are full of eggs. If it had not been for me all the people would have starved.'

'Who speaks to us?' asked the salmon. 'Your uncle, skunk cabbage,' was the reply. Then the salmon went ashore to see him, and as a reward for have fed the people, skunk cabbage was given an elk-skin blanket and a war club, and was set in the rich, soft soil near the river.

There he stands to this day, wrapped in his elk-skin blanket and holding aloft his war club.

GUNTHER 1973

PERSONALITY TRAITS

Lysichitum takes its generic name from Greek where it means "loosed chiton," referring to the shedding of the giant spathe.

Now the chiton was one ancient Greek equivalent of a tunic. It could be made of homespun cotton, of sturdier or more expensive linen, or, on a prostitute, it might be of the flimsiest gauze.

If an Athenian citizen or a slave in the 5th century city wore too loose a chiton, local prudes would tsk-tsk and declare it an outer sign of an inner moral laxity.

Wearing a loose chiton meant the wearer could simply flip it up over his or her head for a quickie nooner in the boscage by the portico. After such a carnal connection, one nipped into any nearby temple of Athena for a thirty second prayer to the virgin goddess, and, all sins absolved, went merrily on one's way, sandals flip-flopping on the cobbles.

CASSELMAN

The plant and flower are some kind of huge throwback to a time when dinosaurs ruled the land. There is a silence that reigns where skunk cabbage grows. The mind quiets as it nears the plant, becoming more silent than even the stillness coming from the forest that surrounds you…Involved in ancient things, the plant takes a while to awaken to your presence. But stay with it, asking for help, for its acquiescence in coming with you as medicine…The root is huge and the rootlets like Medusa's hair, a swirling, moving set of tendrils wriggling out from the bottom of the plant. It almost seems as if they *are* the plant. The whole of your attention focuses upon them. You almost want to turn the plant upside down, as if the roots are the head, the leaves the root. So eventually, you do. You feel yourself then looking at some ancient being, find yourself in some ancient story whose telling began long ago…As you look at the roots you feel something odd happen to your brain. Some older part, some ancient, reptilian part, is being stirred into life.

BUHNER

In leaf and blossom Skunk-cabbage resembles the arum lily only her leaf is rounder and her trumpet does not flare, the top is closed but there is a slit down one side of the flower through which you see emptiness and a greeny-brown coarse core. The bog about her stinks; a rank smell as if this clear freshed radiant flower were sucking all impurities, brown ooze, stagnant scum, seepage from putrefying foliage, rotting wood, slime of slug, poison of mosquito; were pulling these foul things into herself collecting them, filtering them through her own purity holding the bog's evils in her own emptiness to clean it, flinging it's vile effluence to the winds.

EMILY CARR

The odour that *lysichitum* gives off probably imitates the sex pheremones of several swamp insects that pollinate the plant. The aroma is one of fresh, primal fertility, of the vernal surge of life. Why, I immediately began to hum the opening bars of Stravinsky's *Rite of Spring*, and kept looking over my shoulder expecting the arrival of husky Neanderthal maidens all in a circle pounding out their ring dance and some guttural hymn to wet fecundity.

BILL CASSELMAN

To heat up, aroids burn stored carbohydrates and consume large amounts of oxygen. The heat causes scent components to become volatile and airborne to aid dispersion, in order to signal the plant's receptivity to pollinators. To induce and maintain thermogenesis enormous amounts of energy are expended over a very short period of time. This then limits the amount of time and effort that can be spent on blooming.

VERMEULEN

Forget the name; disabuse your mind of any connection with the mephitic animal and the plebeian vegetable, and see this swamp for what it really is—a veritable "field of the cloth of gold." Think of what the name *Lysichitum* means—a loosened mantle (chiton).

Think of a cloak of golden weave thrown carelessly over the shoulders of a water-sprite, or of fairy boatmen in coats of gold who have gathered to honor the coming of spring with a water fete. Thus only may you see this glorious plant in its true person.

LESLIE L. HASKIN

RECIPES

TINCTURE- 30-60 drops four times daily. A fresh root tincture is much better and made with a 1:2 ratio of root to 90% alcohol by weight. Dry root tincture, from the entire root, recently dried, is made 1:5 at 40% alcohol.

COLD INFUSION- Take one tsp of the grated dry root, to one cup of water. Let sit over night. Take one half cup, gently warmed as needed.

CAPSULES "OO"- Two or three dry powder capsules up to three times daily with warm water. The root deteriorates rapidly in a dry form, and must be refrigerated or frozen to keep any medicinal activity at all. Fresh root tincture is best.

SYRUP- Take one part freshly dried chopped root to four parts of honey. Simmer for several hours at low heat, try not to gag over the smell, strain and bottle. One tsp as needed, for the anxiety related "asthma" common to many children. If using dry powder, the ratio is 1:8.

SMOKER'S TEA- Take two cups of dried Sweet Coltsfoot (*Petasites species*) leaves, one cup of dried nettle leaves, one half cup of dried horsetail, and one quarter cup of dried swamp cabbage root. Place in blender until ground fine. Steep one teaspoon to one cup of boiling water for five minutes. Strain and serve.

NOTE: In many herbal books, you are warned to avoid the fresh root. If you are simply making an infusion or decoction that is pretty good advise, as the root has an acridity and pungency. In tinctures, the alcohol takes care of this for us.

CAUTION- The fresh root can cause skin blisters. Do not use in pregnancy or breastfeeding. It may cause uterine contractions or alter menstrual cycle. Maybe. It may also interact with benzodiazepines, narcotics, anti-depressants, etc.

SNEEZEWEED
SNEEZEWORT
(**Helenium autumnale** L.)
(**H. montanum** Nutt.) not accepted
PARTS USED- roots, petals

The road to it (Sutter's Mills) after passing the first four or five miles runs through a sandy soil, covered at present with what we call 'Sneezeweed'.

J W AUDUBON

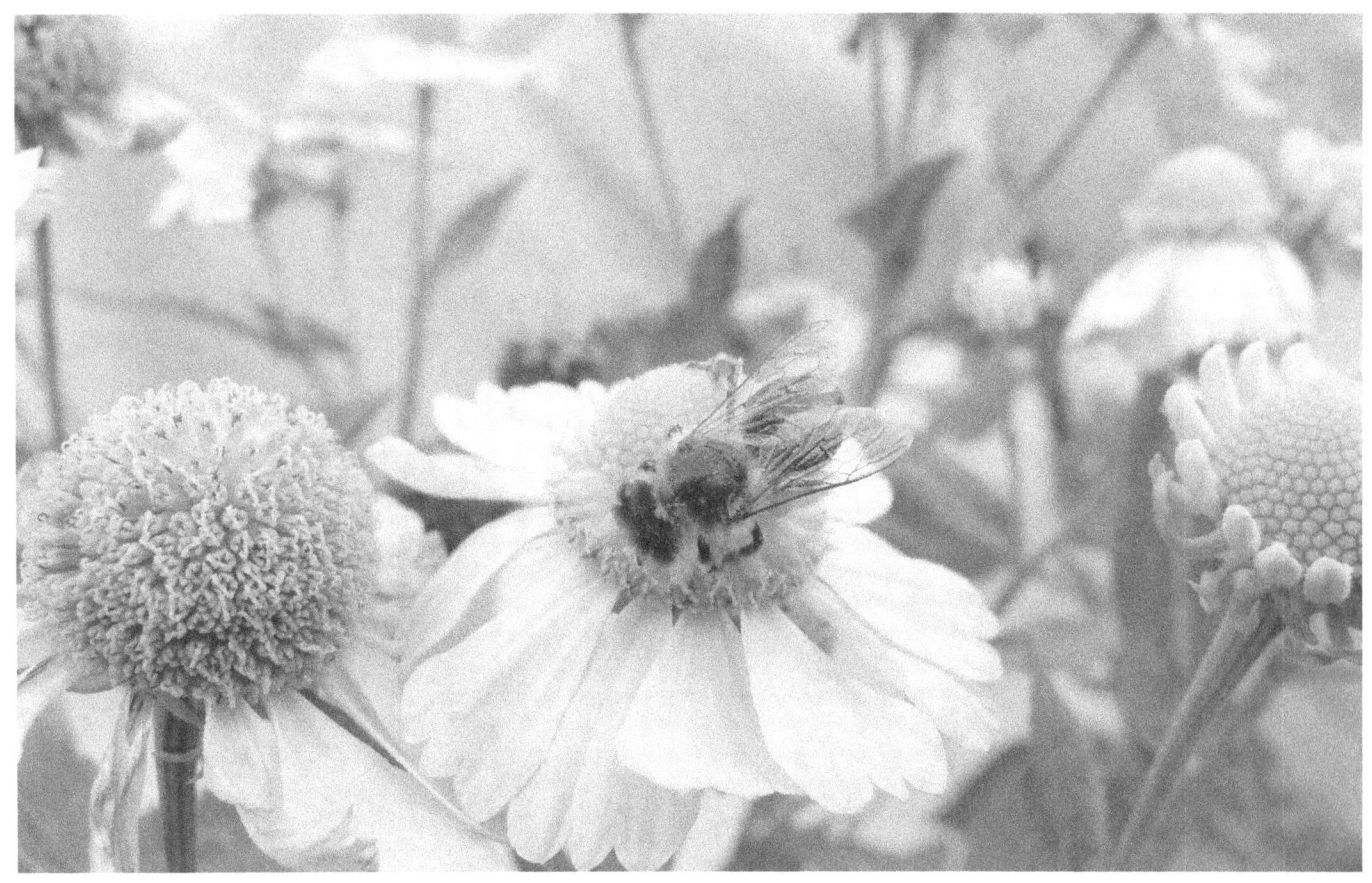

SNEEZEWEED

Helenium is from a Greek word **HELENION** for another plant named after Helen of Troy. She was the daughter of Zeus and Leda, and the wife of Menelaus. Her affair with Paris began the Trojan War.

Autumnale means, "related to autumn", perhaps in reference to its late flowering.

The flower symbolizes tears, probably with regards to Helen; and birth date of November 28th.

Sneezeweed is a common yellow perennial compositae on the prairies. It is often found in moist meadows, or riverbanks in large colonies; and occasionally in the boreal forest.

Sneezeweed is often found in places with wet feet, growing up to four feet tall.

Sneezeweed comes from the Native use of the crushed dried petals as a snuff for combating hay fever; and clear nasal passages during sinus colds and headache. In fact, the Cree name, **CACAMOSIKAN** means, "it makes you sneeze".

Others believe it is the source of their discomfort, and well deserving of the Noxious Weed designation.

It is, to some observers, an unattractive perennial with an abundance of daisy-like flower heads ranging from russet to bright yellow.

They can be hung and dried for winter arrangements.

Sneezeweed is responsible for livestock poisoning in the United States; with the glycoside dugaldin believed partly responsible for this toxic effect.

The Blackfoot of southern Alberta crushed the flower blossoms to use as an inhalant for hay fever. They call it **ES QUE BOIS**.

Other tribes used the plant to clear blocked sinus cavities, or held the root in mouth to relieve toothaches.

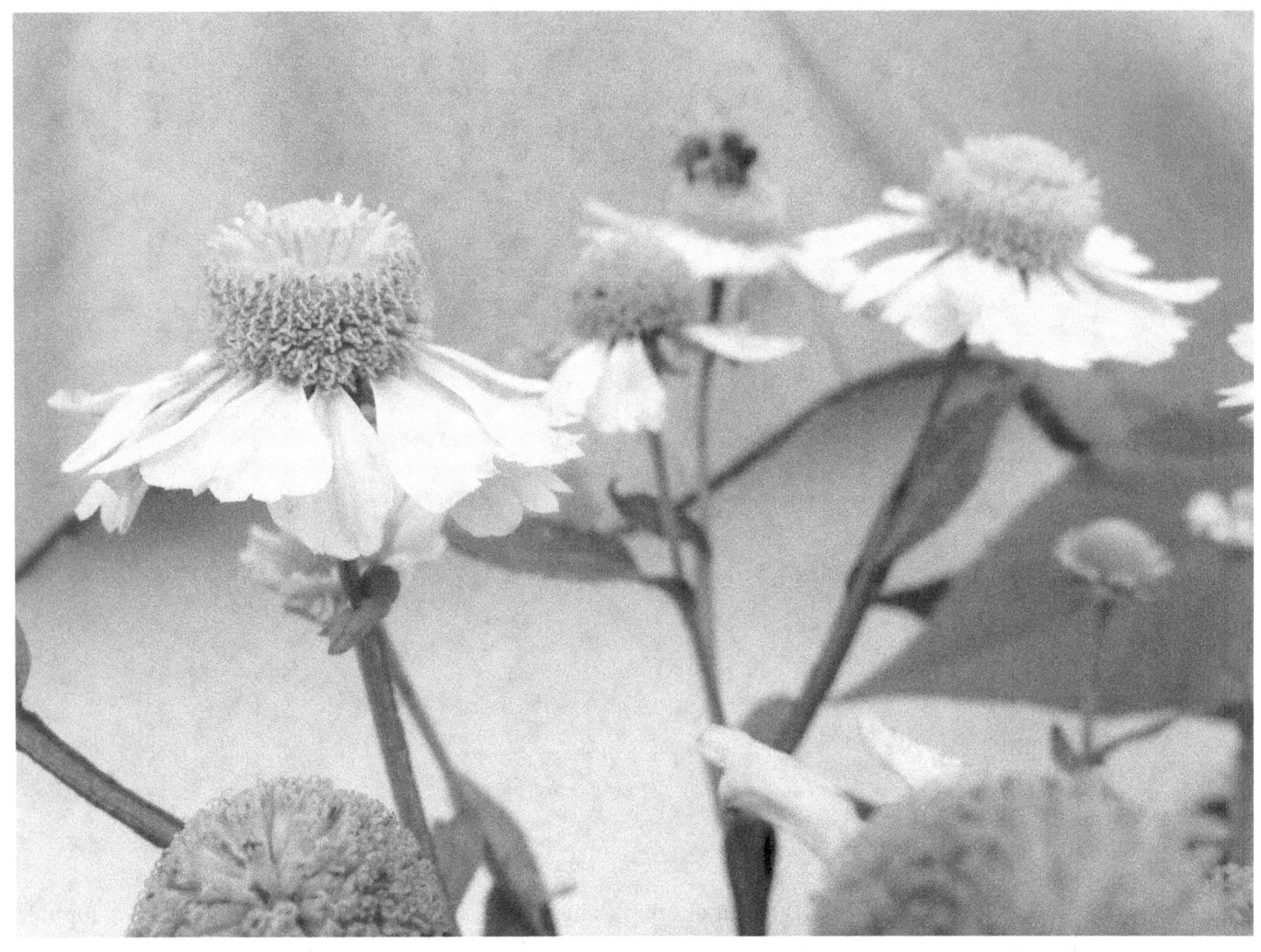

SNEEZEWEED- NOTE DISTINCT CONE SHAPE

A tea can be made of the flower heads to relieve colds.

The Mesquakie call it Inhalant, or **TEATCAMO'SIKANI**, and used the dried flower as a snuff for both head colds and catarrh. They used it as part of a snuff combination that included buttercup and wild bergamot. A flower tea was used for stomach catarrh.

The Cherokee gave compound infusions of the plant to prevent menstruation after childbirth for up to two years. The combination may have been Sneezeweed leaf and Ironweed (*Vernonia novebotacensis*) roots.

The Comanche infused the stems, as a wash to treat fever; while natives of Round Valley, California, used it as a specific for treating venereal disease.

Two related species from Texas have a soft sweet perfume.

MEDICINAL

CONSTITUENTS- halshalin, akhalin, plenolin, balduilin, hakihalin, sulferalin, florilenalin, helenalin, and autumnolide. Carolenin and carolenalin (guaianolides),various glucosides, and various flavonoids including saponaretin, vitexin, orientin, and isoorientin. Helenien is a carotenoid.

Helenalin is an anti-tumour sesquiterpene lactone found in Helenium species.

Studies conducted in 1967 showed helenalin to be the most active anti-neoplastic substance discovered in that year by the *National Cancer Institute.*

Work by Pettit GR et al, *J Med Chem* 1974 17(9): 1013-6 identified the anti-neoplastic agents in sneezeweed.

Helenalin is a sesquiterpene lactone also present in arnica, and believed responsible for some of its anti-inflammatory activity. Other studies by Robles et al, *Planta Medica* 1995 61:3 appear to indicate cardio-tonic activity for this compound.

Helenalin appears to inhibit 5-lipoxygenase and leukotriene C(4) synthase, suggesting a possible pathway of reducing inflammation. Tornhamre S et al, *Biochem Pharmacol* 2001 62(7):903-11. Its action is different from NSAIDs, such as indomethacin and aspirin.

Helenalin suppresses cell proliferation and promotes apoptosis of fibroblasts, suggesting benefit in peritendinous fibrosis and tissue adhesion. Chen S et al, *Cell Death Dis* 2017 8(3):e2710.

Helenalin is cytotoxic to THP-1 cells (acute monocytic leukemia). Zwicker P et al, *Toxicol in Vitro* 2017 40:45-54. It also induced apoptosis in renal cell carcinoma in studies by Jang JH et al, *Toxicol in Vitro* 2013 27(2): 588-96.

In studies conducted by Powis et al at the University of Arizona in Tucson, helenalin caused a marked potentiation of the increases in intracellular free Ca@+ concentration.

It is felt the potentiating effect of helenalin on mitogen stimulated (Ca2+) responses was due in part to an increase in the inositol-(1,4,5)-triphosphate-mediated release of Ca2+ from these stores. In other words, helenalin inhibits phosphodiesterase activity, increases the concentration of cyclic adenosine monophosphate, causes Ca2+ influx and thus enhances the contractibility of the myocardium of the heart. It is a cardio-tonic.

In studies by Merrill et al at Texas A&M, it was found helenalin administered to immature mice caused a rapid decrease in hepatic glutathione. This is not good, as glutathione is an important detoxifier of the liver.

Itoigawa et al, investigated the effect of helenalin on the ventricular myocardium of guinea pigs. Their results conclude that helenalin produces an elevation of cyclic AMP; and increased the force of rested state contraction.

Orientin, also found in barley and some Silene species, is goitergenic, anti-thyroid and anti-oxidative. Iso-orientin, also present in some Gentian species, is anti-oxidant and inhibits pectic trans liminase.

Early Eclectic physicians believed the plant to possess tonic, diaphoretic activity, useful in treating chills, colds, fever and other febrile conditions.

The whole plant, but particularly the florets of the flower disk are active as a snuff, for headache, flu, catarrhal deafness, and other affections of the nose, throat and ears.

The leaves and flowers are active against *Staphylococcus aureus.* Borchardt et al, *J Med Plant Res* 2008 2:4-5.

Florilenalin derivatives may have potential for treating nasopharyngeal carcinoma. Su M et al, *Molecules* 2009 14(6): 2135-46.

The Cree healer, Clifford Cardinal shared a formula with me, treating diabetes with plants growing in Alberta. Some plants, in the dried, powdered mixture, I could identify, including sneezeweed, that he called yellow pipe, due to its distinctive yellow cone.

Others were stove pipe, or horsetail (*Equisetum fluviatile*); Labrador tea (*Rhododendron groenlandicum*), sphagnum moss, diamond willow fungus (*Haploporus odorus*) and something called horse root, possibly Lomatium species.

Recent work has found orientin, vitexin and saponaretin, all found in sneezeweed, may be useful for reducing both high blood sugar and lipids. Gong J et al, *J Ethnopharm* 2016 194: 260-8. All three of these compounds are also found in fenugreek seed.

Helenien is a carotenoid studied for its benefit to eye health. It was never commercialized.

FLOWER ESSENCE

Helenium essence acts as a super highway for the flow of information- energy throughout our entire system. Dissolving the cobwebs of shame, it increases circulation between the upper and lower chakras as it ripples through the etheric bodies.

RAVEN ESSENCES

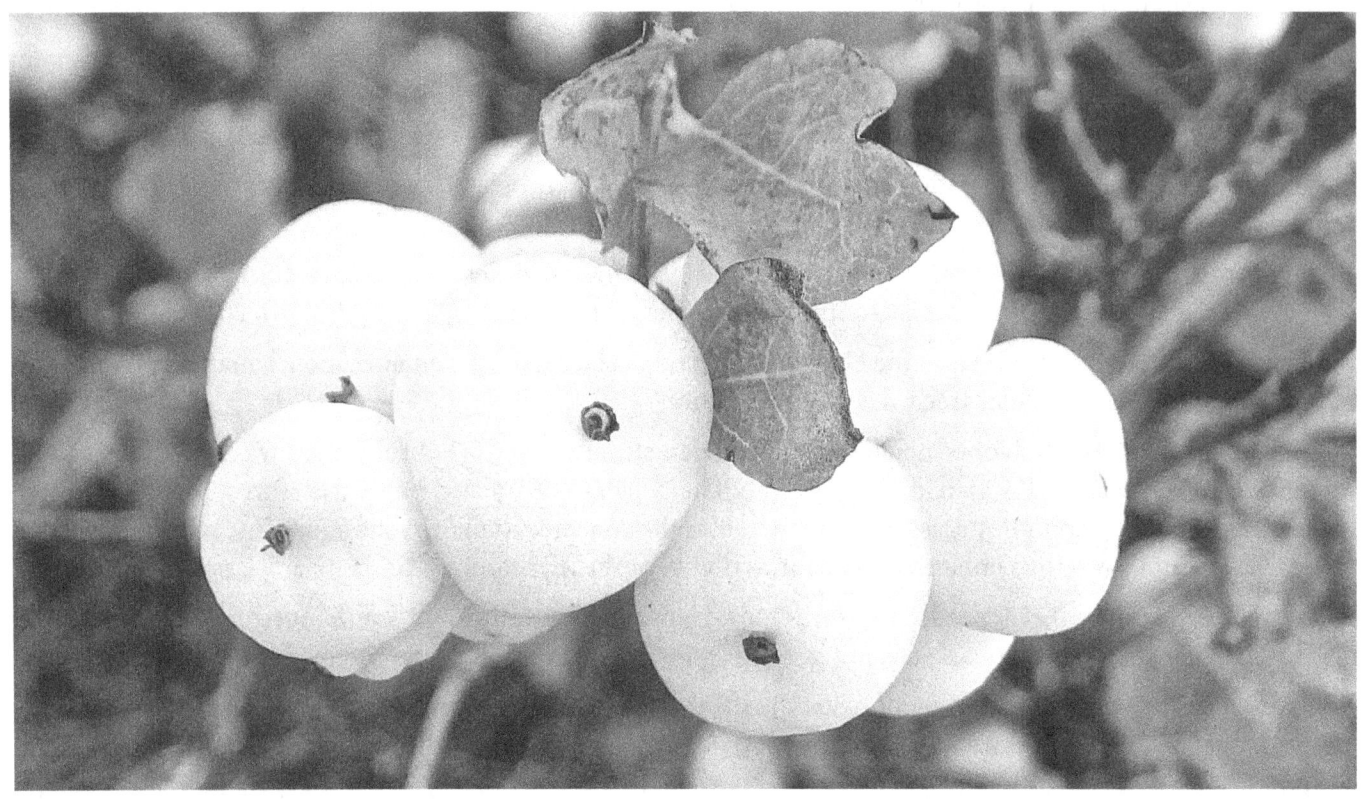

SNOWBERRIES

SNOWBERRY
WAXBERRY
(*Symphoricarpos albus var. albus* [L.] S. F. Blake)
(*Symphoria racemosa* [Michx.] Pursh.) not accepted
(*S. racemosus* Michx.) not accepted
(*S. racemosa ssp. alba*) not accepted
BUCKBRUSH
WOLFBERRY
WESTERN SNOWBERRY
(*S. occidentalis* Hook.)
CORALBERRY
INDIAN CURRANT
(*S. orbiculatus* Moench.)
(*S. vulgaris*)
PARTS USED- inner bark, twigs, flowers and root

I made him gather me wet snowberries, On slippery rocks beside a waterfall.
I made him do for me in the dark
And he liked everything I made him do.

ROBERT FROST

64

Symphoricarpos is derived from the Greek **SYN** meaning, together, **PHOREIN** to bear and **KARPOS** meaning fruit.

ALBUS means white and refers to the bright white berries. **RACEMOSA** means branched and **OCCIDENTALIS** means of the west. It may also derive from the Greek, **SYMPHOREO**, to accumulate, but accumulate what?

The Snowberry occurs in wooded habitats, and is a slender shrub up to one metre tall with white flowers and berries, that are juicy and slight acidic when ripe, but tasteless when past this stage.

Buckbrush, or Wolfberry, is found mainly in aspen parkland, ravine and coulees. The greenish white fruit are in dense clusters that turn purple when dry. Snowberry's common name is because the berries remain snow white, and stay on the bush all winter.

In Kent, England, it was believed that the juice of the snowberry fruit caused warts. An author tried this in 1985, by rubbing it on his thigh and sometime later, three warts appeared. Interesting?

Indigenous people believed that snowberries were ghosts of Saskatoon berries and part of the spirit world, and not to be eaten by the living.

This relates to the European symbology of "thoughts of heaven", attributed to snowberry. The birth date of November 7th has been attached to the plant.

The berries are astringent, and in large doses induce vomiting. The Thompson of British Columbia call them Ghost berries, or Saskatoon berries of the dead.

The Okanagan-Colville call the plant **STEMTEMNIHILPH** meaning, Corpse's Plant, also suggesting poisonous aspects, or perhaps alluding to "ghost-like" color of berries.

Decoctions of the berries, bark or leaves were used traditionally to wash the breasts of nursing mothers; acting as an antiseptic. The branches were decocted to help remove afterbirth, and as a wash for skin sores. The Saanich infused the bark for external wash for skin itching.

The sap, from young shoots, was used as both a laxative and tonic for the stomach.

One or two berries were eaten by the Stl'atl'imx to settle the stomach after eating too much fatty food.

The Cree call it **MEHEEKKUMWATIT** meaning, horse medicine. They boiled the leaves for their animals suffering water retention. The roots and stems were decocted for fevers with teething pain.

The Cheholi rubbed the snowberries into their hair as a shampoo. Like the Wood Cree and Bella Coola, they decocted the root and stem bark for venereal disease. The Kagit used plant infusions for "babies with coated tongues" and bark decoctions for tuberculosis.

The Lillooet of British Columbia would eat two or three berries after fatty foods, to help with digestion. The Wet'suwet'en living further north decocted the plant as an eye medicine. They call the plant **C'ITSIT MI'**.

The Fox tribe used root decoctions to cleanse the new mother of afterbirth; and to aid her recovery. The Chippewa made strong root decoctions for severe constipation; or combined with bluestem for stoppage of urine.

Tribes like the Nlaka'pmx of BC used the berries as a cure for diarrhea, while the St'at'imc squeezed ripe berries into sore eyes before sleeping.

The Pomo of California used the pithy stems for pipes, and named it wood for tobacco, or **SA-KA-HI**.

Snowberry was quite popular in the late 1800s, as a remedy for pregnancy vomiting and morning sickness.

There are reports of snowberry poisoning documented in the US, Britain and Poland. In Britain, just three berries caused a child to vomit, experience dizziness and mild sedation.

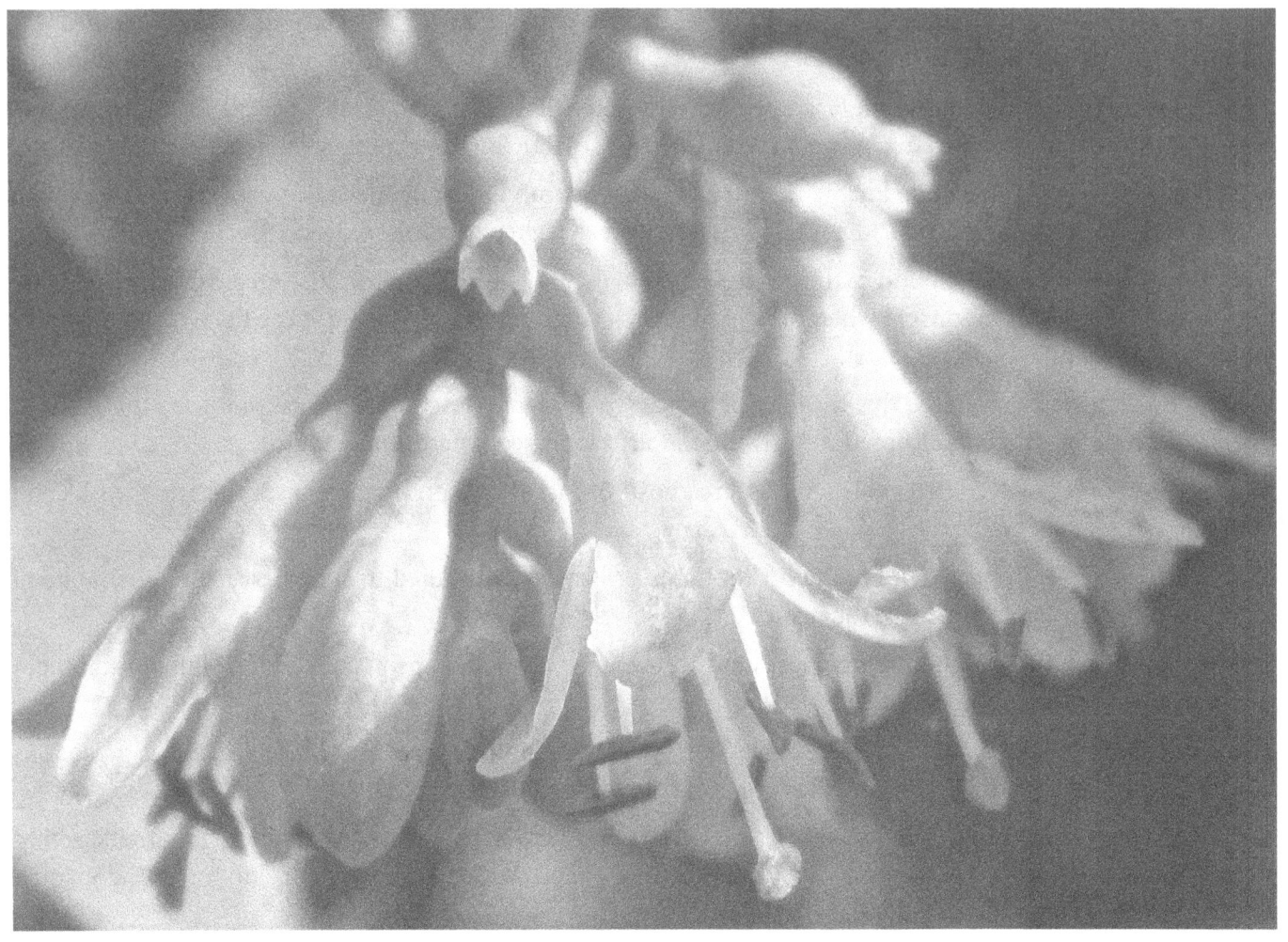

BUCKBRUSH FLOWERS

The Woods Cree of Saskatchewan know Buckbrush as Wolfberry, or **MAHIKANIMIN**. The fruit was infused to treat sore eyes; while the root and stem were ingredients in a decoction for fevers associated with teething sickness and venereal disease. The root bark was decocted for stomach troubles.

The whole plant was infused for skin rashes, and used internally and externally at the same time.

The Cree of southern Saskatchewan know the shrub as Wolf Berry Plant. The leaves were decocted and used for both horses and humans as a diuretic and kidney problems.

Buckbrush is known to the Alberta Cree under the name **MA-HE-HUM-NA-NA-CHE-KUS**. The inner bark was steeped and used as eyewash.

The Blackfoot use it for similar purpose, and call it Whiteberry or White Weasel Eyes or **AP-INI-KUN**. They gave the boiled berries to their horses as a strong diuretic; as did the Crow and Sioux tribes further south. The yellow roots were decocted to stop heavy menstrual bleeding.

The Flathead would simply chew up the fruit and place the juice on an injured eye. At first the eye muscles would tighten up, but soon felt better. A tea of Buckbrush leaves and Wild Rose bark was used as eyewash.

The mashed berries were applied to cuts and burns; while the crushed leaves, fruit and bark were poulticed on scabs and burns to promote healing without scars.

They used a stem tea to remove afterbirth, and in potent mixtures for venereal disease. Kutenai women brewed small branches for menstrual problems.

The Mesquakie used the root tea for cleansing uterus of afterbirth, and call the plant **TATEPA'SIKI**, meaning twisted.

Both the Omaha and Ponca call the plant **INSHTOGAHTE-HI**, meaning eye lotion plant. The Dakota used a tea of the leaves for sore eyes, and call the plant **ZUZECHA-TA-WOTE SAPSAPA**, or black snake food.

The Crow of southern Montana call it **BITDAJA**. Alma Snell tells a story of using 4-5 berries internally to clear the sinuses.

Further east, the Mi'kmaq tied the plant into bundles that were sniffed for headache. Wallis, in *American Anthropologist* 1922 24 mentioned the plant was utilized by the same tribe as a tonic.

The green twigs were burned to blacken the surface of newly made pipes. These were then greased and polished with a piece of tanned skin.

Smaller twigs can be tied together to make brooms.

Early settlers called them Water Brush, suggesting they indicated a good place to drill or dig a well. Maybe.

The toxicity of snowberries has been greatly exaggerated. One of out eight cases of vomiting in children cited in one study, and 5 out of 39 in another. Three to four berries will cause no problem. The LD50 of a fresh berry water extract is 435g/kg in mice, not worthy of concern.

The introduced Coralberry (*S. orbiculatus*) is hardy to zone 2, and produces red fruit that cluster like small raspberries. The related *S. utahensis, S. oreophilus,* and *S. mollis* are hardy as well.

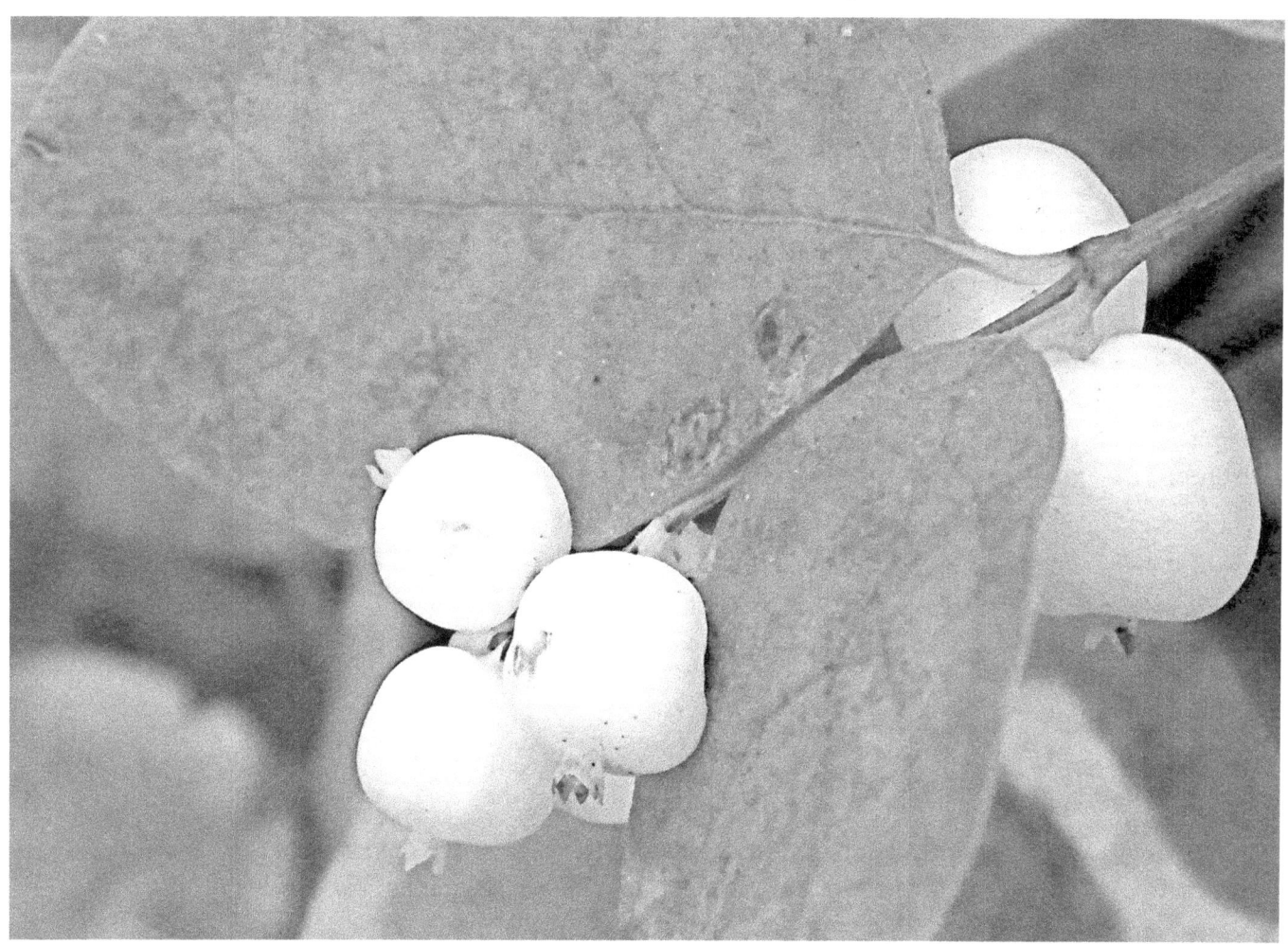

SNOWBERRIES

MEDICINAL

CONSTITUENTS- *S. albus-* chelidonine (major leaf and root alkaloid), various terpenoids including lanosterol, 31-norlanosterol, cycloartenol, butryospermol, lophenol, lupeol, bauerenol, citrostadienol, obtusifoliol, gramisterol, protocatechuic, ursolic and oleanlic acids.

Fruit- flavonoids including apigenin, luteolin and quercitin glycosides; chelidonine (alkaloid), secologanin, loganin, its aglycone, glucologanin and various sugars. Chlorogenic (33% of phenolics), protocatechuic (19% of phenolics), quinic, aminobutryic, malic, tartaric and citric acids.

Flowers- salicylic acid, alpha resorcylic acid, gallic acid, chlorogenic acid (45% of phenolics).

Basically, the root and bark of Snowberry stems is diuretic, and a stomachache tonic.

The berries are astringent, but can be cathartic or emetic if taken in any quantity. Expressed juice of the entire plant shows activity against both gram negative and positive bacteria.

The fresh leaves, and fruit are useful as poultices for bruises, sores and other ailments of the skin. Dried leaf infusions help relieve cold symptoms, while dried bark infusions help treat lung infections and ease stomach ache and indigestion.

Caffeic, protocatechuic and chlorogenic acids are immune stimulating.

Caffeic, p-coumaric and salicylic acids are anti-inflammatory.

Procatechuic and caffeic acids suggest choleretic and cholekinetic properties.

Chelidonine is a central nervous system depressant that in large amounts can cause dizziness, vomiting, depression, and sedation. It is a narcotic present in Celandine, and other members of the Poppy family.

It produces mild but prolonged lowering of blood pressure, increases urination and inhibits or delays the development of anaphylactic shock. The compound depolymerizes the microtubule network in HeLa and human osteosarcoma U2OS cancer cell lines. Wang X et al, *Molecules* 2016 21(7).

It is found in Celandine (*Chelidonium majus*).

Lanosterol is a selective regulator of macrophage immunity. It increases membrane fluidity and ROS production, potentiating phagocytosis and ability to kill bacteria. It also reduces cytokine secretion and showed improved resistance of mice to *Listeria monocytogenes* by increasing clearance from spleen and liver. Araidi E et al, *Cell Rep* 2017 19(13): 2743-55.

Lanosterol suppresses the aggregation and cytotoxicity of misfolded proteins linked with neurodegenerative diseases. Upadhyay A et al, *Mol Neurobiol* 2017 Jan 19. Lanosterols are found in a wide range of medicinal mushrooms.

31-norlanosterol derivatives show activity against *Leishmania infantum* and *Trypanosoma cruzi*, with selective toxicity. Mazoir N et al, *Z Naturforsch* C 2011 66(7-8): 360-6.

The fruit of Snowberry has been used as a source of carbohydrate and secologanin, with the addition of tryptamine, in the biotransformation of transgenic yeast cultures in the production of indole alkaloids.

HOMEOPATHY

Snowberry (*S. racemosa*) is highly recommended for persistent vomiting during pregnancy. It is useful for all gastric disturbances, like fickle appetite to chronic constipation.

If there is nausea during menstruation, and this is made worse by motion, then snowberry is worthy of a trial. There may be aversion to all foods, and the only relief comes when the patient lies on their back.

Metrorrhagia, or excessive bleeding after abortion, may be reduced.

DOSE- Second and third potency. The tincture is made from the fresh, ripe berries. The 200th has proved curative. Burdick observed the effect of tincture on a number of women. The binomial *S. racemosa* is no longer accepted by taxonomists, and is replaced by *S. albus* var. *albus*.

FLOWER ESSENCES

Snowberry flower essence is for acceptance of life as it is, in the moment. It dissolves resistance to "what is", and gently leads us to acceptance. Situations and experiences may not appear to "make sense". Embracing "what is", even when painful, can lead to that exquisite experience of ecstasy. Snowberry guides us to this place of being fully alive in the moment.   **PACIFIC**

Snowberry flower essence is important for those individuals who seem, or feel invisible to those around them. It is not that they do not have much to offer, but shyness, and low self-worth prevent their participation in groups.

It may also be of help in situations where an individual would like to be less visible such as detective work, media reporter, sports referee, or the like.   **PRAIRIE DEVA**

Snowberry flower essence helps you to stay open to your healing process. It helps to integrate learning from the experience without having to be shocked or traumatized again by remembering the actual event.
                                                                                                        TREE FROG

SPIRITUAL PROPERTIES

The soul is a fragment of the Light. On its journey through life, it encounters shadows and darkness even within itself. Only by acknowledging and embracing the dark we can move again in the Light. If we resist, the darkness intensifies.

In the symbology of the Tarot, the correlation for this (snowberry flower) essence is the Devil. What could be a better symbol of darkness? But as James Wanless points out in the Voyager Tarot, devil spelled backwards is "lived" and marks the potential for full expression of life. He quotes Vivekananada, "See good and evil as the same; both are merely God's play." He also notes that the I Ching hexagram for the Devil is #16- Enthusiasm. This word comes from the Greek **EN THEOS**, which literally means "In God".   **PACIFIC**

PERSONALITY TRAITS

In Finland, Snow was personified as a 300 year-old king, Snaer, the son of Iceberg. He was father to three daughters, Thick Snow, Snowstorm, and Fine Snow.

In Japan, a pale and beautiful snow woman called Yuki Onna preyed on travelers in snowstorms. She was young, with an alluring body, but ghostly white. When she came upon people lost in fierce winter blizzards, she lulled them to sleep, and then blew her icy breath over them.

The Algonquin also had a snow legend, regarding a bridegroom named Mowis. He took a bride one cold night, and then disappeared in the warmth of morning sunlight.

SPINY SOW THISTLE
CREEPING SOW THISTLE
(*Sonchus arvensis* L.)
MOIST SOW THISTLE
FIELD SOW THISTLE
(*S. uliginosus* Bieb.) not accepted
(*S. arvensis ssp. uliginosus* [Bieb.] Nyman.)
SMOOTH SOW THISTLE

ANNUAL SOW THISTLE
PUALELE
PUHA
(*S. oleraceus* L.)
PRICKLY SOW THISLE
SPINY LEAF SOW THISTLE
(*S. asper* [L.] Hill)
PARTS USED- leaf, flower

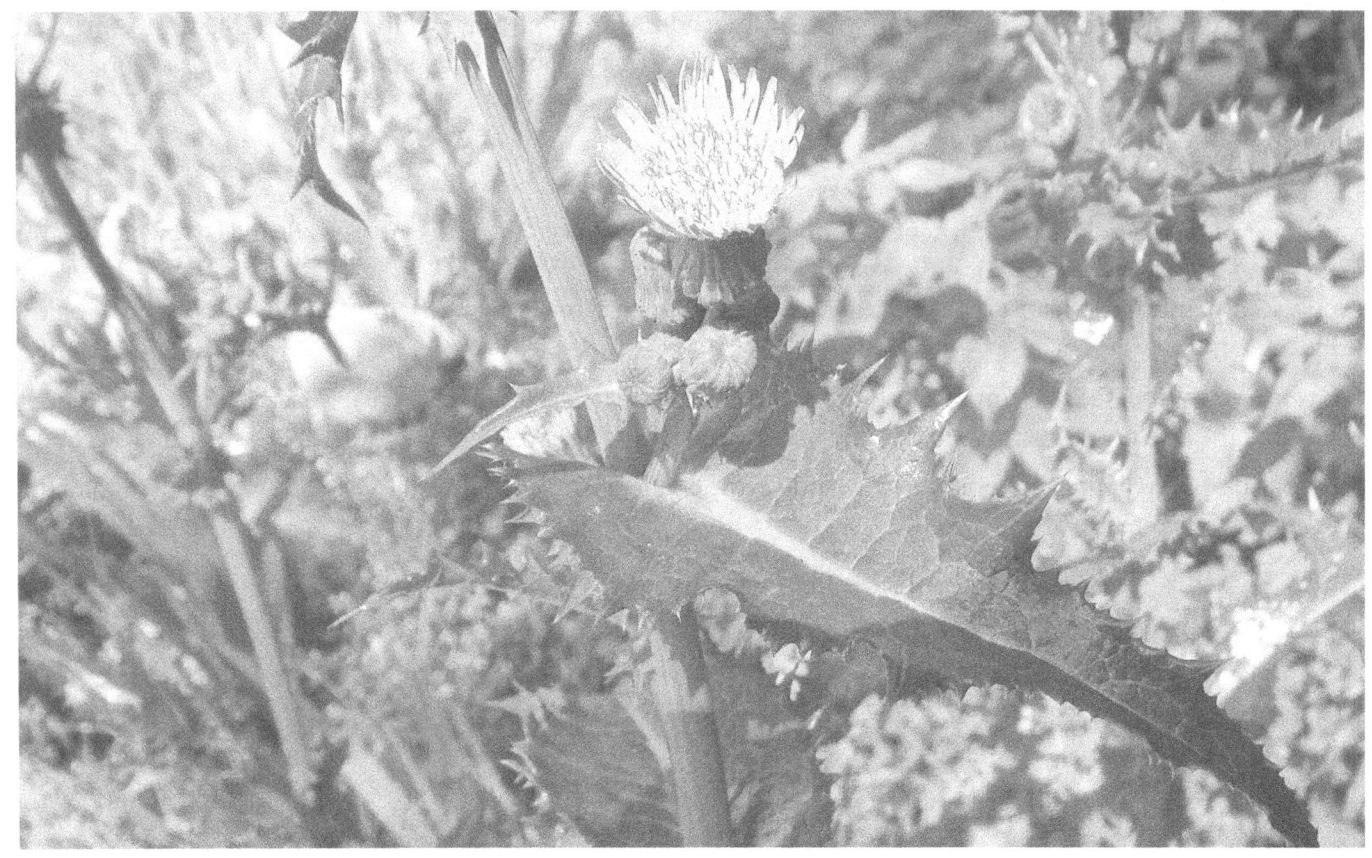

PRICKLY SOW THISTLE

I am fond of pigs. Dogs look up at us. Cats look down on us. Pigs treat us as equals.

WINSTON CHURCHILL

Sonchus is from the Greek **SOMPHOS** meaning hollow or spongy, an obvious reference to the stem. The common name comes from the following quote by Dr. William Cole, a 17th century herbalist. "When sows have pigs, they greedily desire it, because they know by certain natural instinct that it very much increases their milk."

OLERACEUS is from the Latin and refers to the aromatic nature of the plant as an esculent or edible vegetable; of garden origin. Uliginosus means swamp.

Arvensis is from the Latin **ARVENS** of the field; and **ASPER** means rough.

Legend has it that hares chased by dogs will stop and eat the leaves to cool their blood, before they continue. Today, veterinarians and farmers use the fresh plant for reducing fever and heart palpitations in their farm animals.

Both the annual and perennial plants are edible, but somewhat bitter. It was taken as a tea in former times by mothers and wet nurses to increase milk production.

Spiny and Moist are perennial species; the other two are annuals.

Three spoonfuls of the milky juice from stems was dissolved in wine, and fed to expectant mothers to expedite birthing.

The ancient Greeks and Romans used the milky sap for eye and skin ailments. The plant was considered to contain many properties similar to dandelion.

The seed of *S. oleraceus* was said to have supplied the silky down for the baby Jesus to lie down on, and was formally known as Saint Maries.

Because of it's hurtful, prickly stems, sow thistle has long been associated with sorcery, magic and the planet Mars. Russians believed it to be the devil's favorite plant. Culpepper considered that all sow thistles had medicinal virtues, particularly the milky juice.

It was considered to be cooling in nature, and used to ease stomach pain. The juice was given as a drink for shortness of breath, or wheezing.

The juice was applied topically to shrink and soothe hemorrhoids, and used in combinations for catarrhal deafness. The milky juice was often cited for cosmetic and skin clearing purposes in older herbals.

John Lightfoot in his *Herbal Scotica* of 1777 wrote: "An emulsion of the seeds has sometimes been used to thin the blood and cure stitches and pleurises but at present is rarely practiced."

The sap has been studied as a potential source of natural rubber. Buchanan et al, *J Am Oil Chem Soc* 1978 55:9. *S. oleraceus* and *S. arvensis* latex, comprising some 5%, have been investigated as a source of rubber, waxes and energy.

They are a source of pentacyclic terpenes that may be of value to the pharmaceutical industry.

As a forage plant, it is equal or higher in digestible dry matter, crude protein, and macro and micro-mineral content than alfalfa. Lambs are not fond of it, but rabbits readily seek it out.

The Old English Herbarium suggests "for stomach ache, take the upper part of the flower head of the plant we call sow thistle when it is soft and fresh, and give this to eat in sweetened vinegar. It will cure the soreness."

It was said a flower picked when the moon is in Capricorn and carried on your person, will protect one from evil.

Fresh leaves, from *S. arvensis* were applied to caked breasts, by Potawatomi. Various indigenous healers applied the crushed or boiled leaves to swellings.

The Cherokee used infusions of the leaves and flowers to calm the nerves. Opium users in San Francisco later used the plant resin of *S. oleraceus* to help break their addiction. This is probably a version of doctrine of signatures, with milky, white sap.

The Navaho smoked the leaves of *S. asper* for heart palpitations; while the Houmas of the southeastern United States gave infusions of *S. oleraceus* for teething pain in children.

In Caracas, decoctions of *S. oleraceus* are given internally for flatulence; and externally applied to soothe the skin. In Peru, it is considered a stomachic, carminative and anti-spasmodic. In Costa Rica and Yucatan, sow thistle is considered a liver herb, and used for laxative purpose, and increase milk production.

In parts of Albania, the annual sow thistles are made into a cold macerate and applied to sore mouths.

In Indonesia, the bitter leaves are added to curries and rice dishes. The leaves, known as **TEMPUYUNG**, or Kidney Stone Leaves, are an important plant of JAMU, the ancient traditional healing art of that country.

The herb is grown on soil rich in calcium oxalate, and the theory is that organic calcium salts in sow thistle leaf tea help remove calcium build-up in the kidneys. Makes sense to me! Gravel root and Hydrangea root work in a similar manner, but providing ionic phases of minerals to allow for re-creation of more soluble salts that are more easily flushed.

The young leaves are less bitter than dandelion leaves, but best boiled.

The leaves may be useful in fermented vegetable products. In one study, *S. oleraceus* stimulated *Lactobacillus bulgaris*, *L. lactis*, *L. reuteri* and *Bifidobacterium longum* in culture. In same study dandelion leaf stimulated growth in three of four. Kassim MA et al, *Int J Food Sci Nutr* 2014 65(8): 977-80.

The thick upper stems can be used raw or boiled for 2-3 minutes for a flavor of asparagus crossed with artichoke heart, according to wild food expert Dr. John Kallas.

The taproot, with fibrous roots removed, are boiled for five to ten minutes, and used like a potato. They are only good before the stalk has formed.

In China, the leaves are used as a bitter, for liver complaints. They use the stem juice for abscesses, warts and boils, and infuse yellow flowers to reduce fevers.

The plant is dried and powdered for use as a natural insecticide. The Pare Tribe of the former Tanganyika ate the raw root, or boiled it in a meal with bananas to treat roundworm.

In neighboring Ethiopia, the leaf is exposed to fire and the smell inhaled for headache. Work by Al-Hussanini et al, *Molecules* 2009 14:9 found ethanol extracts of the herb exhibit superior activity against *Chromobacterium violaceum*.

The related *S. schweinfurthii* shows activity against *giardia*.

The leaves of *S. asper* are mixed with salt, chewed and swallowed to relieve tonsillitis.

In Nepal, the whole plant is fed to animals for proper development of the fetus, and a paste applied to wounds and boils. The sow thistle has been used traditionally in the treatment of kidney inflammation, hormonal imbalance and impotence.

The juice of *S. arvensis*, known as **BAN RAYO** is given, four teaspoons twice daily, for fevers, indigestion, typhoid and dysuria. The root juice is used to treat bile duct problems.

The Maori of New Zealand make a chewing gum from the white sap. Even the flower heads can be a tasty chew. The roots of *S. arvensis* have been roasted like chicory as a coffee substitute. Studies in Brazil indicate *S. oleraceus* extracts help control spider mites. The seeds can be sprouted and eaten in salads, an ancient name translating as Sprout Thistle.

Rhizobacteria associated with *S. oleraceus* may be useful for bioremediation, particularly zinc and copper sewage sludge soils. Fang Q et al, Front *Plant Sci* 2016 7: 1487.

MEDICINAL

CONSTITUENTS- *S. arvensis*- triterpenes (up to 24%) including alpha-amyrin (9%), beta-amyrin (21%), lupeol (13%), taraxasterol (24%), and pseudotaraxasterol (12%); and two flavone glycosides, quercitin-3-0-alpha-L-rhamnoside, and kaempferol-3, 7-alpha-L-dirhamnoside; various flavonoids including kaempferol, quercitin, orientin, rutin, hyperoside, catechin and myricetin.
latex -rubber and a and b- lactucerols.
pollen- flavanols, leucoanthocyanins, and carotenoids including beta-carotene.
S. asper- sonchusides, pentacyclic triterpenes, like epi-friedelinol acetate, amyrins, taraxasterols, stigmasterol apigenin, luteolin and various 7-glucuronides as flavanoids.
roots- four sesquiterpene glucosides, including various dihydrospermal A componds; and an aglycone.
S. oleraceus- sonchusides, gluco-zaluzanin, crepidiasdie, luteolin, quercimeritrin, quercetin 7-beta-D-glucopyranoside, cynaroside, isocynaroside, macroliniside, picresides B and C, esculetin,vernolic acid, cynaroside, isocynarosides, triterpenes including 3 beta, 25-epoxy-3-hydroxyolean-18-en-28-oic acid.
leaves- provitamin A, 1390 mg/100 grams, omega 3 fatty acids, zinc and manganese, copper and iron. Various polyphenols and flavonoids including apigenin, kaempferol, myricetin and quercitin; ursolic acid, ferulaic acid, villosol and rutin. Novel actinobacterium endophytes NEAU-QY3T, *Plantactinospora sonchi* and *Nocardia caishijiensis*.
flowers- luteolin 7-beta-D-gluoosiduronic acid.
root- loliolide, ursolic acid, lupeol, beta sitosterol-3-o-glucopyranoside, 15-o-beta-glucopyranosyl-11, 13-dihydro-urospermal A; endophytes *Streptosporangium sonchi*, and *S. kronopolitis*.

Today, sow thistle is valued medicinally for many of its traditional purposes.

It is very useful for treating asthma, bronchitis, and coughs, including whooping cough.

It is mildly sedative, and used for insomnia, and withdrawal from stimulants and narcotics.

The fresh juice is used in New Zealand for painful carbuncles and dissolving warts.

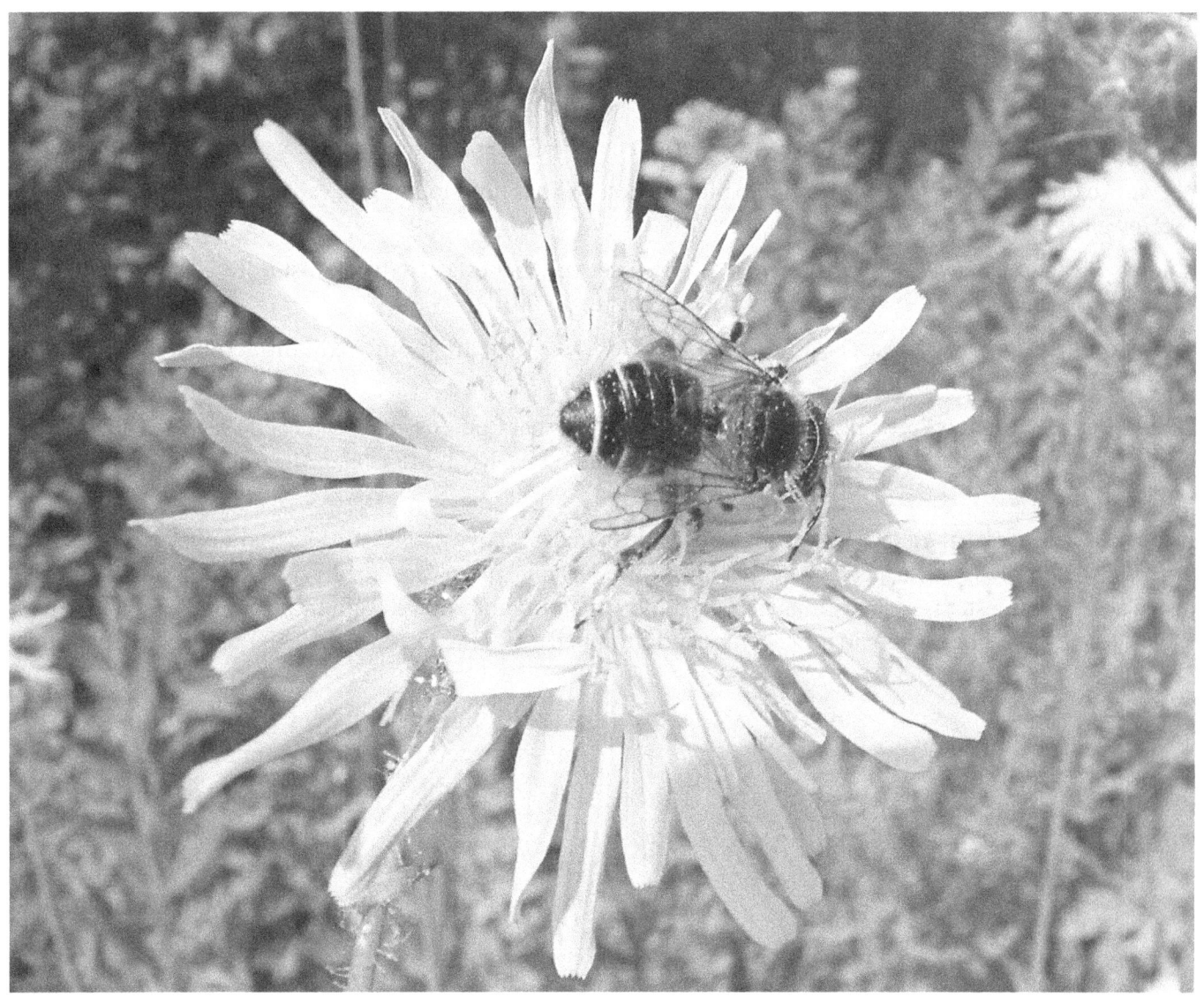

SOW THISTLE AND BEE

Decoctions of plantain leaves, clover blossoms, and sow thistle can be used after birthing to fully expel the placenta.

Sow thistle can be used in veterinary medicine, for animals with fever and heat disorders in form of a decoction.

Annual Sow thistle (*S. oleraceus*) is known as ***KU CAI*** in Mandarin Traditional Chinese Medicine. The herb is a hemostat, excellent for functional uterine bleeding, vomiting of blood, nosebleed, or bloody urine or stool.

It is a strong anti-inflammatory and astringent plant, useful in acute enteritis, appendicitis, mastitis, stomatitis, pharyngitis, tonsillitis, infectious hepatitis and numerous other "itis" or acute conditions.

Work by Vilela et al, *J Ethnopharm* 124:2 with mice, found the herb to possess both anti-inflammatory and anti-anxiety properties. The former was 1/30th the strength of morphine, and the latter 1/60th of chonacepam. Cardoso et al, in same journal issue studied the anti-anxiety effect on mice.

Later Vilela FC et al published a paper suggesting a standardized extract could be of potential interest for treatment of depressive disorders. *J Med Food* 2010 13(1): 219-20.

Taken over time, it is said to quiet the heart, boost Qi, sharpen the senses, lessen sleep and slow aging.

The herb has bitter, cold properties that can be valuable as an anti-tumour agent, in treating breast, skin, liver and stomach cancers.

Other names include **TU CAO**, meaning Rampant Weed, which it certainly can be, and **XUAN**, meaning Choice.

The herb rates high in anti-oxidant activity. Pieroni et al, *Phytotherapy Res* 2002 16:5.

The anti-oxidant activity of leaf is similar to blueberries, and has been found to invade HepG2 liver cancer cells. McDowell et al, *Phytother Research* 2011 24:12.

Studies of the four species found *S. oleraceus* possesses the highest activity against both Gram positive and negative bacteria. Xia DZ et al, *Nat Prod Res* 2011 20: 1893-1901.

The two annual species, *S. asper* and *S. oleraceus* possess very high anti-oxidant activity. Alipnar et al, *Food Sci Tech Res* 15:1.

The former species shows prevention of nephrotoxicity in animal studies. Khan et al, *Food Chem Tox* 48:8-9. And prevention of liver and kidney toxicity in gentamicin treated rats. Khan MR et al, *BMC Complement Altern Med* 2011 11:113.

It appears to be useful in protecting thyroid tissue from oxidative activity, suggesting its traditional use for treating hormone disorders is confirmed. Khan RA, *BMC Complement Altern Med* 2012 12:181. The same author also tested acetylcholinesterase activity in male rats, at the same time and showed significant cognitive enhancement as well as elevated brain antioxidant enzymes and inhibited AChE activity. Khan RA et al, *Behav Brain Funct* 2012 8:21.

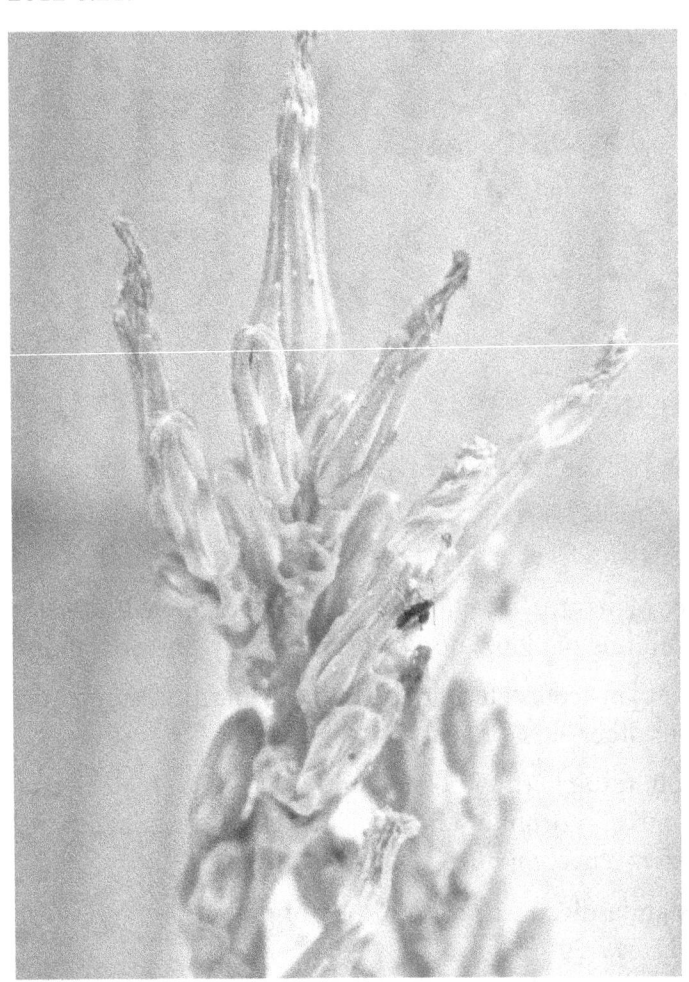

SOW THISTLE FLOWERS GOING TO SEED

Aerial part tinctures show considerable anti-hypertensive activity, supporting its traditional use. Mushtaq MN et al, *Acta Pol Pharm* 2016 73(2): 425-31.

Sonchus asper helped prevent toxicity due to gentamicin in a rat study by Khan et al, *BMC Compl Altern Med* 2011 11:113.

A recent rat study with alcohol extracts of this species found glucose and insulin levels were significantly lower at day 21. The herb is widely used in Pakistan for this condition. Khan RA, *Altern Ther Health Med* 2017 Feb 27.

The latter (*S. oleraceus*) root extracts show cytotoxicity against PC33 (brain) and L5187Y (lymphoma) cancer cell lines, and anti-bacterial activity against *Staphylococcus aureus*, *Bacillus subtilis*, *E. coli* and *Neisseria gonorrhoeae*. Ehab Saad Eikhayat, *Pharmacognosy Magazine* 2009 5:20. Note the reference to treating gonorrhea.

Water extracts show anti-inflammatory effect *in vitro* and *in vivo*. Li Q et al, *Pharm Biol* 2017 55(1): 799-809. The ability to quench free radicals suggests high antioxidant activity, from 70% alcohol extracts. The results were better than vitamin C or chlorogenic acid. Ou ZQ et al, *Molecules* 2015 20(3): 4548-64.

The leaves exert aromatase inhibition, and cytotoxic effect against MCF-7 breast cancer cell lines. Shaban NZ et al, *Cell Mol Biol* (Noisy-le-grand) 2016 62(9): 11-19.

Water extracts of aerial parts inhibit HepG-2 and K562 cancer cell lines, by decreasing cell viability and inducing apoptosis, and inhibiting migration. Huyan T et al, *J Ethnopharm* 2016 185: 289-99.

A study by AbouZid SF et al, *J Med Food* 2014 17(3): 400-6 found hypoglycemic activity in a diabetic model.

An endophyte, Nocardia caishijiensis, isolated from leaf, shows activity against MRSA, *E. coli*, *Klebsiella pneumonia*, *S. aureus*, and *Candida tropicalis*. The mycelium extract contains the compounds stenothricin and bagremycin A. Tanvir R et al, *Microbiol Res* 2016 185: 22-35.

Sow Thistle (*S. arvensis*) is very refrigerant and used to reduce fevers, and calm heart palpitations. It contains sesquiterpene lactones active against *Streptococcus mutans*. Xia Z et al, *Ethnobot Lett* 2009 Dec 16; *Fitoterapia* 2010 81(5): 424-8.

Alcohol extracts appear useful in the prevention of hepatic stress. Alkreathy HM et al, *BMC Complement Altern Med* 2014 14:452.

Work by same author in *Nat Prod Research* 25:20 found alcohol extracts of this herb to possess high anti-oxidant activity, while *S. oleraceus* showed greatest activity against gram-positive and gram-negative bacteria.

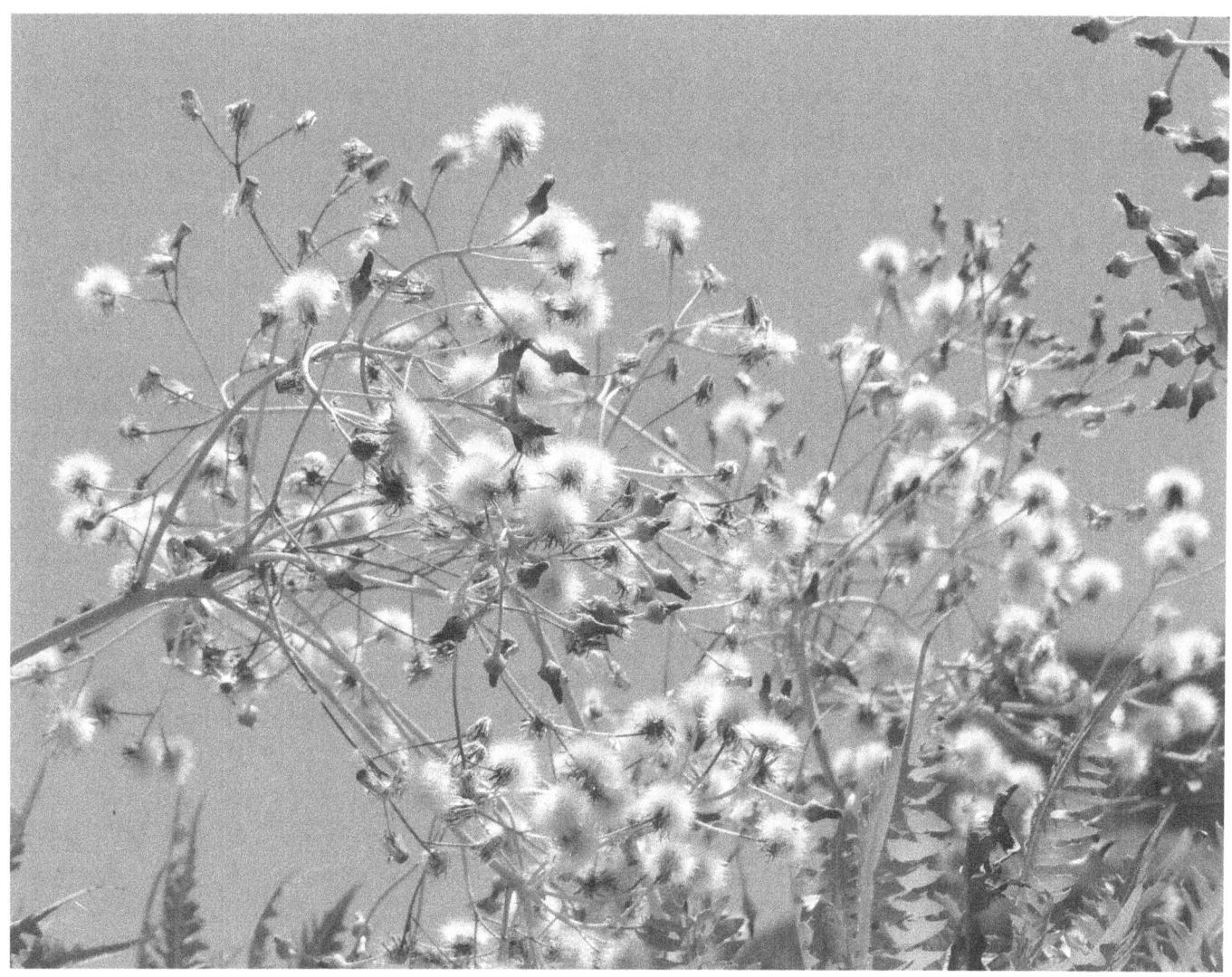

SONCHUS GONE TO SEED

ESSENTIAL OIL

Sow thistle (*S. oleraceus*) has been steam distilled in Egypt by Dr. Sayed. It appears that the non-volatile residue left after distillation contains the triterpene 3 beta, 25-epoxy-3-hydroxyolean-18-en-28-oic acid.

The aerial parts of *S. arvensis* subsp. *uliginosus* have been steam distilled and contain 114 compounds, including heneicosane 28.4%, (Z)-3-hexen-1-ol 19%, (E)-2-hexen-1-ol 11.6%, 1-eicosanol 7.5% and tricosane 5.3%. Radulovic et al, *Nat Prod Commun* 2009 4:3 405-10.

HYDROSOLS

The distilled water of sow thistle is useful for heats and blockages of the liver, and will get rid of jaundice when taken in half gill doses in the morning before breakfast.   **SAUER**

The distilled water is good for all hot inflammations, wheals, and eruptions or heat in the skin, itching of the hemorrhoids.   **CULPEPPER**

SEED OIL

Sonchus seeds contain up to 31.5% oil found useful on swellings and tumours of the skin. In China, the seed oil is used for insecticidal purposes.

FLOWER ESSENCES

Common sow thistle (*S. oleraceus*) flower essence helps develop compassion and gentleness. It revives one after a controversy with another. The essence also helps one come to terms with the death of a loved one; as well as increasing hearing perception, meditating skills, and helps chronic arguers. The disoriented individual is helped by re-establishing contact with the inner self.   **MT. JULIUS**

Thistle (*S. oleraceus*) flower essence is for those who do not love themselves. Often they try to make up for this by trying to please others.   **BAILEY**

Sow Thistle (*S. asper*) flower essence helps us to appropriately deal with obnoxious behaviour, whether our own or others. It also helps us deal with feeling intimidated by dominating personalities.   **DESERT ALCHEMY**

Sow Thistle (*S. oleraceus*) flower essence is for those who are easily discouraged, get depressed and disheartened, for doubt or lack of faith. It is for depression of a known cause and similar to Gentian of the Bach system.   **FLORAIS DE MINAS**

Sow Thistle (*S. arvensis*) was a flower remedy discovered and then abandoned by Dr. Bach. He called the remedy *Arvensis*, and gave it the archetype of "The Destroyer".

"These people are in the depths of gloom; no light; no joy; no happiness". When he finalized the twelve basic types in The Twelve Healers, the pessimistic personality, always looking at the dark side, was replaced by Gentian.   **JULIAN BARNARD**

Sow Thistle (*S. arvensis*) helps us become self-supporting, and reconnecting with our strong, supportive, inner father self, especially after losing one's father or a male partner.   **LIGHT HEART**

Sow Thistle (*S. arvensis*) essence helps promote sleep relaxation and peace in turbulent times.   **MIRIANA**

SPIRITUAL PROPERTIES

Sow Thistle has many noble qualities it can offer the human family.

It can clear the heart of old hates and resentments. It allows one to release emotional negativity that has invaded the astral body and hangs on. Of course, the person must want to rid themselves of the old bitterness and hatred, and must actively try to release it. Simply eat the petals of the raw flower; alone or in a salad.

The key to this potent factor lies in the multitude rays of the yellow petals.

This symbolizes the multi-directionality of the purified heart, and like a miniature sun, it reproduces at the human level, the beating heart of the sun.

The plant is also able to bring a calmness of the soul, especially for those whose recent lives have been filled with agitation or frustration. Such individuals often bring into this life a lopsided vibration which gives rise to friction with those around. For this problem, make a tea of the lower leaves closest to the roots. This tea, made quite weak, should be drunk three times per day for a period of three months. During this time, the individuals can practice deep, slow breathing techniques. This will help induce a calmer spirit into their consciousness.

HILARION

MYTHS AND LEGENDS

Cerridwen was called the white sow goddess of the Celts because the sow was a symbol of divine fertility and she was a symbol of rebirth…In her goddess form Cerridwen had a cauldron of transformation.   **EASON**

RECIPES

INFUSION- One tbsp of fresh or dried leaves to one pint of water. Drink one half cup three times daily.

DECOCTION- One tbsp of dried root to one pint of water. Simmer for twenty minutes. Drink one to two ounces cool before meals up to three times daily.

TINCTURE- *S. oleraceus*- 2-5 ml. The tincture is prepared fresh, in full flower and above ground parts only at 1:4 and 40% alcohol.

SENEGA ROOT
SENECA SNAKEROOT
(***Polygala senega*** L.)
(***P. senega* var. *latifolia*** Torr. & A. Gray)
(***Senega officinalis***)
FRINGED MILKWORT
GAYWINGS
SNOOPY FLOWER
FLOWERING WINTERGREEN
(***P. paucifolia*** Willd.)
WHORLED MILKWORT
(***P. verticillata*** L.)
WHITE MILKWORT
(***P. alba*** Nutt.)
PARTS USED- roots, flowers

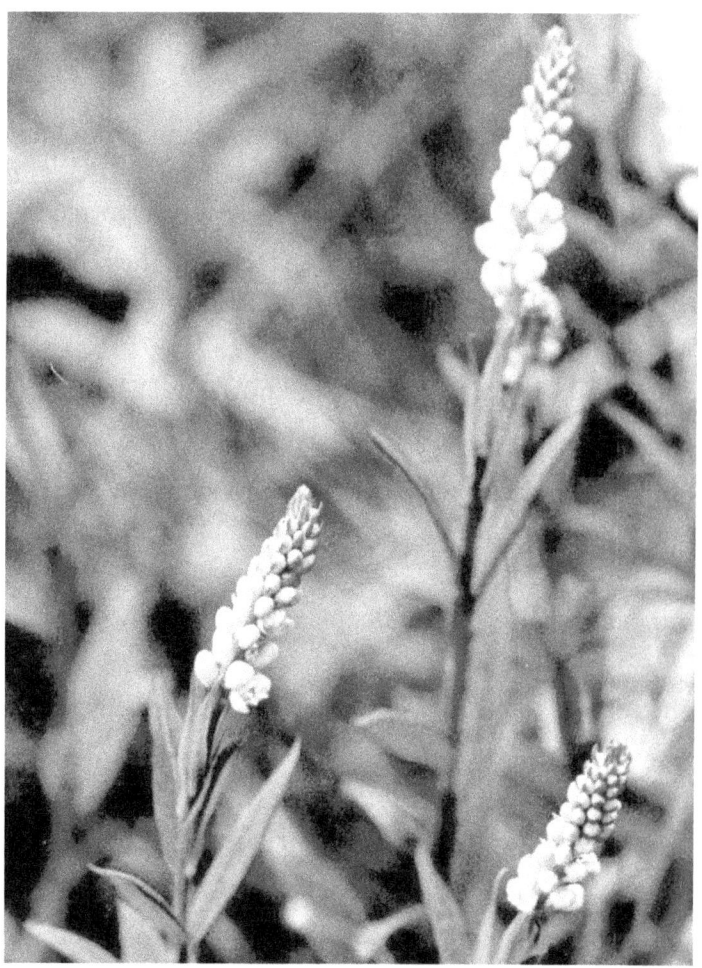

SENEGA ROOT (Courtesy of Dave Haworth)

Polygala is from the Latin **POLY** meaning much and **GALA**, milk. Pliny wrote milkwort "taken in drink… increases the milk in nursing women."

Paucifolia means, "few leafed". Snoopy flower is a name given, due to its resemblance to dancing Snoopy, of Peanuts cartoon fame. Odd.

Seneca was a celebrated Roman philosopher and tutor to the emperor Nero, who later accused Seneca of conspiring against him, and ordered him to take his own life. He opened his veins to bleed to death and later took poison to hasten the process with no effect.

Seneca Snakeroot is derived from the 18th century, when Doctor Tennant, a Scottish physician, learned of the plant from the Senega tribe. He investigated their use of the plant for snakebite, and discovered that an infusion of the dried root promoted excessive saliva, and most useful in chronic catarrhal problems.

The plant is still plentiful in Manitoba and northeastern Saskatchewan, and has been widely wild-crafted for the pharmaceutical industry. The seeds are difficult to germinate, and then it takes about four years for maturity. See below.

Kahlee Keane, and groups such as Save Our Species (SOS) have been working to discourage intensive wild crafting, as well as regulate international trade.

Japan, for example, produced about 10 tonnes of commercial senega root (*P. senega var. longifolia*) in 1993; but prefers the more potent Canadian variety. It is grown commercially, as well, in India and Brazil.

The most desirable root is the Northern or Manitoba Seneca, with larger, dark brown roots, up to 15 cm long and 12 mm thick, and purplish near the crown. Harvesting peaked in the 1930s at nearly 730,000 pounds of dried root annually.

Three-quarters of the world's wild supply came from Manitoba's Interlake District in the 1950s. In the late 1990s about 22,000 pounds of dried roots were harvested on the prairies, a mere 10% of the pre-1960s harvests. In 1995, just 20,000 pounds of dried root were exported to Japan, Europe and the United States from Manitoba.

The Alberta Cree call it **MIYINSIYIKÎYSA**. They chewed the aromatic root for toothache, as well as sore mouth and throat. They used it for various heart problems related to aging, such as irregular heartbeat, coughs, and nervousness.

The Wood Cree of Saskatchewan know it as **WINSIKIS,** while the Chipewyan call it **DLUNE NI.**

The dried aerial parts were mixed with inner bark of Red Osier Dogwood for smoking mixtures.

Both Cree and Chippewa carried the root on long journeys to ensure health and safety. The Chippewa combined senega root, prairie sage (*Artemisia*), buffalo bean, and wild rose root for curing convulsions. They called the plant **BI'JIKIWUCK**, meaning Buffalo or Cattle Herb Medicine.

Bur oak, red oak, and aspen poplar inner bark was combined with seneca root, balsam poplar buds and blossoms for the heart.

The root was a principal war medicine of the Chippewa (Ojibwa), and said to make the men strong.

One warrior custom was to chew the root and spray it from the lips, over both the body and weapons. It was considered useful in counteracting evil directed toward a person, and contributing to building of personal power.

The Blood tribe infused the bloom of senega for unspecified reason, but perhaps the same as the Northern Cree who used flower infusions as a blood medicine.

Both Chippewa and Ottawa tribes used the root as abortifacient.

The Ojibwa infused the leaf for sore throat, and "to destroy water-buds that have been swallowed".

The root is best harvested in the fall, after the tops have died down, but before the first frost. The odour and taste of the root is dominated by the methyl salicylate (like birch oil), initially sweet, but a little later, sour and acrid.

A German plant patent in 1979 was based on senega and other saponoside containing plant extracts for hair care products.

Work by Ishida et al, *Biological and Pharmaceutical Bulletin* 1999 22:11 isolated four active principles involved in hair re-growth; namely senegose A, senegin II, senegin III, and senegasaponin B.

In Japan, the related *P. tenufolia* is used medicinally in Kampo healing. Called **ONJI**, the Asian Senega root, means "profound will".

The root is a warming, bitter herb used for the identical purposes as our native plant. One variation, perhaps, is the use of the root in reducing abscesses and dissipating swellings of the breast.

In combination, it is used for emotional and mental disorientation, resulting in seizure activity; and helps calm the spirit and quiet the heart, relieving insomnia, palpitations and anxiety. It is considered most effective in pent-up or brooding emotions; where a strong will is in denial.

Work by Park et al, *Phytother Res* 2008 22:10 identified activity that may have application for insomnia, neurosis, and dementia.

Japanese researchers are developing products based on compounds in the root that block as much as 90% of ethanol absorption; as well as the rate of absorption. This is based on the work of Yoskikawa et al, in volume 404 of *Saponins used in Traditional & Modern Medicine*.

The closely related *P. sibirica*, also known as *P. japonica*, contains about 4% saponins, and has constituents very similar to *P. senega*. It also contains tenuifolium. In studies it has been shown that *P. japonica* possesses hemolytic effects similar to *P. tenuifolia*.

Our Prairie Senega root is used in veterinary medicine, to treat respiratory problems of horses and cattle.

Fringed Milkwort (*P. paucifolia*) is the only other Polygala species in Alberta.

It has purplish pink flowers, but none of the medicinal benefits of its cousin. It is most common from Manitoba to northeastern Alberta in the boreal forest.

Ditto for the other pink-flowered cousin Whorled Milkwort (*P. verticillata*), an annual found in Manitoba and southward.

Nonetheless, the Iroquois used decoctions of Fringed Milkwort as a wash for boils and syphilitic sores on both adults and babies.

They drank infusions of the plant and applied poultices of the plant to limb abscesses.

Whorled Milkwort was infused as a tea by Cherokee and Iroquois healers, for summer complaint; another way of saying seasonal diarrhea in children.

Rafinesque believed its properties similar to *P. senega*.

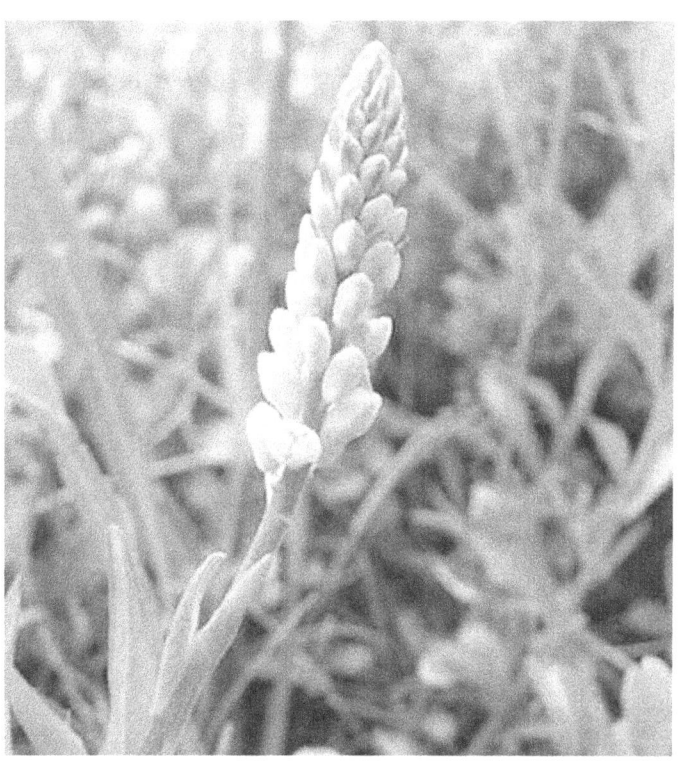

SENEGA ROOT (Courtesy of Karel Bergmann)

"It is stimulant, sudorific, restorative, etc… being milder…it may be very useful when Senega would be too stimulant, and it may perhaps answer all its effects in asthma, rheumatism, dropsy, etc."

White Milkwort is occasionally found on the southern border of the Canadian Prairies, but its natural home is further south.

The Sioux decocted the root and used it for earaches.

MEDICINAL

CONSTITUENTS-root- polygalitol (sorbitol derivative), triterpenoid saponins A, B, C, and D (6-12%), with presenegenin the main sapogenin; bidesmosides (senegins I, II, III and IV) glycosides including senegenin, cinnamic acid derivatives, tenuifolin, valeric ether, methyl salicylate (0.1-0.3%), polygalacic acid, polygalic acid, polygalacins, polygalaxanthone A-B, 1,5-anhydro-D-glucitol, 1,5-anhydroglucitol-2-O-galactoside; various oligosaccharides named senegoses A-O, senegin II-IV, senegasaponin B, senegose A, desmethoxysenegin II, esterfied with acetic, benzoic, p-coumaric, virgineic, and ferulic acids, linked to glucose and fructose; sterols, xylose, mannose, fucose, ribose, D-glucitol, valerianic acid and traces of essential oil.
Aerial- senegenic acid, 1.5-anhydro-(0-alpha-D-galactopyranosul-(1-2)-0-alpha-galactopyranosyl-(1-2), polygalitol.

Senega root is an official drug in Germany and France, where it is highly valued for its stimulating and expectorant properties. The herb is useful in chronic bronchitis, croup, asthma, pneumonia, whooping cough, and other congestive lung conditions.

It was official in the *US Pharmacopoeia* from 1820 to 1936 and in the National Formulary from 1936 until 1960. In Canada, the root is used in about a dozen commercial drug products for cough syrups.

Senega root will exaggerate a feverish state or inflammation, and should not be used at this stage.

Senega acts as a local stimulant in congested, sore throats and is an excellent gargle for either laryngitis or pharyngitis. Both polygalic acid and senegin are irritants to the gastro-intestinal mucosa, and cause a reflex secretion of mucous in the bronchioles.

Many respiratory herbs work in this manner. When you drink an herbal tea, it does not directly act on respiratory tissue, but by irritating the tissue of gut, a reflex action occurs.

I like to remind my herbal students that early in embryonic development, the tissue of our gastrointestinal and respiratory originate from the same endodermic cells. Food and environmental allergies are therefore intrinsically linked, and one influences the other.

A good example is pollen allergies and related food sensitivities.

Rheumatism is helped through both diaphoretic and diuretic influence, as a hot infusion for the former and cooled for increasing urine flow.

The root will bring on a menstrual flow delayed due to cold or fright. It is emetic in large doses, so caution is advised. Combine with wild ginger or angelica root to prevent vomiting.

Crude saponin preparations have been shown to increase the blood plasma levels of ACTH, and corticosterone in mice studies.

Seneca root, the bark of High Bush Cranberry (*Viburnum trilobum*), and sterile conk of Chaga (*Inonotus obliquus*) all possess significant anti-inflammatory effect. Van et al, *J Ethnopharmacology* 2009 125:3.

Work by Estrada et al, at the University of Saskatchewan, on plant saponins, showed increased specific antibody levels to antigens in both mice and hens.

This suggests some potential of senega saponins as vaccine adjuvant to help increase specific immune responses. Katselis GS et al, *Can J Physio Pharm* 2007 85:11.

One study found a wide range of anti-fungal activity in ethanol root extracts.

Japanese studies by Kako et al, *Planta Medica* 1996 62 showed senegin II, the main component of senega root, exhibits hypoglycemic effect on normal and non-insulin dependent diabetes mellitus mice.

A follow up in 1997 in *Journal of Natural Products*, showed senegin II and III reduced blood sugar levels. The relevance of these saponins in non-insulin dependent diabetes is not yet fully understood.

Studies have shown senegins to exhibit hypoglycemic activity in oral D-glucose tolerance tests. Other senegins inhibited alcohol absorption by rats. Yoshikawa et al, *Chem Pharm Bulletin* 1996 44. Senegin II is hypoglycemic and blocks gastric emptying.

Senegins II and III significantly lowered glucose levels, in work by Kako M et al, *J Nat Prod* 1997 60(6): 604-5.

It is also possible that these compounds inhibit glucose absorption by inhibiting glucose transport from stomach to small intestine, or inhibit absorption through villi. Matsuda H et al, *Bioorg Med Chem* 1998 6(7): 1019-23.

Senegin II has been found to possess expectorant and cancerostatic properties. Senegin is identical to a saponin found in Soapwort.

In the same year, Masuda et al, found that the n-butanol fraction of alcohol extracts significantly reduced the blood triglyceride and cholesterol levels of normal and high fat diet mice.

A French company has obtained a patent, indicating that an acid extracted from the plant offers anti-inflammatory properties (Patent# 2,202,683). This includes the use in multiple sclerosis, as well as tissue graft rejection, psoriasis and eczema. Tubery P, *Fr Demande Patent*.

A lesser known, but effective use is in some cases of eczema and psoriasis that do not respond to other therapies. In this case, it is given as a cold root infusion.

One rodent study found root extracts over 98% effective as an inhibitor of stress-induced gastric ulcers. Another study found root extracts reduce blood glucose levels, and another found reduced cholesterol and triglyceride levels. I'm not sure any of these are relevant to human pharmacology, but this is the way things are done today. It will lower blood sugar levels, so caution is advised. Kako et al, *Planta Medica* 1996 62:5.

One clinical trial observed fluid extracts reduced viscosity of mucous in patients suffering bronchiolectasis.

Hong et al, *J Ethnopharmacology* 2002 79:3 found polygala root protective of mucous membranes, in colitis animal models. This protective effect may be due, in part, to the regulation of cytokine production of intra-epithelial lymphocytes.

Scott, Marles et al, *J Pharm Bio* 44:5 found senega root inhibits CYP2C19 but had little effect on CYP19 liver enzymes. Human relevance is unknown.

Ethanol extracts of the root induce apoptosis in lung adenocarcinoma (A549) cell lines both *in vitro* and *in vivo*. Paul S et al, *J Acupunct Meridian Stud* 2010 3:3.

The root extract prevents chemical-induced lung cancer in mice. Paul S et al, *Zhong Xi Yi Jie He Xue Bao* 2011 9(3): 320-7.

When ethanol extracts are nano-encapsulated, the results are enhanced. Paul S et al, *Evid Based Complement Alternat Med* 2011 .

Various triterpeniol saponins possess anti-angiogenic effect. Arai M et al, *J Nat Med* 2011 65:1.

Polygala tenufolia is used widely in China and Japan for medicinal properties above as well as spirit developing essence. See below. Tenuifolin, found in North American and Asian species may be responsible for some of the calming effect on the brain.

Work by Zhang et al, *Phytomed* 2008 Feb 18 found effects on norepinephrine, dopamine and a decrease in acetylcholine esterase in the brain cortex.

Water extracts of *S. tenufolia* block substance P and TNF and interleukin 1 at low doses, suggesting a systemic anti-inflammatory mechanism.

Whorled Milkwort root is a diuretic and mild tonic, used by Eclectic physicians for cleansing the kidneys. Dr. Bastyr used the root tincture as an alternative when treating pleurisy.

The related Milkwort, or Rogation flower (*P. vulgaris*) has been studied for cytotoxic lignans, with *in vitro* studies from roots and aerial parts showing activity against solid tumour LoVo cell lines. Dall'Acqua S et al, *Chem Pharm Bull* (Tokyo) 2002 50(11): 1499-1501. It contains derivatives of aucuparine, methyl sinapate and two xanthones.

The herb has been used traditionally to increase flow of breast milk, and as an expectorant like its more famous cousin.

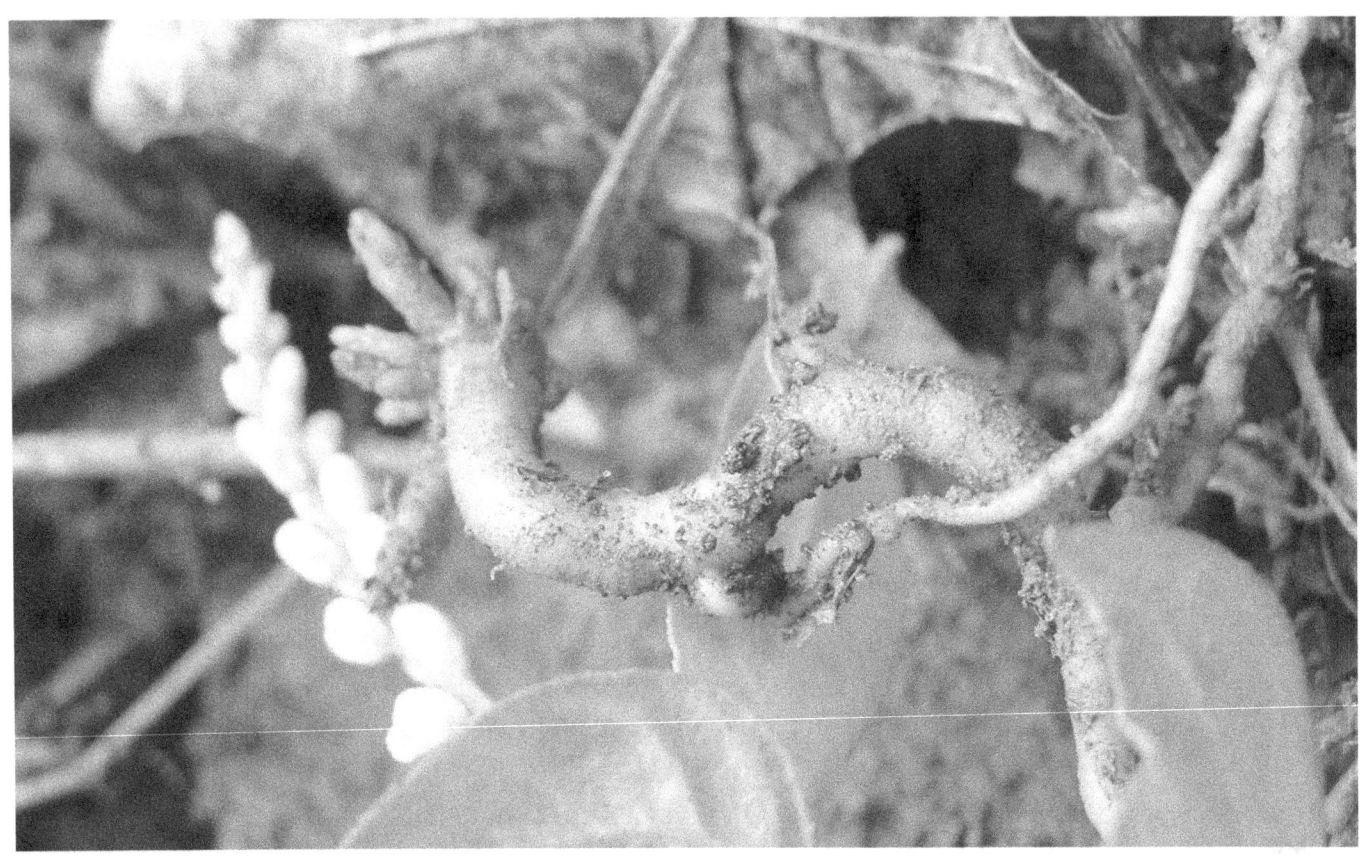

SENEGA ROOT (Courtesy of 7Song)

HOMEOPATHY

Senega is related to distinct symptoms of the respiratory tract. There is a cough that often ends in a sneeze, with a rattling of the chest, and sore, pleural walls. There is a great difficulty in getting rid of the thick and profuse mucous.

Urination may be scanty and full of mucous, and there is often burning before and after voiding. There may be a bursting, distending pain in the kidney region.

Throat may be inflamed and hoarse, with a sensation of rawness and burning.

There may be a feeling that the eyes are too big for the orbits, or they seem to have a haze or opacity of the vitreous humor, similar to cataracts. After an operation, it can help to absorb the fragments of the lens.

There may be a partial paralysis of the left side of the face.

The symptoms are exaggerated by walking in open air, and are made better from perspiration and bending the head backwards.

DOSE- Tincture to the 30th potency. The mother tincture is made from the dried root, equal parts root to alcohol, by weight. The first three attenuations can be made with dried root powder, one grain, to 99 grains of milk sugar.

ESSENTIAL OIL

CONSTITUENTS- *P. senega* root-over 230 components. 54% is made up of carboxylic acids. Hexanoic acid (33.6%), methyl salicylate (26.5%), n-hexanal (5-3%), and o-cresol (3.5%) are the major components. No commercial production at the present time.

ROOT OIL

Oil obtained from the roots yields about 4.5%, and is readily soluble in most solvents. It contains about 13% of unsaponifiables, mostly resins.

The volatile fatty acids contain both valeric and salicylic acids. The saponification value is 193.8 (very high) and has an iodine value of 82.4. Specific gravity is 0.9616.

The fatty acids are 90% oleic and 10% palmitic.

FLOWER ESSENCES

Senega flower essence is for those who want to remember events and places of long ago. It is very useful for those inclined to quarrel and argue for attention. The essence helps individuals manifest their dreams, and aid creative process.   **PRAIRIE DEVA**

Gaywings (*P. paucifolia*) flower essence is for joyful purpose, and moving through doubts and fears to pursue one's dreams. It is for putting oneself "out there" with a sense of freedom and direction.   **WOODLAND**

SPIRITUAL PROPERTIES

Many people claim that *Polygala* (*tenufolia*) enhances dreaming and aids in creative thinking…[and] the ability to manifest our ideas. In fact, the ancient name for this herb is Will Strengthener.

The herb is believed to have the ability to strengthen that part of the psyche we call the will. Daoists have long recommended using Polygala to strengthen the focus of the mind and to empower our thoughts so that they can be made real.

It has the ability to connect the Kidney (sexual) energy with the Heart (love) energy. It opens the Penetrating Vessel, an energy channel that regulates the function of the body-mind. It is called a psychic channel by the Daoists. Commonly this vessel is blocked resulting in a delinking of our sexual energy and our emotional feelings.
                                                                                               TEEGUARDEN

RECIPES

DECOCTION- Add one teaspoon of dried root to one pint of cold water. Bring to simmer, remove from heat and let sit for one half hour. Drink slowly, one half cup up to three times daily.

COLD INFUSION- As above, but with even less heat. Let sit overnight and then gently warm in morning.

TINCTURE- one to two ml. three times daily of a 1:5 tincture at 40% from dried root. Fresh root tincture at 1:2 and 65% alcohol is best. *P. verticillata*- 20 drops three times daily.

FLUID EXTRACT- 10-20 drops as needed

POWDER- 260 mg capsules. Two to three times daily between meals.

CAUTION- Avoid ingesting senega root during pregnancy, and patients with a history of gastritis or IBD. Overdosing will induce vomiting, diarrhea, and CNS depression. Avoid, if allergic to salicylic acid, or while taking blood thinners. Be cautious with stomach ulcers. The LD_{50} is 17 g/kg, suggesting a high level of safety.

Polygalitol (1,5-anhydroglucitol) is a highly sensitive and specific marker for identifying diabetics. Do not use senega root before blood work, or false positive may present. Alcohol may reduce hemoglobin A1c levels, but not this marker.

Note: When wild crafting, leaves a small piece of the root in the ground to encourage re-growth.

PROPAGATION- Cold stratify fresh seed in moist sand for at least two months.

Remove from sand and overnight in warm water. Then, using a sharp razor or box cutter knife, carefully slice open the seed coat, and remove, if possible, the lower half. Do not cut too deeply!

Place seeds on moist paper towel in sealed dish on a warm south-facing windowsill. When seeds germinate, let roots grow to about 1/8 inch. Germination rate may be as high as 60-80%.

Place seedlings into soil and keep soil and air moist. The optimal conditions are 20-25 Celsius, with 12-14 hours of moderate light. Month old seedlings can be grown under lights for four months. They require a cold room at 3 degrees Celsius for two months. When brought back into light and warmth, they will produce side shoots and can go outdoors.

You can also propagate from shoot cuttings of mature plants in early spring. Use only new developed leaves or leaf primordia. Those entering flowering stage will not root well. Use a sharp razor blade, and then rooting compound if desired; and into non-acidic greenhouse soil. Protect from full sun until roots have developed. Repeat winter or cold room as above and plant outdoors.

SNAKEROOT
BLACK SNAKEROOT
BLACK SANICLE
WOOD SANICLE
(***Sanicula marilandica*** L.)
PARTS USED- root

"He who uses Sanicle and Bugle need have no dealings with the doctor."

Who the Sanicle hath, at the surgeon may laugh.

Sanicula is from the Latin **SANUS**, meaning healthy, sound or whole. It may also come from the verb **SANARE** meaning, "to heal". Sanitation and sanitarium are derived from the same root.

A more remote possible origin is derived from Saint (San) Nicoholas, and based on the story Tale of the Tub; and how he obtained the favour of God to restore the life of two children who had been murdered and pickled in a pork tub.

Snakeroot is derived from the traditional use of the root as a poultice for snakebites.

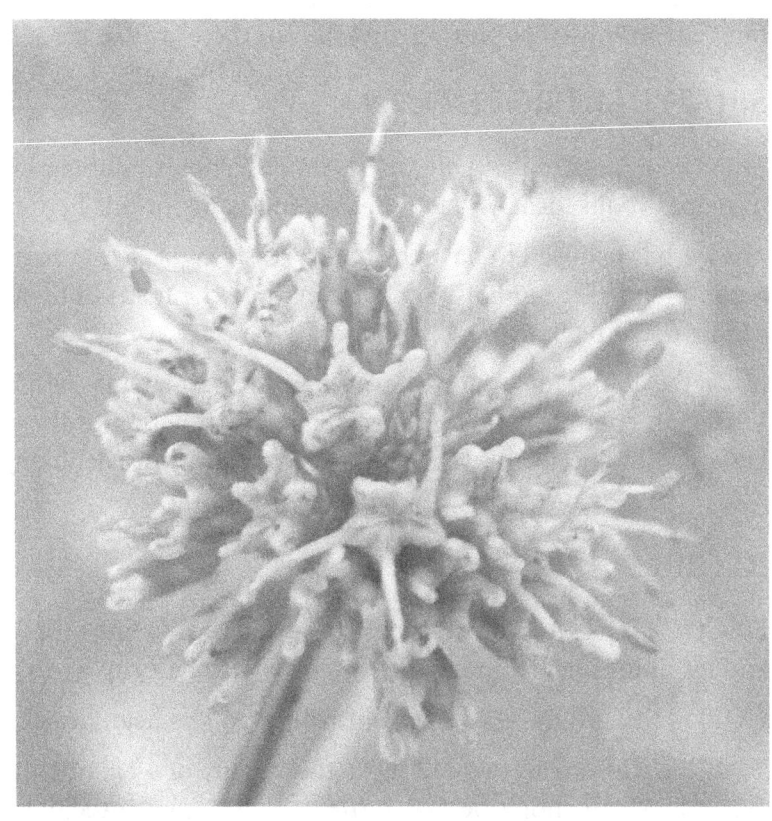

BLACK SNAKEROOT FLOWER

Marilandica is named for the state of Maryland where it was first found.

Snakeroot is a perennial plant of the rich wooded regions of the prairies. It is plentiful where found, and can be identified by its black root, and greenish white ball like flowers.

I've seen the plant in Mill Creek Ravine, in the middle of Edmonton, and quite plentiful near Thunder Lake, where I once owned recreation property.

Snakeroot was worn to attract lovers and placed in bedrooms and added to baths. A piece of the root was traditionally carried to attract money.

The Cree of Northern Alberta call it Blackroot, or **KINEPIKOCEPIHK**, whereas in the southern plains it is **NAMEPIN**.

Snakeroot was used, traditionally, by various natives for its pain relieving, and sedative properties, in a manner similar to Valerian.

For neuritis, the root is used as described in recipes below.

The root is decocted and used in sore throat gargles, due to the tannins and astringent properties.

Various tribes used it for treating kidney and menstrual problems, as well as rheumatic pain and skin conditions in the form of an external application.

The roots were poulticed on snakebites, hence the common name. It also is used in fighting infections, usually in combination with other plants.

Skin problems accompanied with fever call for snakeroot.

The Ojibwa consider **GINE'BIG ODJI BIK** a very potent root, their healers saying that if the root it chewed it will cause eruptions on the epithelial lining of the mouth. Nonetheless, the root tea was used to treat fevers, while kidney troubles, and irregular menstruation, were specifically treated by the Malecite. Harris mentions that the Algonquin used the leaves for swellings and inflammation, "which in almost all cases gave immediate relief."

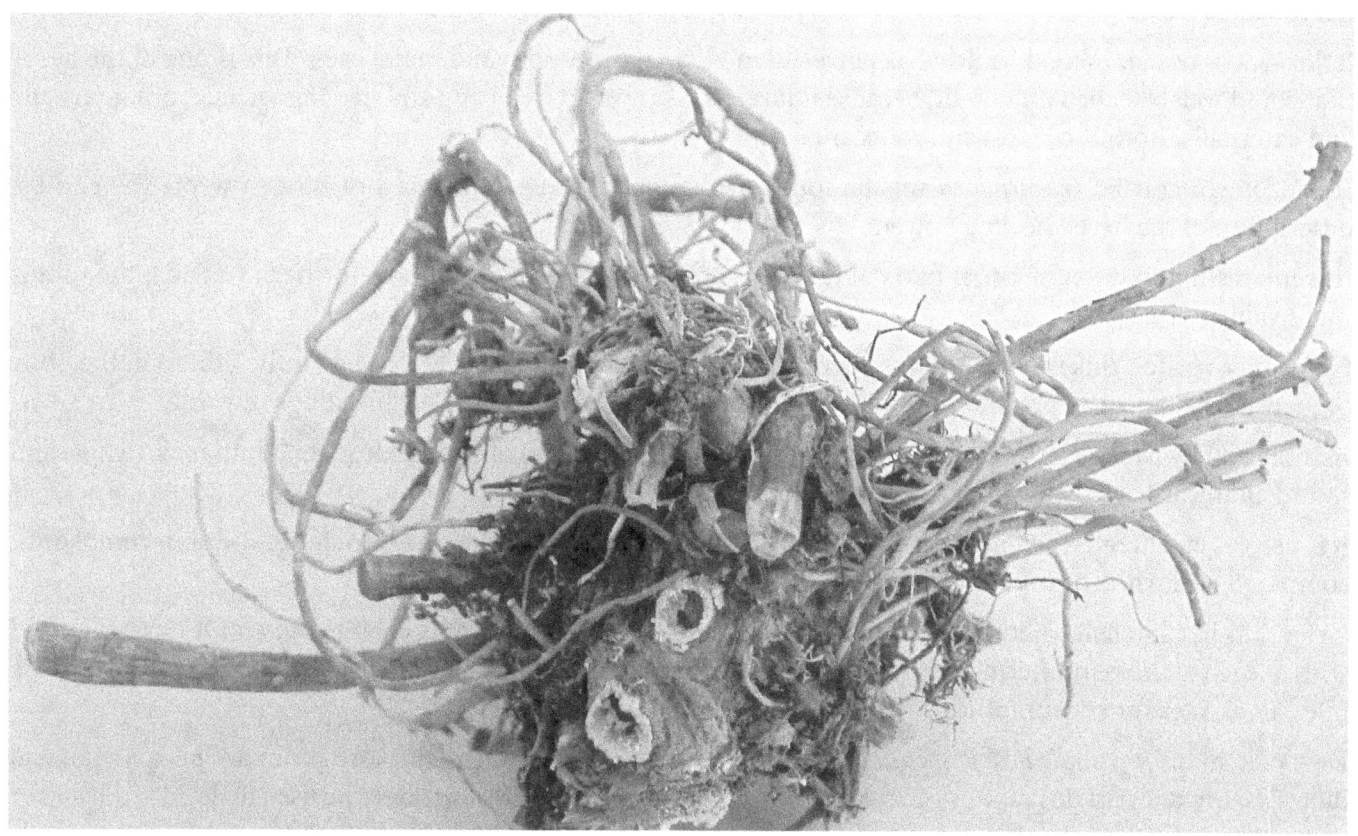

DRY SNAKEROOT

To the Cree, and other indigenous groups, the plant is considered an activator. It is included in nearly all plant combinations found in medicine bundles. This is because the plant is believed to give the herbal blend a "direction", or "intelligence". It is sometimes referred to as Black Root. When freshly dug the root and hairlets are dark brown with a white centre, but turn dark upon drying. The fresh root has no scent, but a pleasant taste with mild bitter aftertaste. As the root dries, a distinct lemon scent is produced.

In the same way that Lobelia is given this ability in the *Christopher School of Herbs*; snakeroot tells the herbal mixture where to go to work.

Kahlee Keane writes. "I find it one of the most reliable tonics to strengthen and enliven either the whole body or individual organs. Snakeroot seems to 'hone' in on the area of the body where it is needed most."

It was used as far south as Alabama by natives for "showing a man's strength and endurance with females in lovemaking."

Dr. Porcher reported, "the Indians used it as we do sarsaparilla in syphilis, and also in diseases of the lungs."

Andre Michaux, a French Botanist, wrote in 1795 that a decoction of *S. marylandica* root was a sovereign remedy for long continued venereal disease.

In general, it was used for sore throat as a gargle, for various skin diseases including erysipelas, a painful strep infection of the skin, and chorea with temporary loss of muscular control.

Rafinesque, in 1830 wrote Black Snakeroot is "subtonic, astringent, anti-syphilitic. Useful for leucorrhea, gonorrhea and syphilis, hemorrhagy, dysentery, etc. Whole plant used in decoction, also vulnerary and balsamic, root for tumors and wounds of horses."

John Gunn relates that Snakeroot "is regarded as an excellent nervine- that is, it quiets, as well as strengthens the nerves. It is also tonic, astringent, and somewhat anodyne, being very similar to Valerian root, and also the Lady slipper root...it is also good in intermittent fevers, as well as croup, sore throat, and hives...and in all nervous diseases."

Jethro Kloss wrote, "Wood Sanicle has powerful medicinal properties and many uses. This is one of the herbs that could well be called a 'cure-all', because it possesses powerful cleansing and healing virtue, both internally and externally. Both the leaves and roots are used."

Its European cousin, *S. europaea* was famous for healing wounds. Hildegard of Bingen wrote the earliest description of the herb's healing powers.

It is interesting to note the aerial parts of this herb are used in Europe, while in northern Canada, the root is more valued.

Culpepper wrote, "this is one of Venus's herbs to cure the wounds or mischiefs Mars inflicteth upon the body of man" and "to heal all green wounds speedily, or any ulcer, imposthumes, or bleedings inwardly."

A 16th century *Niewe Herball* by Henry Lyte records, "the iyce (juice) of Sanicle dronken, doth make whole and sound all inward, and outwarde wounds and hurtes."

It is used as an alterative, combining with other blood cleansing herbs in a variety of lung, and skin complaints, compared well with comfrey and self heal.

Grieve, in her intensive herbal book, says that the root "contains resin and volatile oil, and it has been used with alleged success in intermittent fever and in chorea." In parts of Ireland, the leaves were used for bleeding piles, or as a tea for consumption.

Dr. Cook, in his *PhysioMedical Dispensatory*, suggests Sanicle "used in warm infusion...promotes perspiration and diuresis fairly, and sustains capillary circulation and the nervous peripheries; and may be used to decided advantage in recent colds... and other low forms of fever. By its action on the nervous system, it sustains patients nervously depressed and restless...I have been much pleased at its action in a few cases of measles, and in painful menstruation."

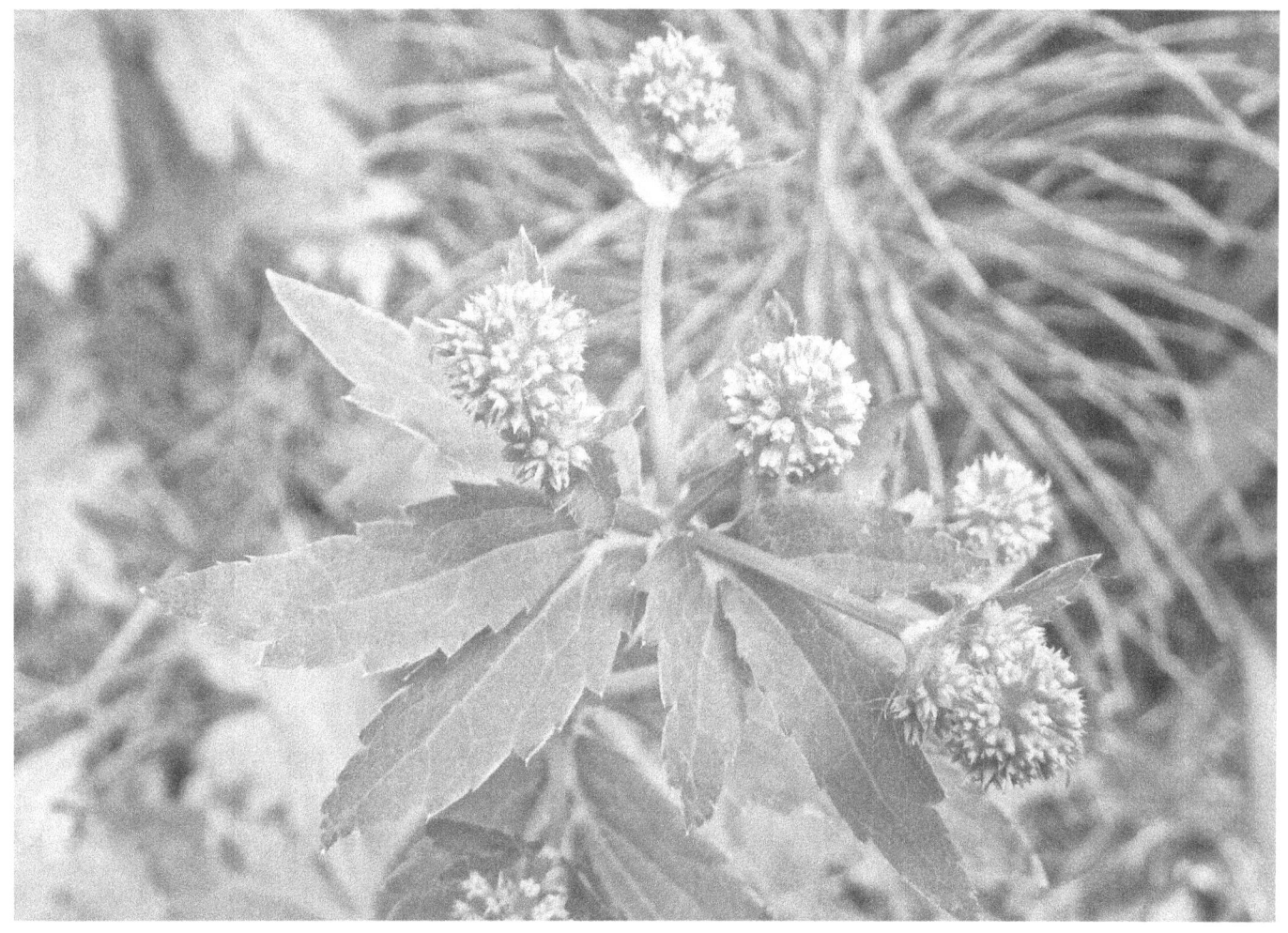

SNAKEROOT

Various Eclectic physicians used the herb for internal wounds, ulcers, hemorrhage, sore throat as well as sore, bleeding gums.

Infusions were used for mucosal congestion of the bronchi.

European Wood Sanicle was traditionally used in France and Germany for profuse bleeding from the lungs, bowels, womb and urinary organs; the fresh juice taken by the tablespoon.

The herb has some similarities to Lady's Mantle, but is not progesteronic nor has any uterine stimulating properties.

The root will however, slow down or stop excessive or in-between period bleeding.

It has a stimulating expectorant quality useful in respiratory infections.

In fact, it was recently revealed water extracts of the aerial parts exhibit significant anti-phage and *in vitro* virucidal effects in the phage-bacteria system. It showed activity against influenza A, and human para-influenza virus type 2. *Phytotherapy Research* 1999 13:5.

An ethanol extract of 50% from the aerial parts exhibits significant activity against HIV. Arda et al, *J Nat Products* 60:11.

Saponins are believed responsible for the anti-microbial, hemolytic and anti-oxidative activity, while hydroxy-cinnamic derivatives, especially rosmarinic acid are responsible for anti-oxidative activity.

Allantoin may explain some of its wound healing and skin disease success.

MEDICINAL

CONSTITUENTS- saniculosides (triterpene saponins), ash, tannin, rosmarinic and caffeic acids, resins, essential oils, and flavonoids including astragalin and rutin.

Snakeroot is a true sedative, in the tradition of Valerian. It is mildly narcotic, and pain relieving; and used for nervous affections.

In the past, it was used in intermittent fevers, sore throats, tracheitis, erysipelas and other skin diseases.

Dr. King considered it very effective in treating chorea, in doses of one half drachm of powdered root, three times daily to children of 8-10 years of age.

J. C. Uphof, *Dictionary of Economic Plants* (1968) writes the plant is astringent, anti-spasmodic and used for malaria.

The root and leaf are both used to cleanse and heal the body externally and internally.

It helps to heal old sores, and wounds very efficiently, through its astringent properties.

The root is considered a tonic for the whole body, and acts as an expectorant of the lungs for heavy mucous build up.

The root is useful when decocted for intermittent fevers, sore throat, kidney problems and stomach and intestinal disorders. The fresh root juice, or decocted leaves, reduced to half, are both effective in cases of diarrhea, and intestinal hemorrhage

Rosmarinic acid is anti-inflammatory, anti-oxidant, antiviral, and cancer preventative; while caffeic acid is analgesic, anti-viral, anti-inflammatory and anti-spasmodic.

Astragalin is present in astragalus root. Pubmed lists 225 clinical studies on the compound, including activity against various cancer cell lines, sedative effects, cardiovascular potential, etc.

This is a valuable, underrated herb, extremely useful in small parts as part of a variety of herb combinations.

MATERIA POETICA

Sanicula, in particular
A candle in the wind
Your moods are going up and down
Easy to offend
Water is not stable
It moves just like a spring
And so it is your symptoms
Change with everything
Also times you're stubborn
And don't want to be touched
You can't complete your homework
You quickly make a fuss
Sanicula, so sweaty
You smell like briny fish
For bacon you are ready
And open air's your wish.

SYLVIA CHATROUX MD

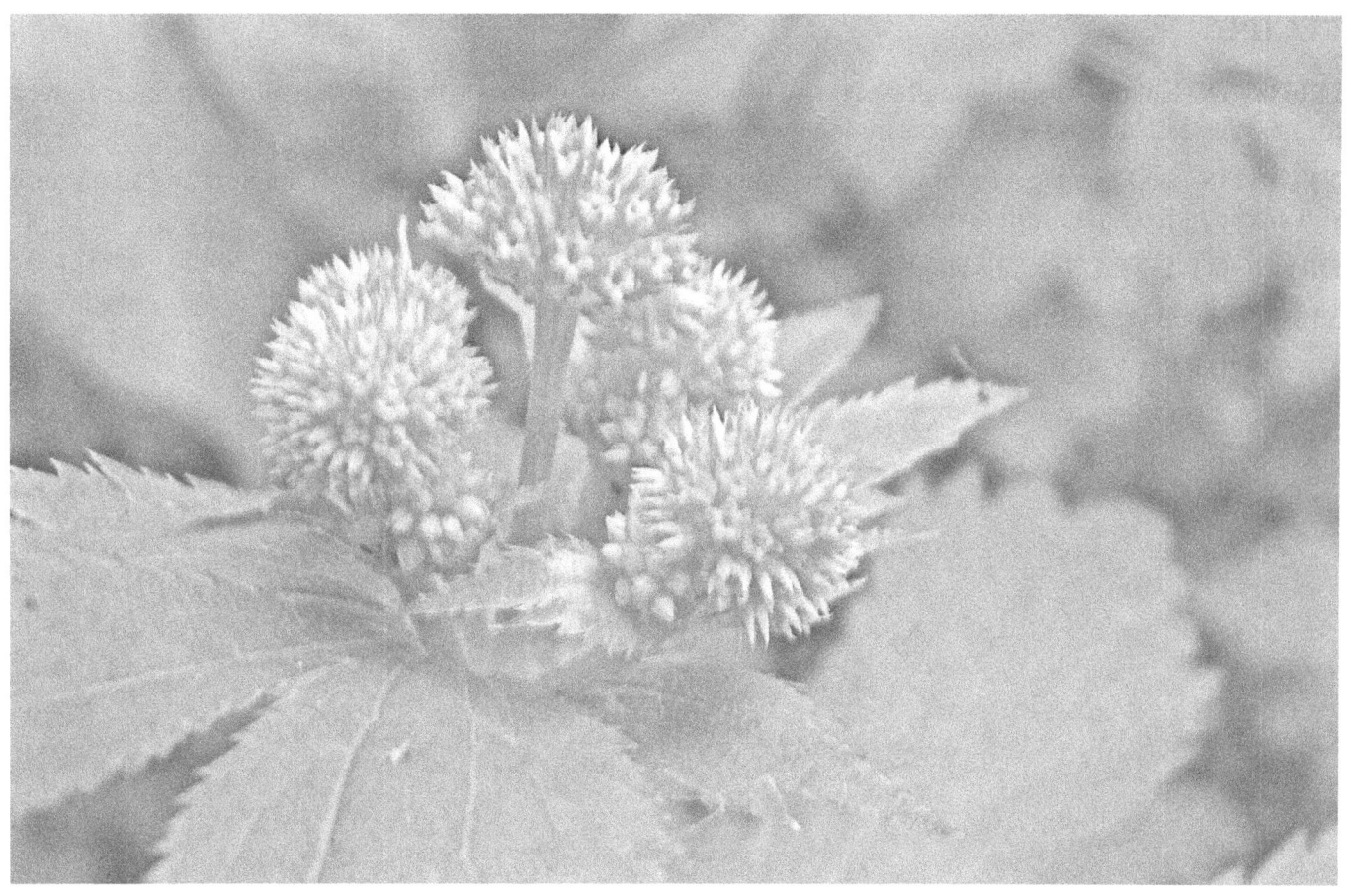

SNAKE ROOT

SPIRITUAL PROPERTIES

Snakeroot is a name associated with several medicinal herbs of North America. Black Snakeroot is an alternate name for Black Cohosh; Rattlesnake Master (*Eryngium yuccifolium*), and Senega Snakeroot (*Polygala senega*) other examples.

To the First Nations people, Snakeroot means more than their usage in treating snakebite.

When a plant is designated a totem of an animal, it means it contains or relays the spirit and meaning of the animal in plant form.

Matthew Woods explains it well in *Planting the Future*, a great book edited by Rosemary Gladstar and others.

"I think we can safely draw analogies between the (North) American Indian Snake medicines and other traditions that use this animal as a psycho-spiritual symbol and see it as a real, active in life power. It would be safe to say that the Native American concept of snake medicine is similar to the concept of kundalini or serpent power in Ayurvedic medicine.

The latter is seen as an energy that rises up the spine, actualizing the intellectual, psychological and psychic faculties but also bringing with it a fierce, magnetic, seductive, sometimes fear-inspiring and nerve-disturbing power that is a challenge to live with and adjust to. When it actualizes the psychic faculties, serpent power allows greater insight and awareness but also brings the challenge of dealing with knowledge and power."

Snakeroot (*Sanicula marilandica*) is a very important medicine to the true indigenous healers of the Cree, and Blackfoot tradition. Only small amounts are added to formulas, but they are considered essential for the mixture to work properly. **PRAIRIE DEVA**

RECIPES

INFUSION- Cut the root into small pieces and when dried, add one tsp to one cup of boiling water. Let it steep for ten minutes. Take up to 4 ounces three times daily.

NEURITIS- Take one tsp. of root tincture in water twice daily to begin, 2 teaspoons the next and so on until you are up to 8 teaspoons in divided doses daily. Continue until relief.

DRY ROOT TINCTURE- 1:5 at 60% alcohol. Fresh root at 1:2 when available.

30-90 drops up to four times daily.

DRY ROOT POWDER- one dram.

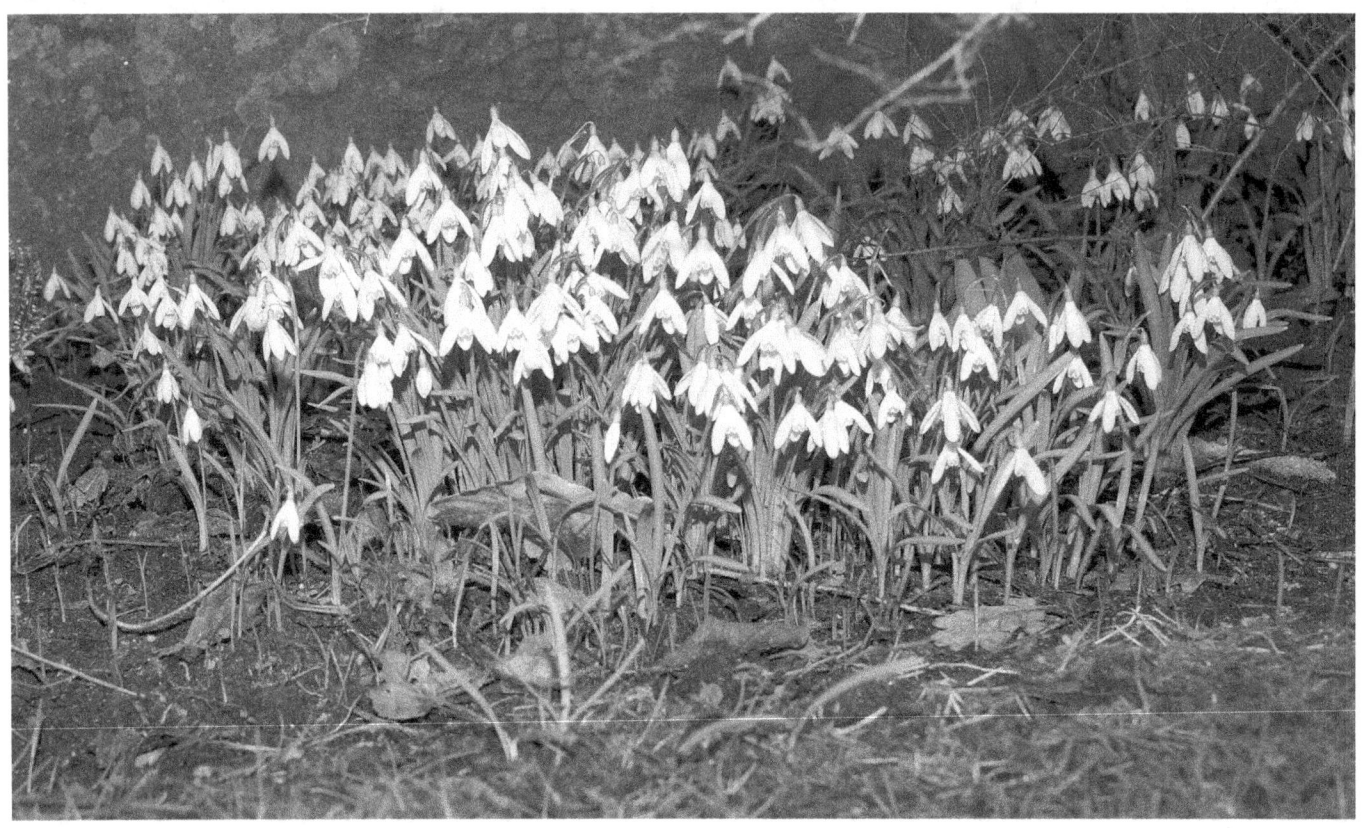

SNOWDROPS

SNOWDROP
(*Galanthus nivalis* L.)
PARTS USED- bulbs

And the snowdrop, wakened by his song,
Peeps tremblingly forth,
From her bed of cold still slumber,
To gaze upon the earth.   **TWAMLEY**

Galanthus is from the Greek **GALA** meaning white or milk and **ANTHOS** meaning, flower. Nivalis means growing near snow. In France it is known as *Perce Neige*.

Snowdrop came into Elizabethan English as a direct translation from the German **SCHNEETROPFEN**, meaning snow droplet, after a style of pendulant earring popular in the 16th century.

Snowdrop is a welcome spring flower that is hardy enough for prairie gardens. There are a multitude of cultivars available, but most are white flowered with green lips or markings at the tip.

The plant is small, only six inches or so, but in the right location, and with quantity, it can really look fine. The flowers have a mossy scent.

Snowdrops were said to have appeared as Adam and Eve were driven from the Garden of Eden. An angel consoled them through the cold, snowy, dark winter, and blew on a falling snowflake that touched the ground as a plant, giving hope.

The common Snowdrop was probably the antidote used by Odysseus to counter the effects of Circe's poisonous drugs in Homer's epic poem, The Odyssey. It was known as Moly as in HOLY MOLY.

If true, this is the first recorded use of galanthamine to reverse central anti-cholinergic intoxication. See below.

It was traditionally known as the Fair Maid of February, and their blooming was considered a sign of good luck for the coming year.

This is connected to the old custom of celebrating the Feast of Purification of St. Mary on February 2nd. At this feast, on Candlemas, young maidens would gather bunches of the snowdrops and wear them as symbols of purity. The flowers symbolize hope, and have been assigned this birth date. It was said, however, that bringing the flower indoors was unlucky if someone in the household was ill.

A few blossoms were sent by mail to warn off a man who expressed intentions.

An old Moldavian legend resembles the tale of Snow White by the Brothers Grimm, in the battle between the Winter Witch and the beautiful Lady Spring. Her name was Snowdrop.

Traditionally the mashed bulb was used as a poultice for frostbite injury.

Grieve wrote that an old manuscript of 1465, called the plant, *Leucis i viola alba*, and classified it as an emmenagogue. "Placed under narcissi, its healing properties are stated to be 'digestive, resolutive and consolidante'."

It has been used in Eastern Europe, as a preparation called Nivalin, for a wide variety of nerve tissue degeneration conditions including poliomyelitis, Alzheimer's disease, muscular dystrophy and myasthenia gravis.

A recent paper in The Lancet, found snowdrop lectins bind strongly to human white blood cell protein.

The experiments were carried out directly on humans who were fed the lectin in Dundee, Scotland. Researchers found that white blood cells, but not red cells, have many proteins that bind strongly to the lectin. The negative implications for the use of snowdrop in GM foods are obvious.

Giant Snowdrop (*G. elwesii*) grows well on the West Coast, but is not hardy enough for the prairie winters. All Snowdrop bulbs should be lifted and divided immediately after flowering.

MEDICINAL

CONSTITUENTS- bulb- galanthamine, hippeastrine, lycorine, narvedine, tazettine, nivalidine, narwedine, ungeremine, hamayne, ismine, and various agglutinin-related lectins.

Galanthamine is a water-soluble alkaloid from snowdrop root and daffodils above.

It is a selective, competitive acetyl-cholinesterase inhibitor that is reversible with time. Individuals with Alzheimer's disease are deficient in the neurotransmitter acetylcholine.

It inhibits erythrocyte acetylcholinase better than brain acetylcholinase; is nearly 100% bio-available and crosses the blood-brain barrier.

It antagonizes muscle relaxation caused by non-depolarizing, curare-like muscle relaxants; and is used post-operatively to reverse the effects of neuromuscular blockers. In other words, galanthamine is strongly analgesic. Schuh et al, *Anaesthesist* 1976 25:9.

In one study of healthy male volunteers, galanthamine reversed central anti-cholinergic syndrome induced by scopolamine. Baraka & Harik, *JAMA* 1977.

Preliminary clinical trials with synthetic galanthamine with Alzheimer's disease have provided mixed results. Dal-Bianco et al, *J Neural Transmission Supplementum* 1991 33.

In one placebo-controlled study by Kewitz et al, *Neuropsychopharmacology* 1994 10 of 95 patients with mild to moderate Alzheimer's disease, clinical evaluation indicates considerably less deterioration in patients after ten weeks of treatment.

And in the *Journal of Pharmacology and Experimental Therapeutics* 1996 227, Bores et al, found acetylcholinesterase inhibitors, including galanthamine useful in Alzheimer's disease.

In addition to being a cholinesterase inhibitor, galanthamine is a non-competitive nicotinic channel activator, which may also be of value in the disease.

According to Frans Vermeulen "the long-term efficacy of galanthamine is attributed to its unique dual mechanism of action. Like other Alzheimer's disease treatments, the substance enhances levels of the neurotransmitter acetylcholine and additionally, unlike the others, it has a modulating effect on the brain's nicotinic receptors, increasing their effectiveness."

Pereira et al, *Jour Pharm Exp Ther* 1993 265. It is interesting to note that the risk of developing Alzheimer's disease is halved in tobacco smokers. Lee, *Neuroepidemiology* 1994:13. This is because nicotine mimics the effect of acetylcholine.

The use of galanthamine as a synthetic drug, is approved in Austria. Common trade names include Jilkon, Lycoremin, and Nivalin.

Work by Snorrason in Iceland treated 49 chronic fatigue patients with galanthamine. Thirty-nine patients completed the trial, and 43% reported 50% improvement in fatigue, myalgia and sleep and 70% reported 30% improvement, compared to only 10% in placebo group. Snorrason et al, *J Chronic Fatigue Syndrome* 1996 2:2-3 35-54.

In the fall of 2001, Health Canada approved the drug Reminyl (galanthamine hydrobromide) for mild to moderate Alzheimer's and related dementia.

Narwedine, a constituent from bulb, was identified by Harborne and Baxter in 1993. It has been found effective in lowering blood pressure, decreasing cardiac contraction frequency and yet raising amplitude, increasing both respiration amplitude and frequency and potentiating the effect of morphine.

Lycorine produces significant sedative activity in lab studies, and increases the analgesic effects of corydalis.

At one time, Snowdrop extracts were being investigated for use in glaucoma.

Extracts of Giant Snowdrop (*G. elwesii*) have been shown to exhibit potent anti-herpes simplex virus activity. Hudson et al, *Pharm Bio* 2000 38:3.

Galanthus species have been found to exhibit cytotoxic activity against cervical, colon and acute myeloid leukemia human cell lines. Jokhadze et al, *Phyto Res* 2007 21:7.

For frostbite or chilblains, make a poultice of the crushed bulbs and apply to the affected area.

Snowdrop extracts significantly reduced salmonella numbers in infected mice. Naughton et al, *J Appl Microbiol* 2000 88:4.

It inhibited the growth of *Chlamydia trachomatis* by binding to a glycoprotein in the organism. Amim et al, *APMIS* 1995 103:10.

Gilljam et al, *AIDS Res Hum Retroviruses* 1993 9:5 found a strong immune response when the glyco-proteins of HIV-1, HIV-2 and SIV were purified with snowdrop extract.

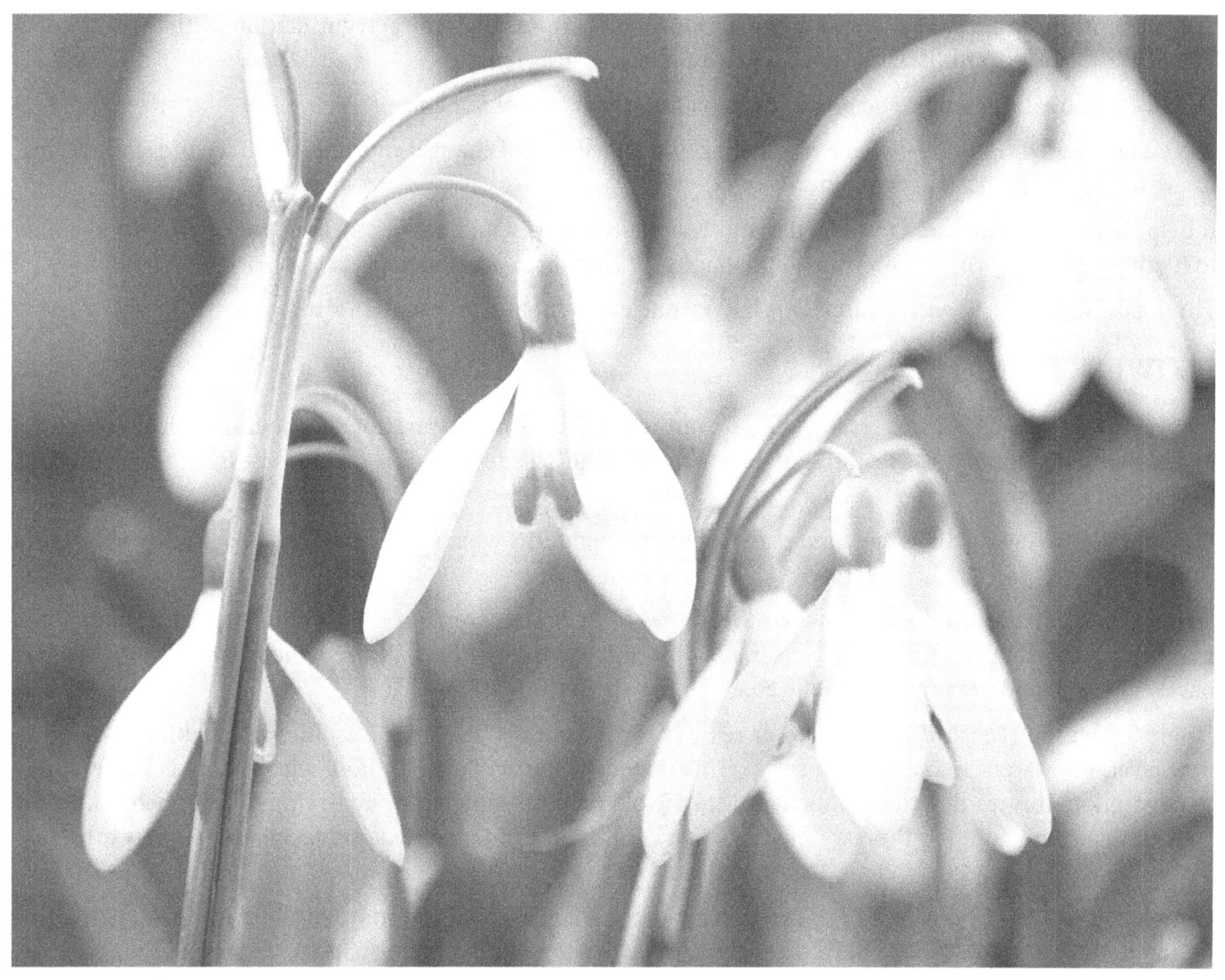

SNOWDROPS

A new and innovative therapeutic approach to the reduction of viral load in patients is a modified plasma filter coated with a lectin derived from snowdrop. Koch B et al, *Dtsch Med Wochenschr* 2016 141(25): 1868-71.

Various lectins possess anti-tumor, anti-fungal and anti-viral activity. They exert anti-viral action by blocking the entry of the virus into its target cells, prevent transmission of virus and force the virus to delete glycan in its envelope protein, and triggering neurtralizing antibody. Wu L & JK Bao, *Gycloconj J* 2013 30(3): 269-79.

Dendritic cells in the skin are the first targets of dengue virus. Snowdrop shows an anti-dengue virus activity against all four serotypes trialed. Alen MM et al, *PLoS One* 2011 6(6):e21658.

Galanthamine may be used as an antidote to atropine poisoning and is antagonist to morphine and other narcotics.

An excellent review of Snowdrop and galanthamine is Heinrich et al, *Journal of Ethnopharmacology* 2004 92 147-62.

HOMEOPATHY

Snowdrop (*G. nivalis*) is indicated for faintness, and sinking sensations. There is a sore, dry throat with dull headache. The patient is half conscious and worried feeling during sleep. The heart is weak with sensation of collapse as if they must fall. Pulse very irregular, rapid and uneven, violent palpitations.

Systolic murmur at apex. Therapeutically, a decided benefit in cases of mitral regurgitation, with broken-down compensation. Myocarditis, with some degree of mitral insufficiency.

DOSE- First to 5th potency. The proving was by Dr. A Whiting of Vancouver, B.C.

A meditative proving by Madeline Evans in England added fear of change, enormous anxiety and stammering, desire to hide, great need of company.

It helps clear deep shock and trauma, nervous complaints, unrest and hunger. Vision is affected, with inability to fix the eyes. It appears to lower blood pressure very quickly in acute situations.

Three case studies, in *Plants* Volume One by Vermuelen and Johnston pages 151-154.

FLOWER ESSENCES

Snowdrop (*G. nivalis*) flower essence helps combine enthusiasm, inspiration and joyful exploration of life experiences. It embodies the qualities of personal power and leadership. It is the flower essence for letting go, having fun and lightening up.

It helps dissolve energy blockages and personal holding patterns which prevent energy from moving freely in the body.

Physically it impacts on disorders where freedom of physical expression is paralyzed or distorted in some manner, such as arthritis, multiple sclerosis, poliomyelitis, or cerebral palsy. It strengthens the will and dissolves paralyzing fear, and helps us get mobilized. **PACIFIC**

Single Snowdrop (*G. nivalis*) is the flower remedy for those experiencing difficulties in breaking through to new levels of awareness and consciousness. This remedy is particularly for those where these is vulnerability to corruption, this leading to a falling back into the old patterns which they are trying to leave behind. At the back of this vulnerability is the fear of letting go of comfortable old identities and facing an apparently bleaker world. **BAILEY**

Double Snowdrop (*G. nivalis* x flore-pena) is for those who need to have more flexibility, who have become frozen in their attitudes…They need the insight to see that everything is constantly changing and that change, however uncomfortable it may feel at times, is a fact of life. It is fear of change that is the main Double Snowdrop characteristic. **BAILEY**

Snowdrop (*G. nivalis*) flower essence allows us to surrender to the end of past events and attachments in life. In the death of the old we find the seed of our eternal inner light and–behold new vistas; immortality. It is indicating in personal darkness and suffering, negative or destructive attitudes, and the fear of death and dying.

It is useful for the depression related to SAD, or seasonal affective disorder, and for the dark night of the soul. The essence of Snowdrop allows us to access deep inner stillness and to surrender to the processes whereby we can release the past. **FINDHORN**

Snowdrop flower essence is for the release of deep pain, tears and old traumas that have been stuck for a long time. Especially when these originate from the handing-in of the heart and you did not stand by yourself and your feelings. When you have done everything for the other and have forgotten yourself. When you do everything the other says, while you know that it should be done differently. To find your own beauty and importance again. To do things you like to do, to feel free. The essence brings a stronger trust, deep down in the base. Joyful refreshing energy after the dark emotional winter. **BLOESEM**

As a flower essence, Snowdrop works on the throat, heart and solar plexus chakra- allowing energy to run unhindered with force from the universe. It creates a surge of energy in the chest to give the momentum to move forward from "issues". It can be taken when you're feeling frustrated or just worn down. **OLIVE**

SPIRITUAL PROPERTIES

When Adam and Eve were turned from the Garden of Eden, it was a cold winter day. They quickly had to find shelter in a cave, learn to find food, and make clothing from animal skins.

But Eve missed the flowers most of all. One snowy day, Eve crept back towards the Garden, hoping for a glimpse of green. But however she approached, a guardian angel would prevent her getting close.

She finally gave up and turned towards home, weeping. The guardian angel saw her pain, and stepping away from the gates held out his hand and caught one of the falling snowflakes. He then raised his hand and gently blew until it turned into a beautiful snowdrop flower.

He presented it to Eve saying, "Let this bloom be a reminder that winter will not last forever."   **FERGUSON**

PERSONALITY TRAITS

In the 19th century, Hans Christian Andersen wrote a tale titled, The Snowdrop. The story vividly tells how excited Sunbeams welcomed the snowdrop and said:

"Beautiful Flower! How graceful and delicate you are! You are the first, you are the only one! You are the bell that rings out for summer, beautiful summer, over country and town."

However, the Wind and Weather said, "You have come too early. We have still the power, and you shall feel it, and give it up to us. You should have stayed quietly at home and not have run out to make a display of yourself. Your time is not come yet!"

But the flower had more strength than she herself knew. She was strong in joy and faith in the summer, which would be sure to come, which had been announced by her deep longing and confirmed by the warm sunlight; and so she remained standing in confidence in the snow in her white garment, bending her head even while the snowflakes fell thick and heavy, and the icy winds swept over her.

The story then compares the snowdrop to a certain poet who came too early, before his time, and therefore he had to taste the sharp winds. And so it is for others who dare to step out ahead of the crowd, who despite having to face biting criticism, confidently chime their bells of hope. Like the little snowdrop, they too can triumph.

G. MOHAMMED

If you listen closely enough you can almost hear the quiet groaning of the leafy earth as the spears of snowdrops split it apart, thrusting their grey-green shoots every upwards…At first one or two shoots peer outwards, inspecting the wintry scene like animals emerging gingerly from hibernation, sniffing the air.

CAROL KLEIN

RECIPES

TABLETS- Galanthamine- Initially, 5 mg three times daily, increasing to 30-40 mg daily. Dosage should reduce acetyl-cholinesterase activity by 35-60%.

IV- 0.3 mg/kg for reversal of neuromuscular blockers.

CAUTION- Do not use with MAO inhibitors, and it is of course, contraindicated in Parkinson's disease and epilepsy. Do not use the raw herb.

Organophosphate fertilizers that inhibit acetyl-cholinesterase and galanthamine should not be used together. In fact, fertilizers with this effect should be avoided by anyone who cares about their health.

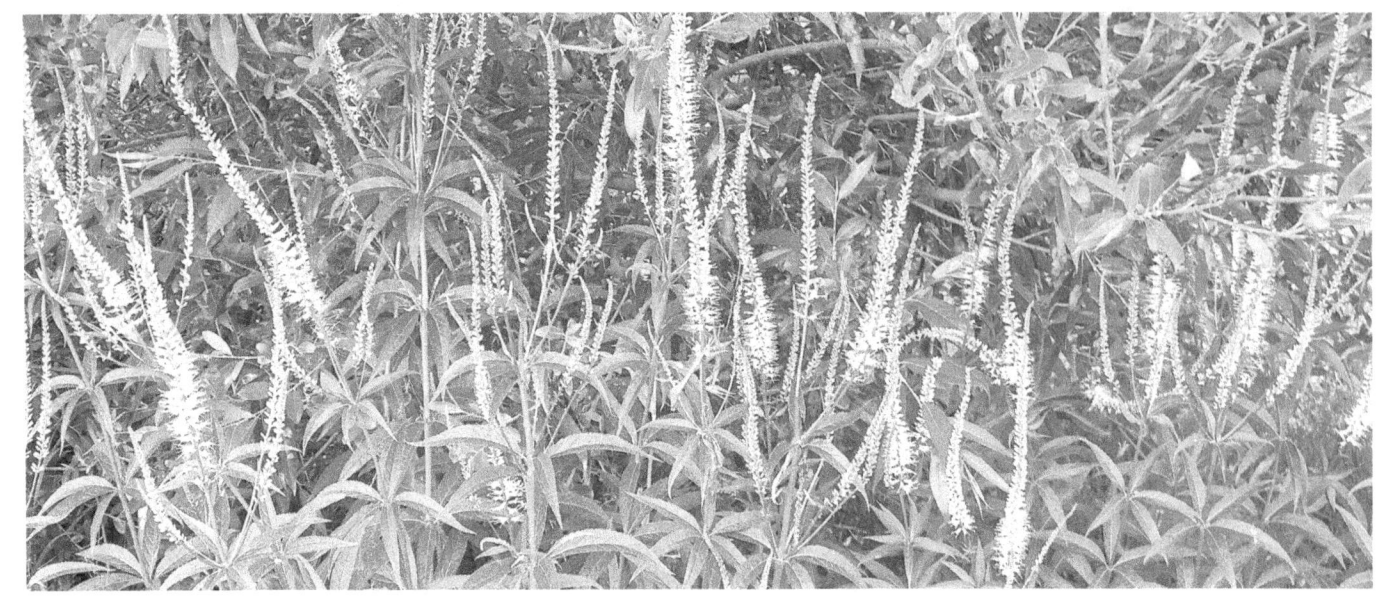

CULVER ROOT- FALSE SPEEDWELL

WOOLLY SPEEDWELL
(*Veronica incana* L.)
COMB SPEEDWELL
(*V. pectinata*)
SPIKE SPEEDWELL
(*V. spicata* L.)
BIRD'S-EYE SPEEDWELL
PERSIAN SPEEDWELL
SCRAMBLING SPEEDWELL
(*V. persica* Poir.)
AMERICAN BROOKLIME
WATER SPEEDWELL
(*V. americana* Schwein. Ex Benth)
WATER PIMPERNEL
BROOKLIME
(*V. beccabunga* L. *ssp. americana*)
COMMON SPEEDWELL
LOW SPEEDWELL
GYPSYWEED
PAUL'S BETONY
FLUELLEIN
(*V. officinalis* L.)
MARSH SPEEDWELL
SKULLCAP SPEEDWELL
(*V. scutellata* L.)
THYME LEAVED SPEEDWELL
(*V. serpyllifolia* L.)
ALPINE SPEEDWELL
(*V. wormskjoldii* Roem. & Schult.)

HUNGARIAN SPEEDWELL
BROAF LEAF SPEEDWELL
(*V. austriaca* L.)
WATER SPEEDWELL
(*V. catenata* Pennell)
BLUE WATER SPEEDWELL
(*V. comosa* K. Richt.) not accepted
(*V. anagallis-aquatica* L.)
PURSLANE SPEEDWELL
HAIRY SPEEDWELL
NECKWEED
(*V. peregrina* L.)
(*V. xalapensis* Kunth) not accepted
ROCK SPEEDWELL
WOODY STEM SPEEDWELL
(*V. fruticans* Jacq.)
DWARF VERONICA
(*V. reptans*)
TALL SPEEDWELL
FALSE SPEEDWELL
LEPTANDRA
CULVER ROOT
BEAUMONT'S ROOT
BLACKROOT
(*V. virginica* L.) not accepted
(*Veronicastrum virginicum* [L.] Farw.)
(*Leptandra virginica* [L.] Nutt.) not accepted
PARTS USED- flowers, leaves, roots

Bring orchis, bring the foxglove spire,
The little Speedwell's darling blue,
Deep tulips dashed with fiery dew,
Laburnums, dropping-wells of fire.

TENNYSON

Veronica is thought named after Saint Veronica, a woman of Jerusalem who wiped Christ's brow with her veil. An impression, such as the Shroud of Turin, was said created on the cloth, leading to her canonization and sainthood. The classic Spanish bullfighting cape movement is called the veronica, as it is swung slowly and close to the bull's face.

July 12th is her feast day, and girls born on this date are sometimes baptized with this name in the Roman Catholic or Russian Orthodox Church.

Some others believe it is a contraction of the Latin **VERA ICONICA**, or true image, from the same Greek root as ICON.

This may be in reference to the flowers bearing markings resembling those on the handkerchief of St. Veronica after she used it to wipe the face of Jesus as he carried the cross, producing a true image. Maybe.

Another version is from the Greek **PHERO** meaning, I bring and **NIKE** meaning Victory, in allusion to triumphing over all illness. This is likely the origin that was usurped by later religions. And, much later by an athletic footwear company.

It may be from an Arabic word meaning "beautiful memory", in reference to the flowers. More likely is named after a person from the Italian city of Verona.

Brooklime originated from its growing in lime, or mud of brooks. It is from the Anglo Saxon name lime, from the Latin **LIMUS**, the mud used to chink stone buildings.

Brooklime comes from Europe, where it grows along brooks with wet mud that entraps birds or "limed" them from an old expression.

Speedwell is an old English blessing, meaning God Speed, or God Bless You. The sister ship of the Mayflower (named after Hawthorn), was called Speedwell, but did not make the trans-Atlantic voyage due to dry rot. It may refer to the colorful corollas falling off quickly after picking, or that the blue flowers seem to speed the traveler along. The leaves of some species were used as an expectorant and cough medicine, and called "spit-well".

Beccabunga is from **BEC**, meaning a beck or brook, or perhaps from the Flemish **BECK PUNGEN** or mouth smart, in allusion to the pungent taste of the plant. It may be from the Old Norse Bekh for brook and bung meaning plant.

Serpyllifolia means, "thyme-leaved. Wormskjoldii is named after Morten Wormsjkold, a Danish lieutenant and member of Kotzebue's first expedition on the Rurik in the early 1800s. Peregrina means immigrant, and refers to its travelling nature.

Veronicastrum means False Veronica. Virginia is the site of its first botanical classification. Leptandra means thin or slender. Dr. Culver used it extensively in his successful medical practice, after learning about it from the natives.

Speedwell is an obvious reference to speedy recovery from sickness, to thrive. Or maybe to the quick manner in which it becomes a lush ground cover. Alternative meanings of speedwell are "get well", "prosper well", or "God speed". It may mean farewell, referring to the speedy shedding of petals after picking.

In the language of flowers, Speedwell means undying love, or constancy, but the blossoms fall quickly, which is not a good emblem of endurance.

An ancient story tells of how a shepherd observed how a stag deer whose hind-quarters were covered in scabby eruptions, laid and roll in speedwell, and ate the leaves as a cure.

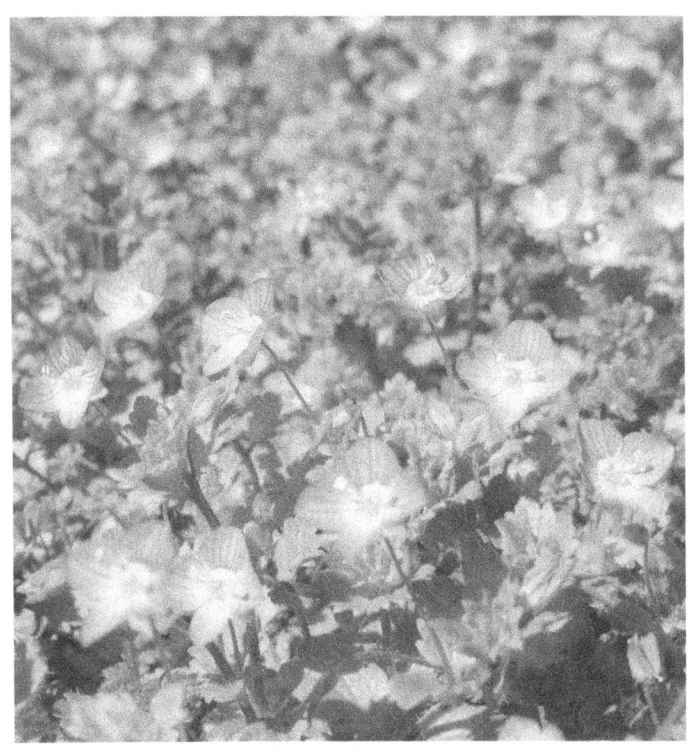

PERSIAN SPEEDWELL (*V. PERSICA*)

In Germany, it is called **GRUNDHEILE**, having cured the King of France of leprosy, which is called grund. In medieval times, the German called it Prize of Honor, making use of the herb for consumption. The Germans named this plant **EHRENPREIS** or prize of honor, suggesting it may have been the original Forget-me-not.

Women drank speedwell tea as a dieting adjunct, and after miscarriage, to help cleanse the system.

Father Kunzle suggested the herb tea for those intellectuals suffering from headaches caused by mental exertion, stress and strain. He advised a week near a mountain stream at the same time.

Persian speedwell can at first glance remind one of ground ivy. The Saints name is based on the Greek **PHERENIKE**, or Victory Bringer, a plant bringing quick victory over disease.

Symbolically, it represents "you are my divinity". The related birth date is April 26th.

In Argentina, the plant is called **CANCHALAGUA**, and used traditionally against weakness and as a diuretic. External use includes wounds and bathing eczema.

The leaves of American brooklime are edible and used like watercress as a potherb and salad vegetable. It is the **BROK LEMPE** of old writers. Use the leaves before flowering for salad, as later plants are slightly bitter.

According to Janice Schofield, the "leaves and stems can be steeped for tea...the taste is reminiscent of Chinese Green Tea."

The bruised plant is used externally for healing ulcers, burns, whitlows, and to soothe swollen hemorrhoids.

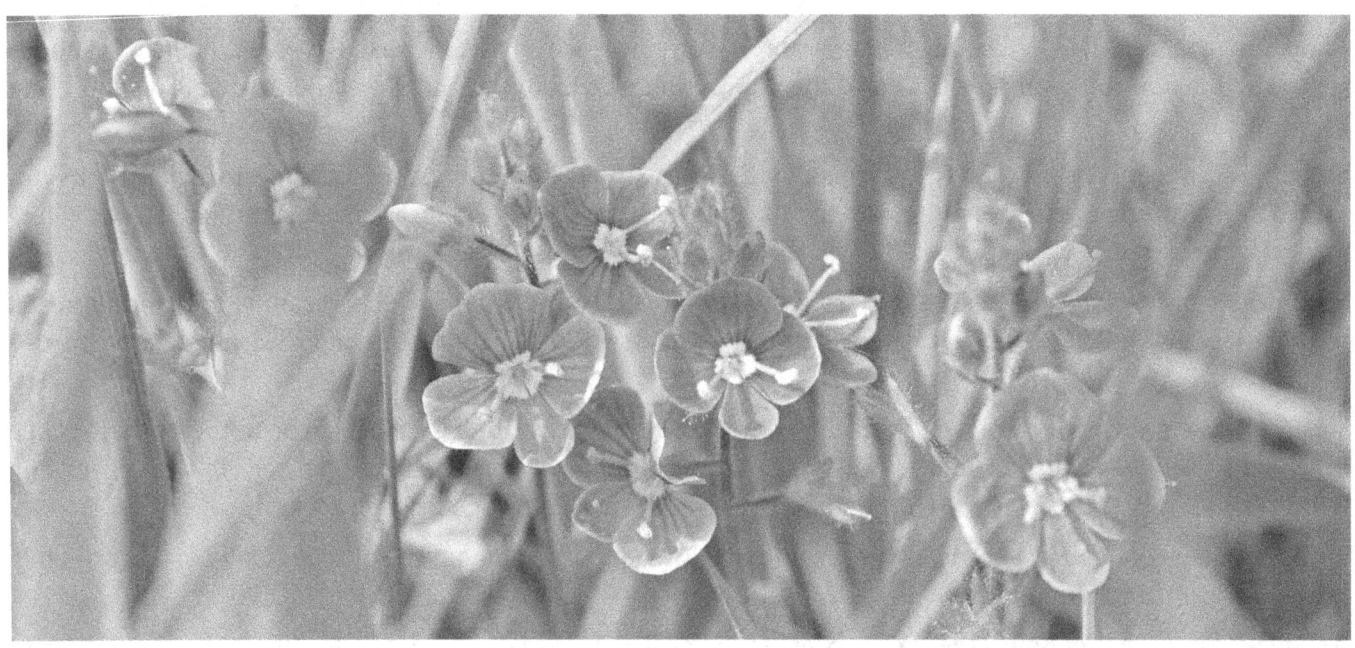

BROOKLIME

The introduced Brooklime (*V. beccabunga*) was used in a similar fashion. Sauer, in his famous Compendious Herbal, says: "Above all else, Brooklime shares in common every virtur of watercress and the broad leaf plantain. When brooklime is boiled in water for use as a plaster, and laid on warm, it checks the pain of hemorrhoids."

Culpepper suggested, "Brooklime and water-cresses are often used together in diet-drinks with other things serving to purge the blood and body from all ill humours that would destroy health, and are helpful to the scurvy.

They all do provoke the urine and break the stone and pass it away...being fried with butter and vinegar and applied warm, it helps all manner of tumours, swelling and inflammations." It has a reputation for healing leg ulcers.

One famous 18th century cure for scrofula was based on this plant in Londonderry, and made the practitioner enough money to buy a fashionable London home. It was mainly used for urinary and kidney troubles, as well as an expectorant.

In Ireland the plant was boiled and sweetened and used as an expectorant.

In Nepal, the plant juice is given for fevers. Gypsies poulticed the fresh leaves on piles and boils.

The European Speedwell (*V. officinalis*) extracts have been found to be effective in healing ulcers of the stomach. Scarlat et al, *Journal of Ethnopharmacology* 1985 13:2.

The plant is common to North America, and is hardy to zone 3.

It was formerly used as a diuretic and expectorant, and commonly used for congestion, coughs, and chronic skin conditions. It was also given to counter nervous exhaustion due to excessive mental activity or concentration.

Dr. Fernie wrote, "it has been asserted that a continued use of the infusion will overcome sterility, if taken daily as a tea."

Its bitter, astringent and tea like smell led to its use as a tea substitute during the 19th century, called *The d'Europe*.

Its original English name was **FLUELLEN**, from the Old Welsh **ILYSIAU LLYWELYN**, meaning the Herb of St. Llywelyn. Shepherds would administer Speedwell to their sheep, in cases of tuberculosis. The leaves were fed to goats and cows to impart a good flavor to the milk.

The European use of this herb was so extensive that botanist Johannes Francus dedicated a three hundred page treatise to *Herba Veronica* in 1690.

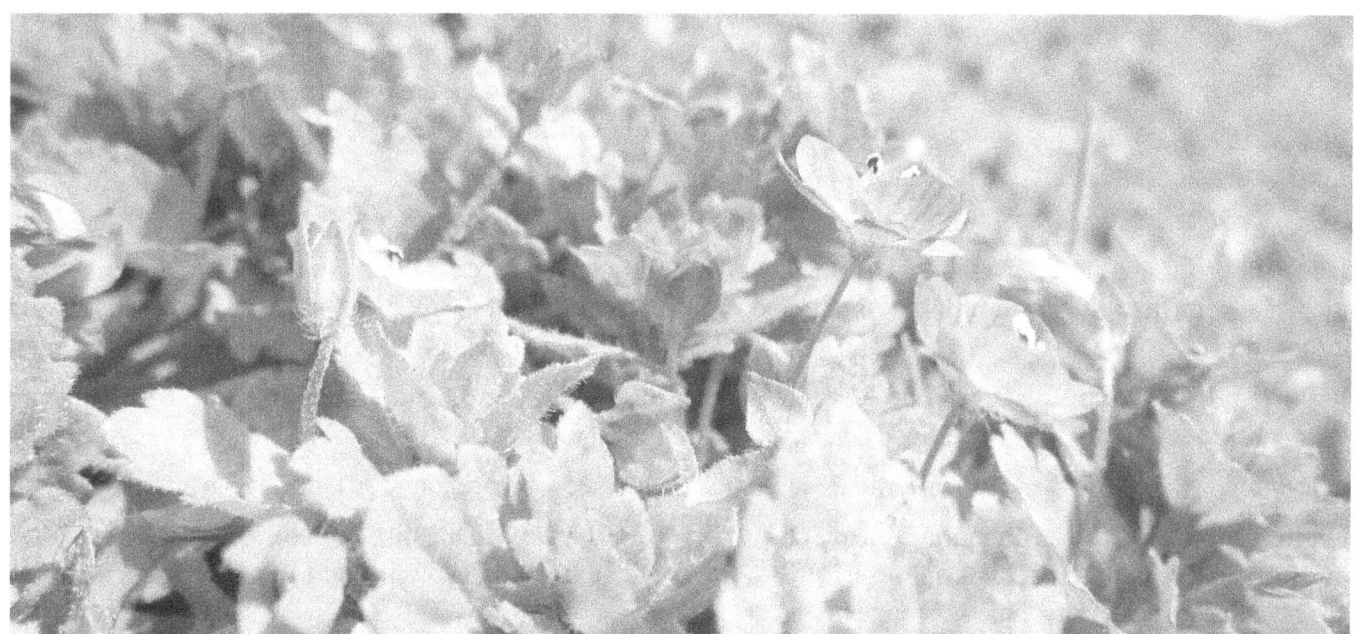

VERONICA OFFICINALIS

Purslane or Hairy Speedwell (*V. pergrina*) is a circumpolar annual more often used in Traditional Chinese Medicine. It is very common throughout Alberta, but less so in the other prairie provinces.

Thyme-leaved Speedwell was well known as Moccasin Weed to the Cherokee. They applied the fresh plant to swollen or sore feet, or "itch and comfort after the long journey". It was used to ripen and resolve skin boils.

Also hardy to zone 3, and a beautiful addition to gardens, is Culver's root. It is obviously related to Speedwell, by observing the shape of the leaves. It grows up to five feet, with white flowers somewhat resembling the spires of Black Cohosh.

Although native to eastern North America, the plant thrives in rich, moist soil, similar to Valerian, and prefers alkaline conditions.

It grows in Tall Grass prairie, and is native to southern Manitoba, and further south and east.

The Delaware call the plant **QUITEL**, while the Missouri and Osage know it as **HINI**.

Numerous indigenous healers used the dry root as a diaphoretic, including the Cherokee, who also prized it for inactive liver and colic.

The Chippewa combined the root with chokecherry bark to cleanse the blood, in cases of scrofula and skin sores. They called it **WISUGIDJIBIK**, meaning Bitter Root, which it is. The Fox gave it to women in labor, and those who were weak.

The Iroquois used the root for chills and fevers, coughs, biliousness and gallstones, or for those with a bad heart.

Many healers ascribed ceremonial power to the plant as a physic, reviver and witch medicine.

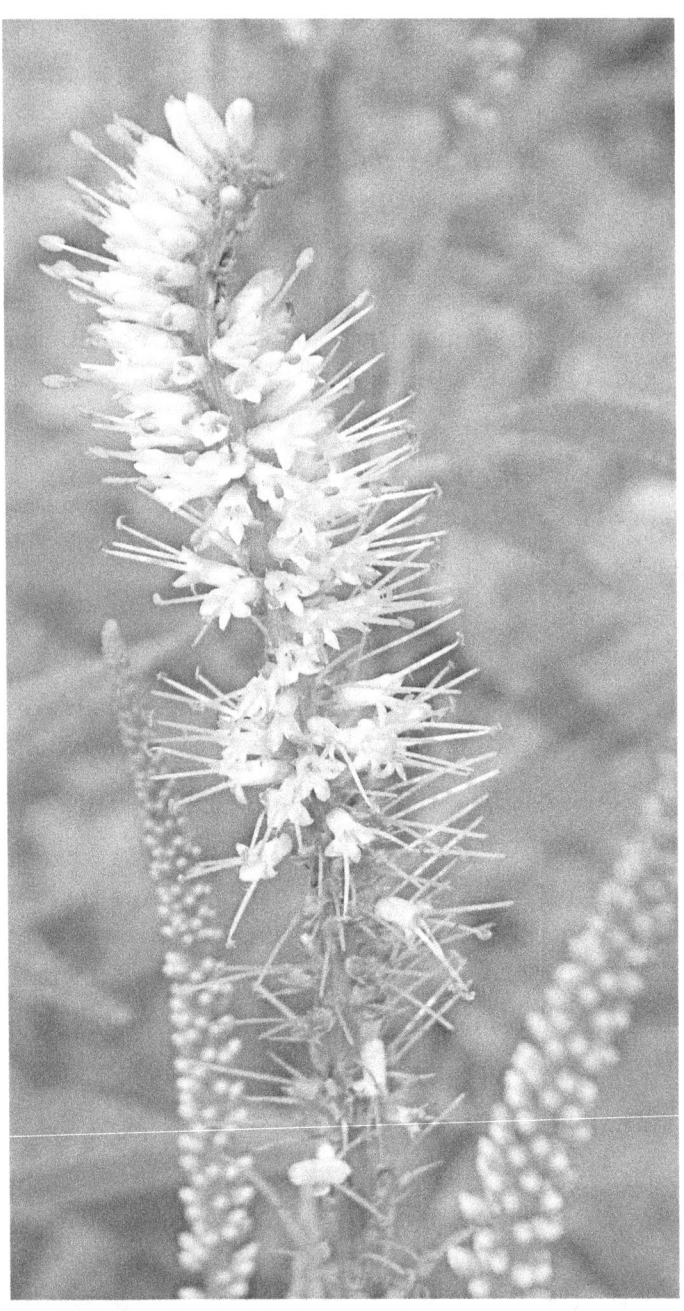

CULVER'S ROOT FLOWERS

Leptandra root was used, by early settlers, as a violent purgative and treat bilious fevers. John Bartram wrote that "one handful of the roots of this plant, boiled in a pint of milk, and drank, is used by the black inhabitants for a powerful vomit.".

"A strong decoction of the fresh root is a violent and disagreeable, but effectual and popular remedy, in the Western States, for the summer bilious fevers," according to Rafinesque.

Leptandra was a previous generic name, while Beaumont's root, a more obscure common name has an interesting twist.

Dr. Beaumont was a surgeon in the United States Army, stationed in Michigan. A Quebecois trooper was shot in the stomach in action. Beaumont inserted into the open wound a pane of glass, and was the first person to observe the workings of a human stomach.

The herb's value was also recognized by watching its action, and hence the common name.

MEDICINAL

CONSTITUENTS- *V. persica-* persicoside, acteoside, isoacteoside, lavandulifolioside, aucubin, aucubigenin, veronicoside, amphicoside, cataposide, catalposide, verproside, cynaroside, verminoside, catalpol, cosmosiin, 4'-methoxy-scutellarein-7-0-glucoside, 6-hydroxy-luteolin-7-0-glucoside, diglucoside, delphinidin glucoside, cosmosiin, calendin, tyrosol, dulcitol, and benzoic acid derivatives.
V. scutellata- vanillic, syringic, coumaric, caffeic, ferulic and sinapic acids, 4-hydroxybenzoic acid, 4-hydroxyphenylacetic acid, luteolin and luteolin-7-0-glucoside, catalpol, aucuboside and other iridoids.
V. officinalis- about 1% iridoid glycosides including aucubin, catapol, ladroside, minecoside, acetopenone, verminoside, veronicoside and verproside; flavonoids (0.7%) including cynaroside, apigenin, scutellarin, luteolin, mannitol and their glycosides; acetophenone glycosides including pungenin, isopugenin and its 6'caffeate; triterpene saponins (10%), and chlorogenic acid; essential oils, tannins, triterpenes, beta sitosterol, caffeic acid.
*V. virginica-*root- leptandrin (bitter), various cinnamic acid derivatives including 4-methoxycinnamic acid, 3,4-dimethoxycinnamic acid and their esters (active ingredients), glycosides, saponins, mannitol, tannins, citric acid, phytosterols, essential oils, gums, and resins.
V. spicata- various flavonoids including agigenin, agigenin 7-beta-D-glucuronide, cymaroside and luteolin; 20% pectins, 5% water soluble polysaccharides, and hemicellulose comprised mainly of xylose and galactose.
V. anagallis-aquatica- aerial- aquaticoside A-C, veronsicoside, catalposide, verproside, verminoside, martynoside, aquaticol (bi-sesquiterpene), ladroside.
V. beccabunga- aucubin (0.8%), catalpol and various flavonoids including scutellarin glycosides.
V. peregrina- protocatechuic acid, luteolin, verproside, veroniscoside, minecoside, specioside, amphicoside, catalposide, verminoside, and chrysoeriol 7-glucuronide.

Speedwell has an affinity for the skin, and like burdock root can be used in chronic skin problems. It is especially indicated for senile pruritis, gently restoring good digestion.

It is decongestant, and stimulating, making it useful in lung formulas for old, dry bronchitis, and bronchial asthma; due to content of various glycosides. It is considered the classic Irish remedy for whooping cough.

As a gargle, it helps relieve inflammation of the oral and pharyngeal cavity, whether acute or chronic.

Speedwell is expectorating, helping to soothe dry, hot and irritated lung tissue; as well as the chronic, congested phlegm that often requires stimulation. It could be considered similar to primrose in this regard.

It combines well with Lungwort (*Pulmonaria officinalis*), Coltsfoot (*Petasites*), and Plantain (*Plantago lanceolata*) for all lung complaints; and with *Agrimony* in coughs that make you hold your ribs. Combine it with licorice root for respiratory conditions, as the sweet licorice will help mask the strongly bitter flavour of the herb. In Germany, the plant is greatly admired for treating pulmonary tuberculosis, and enlargement of duct glands.

As well, Speedwell is astringent and hemostatic, and may be used internally for bleeding urine and stools; and externally to help close and bind cuts and wounds.

It has been compared to pipsissewa; but differs in that it is not useful for pain relief, and addresses skin issues; not complaints of the joints and muscles.

In tubercular children, skin conditions such as chronic eczema and dermatoses are found. Such children often suffer from recurrent running nose, which should be regarded as an excretion of homotoxins and not suppressed. Serous rhinitis is helped by veronica.

Harald Tietze recommends speedwell "for any skin disorders. The fresh plant juice has proved itself best for chronic disorders of the skin. To rub the tincture into the skin is good for rheumatism and gout…Speedwell should be taken in the evening to calm the nerves and to give a peaceful sleep."

Add to this, feet sweating, skin itching, boils, chronic skin complaints.

Speedwell can be very helpful in nervousness caused by too much mental exertion, especially recommended to those who require thinking as their work.

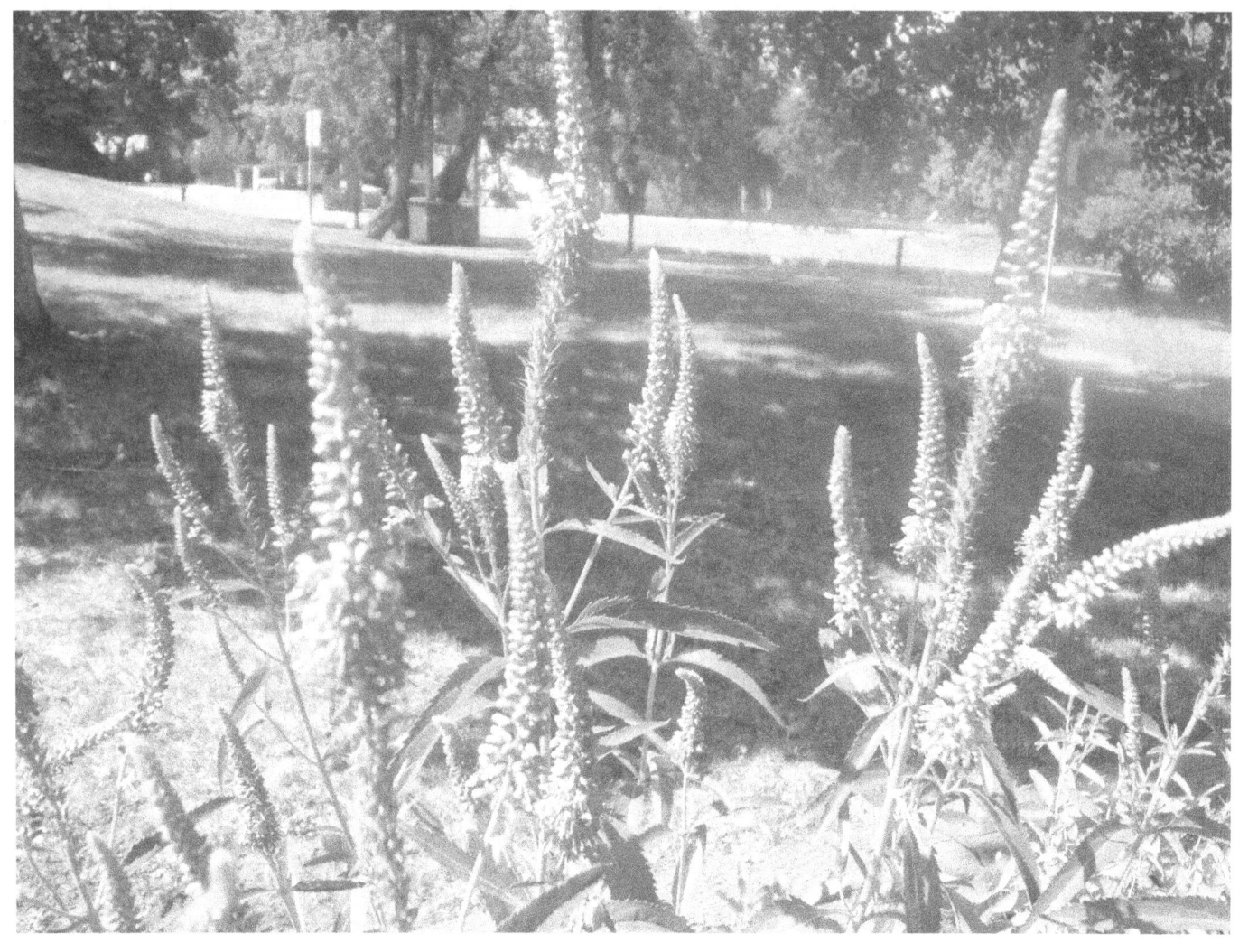

SPIKE SPEEDWELL

Studies in the former USSR indicate speedwell (*S. officinalis*) has a depressant activity on the central nervous system of mice.

John Tobe mentions Speedwell as recommended in Grave's disease, hyperthyroidism, and exophthalmic goiter.

Maria Treben suggested Speedwell in cases of high cholesterol, and arteriosclerosis, by helping to both purify and give new elasticity to arteries and veins. For this purpose it combines well with horsetail. Father Kneipp, famous for his water cures, recommended the herb for consumption and gout, as it helps move phlegm from the body.

Recent work confirmed xanthine oxidase inhibition, and its use for gout. Owen et al, *J Ethnopharmacology* 1999 64 149-60.

Extracts of *V. officinalis* leaves and flowers have significant activity against indomethacin induced ulcers in rats.

In ulcer healing experiments by Scarlat et al, from Romania 1985, reported in the *Journal of Ethnopharmacology*, the plant extracts enhanced the regeneration of gastric mucosa. This is believed due to both saponins and tannins.

Earlier work showed activity against *Staphylococcus aureus*.

For softening the hardened skin on elbows, knees and feet, use the fresh leaf, and rub vigorously into area. The leaf juice will soften dry and callused skin, making a pumice stone treatment much more effective.

Older and non-healing wounds, especially around the shinbone, respond well to fresh fomentations.

I find this interesting because in 1935, the French medicinal plant therapist, LeClerc stated "the infusion has no more virtue than the hot water used to prepare it". Maybe he used older plants!

Work by Bubenchicova at Kursk State Medical University in Russia, looked at Spiked Speedwell and confirmed water-soluble polysaccharides and pectins are responsible, in part, for the expectorating, anti-inflammatory and digestive properties of the herb.

Persian, or Bird's Eye Speedwell contains persicoside and acteoside, both of which exhibit radical scavenging activity. Harput US et al, *Chem Pharm Bull* (Tokyo) 2002 50(6): 869-71. Acteosides are commonly found in a number of medicinal plants.

Persicosides show activity against a range of fungi. Sadeghi M et al, *Food Chem* 2013 141(2): 1512-21.

Lavandulifolioside affects coronary issues, including significant chronotropism, prolongation of the P-Q, Q-T intervals and QRS complex; as well as lowering blood pressure. Milkowska-Leyck K et al, *J Ethnopharm* 2002 80(1): 85-90.

Veronicoside, cataposide, amphicoside and verminoside are four iridoid glucosides found in *V. persica* and other speedwells. These compounds exhibit strong anti-oxidant activity and inhibit HepG2 liver cancer cell proliferation.

The latter three compounds show stronger hepatocarcinoma activity than chemo drug 5-fluorouracil ((5-FU). Yin L et al, *Chem Cent* J 2016 10:27.

Various iridoid glucosides in Veronica species show cytotoxic activity, including verminoside, amphicoside and veronicoside, on various cancer cells line. These include Hep-2, RD (human rhabdomyosarcoma), L-20B (transgenic murine L-cells, and Vero (African green monkey kidney cells (non cancerous). Verminoside induced apoptosis in tested cell lines. Saracoglu I & US Harput, *Phytother Res* 2012 26(1): 148-52.

Neckweed, or Purslane Speedwell is used in Traditional Chinese Medicine and known as **HSIEN-T'AO TS'AO.**

In some books it is known as **CHE-KU HSIEN-T'AO TS'AO,** meaning Bone knitting fairy peach grass.

The herb is warm and bitter to taste with hemostatic and blood activating properties. It helps to knit bones and sinews and promote menstrual regularity. In combination with other herbs, it may also help painful menstruation, or dysmenorrhea.

At one time, it may have been used in tubercular conditions with spitting of blood from the lungs.

Various iridoid glucosides exhibit anti-oxidant activity. Kwak JH et al, *Arch Pharm Res* 2009 32(2): 207-13.

Blue water speedwell contains a number of iridoid glucosides. Verproside and catalposide possess potent anti-noceiceptive and anti-inflammatory activity, supporting its traditional use in Turkey for rheumatism. Küpeli E et al, *J Ethnopharm* 2005 102(2): 170-6.

Catalposide is found in this species and several others. The compound is hypolipidemic by activation of PPARalpha (peroxisome proliferator-activated receptor-alpha). This ligand-mediated mechanism modulates the expression of fat metabolism gene in hepatocytes, regulating lipid uptake and oxidation. In one *in vitro* study, catalposide reduced triglycerides by 21%, while cellular uptake of fatty acids increased by 70%. Lee JH et al, *Biochem Biophys Res Commun* 2012 422(4): 568-72.

Catalposide may be an effective compound for the treatment of conditions associated with mucosal inflammation, including colitis. It appears to down-regulate IL-8, associated with pro-inflammatory activity. Kim SW et al, *Inflamm Bowel Dis* 2004 10(5): 564-72.

The compound is anti-microbial, anti-inflammatory and anti-tumoral. It is also a potent inducer of HO-1 (heme oxygenase-1) a stress response protein known to protect against oxidative injury. Moon MK et al, *Toxicol Lett* 2003 145(1):46-54.

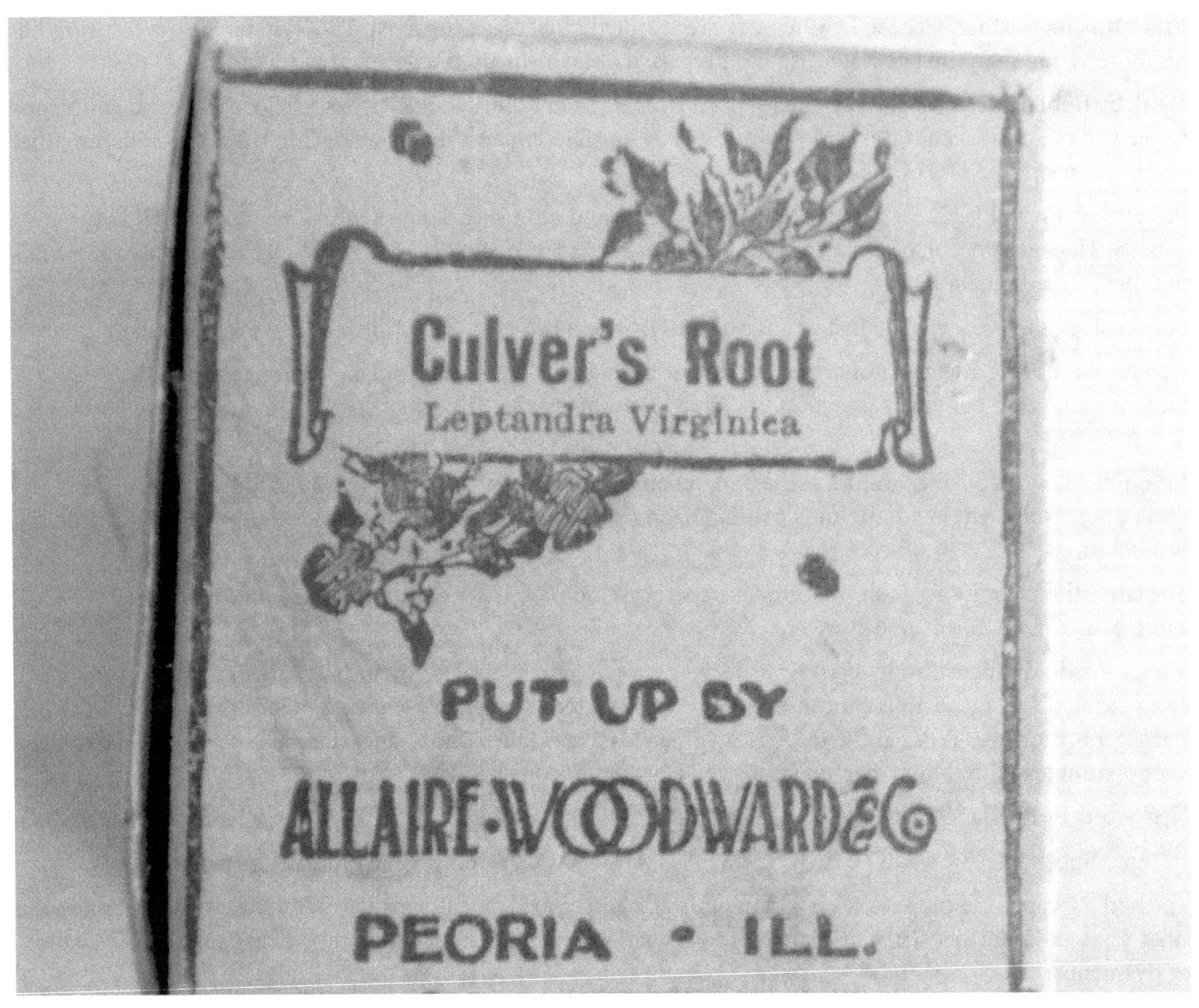

EARLY HERBAL PACKAGE

Another iridoid glucoside, martynoside, strongly inhibits human pancreatic alpha amylase; suggestive of benefit in blood sugar dysregulation.

Brooklime infusions or juice are used to hasten the elimination of urine. It is also used in constipation, liver complaints, and dysentery. As a mouth rinse, it is quite effective for bleeding of the gums; and has been used successfully in various lung conditions.

According to Dr. King, in *American Dispensatory*, *V. beccabunga* is anti-scorbutic, diuretic, febrifuge, and emmenagogue. It is beneficial in amenorrhea, scurvy, dyspepsia, fever and coughs. It relieves the irritation of several chronic skin conditions.

Cynaroside (luteolin-7-glucoside) impairs the nuclear translocation of phosphorylated (activated) STAT3, blocking the IL-22 signaling cascade associated with hyperproliferative and inflamed skin conditions, such as psoriasis. Palombo R et al, *Cell Death Dis* 2016 7(8): e2344.

The compound, also present in olive leaf extract, may be useful for regulating red blood cell production from bone marrow, and inhibiting myeloid differentiation. Samet I et al, *Differentiation* 2015 89(5): 146-55.

Brooklime contains catalpol which protects synaptic proteins from injury. It helps prevent epithelial cell death associated with IBD. Xiong Y et al, *Pharmacol Res* 2017 June 24. Catalpol protects brain cells from beta-amyloid induced injury, and improves cognitive function in aged rats. Xia Z et al, *Oncotarget* 2017 May 17. It may also protect from cerebral ischemia. Liu Y et al, *Int J Biol Sci* 2017 13(3): 327-38; and from diabetic atherosclerosis, via inhibition of oxidative stress. Liu JY et al, *Am J Transl Res* 2016 8(10): 4278-88.

Catalpol suppresses proliferation and induces apoptosis of MCF-7 breast cancer cells, by upregulating miR-1146a and down regulating MMP-16 expression. Liu C et al, *Mol Med Rep* 2015 12(5): 7609-14.

Dr. Prentice mentions he used it successfully in stomatitis maternal and the aphthous sore mouths of children.

Doedens wrote in 1578: "brooklime leaves drunken in wine do help stranguillion [strangury] and the inward scabs of the bladder."

It is taken cold for edema, gout and rheumatic indications.

It is best used as a fresh juice, one to three teaspoons three times daily.

Leptandra root is in some ways, similar to Celandine. They are both warm and restorative; and suited to cold liver syndromes with chilliness, cold extremities and liver congestion.

Both cause perspiration and resolving of intermittent and eruptive fevers; and have a cleansing action on the skin.

However, they differ as well. Celandine is a decongesting and relaxing stimulant. Leptandra is restorative, drying and stimulating. Similar to Milk Thistle, it is used where energy blockage is accompanied by deficiency and cold. In TCM terms it is useful for liver Qi stagnation.

The fresh root is a drastic laxative, and the dried root quite safe and mild, and yet effective for treating constipation, without the griping of *Cascara sagrada* or Senna.

The second year root is preferred, due in part to a better balance of bitter principles, tasting somewhat like raw, green fiddleheads.

It combines well with licorice root, which not only masks the bitter taste, but acts as well as an emollient and demulcent laxative, thus easing some griping properties.

According to Ellingwood, use of this herb is indicated when the tongue is "pale, coated uniformly white, or grayish-white and moist."

It is meant to treat deficient cold conditions of the stomach and intestine, as well as the liver and gall bladder. Christopher Menzies-Trull suggests that when the bile releases, it is more sticky and dark, and leptandra improves the outflow without irritating the intestines. Stools may be clay-colored. If white, consider looking at Fringe tree bark.

It may be useful in ascites, or portal congestion with edema. Consider its use in constriction of the bile duct, with or without chronic emotional stress.

Jaundice and hepatitis, whether acute or chronic, are well suited to Leptandra, as long as due to cold and damp conditions. There is usually little appetite, with inertia and depression of the spirit; with gloominess, foreboding and sleeplessness. The skin may be hot and dry, but the extremities are cool or cold, with palpitation or irregular heart action due to stomach or liver problems.

It will help to reduce pancreatic inflammation, particularly in the hematogenic (brown iris) constitution; and is specific to chronic constipation related to liver and gall bladder disorders, inducing mild cathartic action without debility in the proper dose.

Brent Davis puts it well. The root, "augments bile flow, removes catarrhal and granular detritus from the biliary passages and increases intestinal peristalsis. In delicate constitutions it does not diminish autonomic tone as do harsh laxatives such as cascara, buckthorn, rhubarb, etc. It is indicated in atony of the gallbladder, common bile duct and intestines." He suggests it is for people with gastrointestinal distress who are frustrated and discouraged from their inability to actualize goals.

Mannite and d-mannitol are considered to be osmotic diuretics that work by increasing the movement of sodium and water out of Henle's loop.

Cinnamic acid, another constituent increases bile acid flow by 50% in studies by both Galecka et al, (1969) and Das et al, (1976).

HOMEOPATHY

Veronica-Fleullein/Paul's Betony (*V. officinalis*) is used for persistent bronchial coughing, with running nose.

Great mental anxiety. Delusions that people are distant, and irritability, particularly with alternating moods.

Dramatic increase in energy, frequently associated with an increased clarity of the mental thought processes.

Ear pain, nasal running, abdomen bloating, cramping and pain. Persistant bronchial cough, with little or no mucous production. Burning sensation in the chest, with pounding heart and palpitations.

Stiffness in the lower back, worse from standing. Stitching pain in the hip. Perspiration worse at night, followed by chills and cold sweats after uncovering.

The skin is dry with eruptions.

DOSE- Tincture doses. The mother tincture is prepared from the fresh plant in flower of *V. officinalis*. Dr. David Riley, in 1993, did a proving with 12 females and five males at 12c.

Leptandra/Culver's Root (*V. virginianum*) is a liver remedy indicated for bleeding piles, and clay colored stools that accompany jaundice. Prolapsed rectum with hemorrhoids, or rectal hemorrhage call for this remedy.

Weak portal circulation, with great stomach and intestinal distress, and desire to constantly defecate are noted. An aching in the liver region extends to the spine, and the patient feels chilly.

There is a dull frontal headache, with vertigo, drowsiness and depression; as well as smarting and aching in the eyes.

Pancreatitis is one of its primary indications, and will reduce inflammation of the pancreas, liver and gall bladder.

There is desire for ice water, right side more affected, gloomy and irritable. Sensation as if hair is pulled in when having a dull frontal headache.

DOSE- Tincture to third potency. The mother tincture is prepared from the fresh, two year old roots. Proving by Burt on himself and another man with fluid extract and leptandrin in 1-40 grain doses, as well as 1x trituration in 1856.

ESSENTIAL OIL

The root of *V. virginica* contains essential oils, consisting mainly of the esters of cinnamic acid, methoxycinnamic acid, and dimethoxycinnamic acid.

The related *V. albicans* aerial parts, including flower, produces 39 compounds such as beta caryophyllene (34%), gamma amorphene (19.5), 9-epi-beta-caryophyllene (7%) and alpha pinene (7%).

PLANT OIL

The leaves, stems, roots and flowers of Brooklime (*V. beccabunga*) contain lipids, with flowers containing 12.5%, leaves 9.3% and significantly less in roots and stems.

Of the polar lipids, phosphatydl choline comprises 53% in the leaf; while the flowers contain 2.3% phosphatydl serine.

The fatty oil from *V. thymoides* contains hexatriacontene (21%), linoleic acid (25%) and palmitic acid (20%).

HYDROSOL

The distilled water of Brooklime is celebrated for provoking urine and for breaking up kidney stones, for killing worms in the gut, and in particular for staying disorders of the spleen, provided one drinks a gill (2 oz.) of it regularly in the morning and evening. **SAUER**

The distilled water of Speedwell is highly regarded for jaundice. It also dissolves loin stones, withstands every sort of poison, dispels dizziness, and strengthens the brain. It warms the stomach and encourages digestion, provokes the appetite, and absorbs injurious vapors that arise from the stomach and cause dizziness. Speedwell water also opens obstructions of the liver, spleen and especially the lungs, for it dissolves hard phlegm in the chest and promotes its expectoration. Other uses including the healing of sores in the lungs and the purification of the blood, provided it is taken in two ounce doses each morning and evening. **SAUER**

Water from Veronica is made by steeping the plant in wine and then distilling the entirety. It is used for scabs and blains, opens sweat holes, swellings in the throat, comforts stomach, lightens the tongue and memory. It cures yellow jaundice, especially combined with water of bittersweet nightshade, causes the breast to be large and causes spitting and putting out of phlegmatic matter. It causes increased urination and is good for women that are fat. **BRUNSCHWIG**

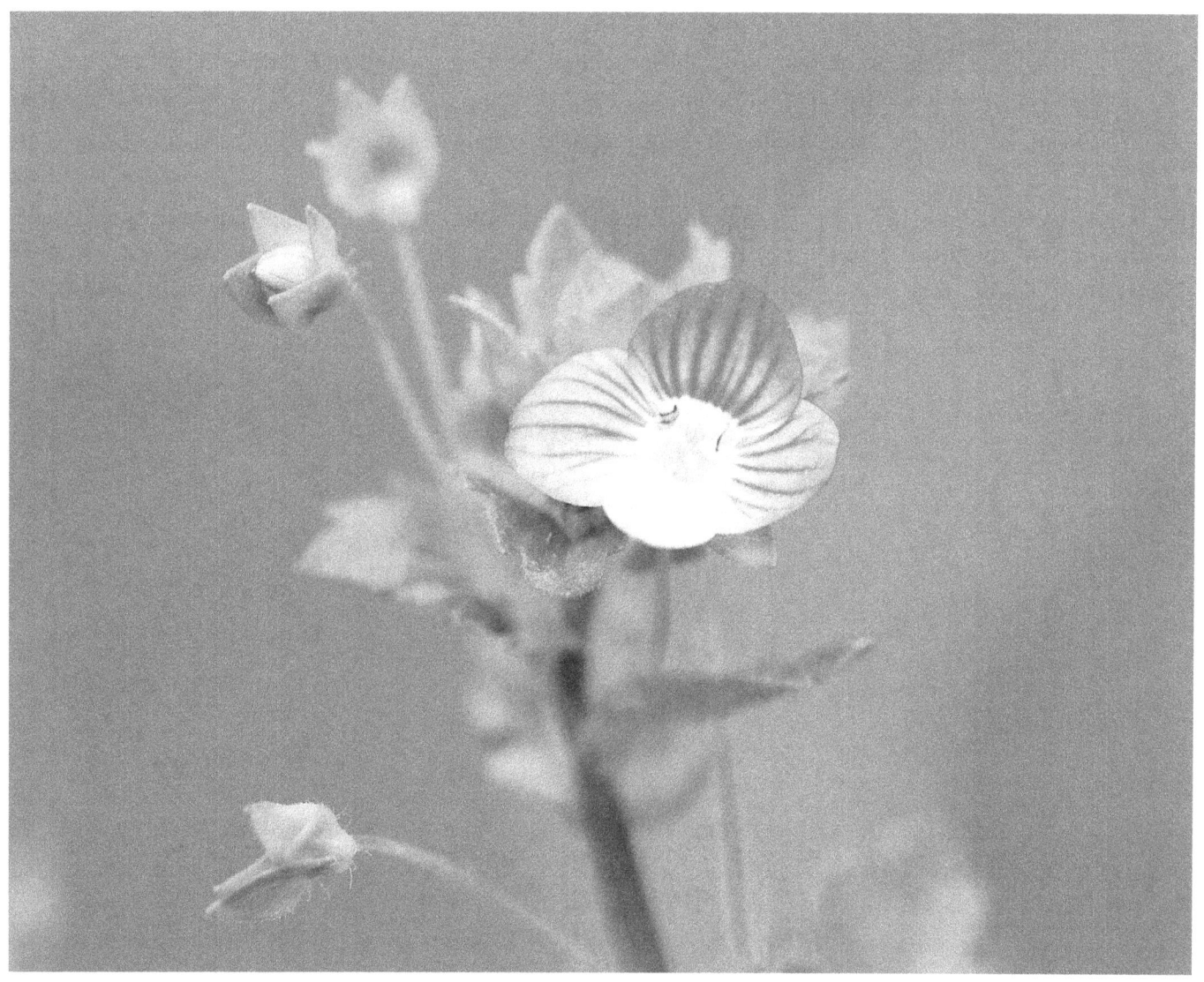

BIRD'S EYE SPEEDWELL (V. PERSICA)

FLOWER ESSENCES

Speedwell (*V. persica*) is for taking the time we need, timelessness, deep concentration, attention, stillness and focus. **LIGHT HEART**

Persian Speedwell essence helps give the necessary distance to view things so that the lessons learned make it possible to grow. **MIRIANA**

Alpine Speedwell helps release the tendency to overthrow the whole idea if one part is out of synch. **ROCKY MTN**

Scrambling Speedwell (*V. persica*) flower essence is for manipulation, submission for gain, laziness and bargaining. On the positive, it helps bring about united effort, give and take and equality. **NEW ZEALAND**

Speedwell (*V. persica*) flower essence helps past negative influences to lose their grip and be dissipated. **BAILEY**

Spiked Speedwell (*V. spicata*) flower essence allows the psyche to slough off the soul scars that have defined it in a limiting way. It purifies the aura of self limiting beliefs regarding what one is truly capable of, and also what one may have settled for in exchange for true joy.

It sweeps the chambers of the heart to cleanse it of all that does not serve the spirit's unfolding.

Spiritually, it holds aloft the vision that one is spirit manifesting through soul and body, and that nothing can truly hinder the perfection of that manifestation. **HUMMINGBIRD**

Culvers root is for releasing past failure, romantic attachments, judgments, oaths, vows and swearings. **FLORALIVE**

Brooklime (*V. beccabunga*) is for courage in times of adversity. It helps us keep faith and perspective while pushing through hard times. This tiny plant is about fluidity, physically and emotionally. It removes stagnation of all kinds (e.g. writer's block). It combines well with other essences and is effective for addictions. **FREEMAN**

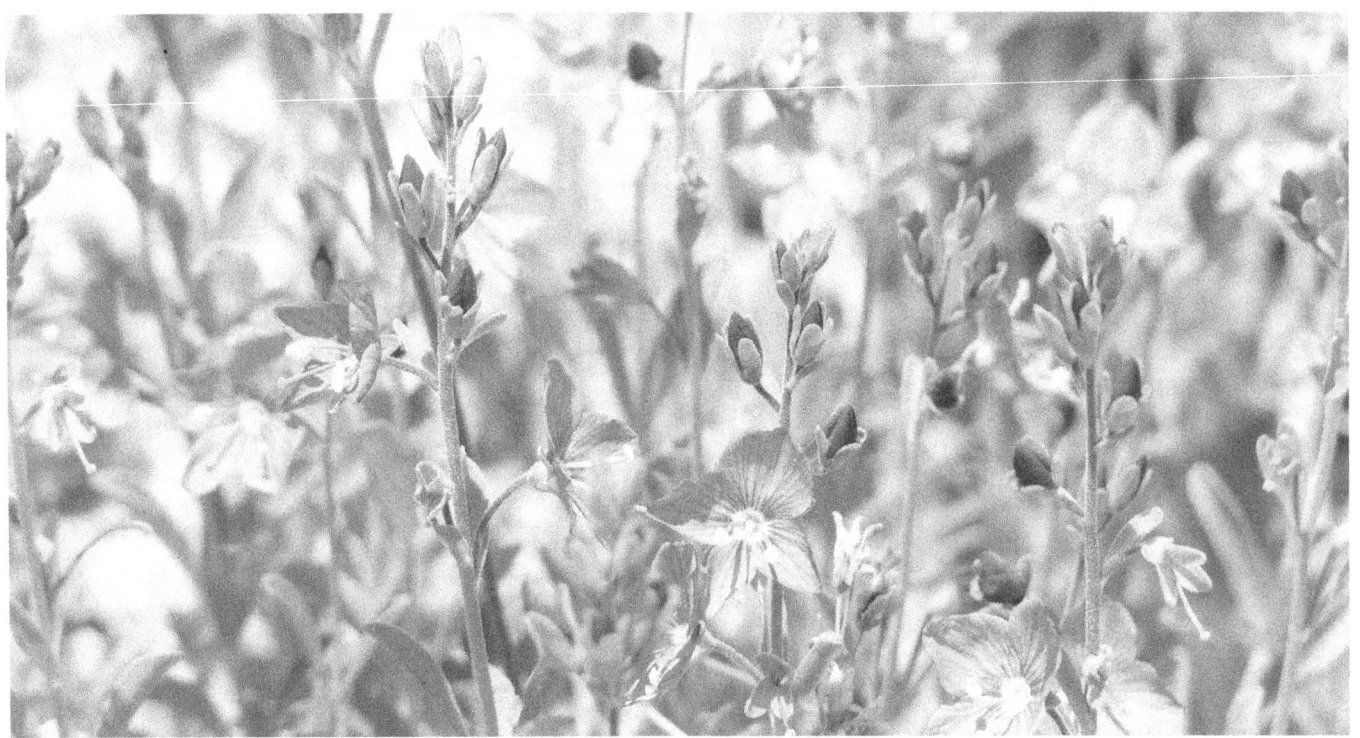

VERONICA FRUTICANS

SPIRITUAL PROPERTIES

There is a singular and interesting tradition regarding the flowers of this plant (*Leptandra*) when cultivated. It is said that those who cultivated it for a religious purpose, believing its flowers to image the face of Christ, produce flowers to a strong resemblance to a human face; while those who cultivate it for its beauty only, produce flowers which, while extremely beautiful, have no resemblance to a human face whatsoever.   **DR. SHOOK N.D.**

Medieval saints and modern fashion models may seem to strive for very different types of perfection- one strictly spiritual, the other physical- but both have traditionally chosen extreme dieting as the surest means to express their divine natures…In his book *Holy Anorexia,* Rudolph Bell postulates hat the two ages' shared obsession stems from out breaks of anorexia nervosa… St. Veronica spent most of her life eating spiders and cat vomit, but eventually settled into a regime consisting of vegetable soup and two ounces of fruit for breakfast. Dinner was a few grapes.   **STEWART ALLEN**

BOTANICA POETICA

Fair flowers, modest, shy, in depths of billowy meadow grasses hiding.
And yet worn footpaths nigh is found the wonted place of your abiding.
To watch with careless gaze the passer-by! Your eyes, wide open, tell in
tones of Saxon blue your heart's warm feeling,
As from the hermit's cell shines midnight lamp his piety revealing, the
fragrant breath of flowers bids me 'Speed well!'

ISACC BASSETT CHOATE

MYTHS AND LEGENDS

The name for speedwell in the Russian language means "Anita's eyes". In folklore, Anita fell in love with a young man who would declare his love to every pretty girl in town only to abandon her later for someone new. Anita had very beautiful eyes and told the man that if he ever found someone new, her eyes would follow him everywhere. The man didn't pay attention to her words and, as usual, told her that she was his only true love. He then went to visit another young woman but felt that Anita's eyes were indeed following him everywhere he walked. He decided to come back to Anita and never strayed again.   **ZEVIN**

It was a shepherd who discovered its worth as a curative, for he saw a deer, wounded by a wolf's bite, rub itself against an oak, then lie in a speedwell patch. The stage remained in its nook for a week, eating of the speedwell from time to time, and when it came forth the wound was cured. Now the king of that country had been smitten with a leprosy and was lying in his bed, so ill he doubted if he should ever again rise from it. To him the shepherd made his way with a dish filled with new-gathered flowers of the speedwell, and related what he had seen.

The monarch applied them to his bleeding skin and also drank a decoction brew from the plant. As a result, he left his bed, sound in health and full of thanks for the blessings that the Lord had showered upon the earth.   **CHARLES M. SKINNER**

RECIPES

TINCTURE- *V. officinalis* made into a fresh plant tincture 1:2 at 60% alcohol. Take 5-10 ml three times daily as needed. Use with caution in pregnancy and avoid use in bile duct obstruction.

Fresh juice is optimal preparation. Take on teaspoon three times daily. Another option is to freeze fresh juice in ice cubes and pop into warm water when needed.

INFUSION- Take 20 grams of dried leaf and flower to one liter of hot water. Steep ten minutes. Drink one cup up to four times daily.

TINCTURE- *Leptandra-* 5-10 drops up to four times daily. A dry root tincture is made from the second year root in ratio of 1:5 at 60% alcohol. The fresh root, like blue flag, is stronger, but is more likely to cause purging and vomiting. Only use dry root. It is cathartic in large doses. Go slow.

Do not use during pregnancy if prepared from fresh root nor with iron supplements, Buscopan, Lanoxin, or scopolamine patches. Care should be taken in acute or severe liver disease including viral hepatitis, septic gall bladder inflammation or obstruction or liver cancer.

The tincture is reddish-orange with an earthy odour, but no characteristic taste.

POWDER- 10-60 grains in juice, or capsules.

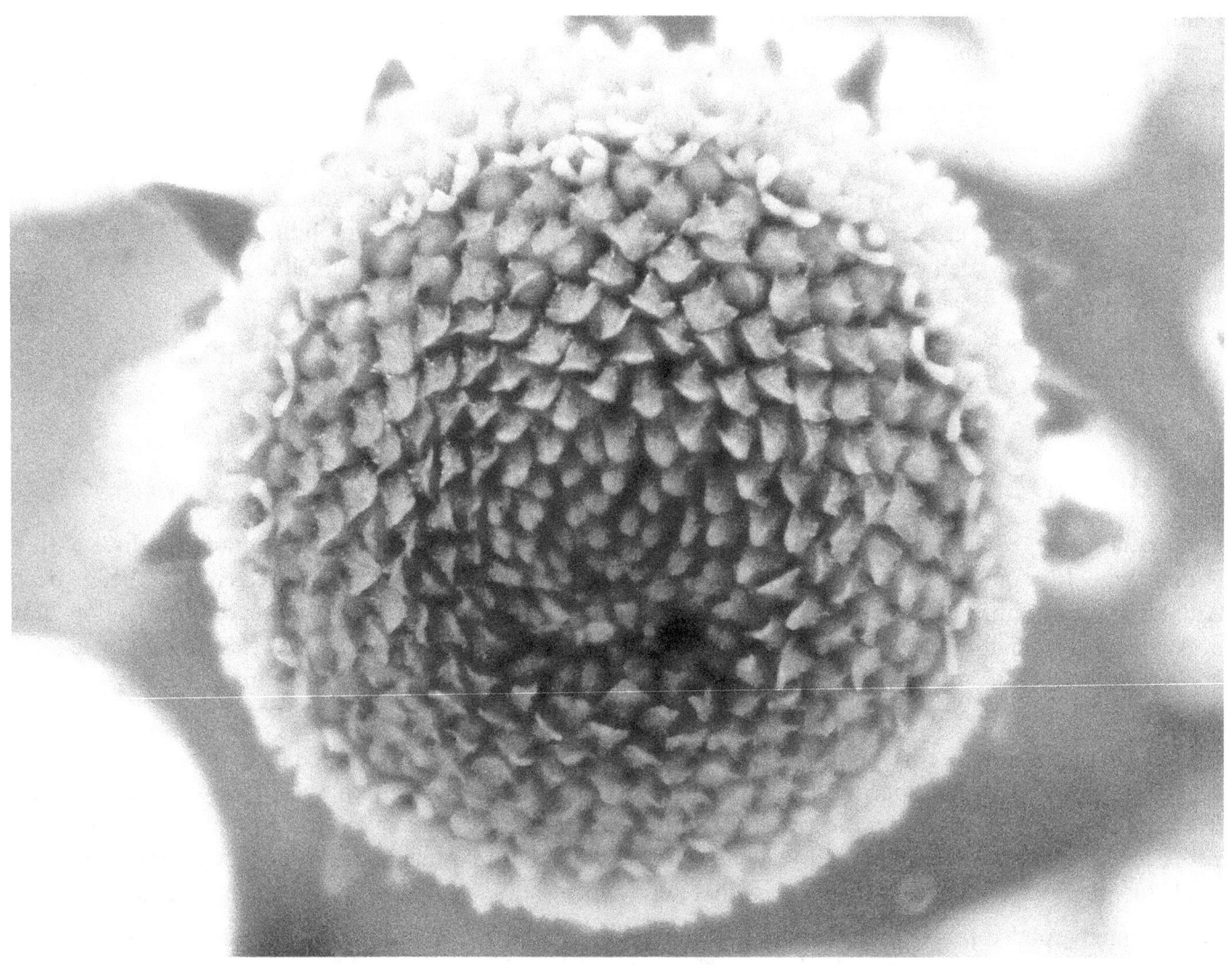

SPILANTHES FLOWER

SPILANTHES
TOOTHACHE PLANT
PARACRESS
(***Spilanthes acmella*** [L.] Murray)
(***S. acmella var. oleracea*** [L.] C. B. Clarke ex Hook. f)
(***S. oleracea*** L.)
(***Acmella oleracea*** [L.] R.K. Jansen.)
PARTS USED- leaves, flowers

110

Spilanthes, or Toothache Plant made its first introduction to me in Peru. It grows in many tropical countries around the world, but as an annual, it can be grown and utilized on the Canadian prairies as well. There is a great deal of confusion regarding the species, and even the proper genus of this plant, but all mentioned above are same plant.

In Peru, it is often eaten as a spicy salad that leaves a lively, tingling feeling in the mouth. The flower heads are used for toothaches, of course.

The flower heads are also known as buzz buttons, Szechuan buttons and electric buttons. When you chew on one, you will know why.

You can add fresh leaves to salads, or add to stews as they do in northern Brazil. A concentrated extract is used as a food flavoring, adding a pungent, cooling, tingling and numbing effect.

Richard Cech, a medicinal herb grower and herbalist writes. "The taste of Spilanthes is pleasantly saline at first, but soon develops and blossoms into an indescribable profusion of stimulatory responses, including profuse salivation and a general tingling buzz of the tongue and lips, as if the teeth have begun to play musical chairs, springing painlessly from their moorage and rioting about in chaotic dance, while the saliva continues to pour." The compound spilanthol is responsible for promoting saliva.

The plant has very unusual flower heads similar to the domed shape of pineapple weed, but with a rusty red dot on the top surrounded by a yellow orange ball outside.

The plant is easy to propagate, but best started indoors from seed, and set outside after frost. The seeds require light to germinate so do not cover with soil.

Space the plants one foot apart. The plant, being tropical likes both heat and moisture. A rich soil (4-5% of organic material) is ideal.

Spilanthol was first isolated from the flower heads in 1903. This compound is toxic and paralytic to houseflies, yellow mealworm, mosquitoes, beet, squash and melons worms, and coddling moths. It would combine well with the pyrethrins of painted, or ox eye daisy and related species.

The fresh flower extract, in dilutions of as low as 1:100,000 is lethal to mosquito larvae.

The flowers are chewed by the Zulu of Africa for toothache, thrush or mouth sores.

In India and Sri Lanka, the herb is used for nephritis, kidney and bladder stones, and to relieve menstruation. The flowers are rubbed on nipples for stimulating breast milk production. It is used to flavor chewing tobacco in India.

The leaves and flowers are infused, strained and cooled as a douche for leucorrhea in Pakistan.

A mound forming annual variety is known in prairie greenhouses as Peekaboo Plant.

In Ecuador, the related *S. leucantha* is chewed for toothache, and known as **BONTONCILLO**.

The fresh plant tincture is useful for various fungal conditions including athlete's foot, lichen planus, vaginal candidiasis, and toenail mycosis.

Spilanthol has been found to permeate the skin and buccal mucosa. Boonen et al, *J Ethnopharm* 2009 Oct 4.

Work by Jondiko, *Phytochemistry* 1986 25 10 found methanol extracts of fresh leaves produced 100% mortality as a mosquito larvicide. The compound believed responsible was identified as N-isobutyl-2E, 4E, 8E, 10Z-dodeca-2, 4, 8, 10-tetraenamide.

Work by Pandey et al, *Parasitol Res* 2007 Oct 7 found *Spilanthes acmella* extract has an LC90 (lethal count 90%) on mosquito larvae. at concentrations of only 7.83 ppm.

A follow up study 108:2 found other bio-larvicidal activity.

Extracts from spilanthes are finding their way into various cosmetics, especially anti-ageing facial skin cream that are a safe alternative to Botox. The herb blocks the micro-contractions of the mimic wrinkles, which results in reduction of wrinkles and improved skin smoothness. Spilanthes, ginger, gotu kola and ferulic acid were used to formulate an anti-age cream with positive results. Moldovan M et al, *Ciujui Med* 2017 90(2): 212-9.

MEDICINAL

CONSTITUENTS- various N-isobutylamides including spilanthol (affinin), acmellonate, undeca-2E,7Z,9E-trienoic acid isobutyl-amide and undeca-2E-en-8,10-diynoic acid isobutylamide; alpha amyrenol, beta amyrenol, myricyl, stigmasterol, sitosteryl-0-beta-D-glucoside. Also contains vanillic acid, trans-ferulic and trans isoferulic acid, scopoletin and various triterpenoids.

Spilanthes aerial parts are used medicinally, like Echinacea, for conditions of the immune system, respiratory tract infections and general winter cold and flu like conditions.

Toothache plant suggests its use in dental health, including gum disease and infection, as well as sore throat and oral pain from any origin.

The plant exhibits anti-viral, anti-fungal and anti-parasite activity, and may be helpful in Lyme's disease, Chagas' disease and other spirochetes.

The flower head is used in Traditional Chinese Medicine, and called **LIU SHEN HUA**. This translates roughly as Six God Flower.

The flower is pungent and bitter in flavour, with a warm, mild property, and tingling effect on the tongue. This is due to the isobutylamides found as well, in Echinacea and Prickly Ash. The initial reaction soon gives way to a throat cooling sensation.

It contains some unknown substances that stimulate saliva flow, as well as secretion of digestive juices. This sialogogue effect increases vaginal lubrication when deficient.

The flowers action removes wind and dampness, helps regulate the flow of chi, invigorates blood circulation, reduces inflammation and strengthens the spleen and stomach.

The plant is vaso-relaxing suggesting use in hypertension. Prachayasittikol et al, *Molecules* 2009 14:2. This work found anti-microbial activity against *Bacillus subtilis* and *Corynebacterium dipthereriae*.

The herb is used in the Amazon to treat drug resistant tuberculosis, but I can find no information on clinical trials.

It is used in treating abdominal pain, rheumatic complaints, and other pains caused by overstrain, as well as internal and external trauma.

Recent work found alcohol extracts inhibit excessive inflammatory response by inhibiting the phosphorylation of MAPKs and NFkappaB. Cho YC et al, *Mol Med Rep* 2017 16(1): 339-46.

Work by Ramasooriya et al, *Pharm Bio* 43:17 found the flower attenuates persistent inflammatory pain and hyperalgesia.

The herb may exert neuroprotective effect, via alternation of calcium homeostasis. Suwanjang W et al, *Asian Pac J Trop Med* 2017 10(1): 35-41. This may very important as other work suggests spilanthol shows high absorbency from the gut, and high blood brain barrier permeation. Veryser L et al, *BMC Complement Altern Med* 2016 16:177.

Spilanthol appears to relieve LPS induced inflammation in macrophage cells due to inactivation of NFkappaB. Wu et al, *J Ag Food Chem* 2008 56:4.

Spilanthol permeates the skin and is a good trans-dermal medium.

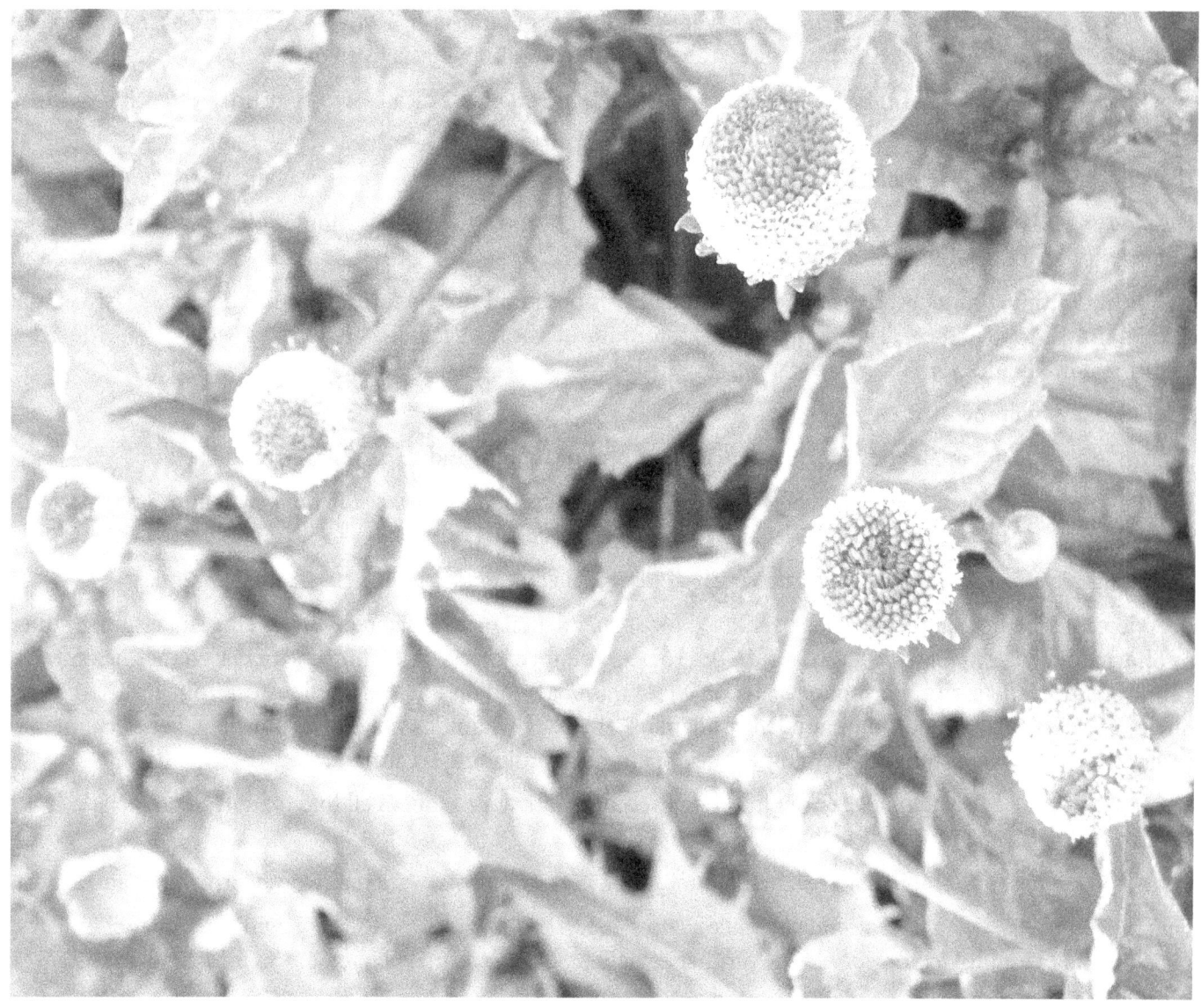

TOOTHACHE PLANT

The herb is used as part of combinations to treat indigestion, anorexia, toothache, as well as reproductive concerns such as in between period bleeding and leucorrhea. In TCM, the herb is used as part of aphrodisiac formulae.

The term Toothache plant is apt in several ways. The herb shows remarkable activity against common root canal pathogens that are responsible for endodontic failures, including *Enterococcus faecalis* and *Candida albicans*. A trial by Sathyaprasad S et al, *Indian J Dent Res* 2015 26(5): 528-32 found it superior to calcium hydroxide.

Spilanthes is used for candidiasis and related infections in South Africa. Masevhe NA et al, *J Ethnopharm* 2015 168: 364-72.

The tincture is useful for thrush, ringworm and athlete's foot.

Flower heads, as a coldwater infusion, show strong, rapid diuretic effect similar to furosemide, with increased sodium and potassium urinary levels. Ratnasooriya et al, *J Ethnopharm* 2004 91:2-3.

The flowers called **AKARKARA**, are used in India and other tropical countries in a tincture form to treat toothache. In Mali, the herb is part of a combination called Malarial-5 for the treatment of this debilitating illness.

They are combined with chewing tobacco for flavor. A study by Skumaran et al, *Mutation Research, Genetic Toxicology* 1995 343:1 found the plant extract inhibited tobacco-induced mutagenesis by over 86%.

Work by Fabry et al, *Chemotherapy Basel* 1996 42:5 found flowers and roots mildly effective against *Helicobacter pylori*, implicated in stomach and duodenal ulcers.

The same author published in *Mycoses* 1996 39:1-2 showing root and flowers active against *Aspergillus* species.

The flower buds have been shown to inhibit lipase production by 40%, suggesting a role in weight reduction and obesity formulas. Ekanem et al, *Phytother Res* 2007 21:12.

Spilanthol (affinin) induces vasodilation and may be of potential use in cardiovascular disease. Castro-Ruiz JE et al, Int J Mol Sci 18(1). This compound is found in the root of *Heliopsis longipes*, a widely used Mexican traditional medicine. And in *Erigeron affinis*.

See Fleabane (volume 2).

Affinin is a powerful analgesic that may be useful in orofacial pain, and trigeminal neuralgia.

For the latter, combine with tincture of green seeds from Cow Parsnip (*Heracleum lanata*). It appears to activate TRPV1 receptors. De la Rosa-Lugo V et al, *J Pharm Pharmacol* 2017 69(7): 884-95.

The analgesic effect is similar to ketorolac. Cilia-Lopez VG et al, *Pharm Biol* 2010 48(2): 195-200.

In Ayurvedic medicine, the herb has been used for sexual deficiency associated with ageing. In a mouse study by Sharma V et al, *Phytomedicine* 2011 18(13): 1161-9, ethanol extracts of the flowers increased mating pattern, penile erection and serum hormone levels. An effect was observed on FSH, LH and testosterone levels. *In vitro* nitric oxide was also noted, comparable to sildenafil. The N-alkylamides may be responsible. What is notable is that the effects were statistically significant even after discontinuing treatment.

The closely related *S. ocymifolia* scored in the top ten of plants with cancer cell line toxicity, in an article from *Revista Brasileira de Plantas Medicinais* 1999 2:1.

Other top ten herbs, found in our area, in this survey of 855 plant species were mugwort, wormwood, and arnica.

Dubey S et al, *Advances in Pharmacological Sciences* 2013 ID 423750 is a good review of the phytochemistry, pharmacology and toxicology of plant. Another review by Prachayasittikul V et al, *EXCLI J* 2013 12: 291-312 is also good.

HOMEOPATHY

Spilanthes may be useful for children who stammer.

DOSE- D3 to 30th potency.

ESSENTIAL OIL

Spilanthes acmella has been steam distilled and contains at least 45 different aromatic compounds, including 25.7% (E)-2-hexenol, 13% 2-tridecanone, 11% germacrene D, 11% hexanol, and 10.8% beta carophyllene. Jirovetz L et al, *J Ess Oil Res* 2005 71:4.

FLOWER ESSENCES

Spilanthes flower essence enhances electric connection to enhance immue system. Increases alertness, vitality and body sensations in context of needs vs. desires. **HUMMINGBIRD**

Spilanthes clarifies issues of man's sexual compatibility and suitability for a particular woman and allows Higher will and destiny to have control. **KANA'I** www.starmen.com

RECIPES

TINCTURE- 20-40 drops as needed. Prepare at 1:4 ratio at 70% from fresh flowers and aerial parts. Culture regeneration of the herb has been optimized, by Yadav et al, *Fascicula Bilogie* 2011 18:1 66-70.

SPILANTHES PARACRESS DROPS- 15-20 drops three times daily.   **VOGEL**

CAUTION- Do not use during pregnancy or lactation.

STAR OF BETHLEHEM
(***Ornithogalum umbellatum*** L.)
PARTS USED- whole plant

The fourth part of a cab of dove's dung was sold for five pieces of silver.   **II KINGS 6:25**

The next akin, a flower which Greeks of old,
From excrements of birds, descended, hold,
Which Britain, nurse of plants, a milder clime,
Gentilely calls 'The Star of Bethlehem'.   **COWLEY**

Flower, that I hold in my hand,
Waxen & white and unwoeful,
Perfect with your race's lovely perfection,
Pure as the dream of a child just descended from the heavens.   **LOUIS JAMES BLOCK**

Ornithogalum is from the Greek meaning "birds' milk", so named by Dioscorides because the flowers, "being opened are like milk." Umbellatum means the flowers spring up on stalks like the spokes of an umbrella. The common name is in reference to the shape of flowers looking like the Star of Nativity, the journey of the Three Kings and their origin in Palestine. In Hebrew and Arabic it is endearingly called "dove's dung".

Star of Bethlehem is originally from the eastern Mediterranean, but is now introduced around the world. It represents the quality of purity.

It is hardy to zone 3-4 in protected areas with some snow cover. The plant has beautiful white flowers that are striped green on the outside.

Once established, the plant spreads quite easily, and in Kentucky is classified as an escaped weed.

It is a bulbous plant, like an onion, that is both edible and nutritious; and in ancient times was either boiled or roasted. William Salmon, a 17th century medical writer, noted, "the root serves for meat or food being roasted in embers, mixt with honey."

It is believed to be the Dove's Dung mentioned in the bible, and being sold at a high price during the siege of Samaria by the King of Syria.

Large quantities of the bulb were dried and stored for long pilgrim caravans to Mecca.

The fresh, cooked bulbs can be eaten by humans, but are considered toxic to cattle.

In Lyte's book *Dodoens*, published in 1578, the bulb is described as "the white filde onyon". Evelyn reported in 1699, the bulbs are "roasted as they do chestnuts, are eaten by Italians with oil, vinegar and pepper."

Gerard named six species. "There be sundry sorts of wild field Onions, called 'Starres of Bethlehem' differing in stature, taste and smell."

Local names in England reflect the fact that the flowers curl up at midday or earlier on cloudy days. Betty Go To Bed At Noon, Shame-faced Maiden, and Eleven O' Clock Lady are some of the most common. The latter relates to the late morning opening of six flower petals.

The Thompson of British Columbia enjoy the introduced plant as an ornamental and call it Wee Little Flowerettes.

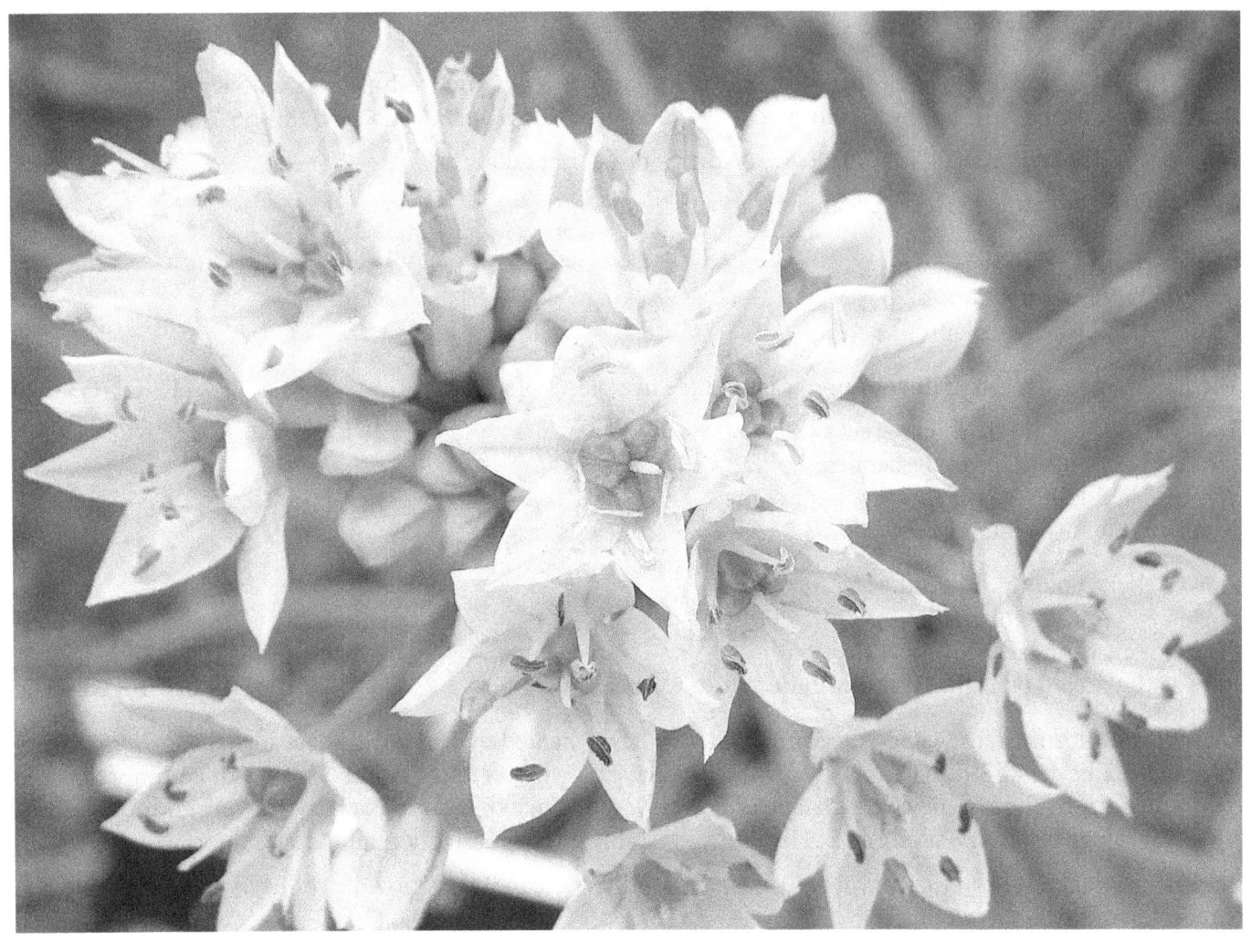

STAR OF BETHLEHEM

MEDICINAL

CONSTITUENTS- bulb- colchicine, eight cardenolide type cardiac glycosides. Mycorrhizal fungi induce the accumulation of various apocarotenoids on bulbs and roots. These include mycorradicin and derivatives; as well as mono-, di- and branched triglycosides of blumenol C, 13-hydroxyblumenol C and 13-nor-5-carboxy-blumenol C.

Dr. Robert Cooper recommended the bulb for the treatment of stomach cancer. Although unproven, it should be examined for potential alkaloids of value in treating this deadly disease.

Its use in gastric and duodenal ulcers is more accepted and of proven benefit. Leyel suggested it has a specific action on the pylorus.

The cardiac glycosides are similar to those in Lily of the Valley, and remain after plant has dried.

The related *O. thyrsoides* was used in Europe traditionally, to treat diabetes mellitus; an infusion of nine leaves to one ounce of hot water.

The related *O. saundersiae* was examined in Japan by Sashida et al. In a paper, presented at the *International Symposium on Plant Glycosides in China* August 1997, the cholestane glycoside showed strong cytostatic activity against human malignant tumor cells. It increased the survival of mice with P388 leukemia by nearly 60% following a single dose of 0.01mg/kg.

116

Follow-up work by Kuroda, Mimaki and Sashida, *Phytochemistry* 1999 52:3 isolated four of these compounds, named saundersiosides. They found all highly cytostatic to human leukemia HL-60 cells, showing IC50 rates from 0.019-0.063; which is as potent as pharmaceutical anti-cancer agents like etoposide and methotrexate.

A cholestane saponin, isolated from *O. caudatum*, induces apoptosis in colon cancer cells, without significant side effects. Zhang Y et al, *Oncol Rep* 2017 37(6): 3509-19.

This plant is known as Sea Onion, or Pregnant Onion and is usually grown indoors, unless you live in zone 8-11. It is native to South Africa. It was recently moved to *Albuca bracteata* by taxonomists.

HOMEOPATHY

Star of Bethlehem is to be considered in chronic gastric and other abdominal indurations, including cancer of the intestinal tract, especially the stomach and cecum. Its centre of action is the pylorus, causing painful contraction with duodenal distention.

There may be depression of spirits, with complete prostration and a feeling of sickness that keeps the patient awake at night.

The tongue is coated, with vomiting of coffee ground looking matter. There is agonizing feeling in the chest and stomach starting from the pylorus with gas that rolls in balls from one side to the other. This is accompanied by loss of appetite, phlegmed retching and loss of weight.

There may be gastric or duodenal ulceration with tendency to hemorrhage.

Pain increases as food passes the pyloric valve, with distention of stomach and a frequent belching of an acidic, vinegar nature.

The skin can have accompanying inflammatory, vesicular condition.

DOSE- Take a single dose of the mother tincture and await action. The mother tincture is prepared from the fresh bulb. Clinical symptoms noted by Cooper and Clarke in 1890s.

FLOWER ESSENCE

Star of Bethlehem is for all forms of shock; sudden and traumatic, long and slow over a period of time, delayed from the past, or the shock of birth.

It helps clear the shock from the system, bringing a sense of well being, centered, soothed and comforted. It helps restore the body's self-healing mechanisms. **BACH**

PERSONALITY TRAITS

The flowers close early and always close in dull weather, hence local names like 'nap at noon', 'peep o' day' and 'eleven o'clock lady'. Additional names referring to the plant's sleeping habits include Jack-go-to-bed-at-noon, John-go-to-bed-at-noon, six o'clock flowers, wake-at-noon and sleepy Dick. Cooper who introduced 'sleepy Dick' into homeopathy, noticed that it caused 'great difficulty in going to sleep owing to a creepy sensation in limbs' and the legs and feet as if going to sleep with inability to keep them still. **VERMEULEN**

SPIRITUAL PROPERTIES

Above the girl's head, shines the Star of Bethlehem, a floral expression of peace and equilibrium. The geometry of this six-pointed flower is made up of two triangles, an upward one representing the Heaven Above, and the downward one representing the Earth Below. The equal proportions of the two triangles allow for the merging of the Above and the Below into a perfect whole.

The central crown within the flower is what holds the two spheres intact. Like the hexagram or the Star of David, the flower resonates wholeness and perfect equilibrium. The fact that this pattern exists in this flower suggests its importance in restoring balance after periods of shock or upheaval. This flower has a soothing vibration that softens and heals and keeps us integrated through sudden changes. **RUDGINSKY**

Star of Bethlehem represents beauty in collective simplicity, and how each element plays its part in the whole collectivity. **THE MOTHER**

Hence we may conjecture that the festival of Adonis was regularly timed to coincide with the appearance of Venus as the Morning or Evening Star. But the star, which the people of Antioch saluted at the festival, was seen in the east; therefore if it was indeed Venus, it can only have been the Morning Star...

At Antioch and elsewhere the appearance of the Morning Star on the day of the festival may in like manner have been hailed as the coming of the goddess of love to wake her dead leman from his earthy bed. If that were so, we may surmise that it was the Morning Star which guided the wise men of the East to Bethlehem, the hallowed spot which heard, in the language of Jerome, the weeping of the infant Christ, and the lament for Adonis. **FRAZER**

WIDE LEAF STATICE
WIDE LEAF SEA LAVENDER
(*Limonium latifolium* [Sm.] Kuntze) not accepted
(*L. gerberi* Soldano)
TARTARIAN STATICE
GERMAN STATICE
(*L. tatarica* L.) not accepted
(*Goniolimon tataricum* [L.] Boiss.)
(*G. serbicum* Vis.)
EUROPEAN STATICE
(*S. limonium* L.) not accepted
(*L. vulgare* Mill.)
CAROLINA SEA LAVENDER
LAVENDER THRIFT
MARSH ROSEMARY
CANKER ROOT
(*L. carolinianum* [Walter] Britton)
(*S. limonium var. caroliniana*) not accepted
CHINESE STATICE
(*S. sinense* Girard)
(*L. sinense* [Girard] Kuntze)
SIBERIAN STATICE
(*L. gmelinii* [Willdenow] Kuntze)
RAT'S TAIL STATICE
PINK POKERS
(*L. suworowii* [Regel] Kuntze)
(*Psylliostachys suworowii* [Regel] Roshk.)
PARTS USED- root

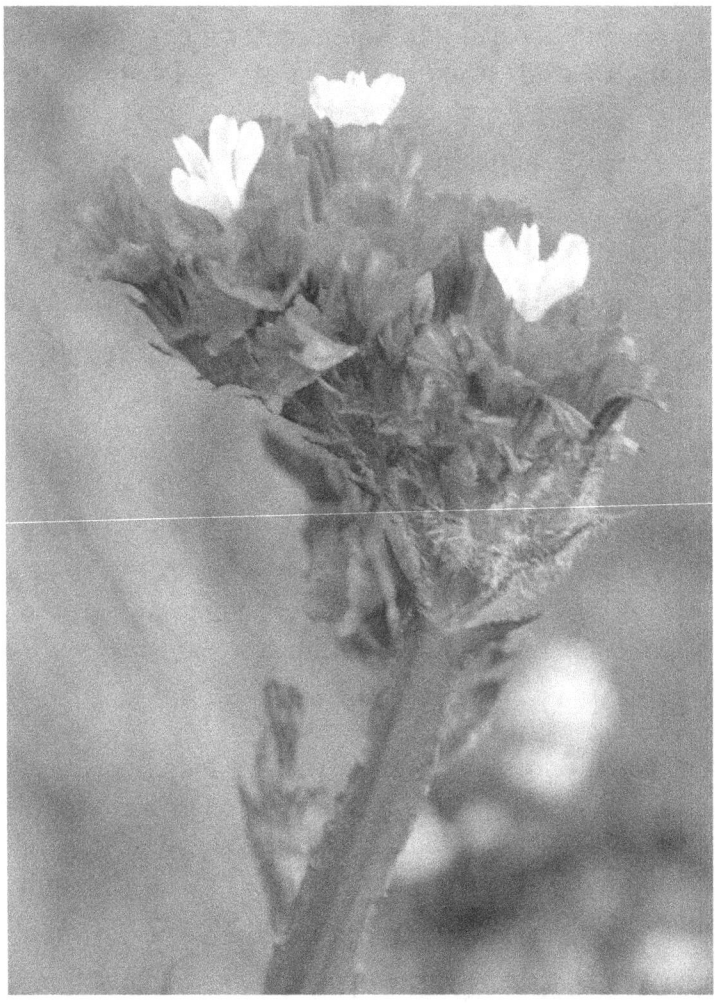

SEA LAVENDER

Limonium is from the Greek **LEIMON** meaning "a meadow". Statice is from the Greek **STATIKOS**, meaning "causing to stand or stop". Gmelinii is named in honor of Johan Friedrich Gmelin, an 18th century German botanist; or Karl Christian Gmelin, also an 18th century German physician and botanist. Sinense means from China. Goniolimon is from the Greek **GONIO** meaning "knee angle", and **LEIMON** for meadow.

118

Wide Leaf Sea Lavender is a hardy perennial for the prairies. At certain times of the year, it looks like Baby's Breath, until you discover the tiny lavender blue flowers.

The flowers start out violet and when they mature, the center becomes pure white.

The root has been used in tanning leather, while the medicinal properties of all are very similar.

Many Statice species have commercial possibilities for the dried flower industry. Both Italian and Chinese Statice are annuals that give high yields, while Tartarian and Sea Lavender are hardy perennials that take a year to establish before flowering.

Chinese Statice is a favorite as it blooms the first year, is quite frost resistant, and has low, dense lower leaves that smother weeds. Growers have several weeks to harvest the slow opening flowers, and perhaps best of all, there are no natural insect predators.

Commercial growers begin eight weeks before the frost date, with greenhouse germination. The flowers are harvested in the cool of day in bundles of 10 or 20, cut to even length and put in water. They do not like refrigeration units, and remain fresh in water for up to 2 weeks. To dry, hang upside down in a dark, ventilated area. Breakage can be used or sold for potpourri.

Average yields are around 15 stems per plant at say ten cents per stem. If you plant 26 beds of 188 plants each, with enough room to walk between on a quarter acre, this will yield sales of over $7,000.

The Mi'kmaq of Nova Scotia used the root of Sea Lavender (*L. carolinianum*) as a decoction for treating tuberculosis with spitting of blood.

The related *S. mucronata* of Morocco is used medicinally for its root. Called **SAFRIFA**, it is decocted as a tea for nervous conditions.

Culpepper wrote that the European Sea Lavender seeds are very drying and binding, stop fluxes and the menses, and help the colic and strangury.

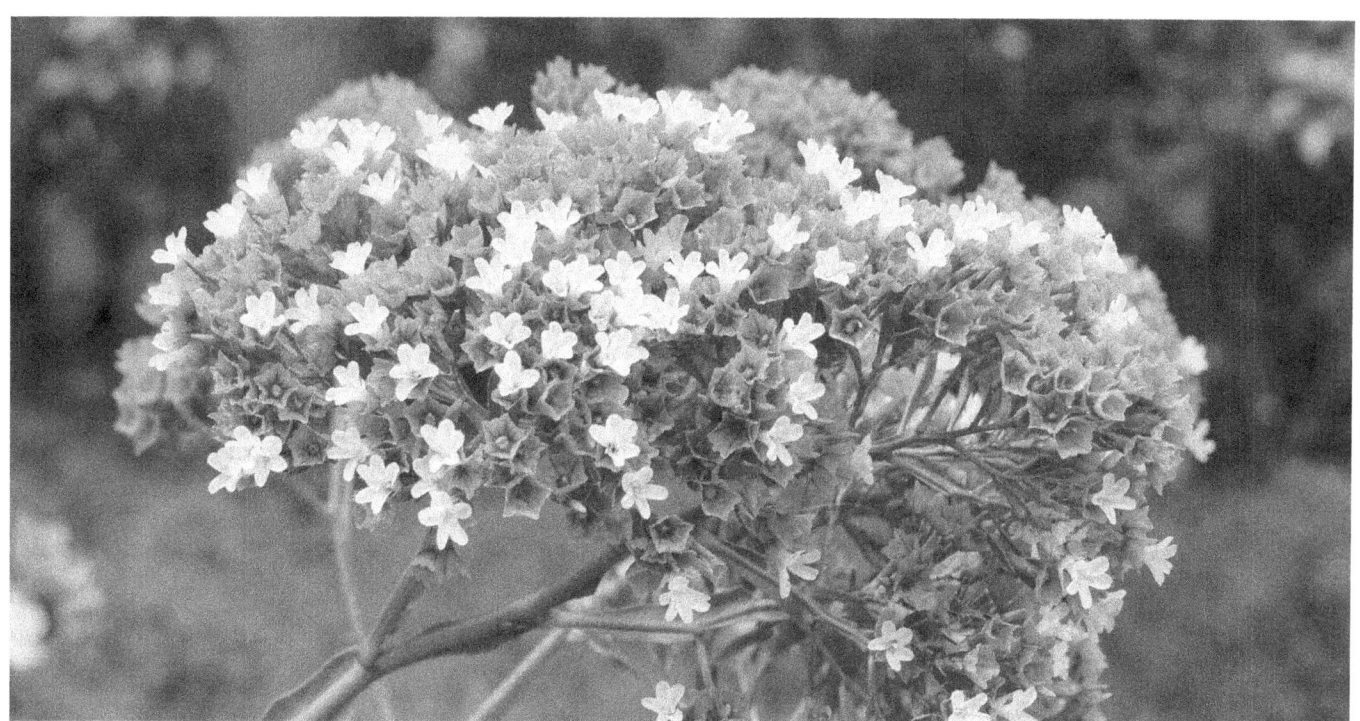

SEA LAVENDER

MEDICINAL

CONSTITUENTS- *L. sinense* root- isodihydrosyringetin, epigallocatechin 3-0-gallate, samarangenin B, myricetin, as well as myrectin and quercetin 3-0-alpha-rhamnopyranoside; N-trans-caffeoyl-tyramine and N-trans-feruloyl-tyramine.

The roots are salty and strongly astringent probably due to the 12% tannins.

Dr. Bigelow reported on Sea Lavender (*L. carolinianum*) medicinal value as an astringent and said that " large quantities are annually consumed... in Boston, it is regularly kept by the druggists, and larger quantities are sold than of almost any other indigenous article".

At one time it was official in the *United States Pharmacopoeia*.

Manasseh Cutler called it Marsh Rosemary. "The roots are powerfully astringent. A decoction of them is given, and used as a gargle, with success, in cankers and ulcerated sore throats".

An essential oil distilled from the root, called Ink Root is used medicinally.

Wide leaved Statice (*L. latifolium*) root was previously used in Spain and Russia for tanning leather. According to Dr. King, the eminent Eclectic physician, the properties are very similar to Sea Lavender.

These include the use in the form of an infusion or decoction as a remedy for diarrhea and chronic dysentery.

"It is not indicated in the acute stages of these affections, but will be found very efficient as an astringent and tonic, after the active symptoms have subsided. It also relieves irritation of the mucous membranes. It is an efficient remedy in atonic dyspepsia, pulmonary hemorrhage, chronic laryngitis, bronchorrhea, and other catarrhal disorders, with profuse secretion.

The decoction is very useful as a gargle or wash in ulcerations of the mouth and throat, scarlatina anginosa, etc."

Externally, the powdered root may be applied to old ulcers, or made into an ointment, as a soothing application for piles. It may be used in all cases where astringents are indicated.

Chinese Statice is similar and can be used interchangeably with other members of the genus above.

The root is known as **HUNG MAO CHA** or **SHIH YEH TSAO**.

The root has a bitter flavour, but is mild and has cold properties.

Decoctions are used to help remove dampness, clear up heat, remove toxins, and control bleeding.

Some of the indications are rectal prolapse, hematochezia, hematuria accompanied by urinary disturbance, menorrhagia, leukorrhea due to dampness and heat, hyperhydrosis, diuresis, diabetes mellitus, edema, cystitis, metrorrhagia, gastrosis, dysentery and bronchitis. It is used for fever, hemorrhage and hepatitis.

The root shows potent activity against hepatitis C virus. Hsu WC et al, *Antiviral Res* 2015 118:139-47. Polysaccharides possess anti-tumor activity. Tang XH et al, *Int J Biol Macromol* 2014 70: 138-42.

Work by Lin et al, *Planta Medica* 2000 66:4 found (-)-epigallocatechin 3-0-gallate and samarangenin B exhibit potent inhibition of herpes simplex virus 1. The latter was particularly potent with IC50 value of 11.4 microM. Cytotoxicity was not involved, as there was no death of the host cells after five days of treatment.

Siberian Statice is known in China as **DA YE BU XUE CAO.**

The related *L. bicolor* is used in TCM. Luteolin and quercitin, derived from the plant shows good cytotoxicity against human colon cancer cells. Kaempferol, derived from same plant, shows growth in inhibition of human breast cancer cells (MCF-7) and osteosarcoma cell lines (U2-OS). Chen J et al, *Pharmacogn Mag* 2017 13(50): 222-25.

Siberian Statice possesses significant anti-oxidant activity. *Prikl Biokhim Microbiol* 2009 45:6.

The related *L. michelsonii* inhibits ACE, or angiotensin 1 converting enzyme, used to improve blood circulation. Jenis J et al, *J Nat Med* 2017 May 26.

Infusions of the flowers of *L. algarvense* possess similar or higher anti-oxidant and anti-inflammatory properties than green tea. Rodrigues MJ et al, *Food Chem* 2016 200: 322-9.

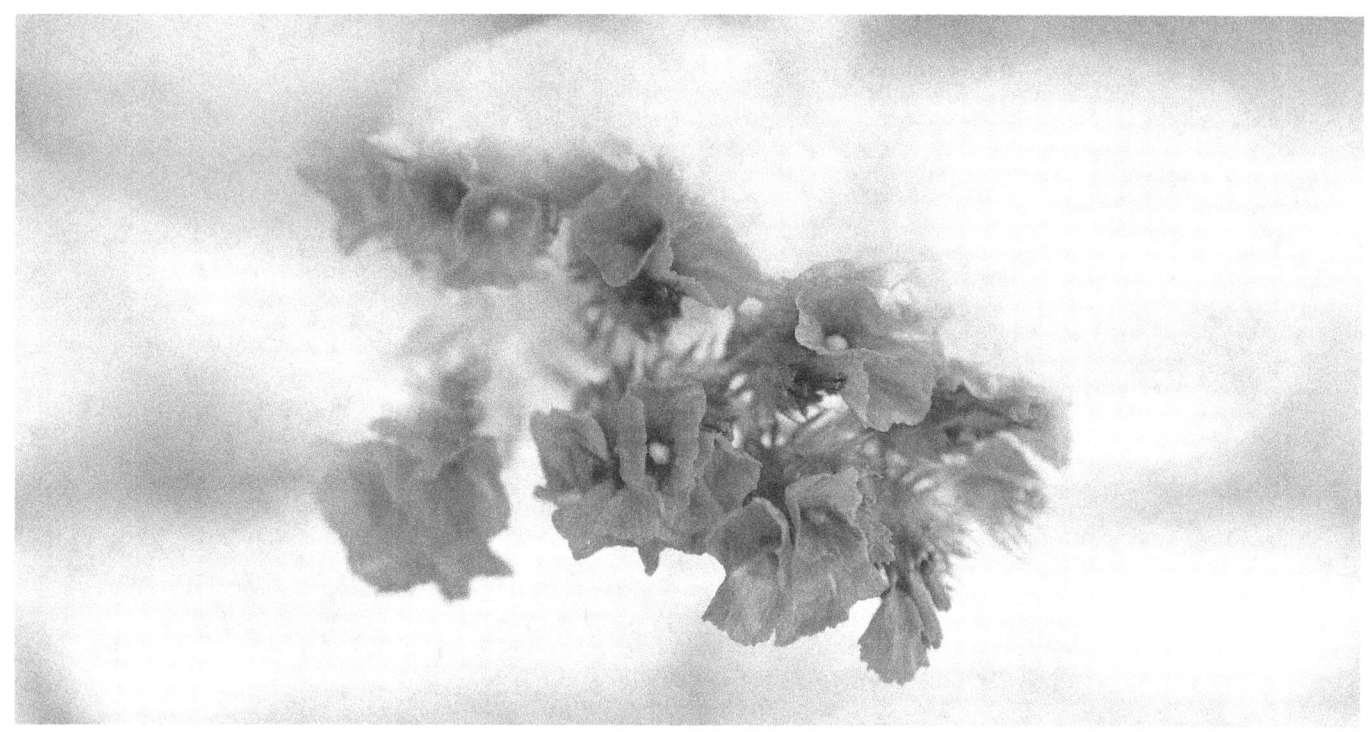

STATICE SINUATUM- CLOSE UP

FLOWER ESSENCE

Limonium sinuatum (*S. sinuatum*) flower essence assists in holding stillness and center when faced with a sense of urgency in transition. In situations of change and chaos, it creates calm in decision-making.

HUMMINGBIRD

RECIPES

TINCTURE- The fresh root tincture is given in doses of 1 to 20 drops. It is prepared from the fresh root at a 1:2 using 98% alcohol.

DECOCTION- root- One half to one ounce three times daily. Use one half to one ounce of root to one pint of boiling water.

SUNFLOWER
(***Helianthus annuus*** L.)
(***H. annuus* var. *lenticularis*** [Douglas ex Lindl.]
　　　　　　Steyerm.) not accepted
(***H. aridus*** Rydb.) not accepted
PRAIRIE SUNFLOWER
(***H. couplandii*** Boivin.) not accepted
(***H. petiolaris* ssp. *petiolaris*** Nutt.)
STIFF SUNFLOWER
(***H. rigidus*** [Cass.] Desf.) not accepted
(***H. pauciflorus* ssp. *pauciflorus*** Nutt.)
RHOMBOID SUNFLOWER
(***H. pauciflorus* ssp. *subrhomboideus***)

NARROW-LEAVED SUNFLOWER
(***H. maximiliani*** Schrad.)
TUBEROUS ROOTED SUNFLOWER
NUTALL'S SUNFLOWER
COMMON TALL SUNFLOWER
(***H. nuttallii*** Torr. & Gray)
JERUSALEM ARTICHOKE
GIRASOLE
(***H. tuberosus*** L.)
FUSEAU JERUSALEM ARTICHOKE
(***H. tuberosus*** L.)
PARTS USED- seed, flower, stem, pith, root

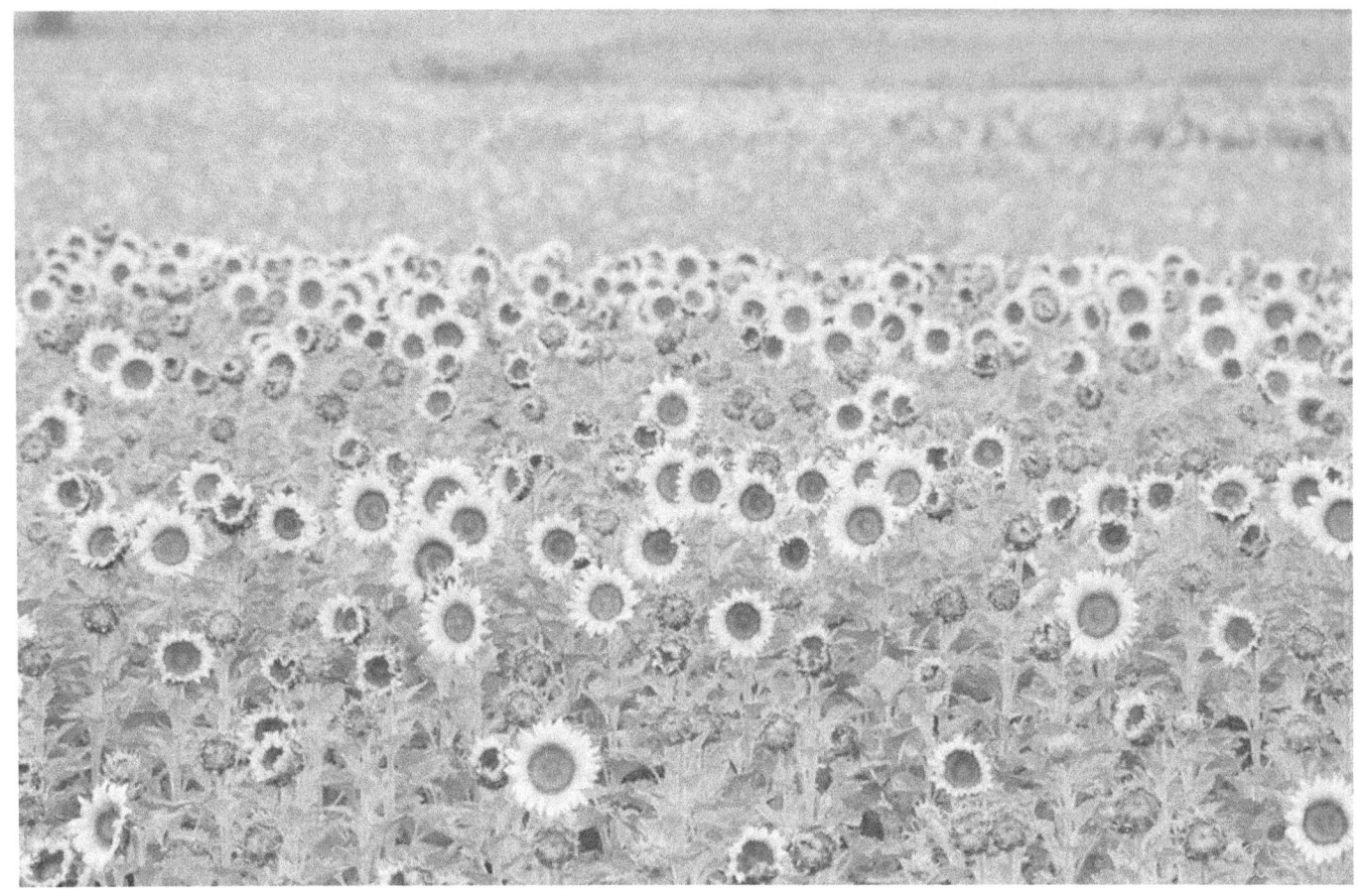

SUNFLOWER FIELD

My summer home is the fairest of all, with a morning glory roof and sunflower walls! **LOVEJOY**

The full Sunflower blew
And became a starre of Bartholomew.

We're not our skin of grime... we're all beautiful golden sunflowers inside. **ALLEN GINSBERG**

Ah, sunflower! weary of time
Who countest the steps of the sun
Seeking after that sweet golden clime
Where the traveler's journey is done. **WILLIAM BLAKE**

These petals (sunflower) are an uncompromising yellow-orange. The color seems to contain all the energy this planet will ever need. This color could power a nuclear reactor. It rings like a carillon. It hits me, with a little punch, in the solar plexus. **RUSSELL**

Helianthus is from the Latin **HELIO** for Sun, and **ANTHOS**, meaning flower. Helios was the Greek god of the sun, who was drowned by his uncles, the Titans, and then raised to the sky. Heliotropism, or following the sun, is a related term. In the case of sunflowers, the buds and leaves display this sun turning behavior, but once it has flowered into bloom, it remains fixed facing east.

Rigidus means rigid, and subrhomboideus, refers to the diamond-shaped leaves.

Annuus means annual, tuberosus suggests tubers. Prince Maximilian Alexander Philipp of Wied-Neuwied, was a major general in the Prussian army, who later devoted himself to natural history and ethnology.

He traveled Brazil in the early 1800s and in 1832 explored North America, spending the winter in Fort Clark, now Bismarck, North Dakota. Accompanying him was Karl Bodmer, who painted landscapes and portraits of the Plains tribes.

Girasole means Sunflower in Italian, from **GIRARE**, meaning to turn around, and **SOLE**, the sun; and is thought the origin of Jerusalem. Others believe that Girasol was term originally used for the fire opal and castor bean long before it was attached to the Sunflower. One suggestion is that Petrus Hondius planted a small tuber in Ter Neusens, Holland and it distributed from there in 1618. They were called Artichoke Apples of Ter-Neusen, and when they arrived in England this somehow became translated to Jerusalem.

Artichoke is so named for the similar in texture to Globe Artichoke heart. In Italy, ironically, the tuber is known as *Girasole di Canada*. Fuseau is from the French, referring to the distinctive spindle shape of the tubers. The uniform shape may provide greater marketing opportunities.

The Sunflower is associated with fire and the sun; and of course, masculine energy.

It grows quickly, taking full advantage the 1,300,000,000,000,000,000,000,000 calories of energy striking the earth each year. Or, put another way, 4.3 pounds of sunlight hit the earth every second.

It was once believed the truth in any matter is revealed sleeping with a sunflower under the bed.

If you cut a sunflower at sunset while making a wish, it will come true before the next sunset. It was once said that sleeping with a sunflower under your pillow, would allow you to know the truth of any matter.

To dream of sunflowers means your pride will be wounded, but to grow them in your garden is good luck.

The sunflower is believed native to the southwestern United States. In Mexico, the plant is known as **CHIMAIATI**, and was cultivated nearly 4600 years ago, according to new research.

It is sometimes known as *Maiz de Tejas*, suggesting it was introduced from the north in exchange for squash, beans and corn. This is uncertain.

The Aztecs have replicated the design of sunflower in body jewelry for the past three millennium. The Mayans made an extract of the petals, which they drank as an aphrodisiac. This may be due, in part to the chlorogenic acid, which has sexually stimulating effects.

Lonicerus suggested cooking the fresh petals in oil and eating them to give "great power to marital works."

Although native to the Americas, it was immediately valued when introduced to Europe. In Holland, the plant is used for marsh reclamation. Russia is the largest producer of sunflowers in the world, due in part to the Russian Orthodox Church, that forbade most oil-containing foods during Lent or the forty days before Christmas.

The radiant petals came to symbolize the sun and usurped the flower language of heliotrope, as a symbol of devotion.

Oscar Wilde took on the flower as his personal symbol and emblem of the Aesthetic Movement. This was a reaction to the industrial age, resulting in the flower's image being carved into chair backs, glazed on vases and added to iron railings.

Sunflower is the floral emblem of both Russia and Peru, where I spent a few years studying plant medicines; and the state flower of Kansas. Only the unopened flower buds track the sun back and forth.

Ironically, an adjoining state, has declared it a noxious weed. It makes a good companion plant with calendula, or angelica.

In ancient Peru, the Maidens of the Sun- the virgins of the Inca, wore large gold suns to cover their breasts. This is interpreted by some authors, as a representation of sunflowers, but there is no evidence it was cultivated in Peru, or any part of South America until recent times.

The juice, expressed from the fresh stems, was used for anointing oneself, if they wished to be virtuous.

The Cree of Alberta call the Wild Sunflower, **PISIMONEPEHKAN**.

They, and many other indigenous people, used the native sunflower for its seeds. They were dried over a fire, and ground lightly to remove the shells, and then ground into a meal or flour for making porridge by boiling, or flat breads in grease, or bone marrow.

The small, flat sunflower cakes were often carried as a lightweight and high-energy food source.

Seeds from about 2850 years ago were approximately one half the length of present day seeds.

The seeds were boiled for oil that was rubbed on the body and used to groom hair. The leaves have been used for treating kidney problems.

The Omaha Ponca call the plant **ZHA ZI** meaning yellow weed. The Teton Dakota boiled the sunflower heads, without bracts, as a remedy for pulmonary disease and chest pain.

The Pawnee pounded the seeds together with unidentified roots, and this was taken in a dry form, by a woman who becomes pregnant, while still nursing a child. This was done so the young baby would not become sick.

Samuel de Champlain observed cultivated sunflowers in eastern Canada as early as 1615.

The Ojibwa crushed the root and applied it as a wet dressing to draw blisters. Some Plains tribes mixed the ground seed with buffalo bone marrow to make a type of firm pudding. The Cochiti smeared the sticky juice of fresh stems on wounds to prevent infection.

The Navajo used the sunflower for prenatal problems believed caused by an eclipse of the sun. The Hopi cultivated a purple seed Sunflower that was boiled for dyeing textiles and baskets.

In Mexico, the leaves and stems are tinctured to treat arthritis and sore muscles externally, while an infusion is given to relieve catarrh, and fevers. The dry or green leaves are decocted and the liquid added to baths for rheumatism or pain in the bones.

The flowers and seeds can be juiced and taken on an empty stomach for intermittent fevers, edema, cancer, palsy, and is considered a specific for bladder and kidney stones.

While traveling in Venezuela, I often found the leaves and flowers sold separately by street herbalists. The flowers are decocted for heart weakness, while leaf poultices are applied to the abdomen in cases of distress, or to relieve rheumatic pain.

Sunflower is an annual grown commercially on about 150,000 acres across the three prairie provinces, mainly for the birdseed and confectionary market. The tallest sunflower recorded in Guinness World Records, grown in 1986, was 7.7 metres tall. At peak of growth, they can grow up to 30 cm a day. The record for most heads is 129, produced in Michigan in 2000. The shortest bonsai mature sunflower measured just over five cm. The record diameter sunflower head was grown in Maple Ridge, BC and measured 82 cm.

Manitoba and Saskatchewan are the primary producers, with any sunflowers for vegetable oil contracted to US companies. A plant in Altona, Manitoba closed its doors in 1996. Yields of about one ton of seed per acre can be expected on average, and worth about $300.

The larger seed is used for the confection market and is 20/64th of an inch or larger (known as the 20s in the industry). This can bring 23 to 24 cents a pound, with average yield of 2000 pounds per acre. The hull accounts for 46% of the weight of in shell product. The kernel is 47% fat, 23% protein, and 18% carbohydrate.

New hybrids, collectively called NuSun, produce sunflower oil that is several times higher in oleic acid than traditional sunflower oil.

Bees help pollination and produce a sunflower honey much in demand.

Sunflower milk, long popular in the Far East and Japan, is manufactured similar to the process for soymilk production.

Sunflower seed butter is slightly greener and more plastic than peanut butter, but shows good nutritional value.

The seeds can be roasted and ground as a coffee substitute, or sprouted for their edible, tasty green that takes approximately ten days to fully mature. Use the black oil sprouting variety, as 99% of the shells fall off naturally.

In Turkey and Persia, a tincture is prepared from the seeds with wine as a substitute for quinine for intermittent fevers. In China, the seeds are used to treat dysentery, in Brazil the leaves are infused for asthma, and in Cuba, a decoction of flowers is used for the common cold.

The un-opened flower buds can be steamed and eaten like artichokes.

A sunflour was produced and marketed many years ago. It had to be mixed with wheat flour because of the high oil content, but made superior bakery goods.

Gonzalez-Perez et al at Wageningen University, in The Netherlands, found a method suitable for producing sunflower seed protein isolate free of chlorogenic acid, which reduces digestibility, functionality and a dark colour. *J Agric Food Chem* 2002 50.

Three years later, the same authors in same journal, reported on the formation and stability of foams from sunflower protein. The work continues.

Soapstock is produced when hexane and other chemicals are used to extract and refine edible oil from sunflower and safflower seeds. It is presently added to animal feed, but could have new uses.

First, researchers had to rid soapstock of its water and hexane, without eliminating desirable properties. Then they spread the soapstock paste onto glass plates and spheres to form thin, flexible films.

This gummy, amber colored byproduct could become a new biodegradable film for encapsulating fungicides and slow-release chemicals, and packaging fresh produce, such as bell peppers. They are testing soapstock gel for hair styling and colouring.

Sunflower seed protein has visco-elastic properties that lend themselves to biodegradable product production.

The inflorescences of cultivated sunflowers contain a highly active anti-feedant for western corn rootworms. Germacranolide angelates exhibit structural features similar to picrotoxinin, a gamma amino butyric acid (GABA) gated chloride channel antagonist. Two diterpenoid acids, 16-kauren-19-oic acid and trachyloban-19-oic acid, have been isolated from the florets of *H. annuus*. They have been shown to inhibit the growth of the sunflower moth, and other insects.

Virgin female sunflower moths, when exposed to the odor of pollen, begin signaling for males more intensely.

Sunflowers have been observed to accumulate scopoletin and ayapin around wound tissue. These compounds show strong fungicide and insecticide activity.

Somaclonal variants of sunflower containing elevated levels of ayapin have shown improved anti-feeding resistance.

The leaves, if carefully dried, can be used as a substitute for tobacco in cigar making; the flavour is said to greatly resemble mild Spanish tobacco.

Work by Macias et al, *Journal of Natural Products* 1999 found heliannuals isolated from sunflower leaves possess phytotoxic activity and potential as a natural herbicide.

Work by Harris et al, at Oregon State University looked at the feeding habits of rabbits on 14 different fresh greens. Out of 100 grams offered, the rabbits ate 98.4% of sunflower leaves, followed by red clover, carrot tops, cauliflower leaves (all 90+%), dandelion (83%), white clover (80%), Swiss chard (78%), corn leaves (66%), and amaranthus (65%).

Sunflower leaves contain fumaric acid, which substitutes for tartaric acid in beverages and baked products.

The leaves and stalks are infused in vodka in Russia for gout.

The left over stem fiber and seedless heads can be used for paper. The Chinese have used the fiber to make thread and weave into silk fabrics; while the Russians have made them into lightweight acoustic ceiling tile. Research by Marechal et al, in *Industrial Crops and Products* 1999 10 shows that sunflower fiber is suitable for cardboard.

The pith of the stem was used at one time for life preservers in Russia, having a greater buoyancy than either cork or reindeer's hair, and specific gravity of 0.028. The pith is like polystyrene and could find application in packaging and packing materials.

This pith is used as a mounting medium for microscope study.

They make great kindling for starting fires. They contain high amounts of phosphorus and potassium and can also be returned to the soil as fertilizer.

Sunflower meal contains 9.7% of di- and oligosaccharides, mainly sucrose, trehalose, and raffinose. Arabinans and arabinogalactans are 9% and 13% respectively in the flour and protein concentrate.

Scientists at North Dakota State University have extracted various anthocyanins from sunflower hulls that have potential as red food colorants.

The hulls were at one time discarded or used for poultry litter. They can be used to produce blotting paper, and fiberboard.

Co-op Vegetable Oils, a Canadian firm, press the hulls into logs, superior in heating units to coal for cook stoves and furnaces.

Today, in Russia, the hulls are used to manufacture ethyl alcohol and furfural, in lining plywood, and in growing yeast. Nitrated or oxidated hulls are a rich source of organic nitrogen fertilizer. Efanov et al, *Chem Nat Comp* 2002 38:6 indicate sunflower hulls then stimulate pea growth.

The hulls may be useful in the removal of color dyes from dilute industrial effluent. Thinkaran et al, *J Hazard Mater* 2008 151:2-3. The petals yield a yellow dye.

The white central pith of the stalk contains nitre, which has been used in the past as a diuretic. It can be gathered like the white fuzz of mugwort as a form of moxa, something practiced by the Portuguese. The cones are burned on acupuncture meridians.

Flower infusions and decoctions are used as fly killers. Water extracts of the flowers have been shown to kill mice, but not rabbits in a most important laboratory experiment!

A University of Alberta professor and bio-organic chemist has recently received a grant to see if sunflowers stems can be bio-engineered to produce natural rubber. John Vederas hopes that by inserting genes from the Brazilian rubber tree into sunflowers he can increase the latex production of the stems from around 50 pounds per acre to around 800 pounds.

"At $1 US a pound, that's a fairly high-valued crop", he says. The southwestern Guayule bush may also be a source of genetic material for the project. The United States demand alone for rubber-derived finished goods is $28 billion per year.

Sunflowers help remediate areas of chemical and radiation pollution.

Near Chernobyl, in the Ukraine, where a nuclear reactor had a meltdown many years ago, sunflowers were grown on floating rafts in ponds full of cesium, and strontium. The plants flourished and absorbed 90% of the radioactivity from the water in the first generation. These radioactive minerals are then concentrated thousands of times greater than the surrounding water.

At the same time, be careful with cadmium rich soils. Sunflowers tend to accumulate the heavy metal in the seeds, at levels exceeding health standards. In one experiment conducted in Germany, the seeds were found to contain 1.1 mg/kg, even when the soil cadmium level was below the 3mg/kg widely accepted for agricultural use.

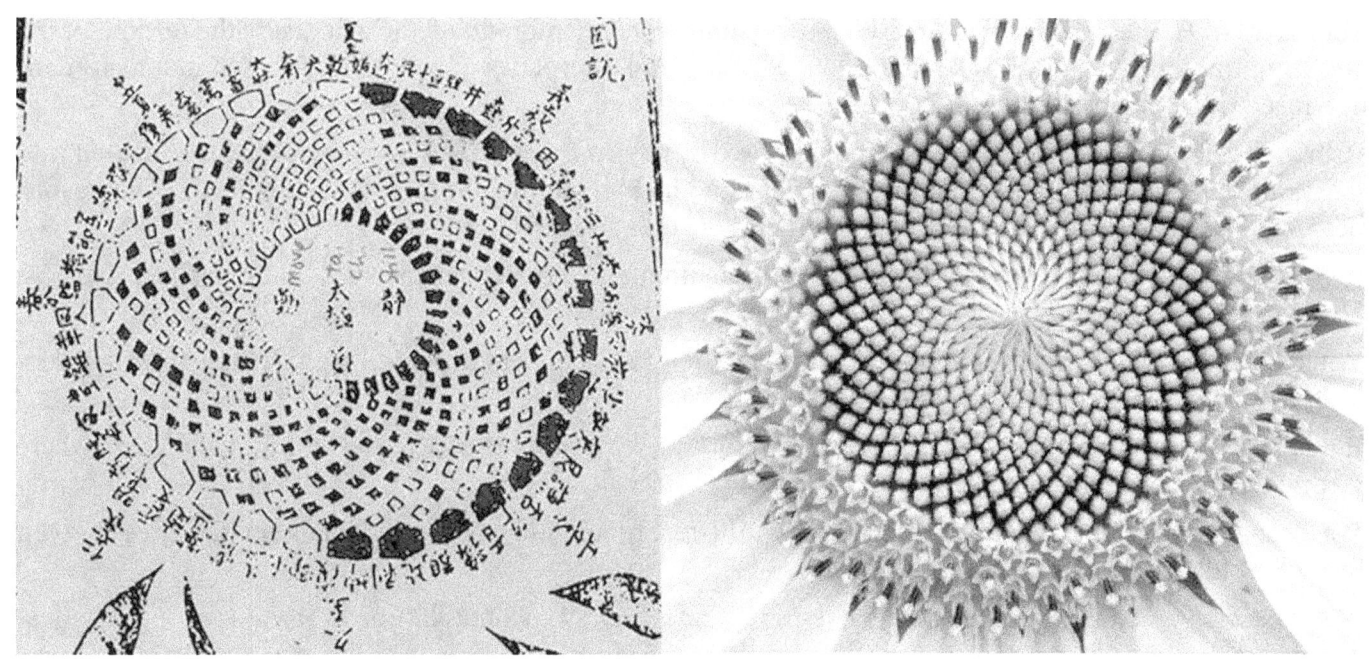

SUNFLOWER AND I CHING

Sunflowers extract heavy metals such as lead, uranium, strontium, cesium, chromium, copper, manganese, nickel and zinc. They also show promise in degrading PAHs in soil.

Sunflower uses a lot of carbon dioxide, each plant requiring 14 ounces per month. Industries requiring carbon credits need look no further.

Sunflower seeds, de-hulled, are used in veterinary medicine for horses suffering respiratory distress, coughs, and heaving of flanks.

In one study, researchers found that feeding dairy cows on kilogram of whole sunflower seed daily, increased milk yields substantially with little or no loss of protein or milk fat, and revenue increase of $2 per cow per day.

The sunflower grows in spirals of 21, 34, 55, 89 and 144 seeds, each number the sum of the previous two numbers. This pattern is found everywhere in nature, from pine needles, sea shells, parrot beaks and spiral galaxies. It is related to the golden mean, a basis for Egyptian pyramids and the Greek Parthenon, as well as art and music.

Even in our own ear's spiral-shaped cochlea, musical notes vibrate to this same ratio. Fabonacci numbers and the golden mean are common in nature and art.

Sunflower buds tend to follow the sun, but once opened, tend to face east, possibly to protect them on very hot days. This heliotropic movement called nutation results from the stems bending toward the sun. Growth is equalized at night, the stem slowly straightening out and at dawn again face east.

On cloudy days they remain facing east. The leaves are heliotropic and if removed the sunflower's head no longer follows the sun. Once the ray flowers are fully developed, movement ceases.

Bears and other animals feed on the tuberous roots of Nuttall's Sunflower, a perennial very closely related to Jerusalem Artichoke. The Cree call this particular Sunflower species, **OWTIYHIYMESKIYHKIY**, or sometimes **MITIYHIYMESKIYHKIY**.

The Cree of Alberta would use the mature root decoction to treat heart problems. The Navaho made an infusion of the dry crushed leaves for stomach troubles.

The leaves of *H. maximiliani* contain 8-beta-sarracinoyloxycumambranolide, which deters the feeding of the sunflower moth larvae. Various sesquiterpene lactones and diterpenes in all species are rich in anti-feedant and insecticidal potential.

Prairie Sunflower (*H. petiolaris*) was traditionally used by the Hopi as a "spider medicine". The Navaho used cold infusions of the flowers sprinkled on clothing for good luck in hunting. In British Columbia, the Thompsons powdered the leaves either alone or in an ointment for sores and swellings.

A tincture of the seeds can be used to treat sub-acute lung infections, as well as allergy related coughs. The tincture is also slightly diuretic.

When I lived near Joussard in the early 1970s, my mentor Jean Chancelet introduced me to Jerusalem Artichokes. They are neither from Jerusalem nor Artichokes.

It was early spring, the ground still frozen, and the snow barely gone. I took a shovel and started digging where directed, and out popped these numerous tubers.

We cleaned and steamed them later that day, and the rest I took home to plant. By fall, they had reached ten feet, with small sunflower-like faces.

The tubers have a crisp texture like water chestnuts, and a slightly coconut flavour.

They can be baked, boiled, roasted, or eaten raw, but in large quantities will cause gas and bloating.

The unopened buds of all these plants can be steamed and eaten like globe artichokes. The French explorer, Champlain, wrote that the roots tasted like artichokes, explaining half the name.

Various native tribes ate the roots. The Chippewa called them raw thing or **A'SKIBWAN'**. Champlain reported seeing them under cultivation near Cape Cod in 1605. The Cree name for the root was **ASKIPAW**, which was corrupted by Europeans into Esquebois. This is very similar to the Cree name for potato, **ASKIPWAW**.

The Cheyenne name is **HOHINON**, and the Pawnee name is **KISU-SIT**, meaning long or tapering.

When introduced into England, it became known as Potato of Canada. The juice squeezed from the plant blossoms was formerly used to restore hair growth.

In the United States, both the tubers and above ground parts are used for livestock feed. The leaves contain a protein isolate rich in lysine, and an amino acid profile comparable to major cereal proteins.

Potential protein yield, from three monthly cuttings, is estimated to be 800 kg/hectare.

In studies by Rawate and Hill at the University of Minnesota in 1985, a protein isolate obtained by water extraction from the tops contained 67-76% protein, also rich in lysine.

The tubers are rich in protein, with methionine the limiting amino acid, containing 58% of that found in eggs.

The tuber can be used in the manufacture of syrup, containing 70-80% fructose, and 20-30% glucose.

The tubers can be sliced and roasted in an oven as a coffee substitute. Combined with the roasted sunflower seed, you have a healthy, sweet beverage from two members of the same genus.

Methods to give high extraction rates of inulin (21%) from the dried tubers has been achieved.

Inulin demand as a prebiotic is increasing worldwide. A new Inulin plant, Asia's largest, has recently been completed in China. The first crop of 50,000 tonnes of tubers was expected to produce some 4500 tonnes of inulin in 2005.

Inulinase is present in inactive form, except during the germination period, one at pH 3, and the other at pH 6.

Inulinase is activated when the pressed juice is treated with trypsin, pepsin, papain or pressed juice of the germinating shoot.

Jerusalem artichoke flowers mature late in fall and are a valuable source of nectar and pollen.

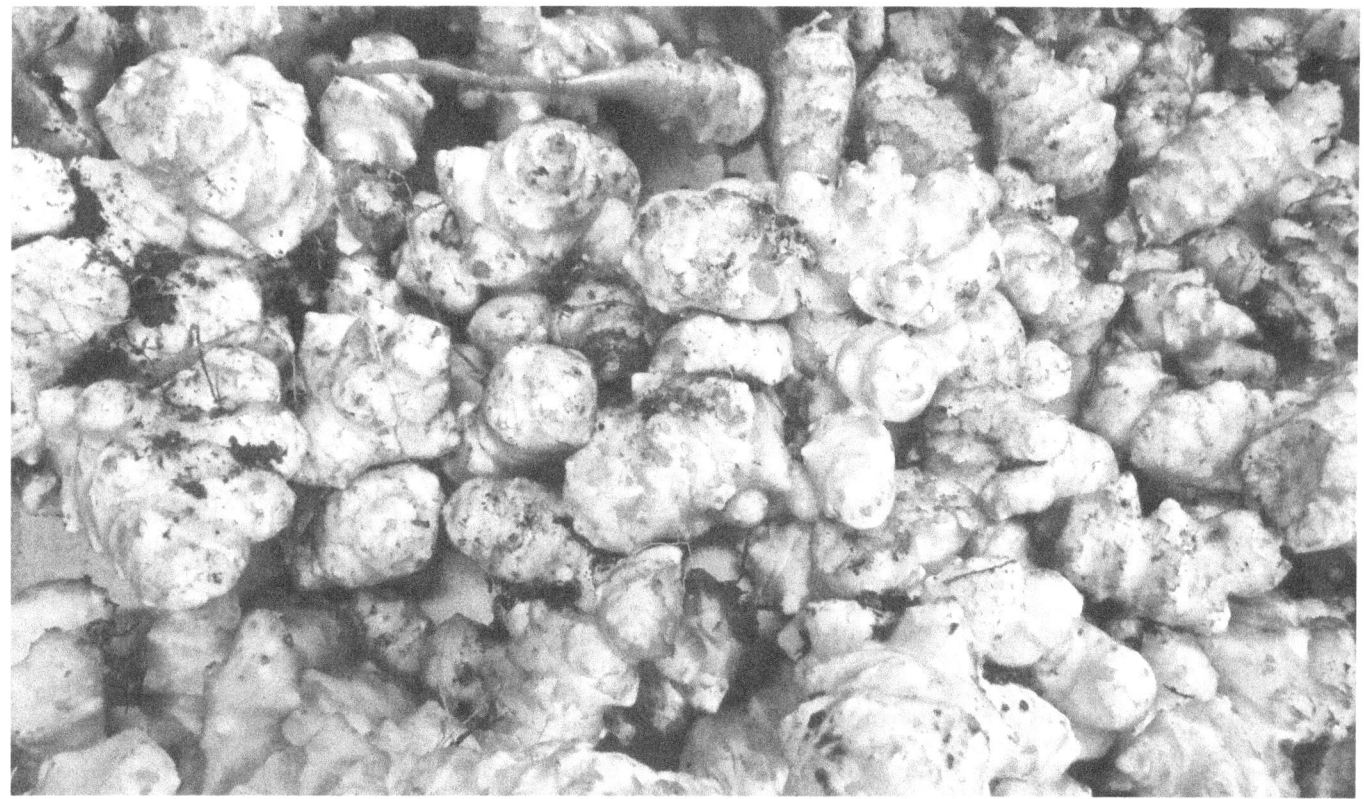

FRESH JERUSALEM ARTICHOKE TUBERS

Sugar yield ranges from 0.09 to 0.3 mg/flower and honey production from 30-60 kg/hectare, in 1988 studies by Cirnu from Romania.

Recently, genetic engineers in Holland have altered the sugar beet by introducing genes from the Jerusalem artichoke. If this is commercially viable, it will change the economics of inulin as both beets and chicory use similar machinery and technology.

This creates a high tech sugar beet that produces fructan, instead of sucrose.

Fructans are polymers of fructose that cannot be digested by humans, and are therefore sought by low calorie food manufacturers.

Jerusalem artichoke naturally converts sucrose to fructan, and the genetically altered sugar beets grew normally and converted virtually all sucrose to fructans.

High fructose syrups are another possibility, with a greater sweetening effect than sucrose or D- glucose. Optics are not favorable, however, as high fructose corn syrup has fallen into disrespect amongst nutritionists.

A fermented beer can be produced form the root sugars, and is said to be better than that from sugar beets.

Spring harvested tubers containing low molecular weight inulin are suited for fermentations or isolation of oligosaccharides; while fall harvested tubers not exposed to frost contain high molecular weight inulin and are better for production of high fructose syrup.

In China, the tubers are dried and pickled as a relish.

Both the tubers and tops can also be used for producing ethanol that is competitive with corn. During World War II, the French set up ten factories where fuel alcohol was made from Jerusalem Artichokes. One ton of tubers yielded 19 gallons of alcohol. The residue was then used as cattle feed. Bio-ethanol is another possible application.

Several cultivars have been examined at Morden Research Station in Manitoba for production, including Columbia, Challenger and Sunroot 1000, which has red-colored roots.

Average yields of 16,000-20,000 kilos per hectare can be expected, with production costs similar to potatoes. At a conversion rate of 80-90%, ethanol yields of 3900-4500 litres per hectare could be achieved. This translates into 1.7, 2.0 and 3.7 times more alcohol per hectare than sugar beets, corn and wheat respectively.

While processing for ethanol, the protein can be extracted. Work by Curt et al, *Ind Crops and Products* 2006 24:3 found the potential of stems for bio-ethanol was 38% that of the tubers.

Content of sucrose and FOS has been found highest in the stalk in August, at least when grown in Norway. Slimestad et al, *J Sci Food* Ag 90:6.

And as a bonus, it has been found that roots grown in nematode-infested soil can reduce the population by 45%, in studies by Kay in 1973.

Jerusalem Artichoke juice has been found to provide the same protection for weaner pigs as in feed antibiotics. For two weeks after weaning, four ml of juice daily were recommended, and two hours after the meals, the lactic acid concentrations in the hindgut showed no increase.

Flower infusions have been used to kill flies. Tests have shown water infusions of the flowers are toxic to mice but not to rabbits.

An old remedy for baldness involved rubbing a cut tuber on the hair roots.

Fuseau, or tophinol, is thought to be a cross species hybrid of Jerusalem Artichoke and the Wood Sunflower (*H. strumosus*). This has not been substantiated, however. Fuseau, shaped like a spindle, is a popular cultivar, due to its easy peeling shape.

Breeding specialists have used hybridization to breed resistance into its close cousin, the sunflower. In fact, the two will produce fertile offspring.

MEDICINAL

CONSTITUENTS- sunflower seeds- high in vitamins A, B, D (92 IU/100 g) and E, zinc, protein (24%), oil (47%), albumin, betaine, calcium, chlorine, flourine (2.6 ppm), copper, choline, histidine, iron, lecithin, as well as fatty acids; quinic and isochlorogenic, citric, tartaric, caffeic, and chlorogenic acids; SAM (S-adenosyl-methionine), Urease; helianthic acid; 270 mg/100 grams of phytosterols, composed mainly of beta sitosterol and lesser amounts of campesterol and stigmasterol. Trehalose is a unique sugar.
Seed sprouts- vitamin D
flowers- bisdesmosidic triterpenoid saponins (helianthosides), lutein (dried petal, 0.078%), sterols, syn alkane-6,8-diol; maniladiol, 24-methyl-enecyclo-artenol, various diterpenes such as grandifloric acid, ciliaric acid, several ent-kaurane derivatives.
sepal- sterol like substance (C21H3602)
corolla- 0.266% quercimeritrin.
root- inulin
young plants- asparagin, potassium nitrate, potassium carbonate, tannins, quercimetrin (flavonic glycoside)
leaf- citric and malic acid (1mg/gram), as well as malonic, lactic, succinic, aconitic, chlorogenic and fumaric acids, urease; heliannuols, three 7,10-heliannanes, nevadensin, a natural aglycone lignan, tanegool, as well as pinoresinol, lariciresinol, and di-hydro-dehydroiconiferilic alcohol.
pith- uronic acid (galacturonic complex). quinic and chlorogenic acids; as well as 53% sugars; potassium nitrate, potassium carbonate
receptacle- benzopyran derivatives.
galls- histopine
pollen- 8 fatty acid esters of triterpene alcohols, 4 free triterpene alcohols, 4 diterpene acids, six 3,4-seco-tirucallane-type triterpenoids, two tocopherol compounds, 4 estolides, 3 syn-alkane-4,6 diols; 1,3-dioxalkanoic acid, and an aliphatic ketone, and free fatty acids.

H. tuberosus- polysaccharides, in particular inulin (fructosan), diterpene acids, saccharose, pseudo-inulin, inulenin, helianthenin, synanthrin and a volatile oil including some beta bisabolen. The ripe tubers also contain levulose and dextrose, and 0.008% betaine hydrochloride.

Glutamine is the richest amino acid at 27.8 g/100 grams of protein. Methionine is also high. Also contains iron, silicon, and spermine. Tubers of some varieities contain over 6% protein.

stem- 14% cellulose.

leaves- deactylviquiestenin, erioflorin, chlorogenic acid

H. couplandii- kauranoic acid esters

H. nuttallii leaf- grandifloric acid, ciliaric acid, furanoheliangolides; 12,8-cis-lactonized eudesmanolides

H. petiolaris- leaves and flower heads- 5 kaurane and trachylobane type diterpenes, four 3,10-furanoheliango-lides; 5,10-epoxygermacranolide helivy-polide; 11alpah, 13-dihydrooxyde-hidrocostus lactone; the unusual 5,10-epoxy-germacranolide; and 3-methoxy-1,2-anhydridoniveusin A; niveusin B; ciliaric acid.

H. maximilianii- cumambranolide-8- (angelate); (2',3'-epoxyangelate); (2'-hydroxyethyl)acrylate; and sarracinate; 3-hydroxycostunolide-8-sarracinate; 2-hydroxycostunolide-8-(2',3'-epoxyange-late); desacetyl-eupasserin; tifruiticin; acetyl-tifruiticin; mollisorin B; deoxy-tifruiticin; acetyledeoxy-tifruiticin; an orizabin derivative; and an ent-labdane diterpene acid.

Sunflower seed and leaf infusions are used as a mild expectorant, useful for bronchial and laryngeal complaints. At one time roasted seed infusions were used for whooping cough. For asthma, the boiled seeds are decocted to half water and made into honey syrup.

The seeds combine well with comfrey and licorice root for this purpose.

A 10% tincture of the flower, made with 70% alcohol, is a recommended febrifuge.

Sunflower seeds are good for the muscles, nerves and blood vessels. The seeds are rich in arginine, an amino acid deficient in men with low sperm count. Arginine has potential cardiovascular health benefits, and is a precursor to nitric oxide.

Habitual eating of the seeds is said to build up physical endurance and resistance against disease. They are deficient in lysine, and when the seeds or flour is supplemented with lysine is a more complete protein, practically equal to that of casein. Sunflower seed combined with grain is a complete protein, high in biological food value.

They are said to help preserve natural sight for a long time without glasses.

Sunflower seeds contain SAM-e (S-adenosyl methionine) a compound used today for treating depression.

SAM-e has pain relieving and anti-inflammatory properties similar to ibuprofen. Much weaker, of course, it would take 250 grams of seed to equal the effect of a single dose of ibuprofen. One study of 20,641 patients with osteoarthritis found SAM-e as effective as OTC pain relievers. Berger & Nowak, *Am J Med* 1987 83.

Furthermore there are very few side effects. A two-year study by Konig, in the same journal, found no significant side effects.

It appears that SAMe increases chondrocyte activity, which involves destroying old cartilage to make room for new, or recycling and renewing. It increases concentrations of synovial fluid 3-4 times, helping lubricate joints.

It prevents the breakdown of proteoglycans, cartilage molecules that retain water, and make the joints flexible and moist.

Najm and other researchers at U of California, Irvine *BMC Musculoskel Disord* 2004 5:1 found "SAMe…is as effective as celecoxib in the management of the symptoms of knee osteoarthritis". In this randomized, double-blind crossover study, researchers assigned 56 patients either 1200 mg of SAMe or 200 mg celecoxib daily for four months. The drug works more quickly, but SAMe was found equally effective over time.

SAMe undergoes methylation and during breakdown releases homocysteine, which can cause cardiovascular harm. In the presence of B vitamins, especially B6, B12, and folic acid, the homocysteine remethylates into methionine or is converted to glutathione, a useful anti-oxidant. Fortunately, sunflower seeds are rich in B vitamins.

Sunflower seeds are a rich source of phenylalanine, which helps reduce pain by inhibiting the breakdown of enkephalins, chemicals involved in pain perception. In laboratory rats, phenylalanine enhanced the effect of morphine and prolonged its action. In humans, it makes acupuncture for reducing pain more effective.

It is involved in the methylation of monoamines, neurotransmitters and phospholipids.

Normally, the brain manufactures all the SAM-e it needs from methionine, but in depressed patients the synthesis is impaired. Added SAM-e results in increased production of serotonin and dopamine, and improved binding of neuro-transmitters to receptor sites.

Matthew Wood notes that sunflowers are Bear medicine. The root is brown and furry, and the seeds contain oils that build up the adrenals and kidneys.

Sunflower kernels contain choline, lecithin and betaine, the latter reducing homocysteine levels in the blood and protecting against heart disease. Choline and lecithin are precursors to phospholipids needed to nourish and insulate neurons of the body and brain.

Betaine is a minor component of red wine, and yet may be part of the French Paradox of a highly saturated fat diet, and yet low national cardiovascular disease rates. Betaine is rich in beets (see Liver) and is a pre-cursor of dopamine production.

Sunflower seed proteins, when hydrolyzed with pepsin and pancreatin, are a potential source of ACE inhibitory peptide. Inhibition of the angiotensin-I converting enzyme leads to reduction of hypertension. Cristina Megias et al, *J Ag Food Chem* 2004 52 suggested defatted sunflower meal may be a useful supplement source of bioactive peptides with anti-hypertensive properties. Why de-fat, the oils are good?

Secoisolariciresinol, a lignan found in flaxseed, with phytoestrogenic and anti-oxidant activity, is found in sunflower seeds, but in much lower amounts.

Sunflower seeds in a water extract have been found to exhibit anti-asthmatic benefit, *in vivo*. Work by Heo et al, *Int J Mol Med* 2008 21:1 found the extract decreased CD4+ and IgE levels, and changed the IL-4/IL-13 expression in mice.

The seeds are rich in chlorogenic and caffeic acids, anti-oxidants with anti-carcinogenic activity.

A derivative of chlorogenic acid from sunflower seed is an inhibitor of arginase and the seeds also contain trypsin enzyme inhibitors.

Work by Moller et al, *Phytother Res* 2008 Nov 11 found ethanol extracts of sunflower and flax seeds possess strong lipase inhibition.

The pectin found in seeds helps give protection against radiation poisoning, according to Dr. Eugene Zampieron and Ellen Kamhi, in *The Natural Medicine Chest*. Not sure.

The seeds contain a unique sugar, trehalose, previously known as mushroom sugar or mycose. It is found naturally in sugars produced by Douglas fir and other conifers.

In Huntington's disease, a huntingtin protein binds to a transcription regulator within a cell, and the genetic activity is disturbed and the cell's control of protein synthesis breaks down. This leads to glutamate remaining between neurons, acting as an excitotoxin.

The elongated huntingtin protein chain causes the neurons to kill themselves.

In 2004, researchers at the RIKEN Brain Science Institute inhibited the aggregation of the proteins with trehalose. This blocking of clumping delayed the disease's onset in mice. Harper et al, *Proceed Nat Acad Sci* 2005 102 16.

Trehalose and hyaluronic acid eyedrops were tested in a phase III, randomized, multi-centre study involving 105 patients with moderate to severe dry eye disease. It proved highly effective. Chiambaretta F et al, *Eur J Ophthalmol* 2017 27(1): 1-9.

This is interesting as Matt Wood points out, J. I. Rodale of organic gardening fame, found sunflowers useful for eyesight in sunny, snowy weather. Alpha crystalline aggregates precipitate lens opacification (cataracts) and vision impairment. Trehalose stabilizes this structure and inhibits alpha crystallin aggregation. Attanasio F et al, *Biochem Biophys Res Commun* 2007 354(4): 899-905.

Sunflower seed sprouts are a rich source of vitamin D, and high in antioxidant activity.

The sprouts contain high levels of cynarin, and exhibit inhibition of advanced glycation end products, in a manner stronger than aminoquandine. Sun, Z et al, *J Ag Food Chem* 2012 60:12 3260-5.

In Traditional Chinese Medicine, the sunflower seed is decocted to treat constipation, and to promote eruption of measles. It is known as either **XIANG RI KUI ZI** meaning facing sun flower seed; **YI ZHANG JU**, meaning ten-foot chrysanthemum, or simply **KUI HUA ZI**.

Dr. Cook considered sunflower seed, burdock seed and Bittersweet (*Celastrus scandens*) to be the only remedies that effectively increase sebaceous sweat from the skin.

The seeds act "efficiently upon the kidneys—promoting the flow of urine, and soothing inflamed and irritable conditions both of the kidneys and the bladder."

This may be true. But a recent randomized controlled trial of 50 patients (15-30 years old) with *acne vulgaris*, suggests sunflower seeds aggravate the troublesome skin condition. Mohebbipour A et al, *Iran Red Crescent Med J* 2015 17(9): e16544.

The sunflower seed shells are used for tinnitus in the form of a decoction.

The leaves are considered bitter, stomachic and useful for treating high blood pressure.

The stems can be cut and dried and infused for intermittent fevers, and are diuretic and useful in inflammatory conditions of the urinary tract.

The flower receptacle is used in folk medicine in China and known as **HSIANG JIH KUEI HUA PAN**.

It is decocted for its sweet, warm property and used to promote urination, reduce heat of headaches, dizziness and toothache. The flowers are used for stomach and abdominal pain, inducing labor and relieving menorrhagia.

Ethanol extracts of the flower head have been shown to reduce blood pressure in cats, due to the dilation of blood vessels.

The flower petals contain syn-alkane-6, 8-diol, shown to inhibit tumor-promoting activity and possess remarkable anti-inflammatory activity. Ukiya et al, *J Agric Food Chemistry* 2003 51.

Flower petals of *H. angustifolia* exhibit activity against leukemia, breast, glioblastoma, and colon cancer cell lines. Kretschmer et al, *Planta Med* 77:17 1912-15.

Various diterpenes, from flowers show moderate cytoxicity against SF-268, MCF-7, and HepG2 cancer cell lines. Suo MR et al, *Yao Xue Xue Bao* 2007 42(2): 166-70.

Sunflower pollen showed potent inhibitory effect (97-100%) on Epstein-Barr virus early antigen, in the same study. In a later study in *J Nat Products* 66:11 the author identified sunpollenol and other 3,4-seco tricallan type triterpenoids in the flowers.

The fresh roots are used for treating stomachache, urinary problems, constipation, traumatic injury, and hernias. In southern China, the fresh root is decocted for treating pain in the penis due to gonorrhea. For hernias, the decoction is mixed with brown sugar.

The pith is used for urinary troubles, including milky or bloody urine, as well as stones. It is used for whooping cough and external bleeding.

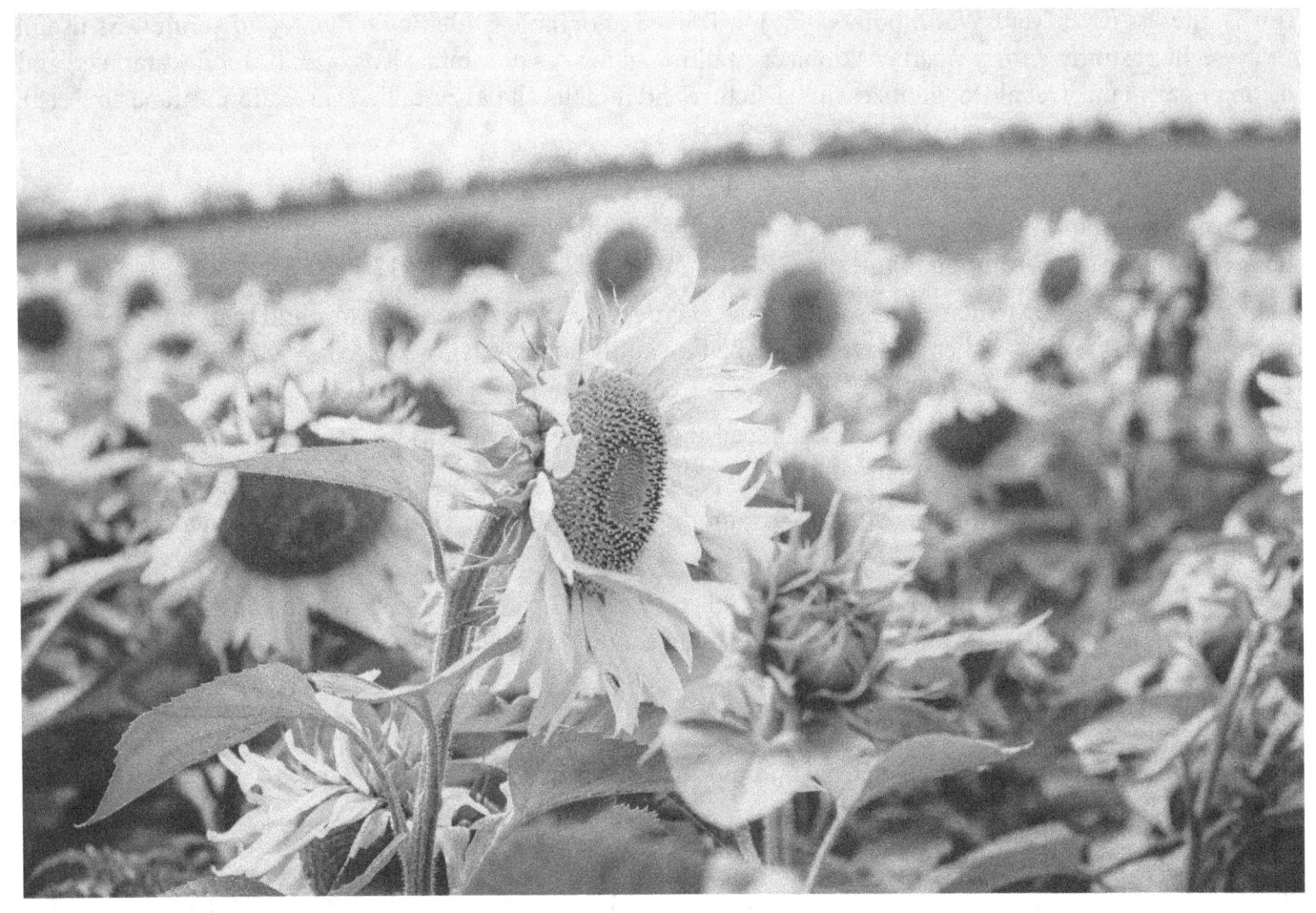

SUNFLOWERS

For stones of the urethra or kidney, a meter of pith is slowly boiled down to one-quarter of the original volume and taken once daily for one week.

In Mongolia, the fresh pith is mashed and applied directly to wounds and cuts to stop bleeding.

The flower receptacles are decocted to treat headaches, dizziness, toothache, stomachache, menstrual pain, sores and swellings.

Recently in China, the fresh receptacles have been boiled until a sticky mass remains. This is applied to affected arthritic joints with all patients showing some improvement.

For mastitis, the receptacles are cleaned of seeds, and dried, chopped and roasted until powder. Nine to 16 grams are mixed in white wine, with all 122 patients reporting satisfactory results.

Helianthoside A, a bitter saponin from the petals, has been shown hemolytic.

In Russia, the seeds are used for bronchial infections, and the stems and heads macerated in vodka (what else?) for tuberculosis and malaria.

In Italy, the aerial parts are used as a diuretic, febrifuge and stimulant.

The well-strained water can be used to ease acute eye inflammation.

The whole plant can be decocted and added to bath water for arthritic pain and joint swelling.

The crushed root is applied to bruises. Heated, the roots relieve rheumatism; when applied cold are good for blisters and headaches.

The root contains inulin, which scientific research has shown to be effective against the wheezing associated with asthma and other bronchial conditions.

Early Eclectic physicians, such as Dr. Howard suggested western sunflower root for medicinal purpose. "A strong decoction of the root, drank freely, will operate as an emetic, and by continuing its used more moderately, relaxes the bowels, promotes perspiration, and effectually cures fevers."

Medicinally, the seed oil is specific for coughs as well as inflammation of the bladder and diseases of the kidney.

Sunflower leaves are astringent in nature, and have been infused for intermittent fever associated with malaria and other such conditions, and confirmed by Danzel.

This may be explained, in part, by the fact that flower infusions have weak insecticidal properties.

The green leaves and stems show positive for *Staphylococcus aureus*, while the roots show activity against *Micrococcus tuberculosis.*

The leaves contain various sesquiterpene lactones with activity against various Gram positive and negative bacteria, and several fungi.

One compound, 15-hydroxy-3-dehydrodesoxyfruticin, shows cytotoxicity against myeloma cells, and Ehrlich carcinoma. Spring O et al, *Z Naturforsch* C 1982 37(11-12): 1087-91.

Trachlboban-19-oic acid and (-)-kaur-16-en-19-oic acid are both anti-microbial agents found in sunflower.

Stem extracts, in tincture, possess activity against *Mycobacterium tuberculosis*. This study was based on observing traditional usage by Mayo of southern Sonora, Mexico. Coronado-Aceves EW et al, *J Ethnopharm* 2016 190: 106-15.

Laboratory tests indicate flower extracts are very stimulating to intestinal contraction, and may be of use in intestinal atony.

Nevadensin is found in the leaves and glandular trichomes of several sunflower species. The compound shows activity against tuberculosis at the rate of 0.2 mg/ml-1 in vitro. Reddy GB et al, *Int J Pharmacognosy* 1991 29.

The same study found significant anti-inflammatory and cytotoxic activity. The compound was more effective than wogonin (see Scullcap species) in Dalton's lymphoma and Ehrlich ascites carcinoma cells. Dong et al, *J Nat Prod* 1987 50.

Nevadensin exhibits hypotensive effects, both central and peripheral, in nature. Song et al, *Acta Pharm Sin* 1985 6.

It exhibits activity against *Escherichia coli* and *Staphylococcus aureus*. Brahmachari et al, *Open Nat Prod Journal* 2008 1. A more complete review of nevadensin can be found by the same author in *Int J Green Pharm* 2010 4:4.

Niveusin C, in common and narrow-leaved sunflowers, has proven cytotoxic and anti-tumour activity.

Sunflower, like nettles and spinach, contains choline acetyltransferase, a form of acetylcholine for the brain.

Triterpenoid saponins derived from sunflower, Plohmann et al, University of Regensburg, Germany (1997), showed immune-modulating and anti-tumour effect.

Helianol, a triterpene alcohol present in *H. annuus* flowers showed marked anti-inflammatory activity. Akihisa et al, *Nihon University* in Tokyo, 1996.

Cosmos, safflower and Chinese chrysanthemum all contain levels of helianol.

Sunflower petals contain maniladiol and other compounds that reduce inflammatory response. Other triterpene glycosides may also be responsible for anti-inflammatory properties. Ukiya et al, *J Nat Prod* 70:5.

The sunflower receptacles have been analyzed for anti-microbial substances. Satoh et al, Hokkaido University, Japan 1996. Two anti-fungal benzopyran derivatives have been isolated and evaluated.

In the mesophyll cells of sunflower cotyledons, are found high catalase concentrations.

Crown gall tumors on sunflower contain histopine, an unusual amino acid derivative of histidine.

Jerusalem Artichokes are a medicinal food, rich in inulin, an invert sugar without need for insulin, and suitable for diabetes, atherosclerosis, and obesity diets.

Jerusalem Artichokes can be juiced, for example, along with carrot, beets, celery and other vegetables to satisfy "our sweet tooth", and satiate flavor centers of the brain, by triggering taste buds on the sides of the tongue. This is very helpful in weight loss programs, where the brain is constantly seeking pleasurable foods.

Work by Burkova et al, in 2004 studied the tuber powder in a controlled study on obese spa patients. Studies found those patients taking the powder improved their carbohydrate and lipid metabolism as well as blood and hormonal factors such as cortisol thyroxin, and insulin.

Various animal studies find the tubers improve glucose tolerance and lipids profiles.

Fructo-oligosaccharides (FOS) present in the tubers have been found to enhance and promote the growth of healthy bacteria in the human intestine. This is significant and could be a very helpful tool, in those immune compromised individuals needing to restore normal bowel flora. Chicory, burdock and dandelion roots all contain inulin.

Inulin derivatives possess anti-arrhythmic, anti-tuberculosis, anti-carcinogenic, anti-coagulating, and fibrinolytic properties.

Dr. Vogel suggests the tincture is "favorable to men's libido and to the production of spermatozoids."

The leaf and stalk can be prepared as an infusion for the relief of rheumatism. Afro-Americans of South Carolina, traditionally steeped the leaves in rum as a remedy for dropsy, and kidney tonic.

Both the stem and root give positive antibacterial results against various gram positive and negative bacteria like *Staphylococcus aureus* and *E. coli*.

The leaves contain chlorogenic acid, which has a structure similar to the anti-viral, anti-flu drugs Tamiflu and Relenza.

The plant is known as Topinambour, in France and parts of Europe. In 1613, six natives from the Topinambous tribe of Brazil were brought to the court of King Louis XIII. The new vegetable had just been introduced but lacking a novel name, put the two together, figuring they both came from the same part of the New World.

A recent paper by Bobrovnyk et al, from Kiev, was delivered at a *Precision Agricultural and Biological Control* conference in Boston in 1998. It articulates other medicinal and bioactive substances in the plant. Spermine, for example, is used in biochemical research.

Experiments by Reshetnik et al, *Voprosy-Pitaniya* 1998 1 found the tubers have very low ability to absorb heavy metals, including lead, cobalt, nickel, strontium, and caesium.

A list of possible applications for inulin, derived from Jerusalem artichokes, include prebiotics, dietary fiber, sweeteners, high fructose syrups, and purified inulin for medical use.

Non-food uses include furfural, mannitol, glycerol, ethylene glycol, acetone, butanol, succinic acid, lactic acid and a range of complexing agents for precipitation of heavy metals.

Ten patents for medical/veterinary application have been filed, including treatment of calcium deficiency, diabetic hepatosis, synanthrin (blood stabilizer), as well as a cell growth factor with anti-tumor and anti-cancer activity.

As of 2008, over 150 applications for use in food, drink and nutraceuticals have been filed, as well as animal feeds and various industrial uses.

The book by Kays and Nottingham in the bibliography is a definitive text on this plant.

HOMEOPATHY

Sunflower (*H. annuus*) is used in cases of intermittent fever. It is for nasal congestion, catarrh, as well as nasal hemorrhage and thick scabs of the nose.

It is specific to rheumatic pain of the left knee, and is used externally as a vulnerary like Arnica and Calendula.

It is indicated for vomiting, black stools, congestion of the mouth and pharynx, and redness and heat of the skin.

The symptoms are aggravated by heat and relieved by vomiting. It is considered a spleen remedy, with marked effect on the stomach, whenever there is nausea and vomiting, and dry mouth.

DOSE- Tincture and low potencies. The mother tincture is prepared from the freshly and coarsely powdered seeds.

These provings are based on two males and one female taking expressed juice of the flowers and one woman eating excessive amounts of seeds in 1848.

Jerusalem Artichoke (*H. tuberosa*) is used for constipation, obesity, and as a therapeutic aid in the treatment of diabetes mellitus.

It is also helpful in helping achieve gradual weight loss without the rebound effect. It curbs the appetite and provides a source of energy at the same time.

DOSE- Mother tincture and low potencies. Intake of larger quantities of the partially hydrolyzed pressed must (with its high fructose content) can lead to elevated serum triglyceride levels in men.

Quantities that exceed 50 grams of fructose per day should be avoided, particularly in cases of hyper-triglyceridaemia or kidney insufficiency.

SEED OIL

Traditional sunflower seed oil is 69% linoleic acid. Hybrid breeding is changing all that, however.

Oleic acid is a mono-saturated fatty acid that can lower serum cholesterol and the risk of coronary heart disease.

NuSun hybrids, mentioned above, can produce oil with nearly 30% less saturated fatty acids than traditional hybrids. Potato chips fried in such an oil could be labeled as low in saturated fat. However, they are still junk food.

Mid-oleic oils (60-75%) require no hydrogenation and are low in saturated fats, creating new demand in the marketplace.

High oleic sunflower oil appears to increase the post-prandial response of circulating oleoylethanolamide and reduce energy intake at subsequent meals in humans. It is well known that dietary fat influences endocannabinoid response. Mennella I et al, *Food Funct* 2015 6(1): 204-10.

The costly and unhealthy step of bubbling hydrogen into polyunsaturated oils- partial hydrogenation won't be required to protect against flavour deterioration.

No hydrogenation means no creation of trans-fatty acids that are harmful to health.

A randomized study compared coconut and sunflower as cooking oil for two years, and found no change in lipid-related cardiovascular risk factors. Vijayakumar M et al, *Indian Heart J* 2016 68(4): 498-506.

The sunflower oil can be used internally to relieve constipation, acting as a lubricant. It can also be used externally as massage oil, or for poorly healing wounds in the form of an oil dressing. Numerous cosmetic companies, including Revlon, L'Oreal, Clairol, Avon and Vaseline, use sunflower seed oil in gels, creams, and hair product formulas.

It has been used in the past for skin sores, rheumatism and psoriasis.

Sunflower oil is an effective diuretic and can help to build healthy teeth in young children. Again, however, the quality of processing is all important. When oils were heated over 110° C, and fed to lab rats, the oil was found to cause liver damage and enhance effects of carcinogens.

A study was conducted by Prottey et al in 1975 on three patients suffering essential fatty acids due to chronic mal-absorption, and scaly dermatitis.

Cutaneous applications of sunflower seed oil to their right arms for two weeks led to major increases in the level of linoleic acids in the epidermal lecithin, significant lowering in the rate of transdermal water loss and the disappearance of scaly lesions.

Ozonized sunflower oil demonstrates significant anti-microbial activity as well as anti-inflammatory and wound healing problems. Topical application to preterm infants, in a randomized, controlled clinical trial, showed a significant reduction of nosocomical infections. Darnstadt et al, *Ped Infect Dis J* 2004 23.

Rodenas et al, *J Am Coll Nutr* 2005 24:5 found a mixture of sunflower and olive oil decreased total cholesterol, LDL and a lipoprotein in fourteen post menopausal women over four weeks. This suggests that a human trial of canola and sunflower oil may produce similar findings and a potential market opportunity.

Sunflower seed oil is a good substrate for production of CLA, or conjugated linoleic acid.

CLA is found naturally in milk, butter, cheese and meat, due to bacterial fermentation in the rumen, and is used in supplements, dietetic foods, as well as skin care and cosmetic products. Areas of interest include weight loss, and potential anti-cancer activity.

Its value in weight loss does not seem to bear out, in a recent DB, randomized PC trial of 74 women over twelve weeks. However, a decrease in hip circumference was noted in CLA group. Madry E et al, *Acta Sci Pol Technol Aliment* 2016 15(1): 107-113.

CLA may, however be useful for patients with rheumatoid arthritis and related auto-immune and bone disease. A randomized, double-blind trial of 52 patients found a significant different in activity of telopeptides C, osteocalin and IGF-1. Aryaeian N et al, *Lipids* 2016 51(12): 1397-1405.

In Ayurvedic medicine, sunflower seed oil is held under the tongue for twenty minutes and then spit out. Matthew Wood mentions it is an old Cherokee recipe for alcohol poisoning. The mouth is later rinsed out to remove the toxins.

He writes of a client poisoned by dental work. He had her hold sunflower oil under the tongue three times daily. After about ten minutes, the oils was burning, the same effect caused by the dental materials, and then she spit it out. She continued until the burning stopped, tapered off and recovered.

Sunflower oil is a reliable source of mixed tocopherols of vitamin E, making it the only vitamin E containing beta sitosterols, stigmasterols and campesterols.

An interesting, unusual study by P. Whitten, *Biology of Reproduction* 1993 49 had rat mothers fed sunflower seed oil, rich in coumestrol. Transferred through milk to newborn pups, the estrogenic effect of only ten days profoundly affected ovulation and sterility in females, and less mounting and fewer ejaculations in the juvenile males.

Low birth weight pre-term babies were given massage with or without sunflower oil. This single blind randomized clinical trial of 54 babies with birth weight of less than 2 kilos, found the sunflower group had greater weight gain. Fallah R et al, *Early Hum Dev* 2013 89(9): 769-72.

A mixture of 10% birch bark extract (betulin) and 90% sunflower oil was tested in a randomized phase III clinical trial on 219 patients with burns. It accelerated re-epithelialisation of partial thickness wounds, compared to standard of care. Barret JP et al, *Burns* 2017 April 8.

Sunflower oil is an attractant to leaf cutting ants, and may be useful in poisonous traps.

Prairie Sunflower (*H. couplandii*) seed contains 30% oil composed mainly (65%) of linolenic acid, 26% oleic acid and 5% saturated fats.

Narrow-leaved Sunflower (*H. maximilianii*) seed contains 30% oil, with 73% linoleic, 13% oleic, and just 0.5% linolenic acid.

Wild sunflower seed oil, native to Canada, contains 6% saturated fats; half of Mexican species.

LEAF, STEM & ROOT OIL

Jerusalem Artichoke contains lipids in all plant parts, consisting of fatty acids and unsaponifiable substances.

The leaves contain 2.7% lipids composed of 42% palmitic, 31% linoleic, 20% linolenic, and small amounts of oleic and stearic acids.

The stems contain 1.2% composed mainly of 45% palmitic and 40% linolenic acids.

The tubers contain 54% linoleic and 30% palmitic acid, as well as 12% linolenic.

The stem and leaf oil is dark green, that from the tubers a light brown.

ESSENTIAL OIL

The tubers and leaves of Jerusalem artichoke contain volatile oil with beta-bisabolene, at 63.1% and 70.7% respectively. Helmi Z et al, *Adv Pharm Bull* 2014 4(suppl2): 521-6.

The sunflower heads contain 0.2% of a strong smelling essential oil, composed of 72.6% alpha pinene.

Gerard, in his famous *English Herbal*, wrote the sunflower centre is "like some curious cloth wrought with the needle… from which sweats forth excellent fine and clear turpentine". Parkinson added that in warm weather both the flowers and leaf joints "sweat out a fine thin and clear rosin or turpentine, so like clear Venice turpentine that it cannot be known from it."

And oleo-distillate of the seeds in a 2% ointment has been found useful in a trial involving 20 adults with atopic dermatitis. Eichanfield et al, *Pediatr Dermatol* 2009 26:6.

Sunflower leaf essential oil contains 23% sabinene, 28% alpha pinene, 12% limonene and 7.8% isobornylacetate.

WAX

A wax has been isolated from sunflower seed oil, and found to consist mainly of ceryl cerotate. The hulls contain up to 10% of the same wax.

Ceryl Cerotate melts at 84° C, with the formula $C_{22}H_{104}O_2$. A minor part of the wax is sitosterol. It could be recovered from the whole sunflower seed with a solvent, before pressing, or later from the press cake.

Sunflower seed wax, if derived from supercritical fluid extraction, or another natural process, has use in the cosmetic industry.

Ching T. Hou, a chemist working in Peoria, Illinois found a *Pseudomonas aeruginosa*, in pond water, has the ability to convert the oleic acids in corn, safflower and sunflower oils into an unusual structure.

The compound called 7, 10-dihydroxy-8-(E)-octadecenoic acid is an excellent starting material for creating plastics, lubricants, paints, and new antibiotics.

FLOWER ESSENCES

Sunflower essence heals disturbances or distortions in the soul's relationship to the masculine. This is often associated with a conflicted or deficient relationship with the father in childhood. Sunflower essence brings to the soul the quality of light.

FLOWER ESSENCE SOCIETY

Sunflower essence is for compassion and tenderness; for the expressed love for helpless people, animals and the environment. It may be used with children who are selfish, or those who steep themselves in righteousness and superiority. Humility and inter-dependence are better understood.   **NEW ZEALAND**

Jerusalem Artichoke essence helps in the recognition that the knowledge and experience of other people can be very valuable.   **MIRIANA**

Sunflower essence tempers and spiritualizes the male ego. Lessening the impact of the overbearing male ego awakens the male's maternal instinct and desire to have children. This draws the individual closer to a sense of androgyny within the self. It also aligns the superconscious mind's spiritual values with the heart chakra.

Sunflower balances the yin and yang energies, and attunes people to higher wisdom. People demonstrating anger or hostility towards their father experience increased understanding with this essence.

Osteopathic and chiropractic adjustments are augmented. It stimulates the kundalini and aligns it properly along the spine. On the cellular level, absorption of vitamin D increases.

Sunflower dissolves fatty tissue. The ability of plants to receive the afternoon or evening sun will be enhanced.
                                                                                                            GURUDAS

POLLEN ESSENCE

Sunflower pollen essence is for uplifting and strengthening.   **HORUS**

SPIRITUAL PROPERTIES

Sunflower tempers and spiritualizes the male ego, and draws the individual closer to a sense of androgeny. It balances yin and yang energies, and attunes people to higher wisdom.

When people have trouble with their intuition, and want to know if their perception is correct, or if it is just the idle chatter of the material mind, sunflower resolves the problem.

On a cellular level, the absorption of Vitamin D is increased. It eases sunburn particularly if there is heat exhaustion or toxicity in the skin, including skin cancer.

Sunflower dissolves fatty tissue.

Associations with Leo are noted, for instance, the ability of individuals to work with progressed energy through Leo.   **GURUDAS**

These petals are an uncompromising yellow-orange. The color seems to contain all the energy this planet will ever need. This color could power a nuclear reactor. It rings like a carillon. It hits me, with a little punch, in the solar plexus.   **RUSSELL**

PERSONALITY TRAITS

The Sunflower originated in the New World, so any mention of sunflower in ancient Greece probably pertains to a daisy or marigold type flower that turns and follows the sun across the sky.

The Greeks called the Sunflower, Clytie or Kleite (Famous One).

Classical writers made her a water nymph who loved the sun god and followed his fructifying beams with her head. Since her name was also the root of the word Clitoris (Kleitoris), it seems that the myth may have begun with symbols of the divine marriage between Father Heaven and Mother Earth.   **WALKER**

Helios was born of Euryphaessa, the Moon Goddess, and the Titan Hyperion, who fathered Selene and the dawn goddess Eos.

In mythology, Helios was drowned by the Titans at sea, but rose up and ascended into the sky. Helios had a magnificent eastern palace that he left every morning and arrived in the western Islands of the Blessed every evening. He and his horses rested that night, and a golden ferry fashioned by Hephaestus, the Smith God, carried him, via the river Oceanus back east to start the journey anew.

In myth, he had a single round eye with which he observed everything. **PRAIRIE DEVA**

When I hear Jerusalem, I think of a spiritual place, the Bible's holy land; a place close to God that exudes purity and intimacy. In good Christian conscience I would like to change the name of this vegetable to Siberian Artichoke, or Dark side of the Moon Artichoke. **DARYL SHEPPARD**

DOCTRINE OF SIGNATURES

The deep root system of sunflower is far reaching, giving it the ability to draw trace minerals that may not be found in the topsoil.

The flower head's ability to follow the sun throughout the day is also a signature of the plant's amazing talents. Along with the vitamins and other nutrients found in sunflower seeds, these signatures symbolize the wealth of nutrients the plant has to offer us, and its incredible relationship with the sun.

The golden-yellow colour and shape of flower head, along with the golden yellowish, purplish disk, is also symbolic of the sun, and represent the fire of life, the will.

The stalk is sturdy and tall and gives a feeling of great strength, endurance, and a desire to reach toward the sun's natural power and light. These signatures relate to the third chakra, will, purpose, power, self-empowerment, and self honour. This is the energy centre that gives us the ability to think and reason, to gather the strength and power from deep within our roots, to find purpose and desire in life, to empower ourselves with who we are. The third chakra or solar plexus centre is sun energy. It is associated with the left side of the brain and its activities, representing the male or yang energy.

This gives us the ability to assert ourselves in the world with positive determination, optimism, and direction. The sunflower's large disk represents an eye. The eye of this plant is open wide and offers a journey of seeing and believing. **PALLASDOWNEY**

MYTHS AND LEGENDS

The people of India used the flower to represent their sun god Surya, and the people of ancient Persia used it to represent their sun god Mithras.

RECIPES

SUNBUTTER- Take one cup of raw sunflower seeds and add 1-2 tbsp of honey, or rosehips syrup and blend. Refrigerate. The seeds contain over 50% protein and are suitable for those needing to put on weight. It is a very rich spread not suitable for weight watchers!

SUNFLOWER SEED CHEESE- In the evening, take one pound of raw, shelled sunflower seeds, and cover with distilled water. In the morning, drain and combine one cup of soaked seeds, with one cup of distilled water, and put into blender or food processor. Pour into large bowl and let set for 4-7 hours. When ready, the surface will be puffy, and the water will have separated from puree, with a mild yogurt like smell.

Strain through cheesecloth, and then tie up corners and squeeze to remove excess moisture. Stored in fridge, it will keep about one week.

Use as a vegetable dip, or sandwich spread. As the protein, fats, and sugars are all predigested, the cheese is a very balanced and nutritious food.

CHOKE COFFEE- Slice the washed, fresh, sliced roots and place on cookie sheet. Slow roast in the oven at 250° F, until dark brown. Grind and use as coffee substitute.

SUNFLOWER BATH- Take whole dried plant, including some stem, and decoct until a beautiful purple gold. This is strained and added to hot baths for rheumatic and arthritic pain.

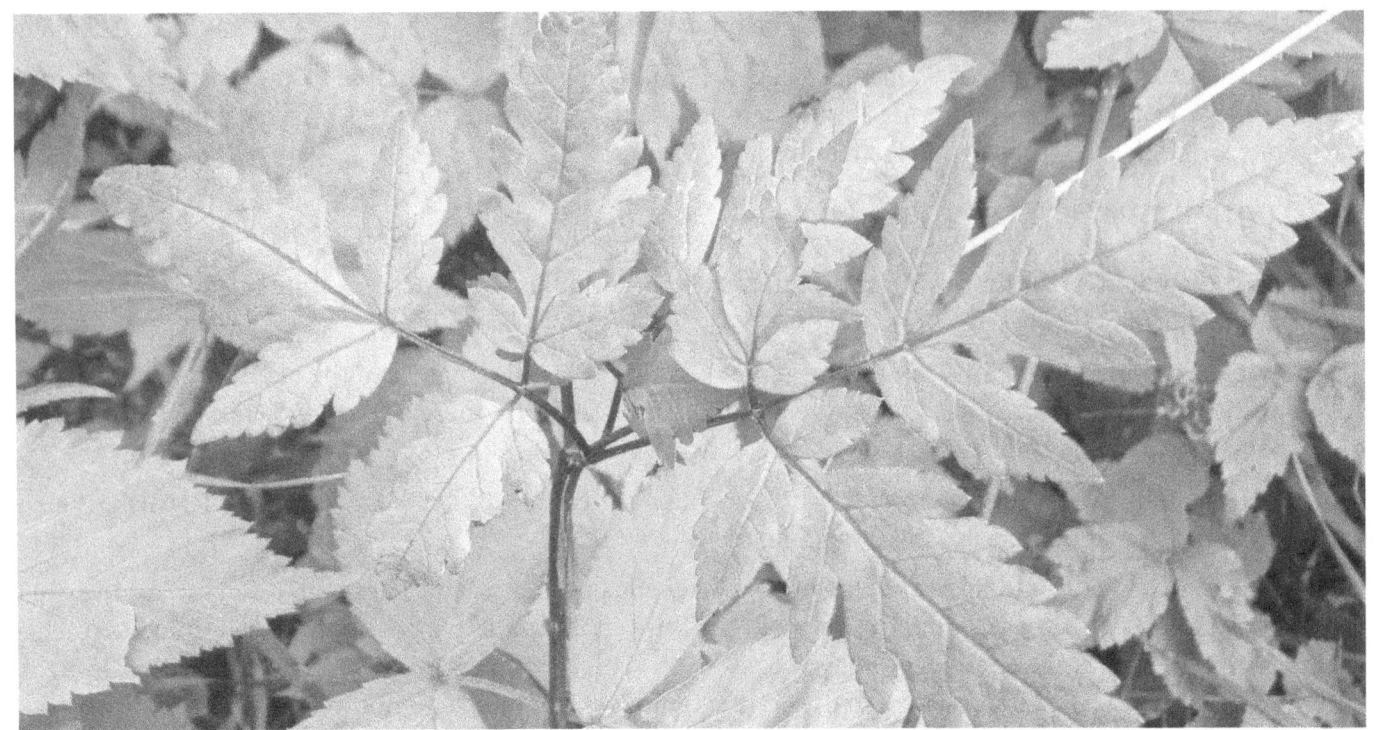

SWEET CICELY LEAVES

SMOOTH SWEET CICELY
SWEET ROOT
(*Osmorhiza aristata* [Thunb.] Rydb.)
LONG STYLE SWEET ROOT
(*O. aristata var. longistylis* [Torr] B. Boivin)
(*O. longistylis* [Torr.] DC.) not accepted
HAIRY SWEET CICELY
CLAYTON'S SWEETROOT
(*O. claytonii* [Michx.] C. B. Clarke)
(*O. aristata ssp. brevistylis* [DC.] B. Boivin)
                                        not accepted
MOUNTAIN SWEET CICELY
BLUNT FRUITED SWEET CICELY
(*O. chilensis* Hook. & Arn.) not accepted
(*O. berteroi* DC.)
(*O. divaricata* [Britton] Suksd.) not accepted

PURPLE SWEET CICELY
(*O. purpurea* [J.M. Coult. & Rose] Suksd.)
SPREADING SWEET CICELY
BLUNT FRUIT SWEET CICELY
(*O. depauperata* Phil)
WESTERN SWEET CICELY
(*O. occidentalis* [Nutt. ex Torr. & A. Gray] Torr.)
SWEET CICELY
(*Myrrhis odorata* [L.] Scop.)
PARTS USED- root, seeds

First let me tell you when her name has sprung,
Cecilia, meaning as the books agree,
Lily of Heaven in our English tongue,
To signify her chaste virginity.

CHAUCER

Cicely is from the Greek **SESELI** for a sweet smelling plant, or a carrot family member used in medicine.

Osmorhiza is from the Greek, **OSMO**, meaning sweet, and **RHIZA**, meaning root or rhizome. The root is sweet and anise- like.

Aristata is from the Latin meaning bearded and referring to the hairy seeds. Purpurea means purple, and depauperata means dwarfed or starved, perhaps due to its lower growing stature.

Myrrhis is from the Greek **MYRON**, meaning perfume or **MYRRHA**, fragrant or scent of plant.

Smooth Sweet Cicely (*O. longistylis*) roots, stems and leaves were infused by the Cheyenne for bloated or disordered stomachaches, and malfunctioning kidneys.

The root alone was taken for amenorrhea, or used as a nostril wash for improving their dog's sense of smell.

The Fox made compound infusions of the leaves to regain flesh and strength, but mainly used it as an eye remedy.

They grated the root and mixed it with salt for horse distemper.

The Ojibwa infused **SEGEDE BWENS** root to ease parturition, to soothe sore throats, and treat amenorrhea.

The Blackfoot used whole plant infusions for coughs and congestion of the nose and eyes. The root was gathered for winter to give a pleasant scented treat, and known as **PACH COI AU SAUKAS.**

Sweet Cicely root, valerian root and dried chokecherry bark was decocted to treat dysentery, and bloody diarrhea.

The Blood tribe of southern Alberta used Spreading Sweet Cicely (*O. depauperata*) root as a love potion. It was believed that a person holding a piece of root in their mouth could not tell lies.

It was in some ways sacred, and ordinary people could not touch the plant.

A charm of the plant was often tied to horses to help them win races.

The leaves were made into ceremonial wreaths to promote birthing of babies; and a wash of the roots used to bath newborn babies.

They used the plant for healing sores, chest and stomachaches, and even hemorrhage.

The neighboring Blackfoot gave various *Osmorhiza* species to pregnant mares in winter to improve their health, and prepare them for foal. This root, and those from *O. occidentalis* were used by women as a feminine deodorant.

A piece of root kept amongst clothing and quivers. Root infusions were used by the women to treat swollen breasts, coughs, ear problems, eyewash and to encourage labour in pregnancy. The volatile oil may play a role in these uses.

The stems were combined with ochre and applied to robes. Even "diapers" were sweetened with an infusion of the root.

Spreading Sweet Cicely is known as Sweetroot, Indian Carrot, or **SHWI TOK**, by the Thompson of British Columbia. The last two names were used for Yampah, another edible root. The nearby *O. claytonii* root is considerably less sweet, but the seeds have slight taste of anise.

Several tribes of interior, used the root of Mountain Sweet Cicely (*O. chilensis*) as food, the licorice-like taste breaking the monotony of biscuit root or yampah.

The Blackfoot made hot drinks of the root for coughs, colds or tickling in the throat. It was called Smell Root, and the symbolic power of a men's secret society that still exists today.

The Cheyenne used the root and leaves for colds; while the Karuk chewed the root for headaches, and placed it under their sleeping gear to prevent sickness.

It was known as *MUHISH* meaning "its seeds, according to Josephine Peters. It was also known as Black Jack, due to the licorice flavor that was similar to a gum once sold in stores.

The Cheyenne chewed the root to "bring one around" if too much peyote was ingested during ceremony.

The Swinomish chewed on the root as a love charm. Both the Omaha and Ponca used the root, according to legend, to attract horses. Other animals, including sheep, cattle, and deer are attracted to the scent.

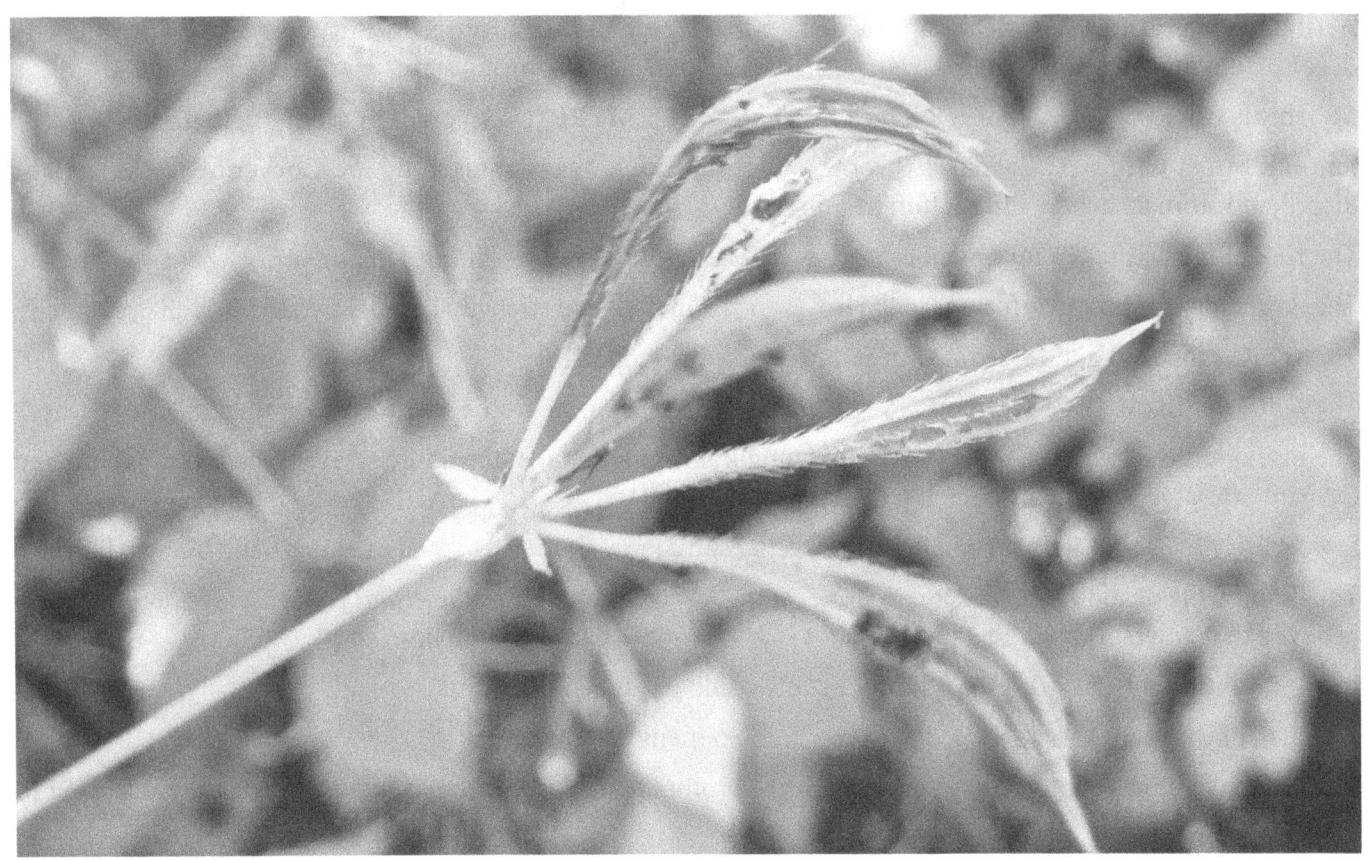

WESTERN SWEET CICELY SEED PODS

The Omaha and Ponca would hold the root in their hands and whistle to horses, ensuring an easier catch.

Human coprolite deposited on the cave floor in Utah around 4400 BC was tested with gas chromatography in 1984. The distinct anise-like smell was associated with one of two plants from the area, Sweet Cicely or Licorice.

Western Sweet Cicely (*O. occidentalis*) is restricted to the southwest region of Alberta. It has distinctive yellow flowers and hairless seeds. The root has a strong root beer or sassafras odor, and a sweet, spicy flavor with tingling aftertaste.

This species was widely used by the Paiute as a root decoction for disinfecting wounds, killing head lice, and an eye wash externally. Taken internally, the tea was good for chills, colds, respiratory problems including pneumonia, and taken both internally and externally in attempts to cure venereal sores and disease.

The Shoshone used Sweet root, as it was known, for similar purposes. The raw root was chewed for toothache, or inserted into the nostrils to relieve headaches.

Both the Okanagan and Thompson of the interior of British Columbia used the root of **XWAYT**, as a cold medicine.

The dried and crushed leaves can be added to salad dressings, and marinades for their tarragon-fennel like flavour.

For beers, root beers and other brews, the root, leaves and seeds can all be used. Michael Moore suggests the root would improve the taste of "potentially insipid wines as Dandelion, mountain ash and service berry (Saskatoon)."

The anti-fungal activity of the root may reduce alcohol content a bit.

Sweet Cicely (*Myrrhis odorata*) is an introduced, commercial perennial from Europe hardy to zone 3-4.

The ancient Greeks prized it for food and medicine, and called it **SESELI.**

Gerard in 1577, mentions "great Cheruill or Myrhhe" for its flavour similar to Garden Chervil. The root, probably due to its resemblance to angelica, was juiced and drunk for protection against the plague.

In the Leech Book of Bald (950 AD), extracts were mentioned as a salve for the treatment of tumours. The herb produces several lignans related to the cytotoxic compound podophyllotoxin.

Leyel mentions its use as one constituent of holy oil of the Tabernacle that Moses used to anoint the sacred vessels.

In parts of Wales, Sweet Cicely is planted around the headstones of loved ones.

The root is antiseptic and was used as an aphrodisiac by ancient herbalists, who also recommended the plant to increase strength, and as a tonic for young girls.

In France, the seeds of the related European species were crushed and added to brandy and Chartreuse to take off the harsh edge. It combines well with tarragon in a number of culinary dishes; as the seeds are quite spicy. When green, they are best in fruit salads, or ice cream and when ripe in spicy herb mixtures for cooking, such as apple pie.

The leaves have a sugary, licorice flavour, and a small commercial production in Europe is geared towards sweet flavourings for diabetics. The leaf is added to cream to give a sweeter, less fat taste. When added to cooked preserves of rhubarb, gooseberries or black currants, the dried leaf helps one use less than half the amount of recommended sweetener.

The root may be cooked as a vegetable, resembling a parsnip with hint of licorice. It is also grated raw and served in salads.

In India, the seeds were used to cure leprosy, the patient sitting in the sun until the affected skin blistered and the new skin revealed a natural colour.

The large brown seeds were ground fine and used in the north of England in the 17th century for polishing and perfuming oak floors, panels and furniture.

Like Angelica, the seeds need to be replanted immediately in fall, or require alternate freezing and thawing to promote germination.

It is an early nectar plant, valued by bees, and their keepers.

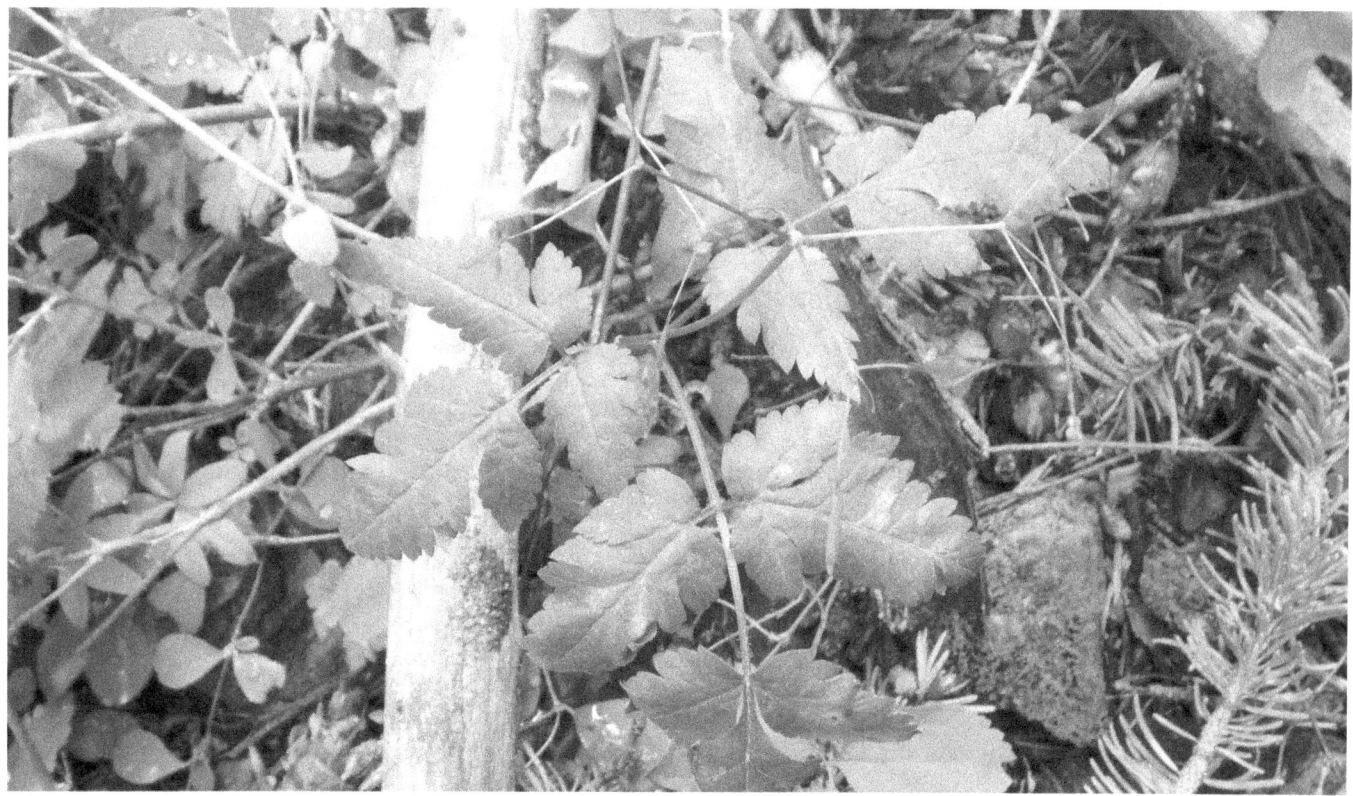

PURPLE SWEET CICELY

MEDICINAL

CONSTITUENTS- *O. aristata-* anisaldehyde, ortho-methyl-chavicol, (E)-anethole, 2,4-dimethoxy-1-allylbenzene, and 2,4-dimethoxy-1-propenylbenzene; phenylpropanoids trans anethole, and estragole.
O. occidentalis- falcarindiol, 3-0-methylfalcarindiol, anethole, phenyl-alanine-derived phenolic esters.
M. odorata- flavonoids including apigenine-7-0-glucoside, and luteolin-7-0-glucoside; peucedanin; essential oils including anethole, anisaldehyde, limonene, chavicolmethyl ether and alpha pinene.

Studies by Hussain et al, reported in Economic Botany 1990, indicate that the sweetness in the root of Smooth Sweet Cicely (*O. aristata*) is due to trans-anethole and estragole (phenyl-propanoids).

The root can be pounded or boiled as poultice for boils. The fresh root tincture can be diluted in 3 parts water as a wash for tinea and other fungal conditions.

It is useful for upper intestinal candidiasis, or low-level stomach infections, and combines well with fireweed leaf for this purpose.

Root decoctions are mildly stimulating to intestinal mucous membranes and gently laxative.

As a warm decoction, it can be a useful douche for vaginitis, or as a retention enema for chronic Candida infections from the rectum to sigmoid flexure.

A good combination is Fireweed leaves, Sweet Cicely root and Water Smartweed (*Polygonum hydropiper*) aerial parts, in equal parts. Decoct root, remove from heat and infuse fireweed and smartweed for 15 minutes, strain and cool down.

For blood sugar regulation make a tea of two parts Wild Sarsaparilla root, one part wild licorice root, and one part Sweet Cicely root. Drink one-half cup one hour before meals three times daily.

The seeds appear to have a stimulating effect on the bowel reflex, and can often trigger a laxative type reflex.

Michael Moore suggests that the root tea of Western Cicely can help "the adrenaline-dominant, stress addicted ectomorph, with gum problems, dry skin, and chronic dry feces".

The tea can be an effective laxative and stool softener, especially in those who have stopped smoking or drinking coffee and are irritable and constipated.

Greg Tilford, another accomplished professional AHG member, believes Western Cicely is stronger than *O. chilensis,* and *O. artista*, in both flavour and medicinal benefit. I would agree.

It is good for all fungal infections including tinea of the skin. The tincture helps indigestion and poor intestinal conditions such as candidiasis.

Michael Moore suggests warm decoctions for vaginitis and enemas for infections of the lower intestinal tract.

"Clarissa Smith, the Wyoming herbalist, recommends chewing a few seeds as a stimulus to the defecation reflex. This would probably be very helpful to those who have stopped smoking or drinking coffee and have gotten very cranky and constipated".

Smooth Sweet Cicely (*O. longistylis*) was recommended by Dr. Cook, as "a mild stimulant, and relaxant of the nervine and anti-spasmodic order, promoting mucous flow, and leaving a gentle tonic impression."

Matthew Wood suggests, "it is a specific for helping the cells pick up more blood sugar in type two diabetes." It is therefore indicated in peripheral neuropathy and retinopathy associated with this condition. He notes it is "a reliable tonic for diabetes mellitus, reduces fluctuations of blood sugar, even in old cases, but does not cure, except adjunctively with dietary changes in recent, adult onset diabetes."

In China, the root of *O. aristata* is called **XIANG GEN QIN** and noted for its acrid and warm properties. It is used to dissipate cold and effuses the exterior, is anodyne, and used to treat common colds and headaches at the vertex.

Thomas Garran suggests Western Sweet Cicely treating "dampness obstructing the middle burner with symptoms such as regurgitation, abdominal pain, nausea, bloating, gas, lack of appetite and fullness and oppression in the chest."

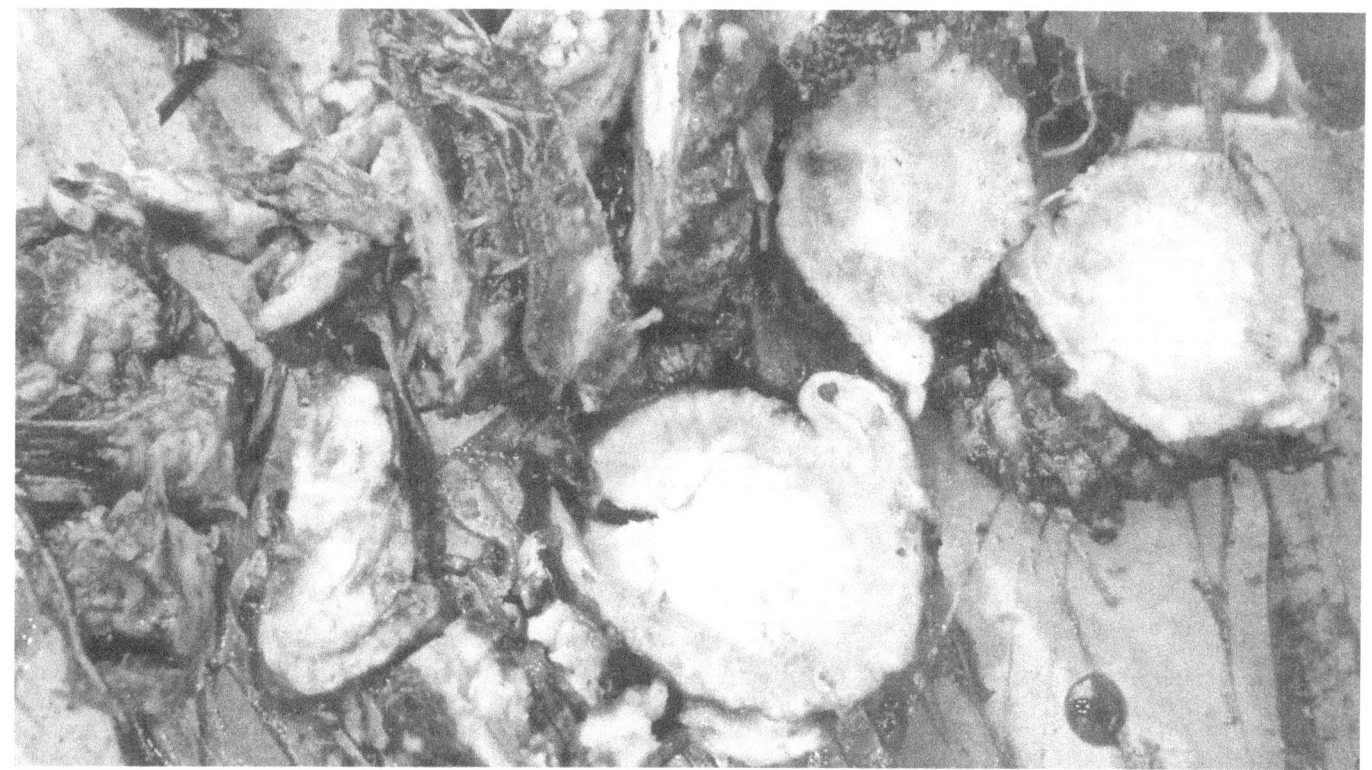

WESTERN SWEET CICELY CUT ROOTS

Combine with Oregon grape root in such cases, or with added heat think of adding marshmallow root.

In Korea, the dried rhizome of *O. aristata* is substituted for various *Ligusticum* species, especially *L. sinense*, or Chinese Lovage root, known in Traditional Chinese Medicine, as **KAO PEN,** or **GAO BEN.** Because it was used as a raw material for perfume in ancient times it was known as **KAO PEN HSIANG.**

The roots are used to dispel wind, disperse cold and control pain. Entering through the bladder meridian, the warm and pungent remedy is used for headaches due to wind cold, hernia and mass formations due to cold damp, abdominal pain, diarrhea and tinea.

Water extracts have proven very effective against various fungal skin problems.

It is often used as a substitute for licorice or astragalus root in formulas.

The leaves, roots and seeds of *M. odorata* are used for improving digestion and for expectoration. They have been used for cases of anemia, as well.

Sweet Cicely strengthens what is known in Traditional Chinese Medicine as **WEI QI**. This makes the root useful in the prevention of colds.

Western Sweet Cicely is useful for treating *Candida albicans*, using the fresh root tincture. A strong root decoction may be used as a douche in combination.

Root and seed tea stimulates appetite, help reduce flatulence, motion sickness and colic in young children, while a fresh root tincture is used for diuretic purpose and as a cold remedy.

Sweet Cicely (*M. odorata*) is used in Europe as a blood purifier, and expectorant. It is useful in cases of breathing difficulties and other respiratory conditions including asthma.

The root is used specifically for chest, throat and urinary complaints while the fresh herb is most useful externally for the inflammation of gout.

Peucedanin is found, as well, in carrot root, and *Pastinacea silvestris*; and possesses anti-neoplastic activity.

ESSENTIAL OIL

The root of Sweet Cicely (*O. longistylis*) has been steam distilled, and yields 0.57-0.63% essential oil, comprising mainly of trans-anethole (95.43%). It has a specific gravity of 1.0114, meaning it is heavier than water and thus requires a reverse clavenger trap, like catnip.

Minor components of limonene, alpha and beta pinene, terpinolene, carene, beta cymene, and beta phellandrene.

The roots of *O. aristata* contain anethole, esdragole, osmorhizole, isoosmorhizole, anisaldehyde, nothosmyrnol, allyl-2,4-dimethoxybenzene, methyl chavicol.

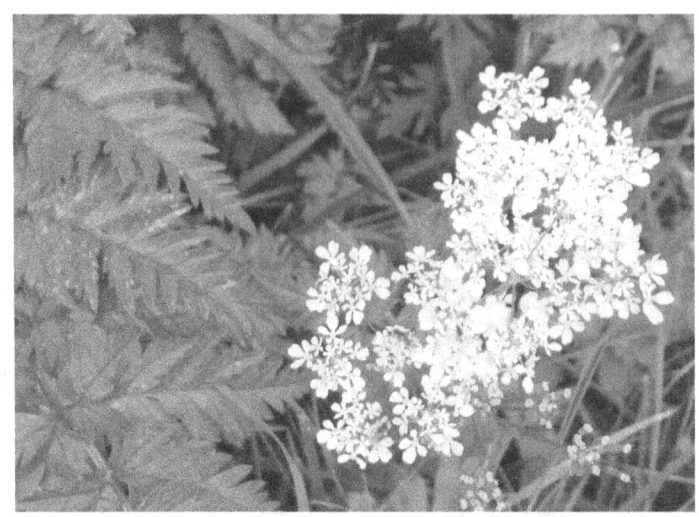

SWEET CICELY (*M. odorata*)

Sweet Cicely (*M. odorata*) seed contains 39 compounds, the major one being (E)-anethole, comprising over 83%. The leaves are rich in (E) anethole, up to 85%.

Anethole has been shown to possess both anti-bacterial and anti-fungal activity. It is strongly insecticidal, and effective against houseflies in laboratory studies.

Anethole is synergistic with polygodial compounds (see Water Smartweed under Bistort), in significantly decreasing fungal infections, including *Candida albicans*.

FLOWER ESSENCE

Sweet Cicely essence helps increase sensitivity of the five outer senses.   **ROCKY MTN**

SPIRITUAL PROPERTIES

Cecilia was a young Sicilian virgin, living and dying in the second century. According to Chaucer, she called her judge blind (Blind Justice!) for not being able to see that a statue was mere stone and not a god.

For refusing to give up her belief in Christ, she was boiled for two days and, when she was still alive after that, an executioner tried to cut off her head with a sword. Three blows to the neck failed to severe it and she was left to bleed to death...She was later canonized as Saint Cecilia and, since somewhere along the line she was thought to have invented the organ as a musical instrument, she became the patron saint of music, and, of course, blindness.

Her Saint's Day is November 22, and one can be certain that every year on the day, someone will play some of the music composed in her honour on CBC radio. Hymn to St. Cecilia with words by W. H. Auden:

Blessed Cecilia, appear in visions
To all musicians, appear and inspire;
Translated daughter, come down and startle,
Composing mortals with immortal fire!

RECIPES

FRESH ROOT TINCTURE- 5-20 drops in warm water three times daily. The fresh root tincture is made 1:2 at 65%; while the dry root is 1:5 at 30% alcohol. Dr. Cook recommended a 30% tincture of the dry root as optimal.

DECOCTION- 3-4 ounces as needed three times daily, made from 2-9 grams of root. Decocting the roots results in significant volatiles being lost. A cold infusion, gently warmed after 12 hours is best.

INFUSION- One handful of leaves, with seeds to one pint of warm water. Steep ten minutes. Drink 1-3 cups daily.

PROPAGATION- Sweet Cicely seeds are difficult to germinate. Like Angelica, it is sometimes best to plant the fresh seed where you want the plants directly outdoors in all. This is assuming you already have a plant with seed, or a seed company that ships fresh in fall.

The second is to take the seed and mix it into peat moss in a plastic bag. Place this in a fridge, and in February check for seeds starting to germinate. Remove and transplant into pots.

Return un-germinated seed back to fridge and observe for irregular germination.

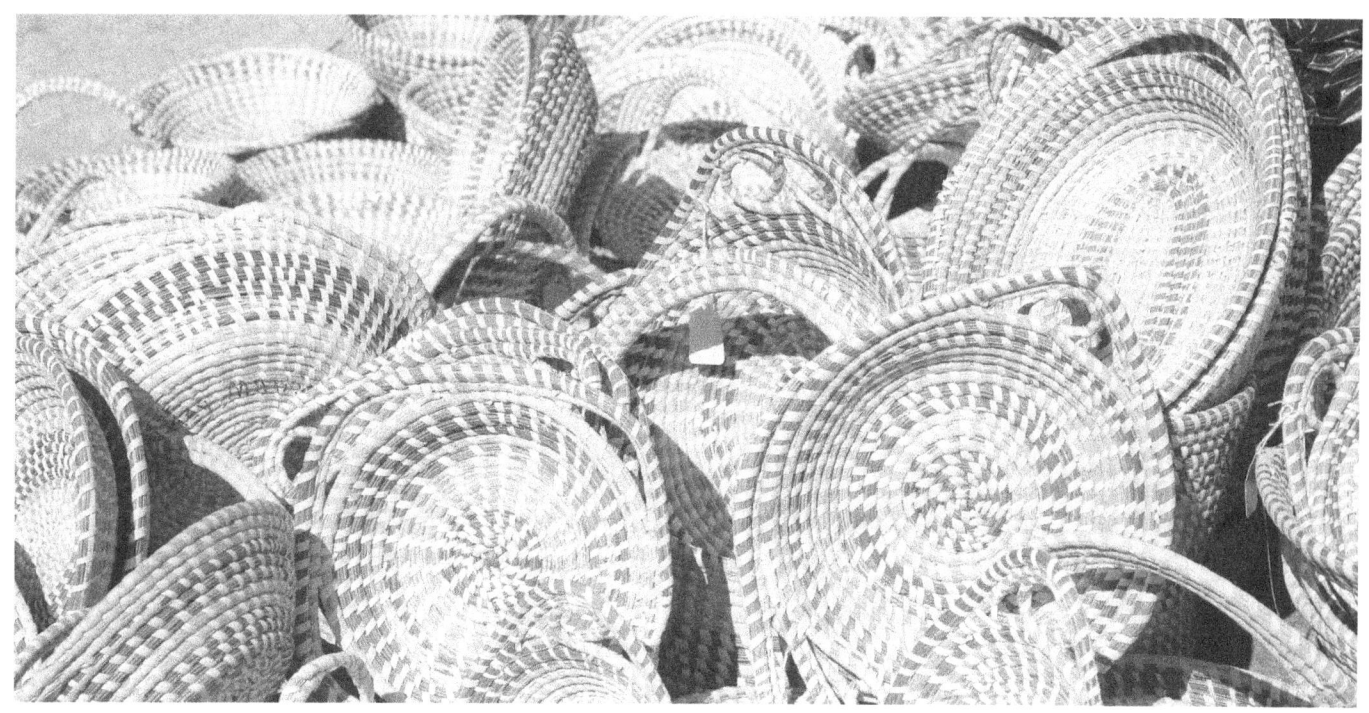

SWEETGRASS BASKETS

SWEETGRASS
(*Hierachloë odorata* [L.] P. Beauv) not accepted
(*Holcus odoratus* L.) not accepted
(*Teresia odorata* [L.] Hitchc.) not accepted
(*Anthoxanthum nitens* [Weber] Y. Schouten & Veldt.)
HOLY GRASS
ALPINE SWEETGRASS
(*H. alpina* Sw. ex Willd] Roem & Schult) not accepted
(*Anthoxanthum alpinum* A. Love & D. Love)
PARTS USED- whole plant, mainly leaf and stem.

"My sweet smoke brings protection and takes your prayers and wishes to the heavens to be heard."

The brown laboring bear
Nohkom, the medicine woman
Alone in her attic den
Smoking slim cigarettes
Wears the perfume of sage, sweetgrass
And earth medicine ties.

SKY DANCER

Hierachloë is from the Greek **HIEROS** meaning holy or sacred, and **CHLOA**, grass, or **KHLOROS**, meaning greenish-yellow. Odorata is obvious. Anthoxanthum means yellow flower. Nitens refers to the shiny leaves.

Sweetgrass has been used as an incense, holy purifier, perfume, and medicine in many cultures.

The Northern Cree know it as **WIYIKASKWA**, sweet scented grass, while other Cree call it **WEHKUSKWA**, or shorten the name to **WEKUS.**

The Chipewyan call it the "grass that smells", or **TLH' OTSEN**, while to the Slave it is simply "Sweet", or **HLEKO.**

Sweetgrass is burned for its spiritually purifying and protective properties. Woven strands are symbols of life's growth and renewing powers. Kahlee Keane says "in plaiting a braid, the three sections signify mind, body and spirit."

Sacred pipes, or battle weapons are all passed through the smoke for strength.

In some Native legends, the little people were so mesmerized by their own reflections in a pool that they pined away, leaving only the memory of their sweet scent lingering upon the grass.

Among the Blackfoot, sweetgrass is used to purify dancers of the Sundance; and is known as **SIPUTS-SIMA**, or **SIPATSIMO** meaning, "fragrant smell".

The leaves were mixed with tobacco and smoked to summon the benevolent power possessed by sweetgrass. It was even braided into the hair, or soaked in water to make a hair wash. The stems were soaked in water to wash chapped and wind-burned skin; or to treat sore eyes.

Sweetgrass was mixed with the gelatin of boiled hooves, and used as a hair tonic.

The Blackfoot used it for medicine, inhaling the smoke for colds. Others, including the Flathead of Montana, made a tea for colds, fevers and nasal congestion, combining sweetgrass and the seeds of meadow rue (*T. occidentale*).

Both indigenous groups used braided material in a sachet in clothing or burned them as incense, air/clothing freshener and insect repellant.

It was drunk as a tea to treat venereal disease with little success.

It is chewed in ceremonies involving prolonged fasting as a means of extending endurance. Sweetgrass is chewed by singers and the juice is spat upon patients in some cases.

The Mi'kmaq chewed the leaf for sore throat or toothache. After chewing it can be applied as a poultice to wounds for its antiseptic and pain relieving properties.

The strained tea was used to stop vaginal bleeding, or to expel afterbirth. Traditionally, a woman would remain apart from her husband for about 34 days after giving birth. Before this return she bathed in water scented with sweetgrass, dressed in new clothes that were smudged four times.

The Cree in Saskatchewan would boil four sweet grass braids and give the decoction to a young girl in difficult labor to speed and assist childbirth.

It was told by one Blackfoot Elder that the Owl and Loon in the medicine pipes owned the sweet grass, and the Bear owned the juniper.

The Cheyenne use sweetgrass in their Sacred Arrow ceremony as a symbol of life's growth. It is said that if your animals are not grazing and producing properly, plant sweetgrass around their pasture.

Before battle, a warrior passes his shield four times through the smudge. A Contrary Warrior always purified his lance in smoke before battle.

Many native people have integrated sweetgrass into the Palm Sunday, carrying it to the Roman Catholic ceremony, and later hanging the braids in their homes.

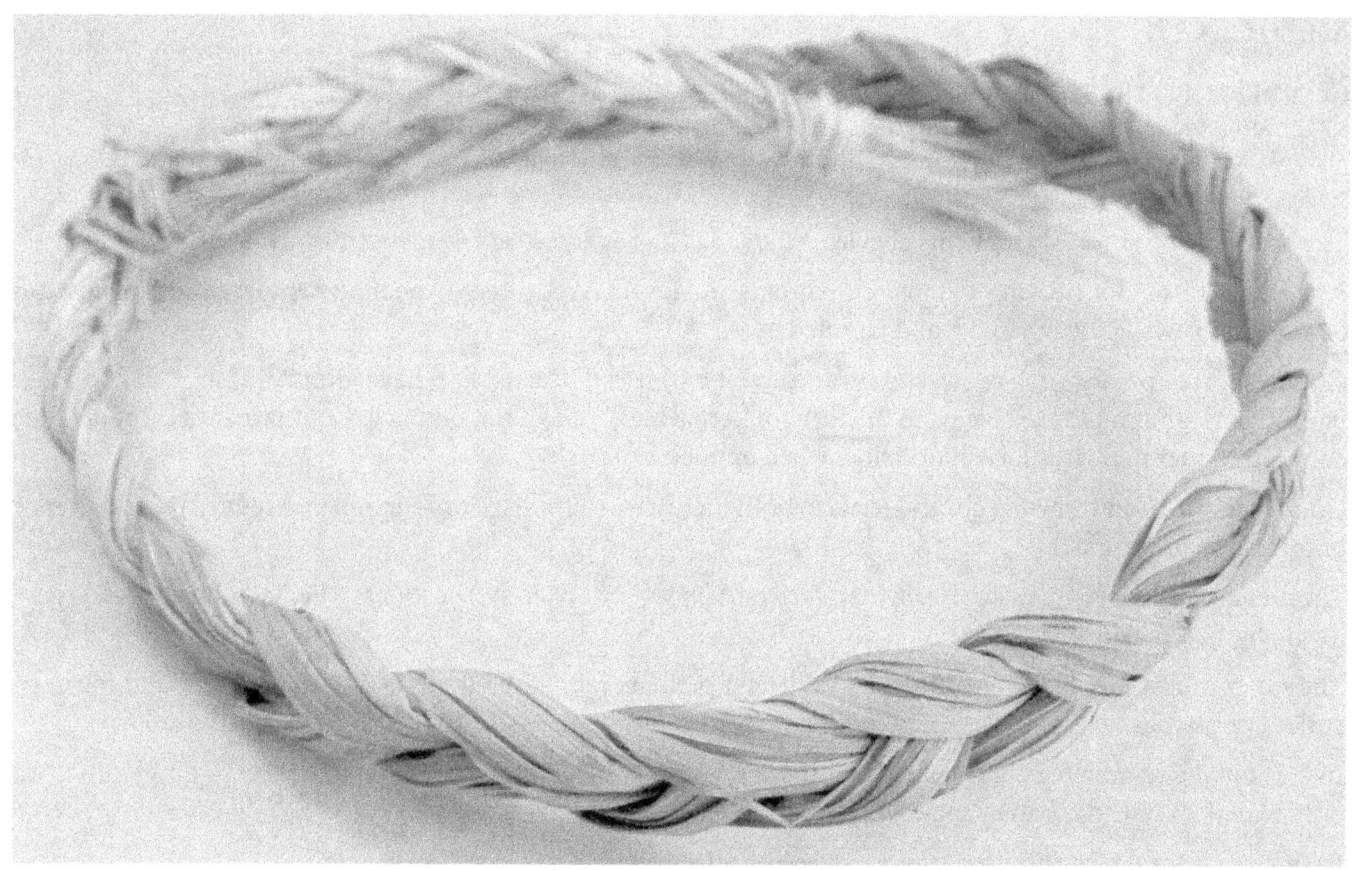

SWEETGRASS BRAID

In Europe, the Slavs used the plant for its fragrance and certain saint's days. In Poland and Russia, the grass is used for flavoring vodka (*Zubrowka*), and liqueurs. Extracts are also used to flavor candy, soft drinks, and tobacco.

The grain is small, but edible.

Sweet grass (*H. odorata*) is the scented grass of Norway. It is known as luktegrass (scent grass), or *Haissasuoidni* to the Northern Sami, or *Hajuheina*, in Finland.

The plant is circumpolar and is known as **MAO XIAN** in Traditional Chinese Medicine. It is used medicinally to treat kidney infection and internal bleeding.

Holy Grass is a shorter species that is more common in arctic and alpine meadows, but otherwise similar.

In Mexico, the grass is used to perfume clothes and burned as incense.

While traveling in Columbia, I noted that the related *H. redolens*, called **ITAMO REAL**, was considered a very valuable medicine and used a great deal by the elderly for a variety of diseases.

The Alberta Research Council in Vegreville recommends sweetgrass as an effective reclamation plant for controlling erosion in moist area, and for stabilizing sandy areas with an underlying water table. The seed is small, 1.6 million per kilogram; and is a poor germinator, yielding only 5% in three weeks with pre-treatment.

A one-inch plug can develop into a dense ten square foot mass in one year, and cover over 50 square feet at the end of the second year. It will help alkalize low pH soil.

A cultivated form, *H. nashii*, produces especially long leaf blades.

MEDICINAL

CONSTITUENTS- coumarin (from z-2-glucosyloxycinnamic acid (3.6%); lauric and palmitic acid; as well as 5,8-dihydroxybenzopyranone, 5,8-dihyroxycoumarin, 5-hydroxy-8-0-beta-D-glucopyranosyl-benzo-pyranone. It contains massoilactone, an active unsaturated lactone, (5-hydroxy-2-decenoic acid lactone) similar to the grasses used in certain Polish vodkas. The ethanol extract is 62% coumarin.

The grass can be smoked and helps alleviate colds.

As a tea, it is used for treating coughs, sore throats and fevers. Well filtered, the body temperature infusion can be used as eyewash for inflamed, and irritated eyes.

Coumarin rich plants, such as sweetgrass and sweet clover can be used to relieve joint pain, sciatica and other painful back and muscle problems in the form of herbal bath, or as a hot poultice. Coumarin is a camphor-like compound that increases local blood flow when applied externally.

Coumarin has been shown in clinical trials to both increase macrophage production and reduce the recurrence of metastatic melanoma.

Thornes et al, *European Journal of Surgical Oncology* 1989 15:5 looked at 27 patients who had undergone surgery for malignant melanomas.

The randomized, double-blind study, had thirteen patients receiving 50 mg of coumarin daily, and fourteen patients a placebo.

In a follow up conducted three years later, there was recurrence of melanoma in 10 of the 14 on placebo and only two of 13 in those patients taking coumarin.

Besides Sweetgrass, coumarin is present in substantial amounts in red and sweet clovers.

Research has shown coumarin helps reduce lymphedema and other high protein edemas.

Sweetgrass aerial parts have been found to contain at least two compounds with free radical scavenging activity. Pukalskas et al, *J Agric Food Chem* 2002 50.

The compound 5,8-dihydroxycoumarin is cytotoxic. Nemeikaite-Ceniene et al, *Z Naturforsch* 2005 60c 11-12.

Recent work on human lymphocytes, in vitro, suggests weak genotoxicity of this compound. Slapsyte G et al, *Molecules* 2013 18(4): 4419-36.

ESSENTIAL OIL

CONSTITUENTS- over 160 compounds, but richest in coumarin, comprising 10.3% of the root oil, and nearly 25% of the aerial parts. Other principal constituents are 3-methylbutanal, 3-methylbutanol, massoilactone (dec-2-en-5-olide), furfural, and aliphatic acid ethyl esters.

Massoilactone has commercial application for providing coconut-like notes in food flavouring and certain aromatherapy and perfume applications.

Several years ago, a Saskatchewan company produced small amounts of CO2, or carbon dioxide extractions of sweetgrass, with a beautiful, true and lasting fragrance. However, the product was expensive, and unavailable to the average retailer, perfumer or consumer.

Hay essential oil is steam distilled in France from several sweetgrass species and available commercially. Known as Flouve, the essential oil or absolute is used in tobacco flavoring, and in perfumes, blending well with fougeres, chypres, oriental bases, ambers and such. It was used in the past to modify maple and other flavours.

HYDROSOL

Several producers associated with the Alberta Natural Health Agricultural Network that I chaired for several years, produce a high quality sweetgrass hydrosol. The advantage of this product, in a spray bottle, is the lack of smoke associated with burning. The scent is authentic and pleasing. It is widely used in regional hospitals as an alternative to burning sweetgrass by native healers.

Sweetgrass water is an excellent after shampoo hair rinse. It will make your hair thick and healthy.

The hydro-distillate contains phytol, coumarin and 2-methyl-4-vinylphenol, that shows deterrence to mosquito biting. Cantrell CL et al, *J Agric Food Chem* 2016 64(44): 8352-8358.

FLOWER ESSENCES

Sweetgrass flower essence cleanses and rejuvenates the etheric body; helps bring one's lessons and experiences to completion on the etheric level.
ALASKA

Sweetgrass flower essence helps create a free flow of energy, releasing blockages and generates a field of protection. **WILD ROSE**

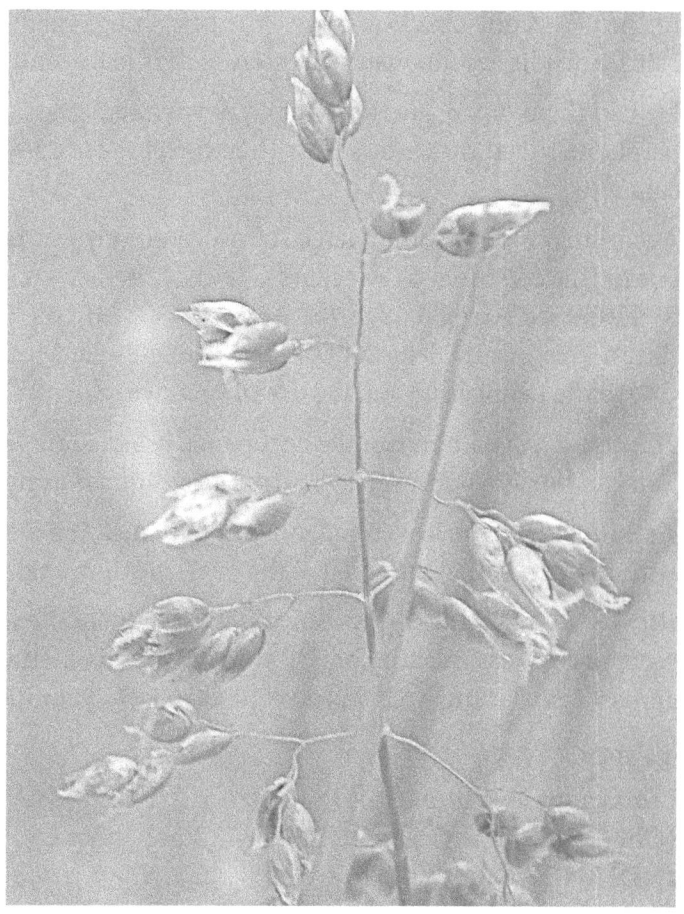

SWEET GRASS SEED HEAD

SPIRITUAL PROPERTIES

Sweet grass once lived in the sky. It came to earth through a hole in the blue lining of the Sun Chief's lodge- a hole that we call the North Star- through which shines the light of the fire in the lodge. The hole was made when an Indian maiden (could she have known Eve) pulled up the sacred turnip Sun had forbidden her to touch.

Morning Star had seen this maiden first in the Blackfoot camp on the prairie and had loved so that he took her to the sky to live with him. She was very happy there until she was tempted (by a serpent in the form of a pelican) to pull the forbidden plant. Through the hole she saw her home again far down against the prairie. Sun, at the same time angry and pitying, sent to back to her people and with her she brought to earth the sacred turnip, the sweet grass and a root digger painted red. When the grass had grown and the prairie was well covered with it, Sun sent another messenger to the people telling them many things.

He sent them the songs and ceremonies of the Sun Dance. He told them how to purify themselves outwardly by using sweet grass incense and inwardly by nibbling the sacred turnip. **A BROWN**

The Sweetgrass trail is explained in terms of the different "roads" that people take on their journey through life. The central road is likened to a tree trunk, and an individual can diverge from it at any time. A person can also veer away for a period, as in drinking or drug use, and later return to the Sweetgrass Trail. There is no guarantee, however, that a person will reach the culmination of his or her journey. A person can make it nearly all the way by attaining the age of seventy or over and still experience a sudden heart attack.

If the proper road is adhered to an individual reaches the age of 80-100, the Sweetgrass Trail has been successfully followed and fulfillment has been achieved. At this point death is not feared. On the Sweetgrass Trail the good years start at about the age of fifty. **DAVID YOUNG**

In the Cheyenne Creation story, "the first things made were the stars, sun and moon. This creator, whom we call Maheo in our language, held out his left hand, and his power being such he got five strings of sinew.

He laid them down, and next he put down sweet grass...then he produced buffalo tallow, then he produced red paint...he rolled that into a ball. Then he blew on it four times...he let it go. And it grew and grew. This is the earth. **SPEAR**

According to history, the Sacred Arrow ceremony was performed at the beginning of time. The thing that stands out in this ceremony is sweet grass itself. It is very sacred to use. It is used to purify the pledger, the members of the Sacred Arrow Lodge, the Arrows, the Medicine Bundle, the Earth. We burn sweet grass on charcoal 445 times. This was the length of time in which Sweet Medicine lived. So we retrace that. We renew the life of the Cheyenne people through the use of this sweet grass. **SPEAR**

To protect your home and its occupants, braid some Sweetgrass and hang it near the entrance to your house. You can purify your home by burning Sweetgrass as incense; it will also call your spirit guides and helpers.

Crushing the fresh leaves and inhaling the smell is a wonderful way to enhance your divination and to connect with the ancestors. The smell of the grass is emotionally uplifting. **SUSAN GREGG**

RESOURCES- Although sweetgrass is plentiful in the wild, it is also being grown commercially for reclamation seed, herbal teas, making braids or for steam distillation. Sweetgrass Farms are people I know that ship plants across Canada, and hold a pick-your-own in July and August. They can be reached at 1-888-384-5683.

TANSY
(***Tanacetum vulgare*** L.)
(**Chrysanthemum vulgare** [L.] Bernh.) not accepted
INDIAN TANSY
(***T. huronense*** Nutt.) not accepted
(***T. bipinnatum*** [L.] Sch. Bip.)
COSTMARY
ALECOST
MINT GERANIUM
MAUDELINE
(***T. balsamita*** L.)
(***C. balsamita*** [L.] Baill. non L.) not accepted
(***Balsamita major*** var. ***tanacetoides*** [Boiss.] Moldenke) not accepted
PARTS USED- leaves, flowers

On Easter Sunday be the pudding seen
To which the tansy lends her sober green. **OXFORD SAUSAGE**

It may be, when my heart is dull, having attained its girth, I shall not find so beautiful the meager shapes of earth. Nor linger in the rain to mark the smell of Tansy through the dark. **EDNA ST. VINCENT MILAY**

(Costmary) is an especial friend to evil, weak and cold livers. **CULPEPPER**

Coole violets and orpine growing still,
Enbathed balme and cheerfull galingale,
Fresh costmarie and healthfull camomile. **MUIOPOTMOS**

Tansy is most likely derived from the Greek **ATHANASIA** meaning immortal, or "not death", or "long lasting", depending on interpretation.

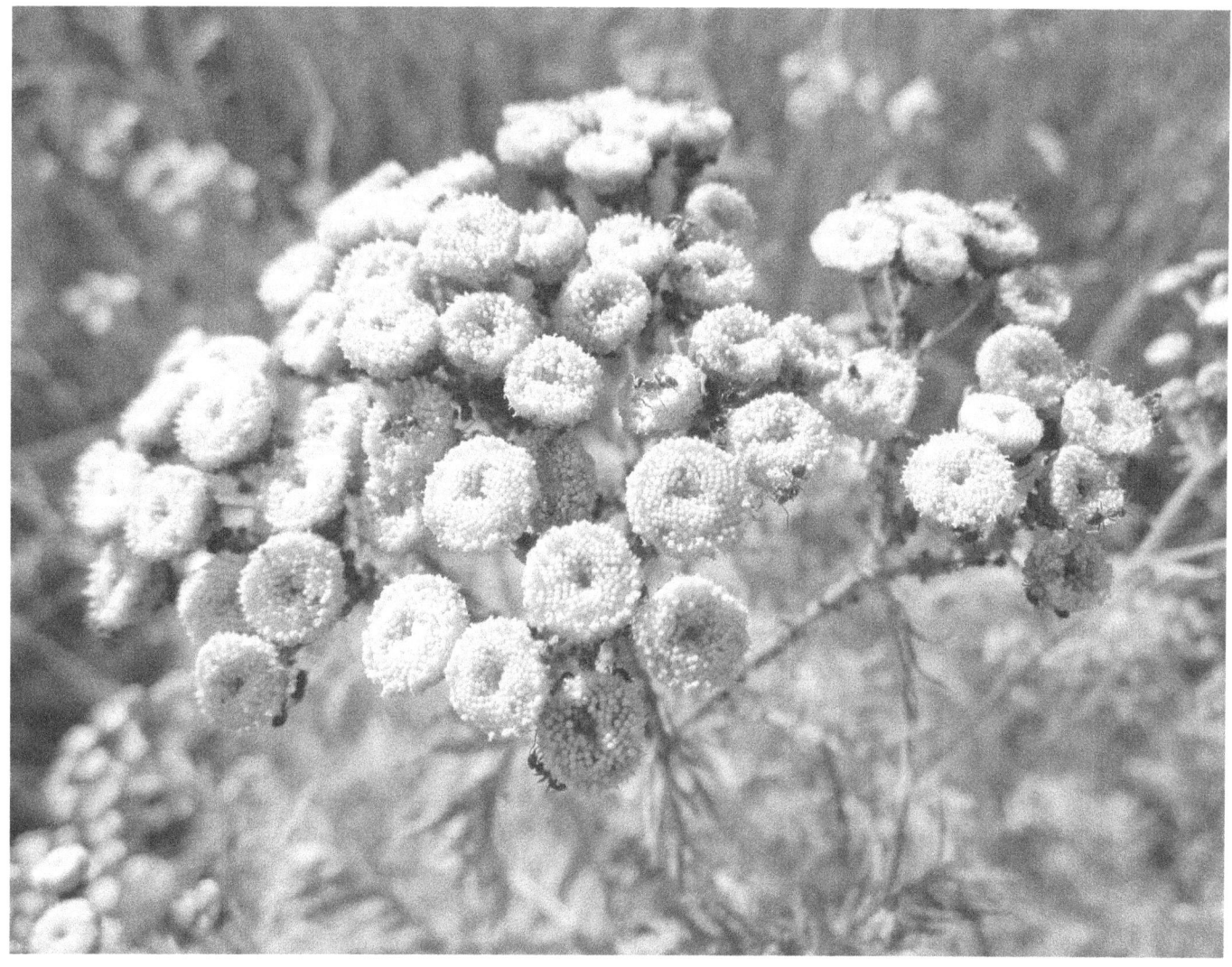

TANSY

The Romans knew it as **TENACETUM** that in medieval Latin of the 13th century became **TANAZETUM** or **ATHANACETUM**.

This became **TANAISIE** in French, and then **TANSIE** to the English. This is either because of the long-lasting flowers, or a good preservative for corpses.

Costmary is said to derive from the Latin **COSTUS** for an "oriental plant" with similar fragrance, and **MARY**, the mother of Jesus. The herb was originally called Costus marie, or Mary Magdalene's balsam, as well as Maudelaine and Maudelinewort. This is the Christian version of events.

There is some speculation that the original name was Costus Amarus, or Bitter Balsam. Alecost is derived from the use in beer. Cost is from the Greek **KOSTOS**, meaning spicy and hence a spicy herb for ale. This makes good sense.

In France, it is known as Herbe Sainte-Marie, and in German either Marien Balsam, or Frauen Mnze, dedicated to the Virgin Mary.

Hildegard de Bingen, the 12th century Abbess wrote, "when one is unable to urinate, because he is constricted by a stone, he should pound Tansy, strain its juice through a cloth, add a bit of wine, and drink it frequently."

155

One Greek legend of Tansy is about Ganymede, a famous young man, who was given some tansy tea to make him immortal; and thus serve as Zeus' cupbearer.

The custom of using tansy for embalming was common to both sides of the Atlantic. Today, it is often representative as a funeral bouquet. In the language of flowers, tansy is the emblem of Saint Anthanasius.

During the hunting season, the tansy leaves are used to keep flies and other insects from dressed deer or moose.

Tansy is a common sight along farm fence lines, and has been since its introduction to this country. *Tanacetum huronense* is our northern, native tansy, and is restricted to the northeastern part of the province on gravel beds and sand dunes. Both are similar in appearance and properties.

The Chipewyan near Lake Athabasca call this native tansy **TLH'OGH TSEN** meaning, "grass than smells."

The fragrant leaves of this tansy were mixed with meat and used as bait for trapping white fox or lynx.

The Haida used the Yellow Beach Tansy (*T. huronense*), also known as **K'ANHLAHL JAHJUU** meaning, "sloppy yellow medicine on the beach", in an unspecified manner.

The Chippewa and other native tribes made use of the introduced plant root decoctions for sore throats and ear pain. Or they simply chewed on the root. The leaves were infused with catnip to induce menstruation in young women.

The Anishinaabemowin name **O'CKINIGI'KWEA ANI'BIC** means "young woman's leaf."

The Malecite and Mik'maq used the whole plant to prevent pregnancy, and the leaves only for kidney complaints.

The Cheyenne called it "Yellow Medicine", or **HEOVE-HESEEO?OTSE**. They pulverized the introduced leaves and flowers and made an infusion for those who felt weak.

The dried leaves have a spicy rosemary-like fragrance and taste that can be added to culinary dishes. One of the more unusual I have seen was a tansy pudding offered in a Chester, England restaurant. Tansy was eaten near the Easter season, as a remembrance to the bitter herbs eaten by the Jewish at Passover, but with a little bacon in the cake so no religious connotations were assumed. In large part it was a form of cultural culinary vermifuge that took on ceremonial aspects.

Stewed rhubarb also benefits from a small addition of the fresh leaves.

In Scotland, the whole plant was infused in whey to treat intestinal parasites, and infusions of the dried flowers for gout. It is used for young children that have temper tantrums, possibly due to irritation from the worms.

Tansy has been used in both England and France for curing ales, and is an ingredient in Chartreuse, the liqueur. Tansy was called **OLKALL**, or Ale Man, in parts of Norway.

In Russia, the flowers are steeped in vodka, and used for stomach and duodenal ulcers. Many believe it one of the 130 herbs in Chartreuse, the liqueur.

The leaves were used traditionally in Europe either fresh or dried for children's colic, abdominal cramps, and even gout. Many Ukrainian and Eastern European settlers of the prairie used tansy for various arthritic complaints. In Scotland, the roots are candied and eaten for gout as well.

The roots can also be gathered, washed, dried, roasted and ground as a coffee substitute like dandelion root. It has the added advantage of reducing high blood pressure, as well as toning the nervous system, depression and those suffering extremes of emotion.

For centuries, tansy has been considered a specific for young girls suffering from slow and painful menstruation.

Matthew Wood relates a story of driving in the countryside with a girlfriend and he stopped and placed a single shoot on the dashboard for decoration. Immediately his companion began to have severe uterine spasms that stopped when the flower was removed.

As a generalization, use the flowers as an antiseptic, the flowers and root as anti-bacterial, the oil as an anti-fungal, and the whole plant for liver and bile stimulation.

Tansy is a stimulating, astringent water for cosmetic use, and makes an excellent steam for those with mature, sallow skin.

Water extractions of tansy deter the Colorado potato beetle, and would be a useful companion plant for the whole nightshade family. The pyrethrins are similar to those found in ox-eye daisy and useful for repelling ants, fleas, and moths. Strong tansy infusions are also useful against aphids, cabbageworms, Japanese beetles, diamondback moths and squash bugs. Mix with small amount of liquid soap for longer activity.

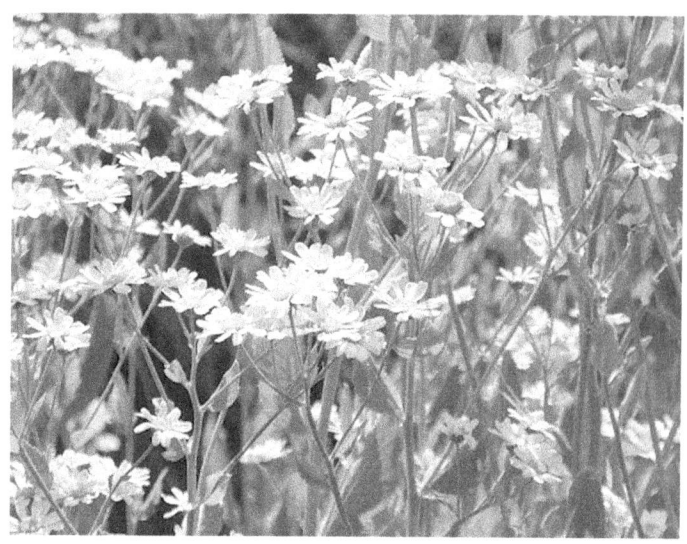

COSTMARY

Although water extracts are toxic to house flies on contact, a buffered solution of pH 4 or 9 is more effective.

Water extracts help protect rainbow trout raised commercially, from ravishes of *Saprolegnia parasitica*. Pirbalouti et al, *J Food Ag Envir* 2009 7:2.

Tansy is said to be a good companion plant for both roses and raspberries.

The flower tincture is a good fly wipe for horses.

The flowers are used in dried flower arrangements; and were given in Victorian times from one woman to another as a signal of esteem.

The roots are mixed with certain chemicals in Finland to produce a green dye, the leaves greenish-yellow and the flowers golden tan. In the past the leaf juice was often used to dye buns and cakes.

Costmary may be originally from the Orient, but was introduced into England in the 1500s. It looks, at first glance, like a daisy or chamomile.

Before that, it was popular in Greece, Rome, and Egypt and by 800 AD was in common use in parts of Europe. It became so popular that by the 16th century, it was being exported into England from Spain.

Although closely related to tansy, it has a more aromatic, balsamic fragrance than its cousin. Hence, its ancient name, Balsam Herb. The leaves have a balsam minty flavor, similar to spearmint chewing gum.

It shares with Tansy, small yellow button flowers, but has a blue green waxy feel to the leaves.

It was a popular strewing herb that helped scent floors, cupboards and clothing.

It is now well-established perennial in parts of Saskatchewan and Alberta, in some areas as an escapee. It likes dry soil.

Parkinson wrote of its use in flavoring ale, from which comes Alecost. Like almost any other aromatic plant of that era, it was used in making beer, and to flavour various wines.

Culpeper says it "provoketh urine abundantly, and moistenth the hardness of the mother; it gently purgeth choler and phlegm...cleanseth that which is foul, and hindereth putrefaction and corruption...and it is a wonderful help to all sorts of dry agues.

It is astringent to the stomach, and strengthen the liver and all the other inward parts; and taken in whey, worketh more effectually...it is very profitable for those...with cachexia (a general wasting of the body), especially in the beginning of the disease."

Sir John Hill also valued its virtues. "It was one greatly esteemed for strengthening the stomach, and curing head-aches, and for opening obstructions of the liver and the spleen."

Gerard recommended the seeds to expel worms out of the belly.

In Colonial times, the costmary leaf was used as a bookmark in bibles and prayer books of Christian churchgoers; and named Bible Leaf. When the sermon grew long, the sleepy listener would nibble on the minty leaf to help stay awake. More likely is that it repelled insects that would eat the paper, as Costmary has been used traditionally as a strewing herb to discourage insects.

The fresh lemony, balsamic leaf can be added to tea, beer, ales, salad, soup, stew and German sausage. Italians swish a leaf in butter being melted to prepare omelets, one leaf again the dominant theme, as the taste is quite pronounced, and unusual.

In parts of the American southwest, the plant is known as Romero de Castilla. It is boiled with crushed meat and shells of pecan for a mouthwash. A handful of the plant is boiled in red wine, and this in turn is poured over a heated brick. The patient suffering uterine hemorrhage stands over the rising steam until it stops.

When dried as a potpourri ingredient, or used to sweeten closets and drawers, the scents is subtle and soothing; minty and yet woven with lavender.

The fall stems can be woven into fragrant baskets, by simply stripping the dead leaves and using immediately.

The roots from commercial crops today are included in very expensive perfumes, with a fragrance similar to a blend of lemon, mint and chrysanthemum.

The perennial does rarely produce seed, and must be propagated from root division. Picking off the seed heads also produces a bushier plant with more leaves.

It is hardy to zone 3 (-29° C) and will spread quickly if not deterred. If prefers dry, rich soil, as it is a heavy feeder. A pH of 4-6 is best, with full sun necessary for flowering.

MEDICINAL

CONSTITUENTS- *T. vulgare*- thujone (up to 70%), tanacetin, borneol, camphor, stearin, lead oxides, gallic, citric, oxalic and tannic acids, vitamin C, pyrethrins, pontica epoxide, l-viburnitol, and crispolide; numerous sesquiterpenoids including longipinane-2, 7-dione, reynosin, tabulin tanacetals; monoterpenoids like chrysanthemyl acetate, and thuj-4-en-2-yl acetate; carotenoids, various sterols, the major one being beta-sitosterol; as well as campesterol, cholesterol and taraxasterol, and 6-hydroxyflavones. Both beta and alpha amyrin are triterpenes, while arbusculin-A, tanacetin, germacrene D, and crispolide are sesquiterpene lactones.
In some tansy, parthenolides are found, along with other sesquiterpene lactones such as matricarin and artemorin; as well as methoxyflavones, jaceosidin, eupatorin, chrysoeriol and diosmetin. The plant is highly variable in its constituents.
shoots- davanone
flower- 1-epi-ludovicin-C; 11,13-dehydroesaacetyl-matricarin; cis-longipinane-2,7-dione; tatridin-A.
root- a spiroketal-enol ether derivative (E)-2-(2,4-hexadiynyliden)-1,6-dioxaspiro[4.5]dec-3-ene.
T. vulgare var. *boreale*- leaves- eight flavonoid glycosides, including 7-O-glucosides ofluteolin, scutellarein, and 6-hydroxyluteolin; and 7-O-glucuronides of apigenin, luteolin, chrysoeriol and eriodicyyol; eight flavonoid algycones- apigenin, luteolin, hispidulin, nepetin, eupatilin, jaceosidin, pectolinarigenin and axillarin.
T. huronense- tanacin.
T. balsamita- C7-C11 alpha, beta-unsaturated aldehydes, various fatty acids and alcohols; sesquiterpenoids including dehydroisoeivanin, and isoeivanin. Also contains parthenolides.

Above all, tansy is a digestive and bitter tonic, with an astringent and toning effect on the mucous membranes. At the same time it has relaxant and nervine properties that are helpful in painful cramps and spasms, notably digestive and menstrual in nature.

As a bitter and pungent digestive stimulant, tansy helps relieve stagnation, lack of appetite and nausea in a manner similar to mint.

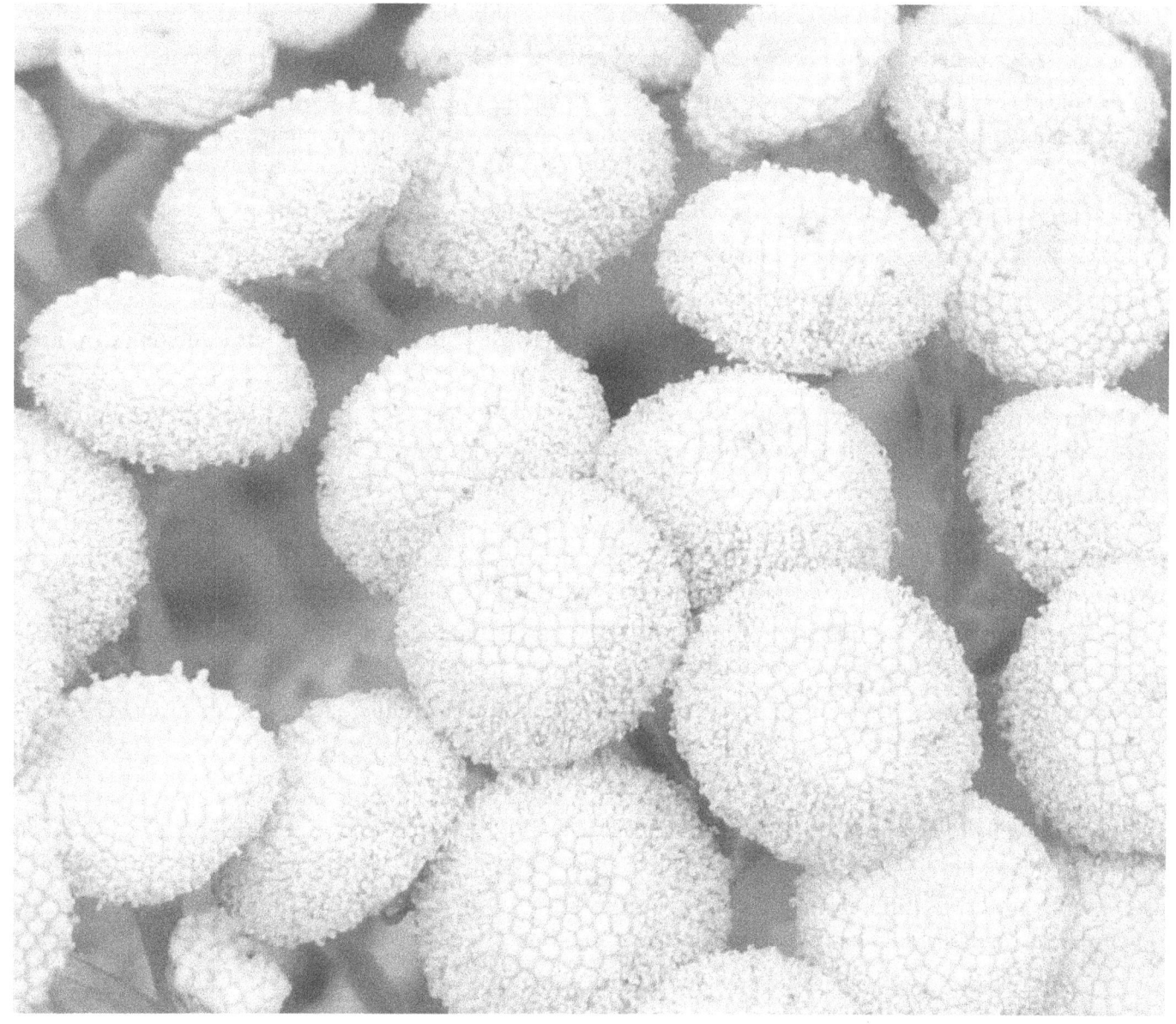

CLOSE UP OF TANSY FLOWERS

A simple cold infusion of the fresh leaves, with a touch of honey, will quickly relieve heartburn, especially related to liver or gall bladder disorders. Caffeic acid is a well- known bile stimulant present in the herb.

Its relaxing effect on spasmodic and painful dysmenorrhea is similar to crampbark, or peony root.

In some ways, it is similar to yarrow as a woman's herb, being useful in reducing estrogen buildup that leads to breast lumps and cysts.

An older herbal formula for prostate enlargement was largely composed of tansy and green flowering oats; suggesting hormonal influence.

As a hot infusion of the leaves and flowers, it gives relief to the emotional holding that leads to nervous unrest. Taken hot, the herb promotes vasodilation and exhibits diaphoretic properties in treating colds, flu, fever, sore throats and other conditions where Yarrow or Linden Flower would be used.

Taken cold, the tea is an effective diuretic, but it does excrete potassium as well as sodium and chloride ions. Nahlou et al, *J Ethnopharm* 110:3.

Jethro Kloss recommended tansy tea for heart palpitations, working in a very short period of time.

The infused tea, taken hot, is an effective febrifuge, while taken at room temperature helps alleviate painful gout.

The seed head is most effective against various parasites, including pin, thread, and round worms; and combines well with mugwort and pineapple weed for this purpose. Take as a water infusion to avoid the alcohol soluble ketones.

Hot leaf fomentations give rapid relief to various swellings, varicose veins, inflammations and rheumatic pain.

Strong decoctions can be used as a wash for scabies, and as an ointment for pruritis ani.

The root has been extracted with ether, and shows activity against gram positive bacteria, and protozoa.

Studies at the University of Saskatchewan by Ramfrez-Erosa et al, have found tansy extracts exhibiting significant cytotoxic activity against colon, breast and lung carcinoma. *Can J Physio Pharm* 2007 85:11.

At the same time, other research suggests various acidic polysaccharides exhibit potent complement fixing activity and immune modulation. Xie G et al, *Int Immunopharmacol* 2007 7(3): 1639-50.

Hybridization research of tansy to produce the active ingredient, parthenolide in feverfew (*Tanacetum parthenium*) is ongoing. Studies conducted by Hendricks and Bos in The Netherlands, have shown tansy containing 0.05-0.46% parthenolide in the leaves, and 0.06-1.33% in the flower heads, was also absent of alpha and beta thujone. Due to the hardiness of tansy, these parthenolide rich specimens hold promise for future study.

Tournier et al, *Journal of Pharmacy and Pharmacology* 1999 51:2 found that parthenolide extracted from Tansy helped prevent gastric ulcer formation in laboratory studies.

Onozato et al, *Phytother Res* Jan 16 2009 found the herb extract and parthenolide both active against herpes simplex virus 1.

Feverfew has shown great promise in controlling some migraines and rheumatoid arthritis.

Williams et al, *Phytochemistry* 1999 51:3 compared the flavonoids of tansy and feverfew leaves and flowers. When tested pharmacologically, they variously inhibited the major pathways of arachidonate metabolism in leukocytes.

There was significant difference in potency, with the tansy 6-hydroxyflavones less active than feverfew 6-hydroxyflavonols as inhibitors of cyclooxygenase and 5-lipooxygenase.

One flavone, eupatilin and at least one sesquiterpene, santamarine decrease NO and inhibits LPS induced macrophage NO production (5-LOX).

New sexual hybrids between Feverfew and Tansy have been produced. Brown et al, *Journal of Experimental Botany* 1999 50:333. Parthenolide content was very low, but a new generation of secondary metabolites, were formed.

Pharmacologically, the leaf extracts inhibited human polymorphonuclear leukocyte (PMNL) activity *in vitro*, despite just traces of parthenolide. This provides further evidence that more than parthenolide is responsible for the pharmacological activity of the genus *Tanacetum*. On a related note, low levels of parthenolide were tested on two tumour cell lines, at the University of Ottawa by Ross et al. The effect from low levels on human lymphoma and mouse fibrosarcoma cells was reversible in 85% after 24 hour exposure at 2.5 μM; whereas at 5.0 μM concentration the activity was permanent.

The flowers of tansy show activity against human acute T leukemia cell lines with IC50 dose of 0.20 mg/mL. Wegiera et al, *Acta Poloniae Pharmaceutica* 2012 69:2 263-268.

In another study, the eudesmanolides, derived from the flowers, showed cytotoxicity against A549 (human lung carcinoma) cell lines. Rosselli S et al, *Molecules* 2012 17(7): 8186-95.

Water extracts of the leaves given to mice for 90 days showed no signs of toxicity, suggesting herb infusions to be relatively safe for humans. Lahlou et al, *J Ethnopharm* 2007 117:2.

Work by the same author, same journal in 2008 120:1, found water extract present NO mediated and NO independent vaso-relaxing properties *in vitro*.

Methanol extracts show anti-thrombin and anti-cancer activity. Goun EA et al, *J Ethnopharm* 2002 81 337-342.

Tansy was one of the few plants, of 1400 tested, exhibiting anti-inflammatory effects on INOS expression and IL-6 at less than 250 µg/ml. Others of note were elecampane root, yerba santa, ashwagandha, feverfew, rosemary, tumeric root, osha root and green tea. Mazzio EA et al, *BMC Complement Altern Med* 2016 16(1): 467.

A combination of rose, stinging nettle and tansy could possess anti-dementia properties, and improved spatial learning and memory in a sporadic Alzheimer's disease rat model.

Daneshmand P et al, *Avicenna J Med Biotechnol* 2016 8(3): 120-5.

Tansy root contains an interesting anti-viral compound that is effective against herpes simplex 1 and 2. It inhibits virus penetration and has a novel mechanism of specific arrest of viral gene expression and thus a decrease of viral protein accumulation within infected cells. Alvarez AL et al, *Antiviral Res* 2015 119:8-18. Earlier work by same author identified anti-HSV-1 activity in aerial parts.

Tansy decreases the activity of the antibiotic ciprofloxaxin by four to eight times. Do not use concurrently in cases of *E. coli* infections. Smirnova G et al, *J Appl Microbiol* 2012 113(1): 192-9.

Indian or Lake Huron Tansy (*T. huronense*) aerial parts contains tanacin. A study by Dissanayake AA et al, *Nat Prod Commun* 2016 11(5): 579-82 found tanacin inhibits glioblastoma derived cell line U-87 MG.

Costmary was official in the *British Pharmacopoeia* until 1788 as an aperient, especially useful in treating diarrhea and dysentery.

It was used in cases of excessive coldness.

Being slightly astringent and antiseptic, it can be used on wounds and in ointments for skin parasites, as well as dry, itch skin.

It was part of the very old remedy, *Aqua Composita*.

The unsaturated aldehydes in Costmary show activity against a broad spectrum of bacteria and fungi. Work by Kubo et al, *J Nat Products* 58:10 found the plant active against 14 microbes.

It possesses anti-oxidant activity. Pukalskas et al, *Food Chem* 122:3.

The related *T. gracile*, native to the cold, alpine deserts of China and elsewhere, has been tested for oil content that induces apoptosis in HL60 human cancer cell lines. Verma et al, *Planta Medica* 2008 74.

HOMEOPATHY

Tanacetum vulgare (Tansy) is indicated when individuals have that nervous and tired "half dead, half alive" feeling. They are mentally irritable and very sensitive to noise. The ears roar and ring, and seem to close up suddenly.

For painful dysmenorrhea with bearing down pains; or to bring on suppressed menses use tansy with benefit.

It is a specific for poison ivy rash, where the homeopathic Rhus Tox does not give complete relief.

Respiration may be hurried and laborious, with frothy mucous obstructing the air passages. Right side more affected. Drowsiness from 11 am until 3 pm.

DOSE- Tincture to the third potency. The mother tincture is made from equal parts of the fresh leaves and flowers. Provings began with Burt, with dose drops of oil around 1865; followed by proving on three females at 12th and 30th dilutions in 1873. Van de Warker self experimented with oil in syrup around same time.

ESSENTIAL OIL

CONSTITUENTS- *T. vulgaris*- thujone (0.2-0.6%), l-camphor, bornyl acetate, monoterpenes including limonene, sesquiterpenes including chamazulene (up to 30%), 3,6-dihydrochamazulene. The yield is from 0.12-0.18% of a rich golden oil with unusual green notes. Specific gravity is about 0.92. Tansy is a plant that produces numerous chemotypes, and some safer varieties could be harvested and distilled for market. In one study in Hungary, 33 different chemotypes were identified, with camphor and thujone dominating.

Studies in Quebec in 1993 by Collin et al, identified four chemotypes with beta-thujone, camphor, 1,8-cineole/borneol; dihydro-carvone; or chrysanthenone dominating each one. Others contain up to 61% umbellone, and another contains up to 79% artemisia ketones.

Rohloff et al, *J Ag Food Chem* 2004 52:6 identified seven major chemotypes in Norway.

T. balsamita- Over 85 volatile compounds have been identified in one form with carvone (51-68%) and alpha and beta thujone (9-16%) comprising the largest single entities. Smaller amounts of beta bisabolene (4.5%), 1,8-cineole (3.42%), and germacrene D (4.24%) and camphor are also present in this minty type.

At least two other chemotypes exist. The first, is rich in camphor, containing up to 92%, while another is 35-47% camphor, 28-41% thujone.

Another analysis of the leaf showed 47% bornyl acetate and 27% pinocarvone, and the flower at 34% of the latter and only 5% bornyl acetate.

The content of sesquiterpenes is more than twice as high in flowers as leaves.

Tansy oil is steam-distilled from the leaves and flowers of the fresh plant. In small doses, it is useful for ridding the body of pinworms and threadworms, but with extreme caution.

Medicinally it can be used in diluted carrier oils like St. John's wort, for rubbing on rheumatic, erythema and sciatic pain.

During an asthma crisis or in emphysema, it can be rubbed into the lung region, or diffused into the air.

In small amounts it is beneficial in couperose type skin, and even more irritating dermatitis. It is used in perfumery in small amounts to add unusual spicy notes.

Research out of France shows that tansy oil shows promise in certain forms of leukemia and is considered an immune stimulant.

The essential oils completely inhibited the growth of *Candida albicans* in lab studies, as well as 92% of gram-positive bacteria like *Staphylococcus aureus*. Lower activity but still good results with *E. coli* and other Gram negative bacteria were also found. Work by Opdyke et al, *Food Cosmet Toxicol* 1976 14 found, *in vitro*, anti-fungal activity against 15 pathogenic and non-pathogenic organisms. The same study found tansy given to rabbits reduced serum lipid levels and inhibited further development of hypercholesterolemia. The recovery of blood sugar concentrations was inhibited in animals given twice daily doses.

The essential oil has been used in treating the Colorado potato beetle as mentioned above. The compounds with greatest deterrent were 1,8 cineole, followed by bornyl acetate, and then p-cymene.

Studies in Sweden suggest the essential oil may be useful as a tick repellant. Palsson K et al, *J Med Entomol* 2008 45(1): 88-93.

CAUTION- The essential oil is strongly abortifacient and is contra-indicated in pregnancy, during nursing, or even sensitive women with endocrine imbalance. Fifteen drops can be toxic. Four mls can induce epileptic-like convulsions, even death. One case in the literature cites a wrong prescription by a general practitioner in Germany. Instead of 10 drops of tansy oil in thirty grams of caster oil, 10 grams were given. The patient immediately suffered severe convulsions and was treated for nearly two months. Effects of the poisoning were observed two years later. Ten to 30 grams of essential oil from flower heads is considered lethal.

Costmary Oil can be produced from both the leaves and flowers. Highest content of essential oils in both is before full blooming at 1.15% and 1.34% respectively.

The essential oil, sometimes called Balsamite oil is clear to pale yellow with a very powerful fresh herbaceous, somewhat medicinal odour. The first top note is reminiscent of wild marjoram, pennyroyal or the light notes of pine. The body notes are similar to basil, hyssop and savin. The savin note is very persistent, with a sweet dry out.

The leaf essential oil possesses insecticidal properties, due in part to content of muurolol and cadinol.

In France, the oil is used for treating chronic bronchitis, due to its mucolyptic and anti-catarrhal properties. The oil is a digestive stimulant, useful in dyspepsia and cases of hepatic insufficiency such as low bile production or promotion.

The essential oil exhibits moderate to high anti-microbial activity. Cytotoxicity on human fetal skin fibroblast and monkey kidney (Vero) cell lines showed IC50 values of 2500 and 1250 microgr/mL respectively. Yousefzadi M et al, *Nat Prod Commun* 2009 4(1).

Liquid preparations and tablets based on Costmary essential oils and waters are produced in Florence.

Original recipes from the Dominican monk, Angiolo Marchissi have been prepared since 1614, for their sedative properties. About 150,000 tablets and 560 liters are marketed each year. Gallori et al, *J Ag Food Chem* 2001 49:12.

The oil is neurotoxic and contraindicated in young children and pregnancy.

Ten drops of the essential oil will produce flushing of the head and face, giddiness and heated stomach. One drop four times daily in water has been used successfully for epilepsy. I don't recommend it.

SEED OIL

The closely related *T. corymbosum* produces a seed rich in novel conjugated acetylenic acid.

The white flowering plant grows up to three feet tall, and is hardy to zone 2.

The seed oil contains 17% of octadeca-8t, 10t-dien-12-ynoic acid, which is a new conjugated trans, trans-di-unsaturated acetylenic acid.

It also contains 10% crepenynic acid. More research is warranted, given the plants hardiness and ease of growth.

HYDROSOLS

CONSTITUENTS- Tansy aromatic water contains small amounts of trace essential oils including nearly 75% carvone, and lesser amounts of alpha thujone and 1,8 cineole.
T. balsamita- This hydrosol contains over 74% carvone as part of the volatile organic compounds, with 6.2% alpha thujone, 3.5% 1,8-cineole and a number of minor constituents.

The distilled water of tansy expels blocked urine, a dead fetus, and worms as well, when a few loths are taken according to taste. When four or five loths are drunk in the morning and evening, and this is kept up for a month, this will prove good for treating the stone and related afflictions.   **SAUER**

Our woemen in Englande and some men that be sunneburnt and would be fayre, eyther stepe this herbe in white wyne and wash their faces with the wyne or ellis with the distilled water of the same.   **TURNER**

Tansy water is good for those that cannot pass a stone or have pain on urination, as well as worms in the belly. The water from root and herb is good for eye redness, and sticky eyelids, or in eye for darkness or spots within the last year. It heals tuberculous wounds, backbone pain, and the whites in women.

The flower water only comforts man in all his members. It is drawn up the nose for catarrh in the head, and put in eye before bed. It is used for confusion in the head and brain.   **BRUNSCHWIG**

Costmary leaf water has been used to improve complexion, as a hair rinse, and as a "sweet washing water" in baths.

Costmary water distilled in May or June, strengthens the liver, helps the yellow jaundice, opens obstructions, and helps the dropsy.   **CULPEPPER**

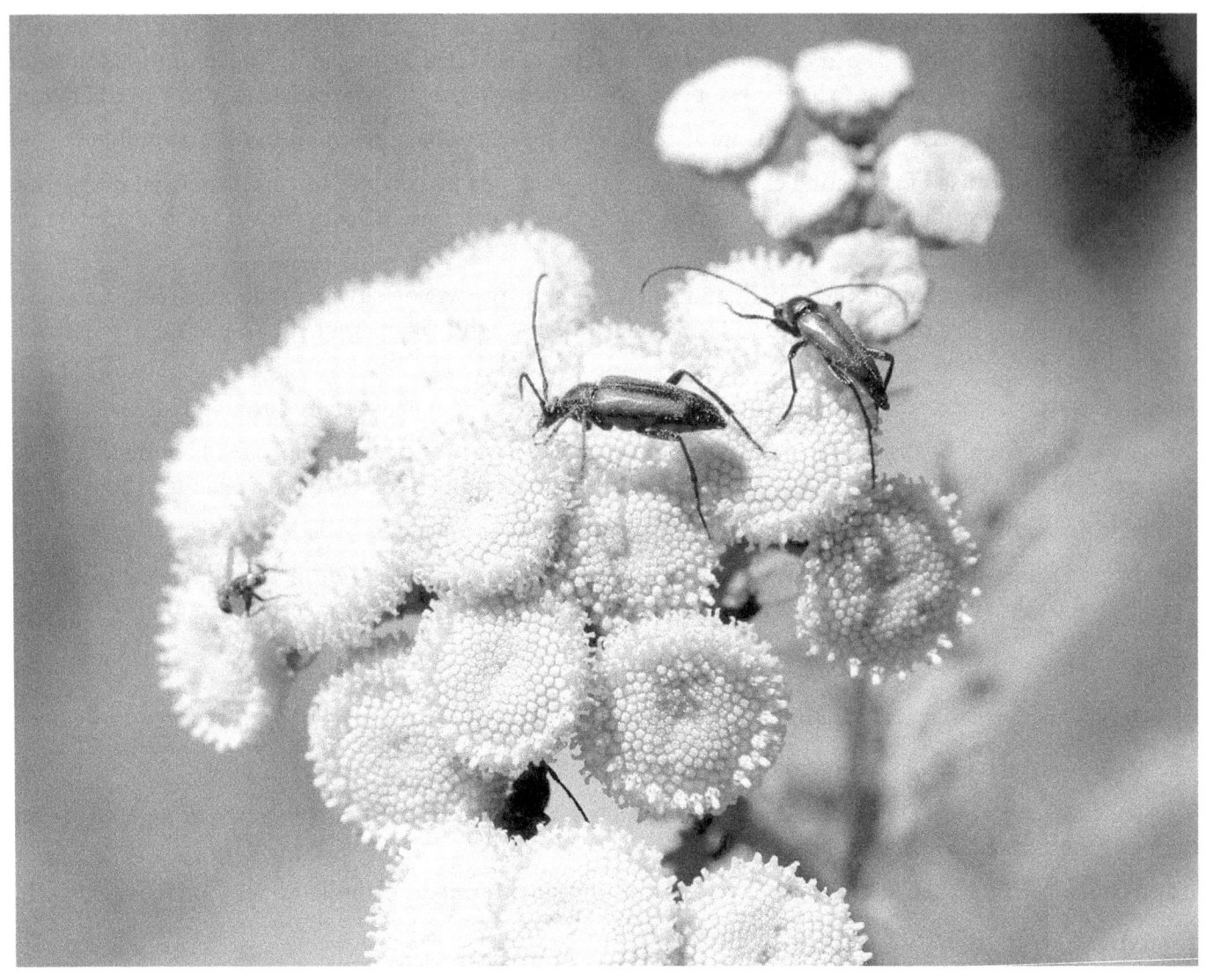

TANSY BLOSSOMS

LEAF AND FLOWER OIL

A carrier oil can be made by bruising tansy leaves and flowers and soaking them in canola oil for seven to ten days. This sun infused oil may be added to insect repellent blends, or to ointments for scabies, or for anal itching created by pinworms in all ages. By adding beeswax, an ointment can be made that is used for skin tumours of the tendons, or wherever an anti-inflammatory and analgesic rub is required.

FLOWER ESSENCES

Tansy flower essence is used for taking decisive action in meeting one's goals. Those individuals who are sluggish and hesitant in action are helped in cutting through lethargy. It can also be used by those hesitant to act, even when they know what they want to do.
FLOWER ESSENCE SOCIETY

Tansy flower essence can repel negative thought forms, and at the same time attune individuals to the purpose behind them.
PEGASUS

Tansy protects the aura of the spiritual warrior. It is indicated for those affected by environmental chemicals and pollution. This may include emphysema, pleurisy and bronchitis.
PETITE FLEUR

SPIRITUAL PROPERTIES

Tansy is a most fascinating member of the vegetable kingdom, for this plant has the double capability from a spiritual point of view, symbolized by the two distinct colors which its flowers show: orange and yellow.

Orange is the color of knighthood in the ranks of the spiritual workers, for it denotes an ability to "know" truth which goes beyond that commonly found. Yellow is the color of the sun, whose love for all creation is so vast as to be unimaginable by man— this being symbolized by the warmth and light which that mighty being floods out upon its surrounding space. Yellow is thus universal or Christ Love in action.

The combination of love and knowledge is a very potent one, and the seeker may move the more quickly in his chosen direction by adding to his other spiritual practices that of eating on of these flowers each day during the blooming season. Flower steeped oil can also be dabbed on the ajna center and left for twenty minutes a day.

HILARION

RECIPES

INFUSION- Take one tsp of dried herb to one pint of hot water. Steep for thirty minutes. Drink one tsp. every three hours- cold when exhausted, and hot for sweating with cold, flu, and menstrual difficulty.

For worms, use one ounce of herb to two litres of boiling water. Steep 90 minutes.

For adults take one half ounce twice daily with food around full moon. For children, use one half tsp twice daily.

Both tansy and Costmary are contraindicated during pregnancy.

SEED INFUSION- As above, but combine with a laxative herb to ensure quick movement through the system. Take on an empty stomach before breakfast.

CAPSULES- two "OO" of powdered herb as above.

TINCTURE- 10 drops three times daily for bacterial infections; 25 drops three times daily for parasites. The root tincture is more useful for Gram positive and protozoal infections including giardia; the flower buds, better for round and pinworms. Prepare either from fresh herb at 1:4 and 60% alcohol.

ESSENTIAL OIL- 2-4 drops as needed

CATARACTS- An old Welsh recipe recorded by David Hoffman. Take tansy and boil in white wine. Remove from the heat, strain and cool. Add some pure camphor and leave until dissolved. Put small amount in eyecup, well diluted with distilled water for eye problems.

TANSY PUDDING- Boil 3 oz. of ground rice in 20 oz. of milk until soft. Then add 4 oz. butter and three well-beaten eggs plus sugar and rose water to taste. Juice some fresh tansy leaves and blend into mixture. Pour into dish and bake at low heat for 45 minutes.

COSTMARY ALE- Boil 1 oz. dried herb, with two pounds brown sugar and 2½ gallons water for half hour. Cool to 70° F, strain into fermenter and add yeast. Ferment until done, siphon into bottles, add ½ tsp sugar and cap. Ready in 10-14 days.

BUHNER

FOOTBATH- Steep two ounces of fresh tansy leaves in one cup of boiling milk for ten minutes. Strain, and pour the scented milk into hot water.

REPELLANT SPRAY- Soak one cup of bruised fresh leaves in a quart of hot water for about one hour. Add tbsp liquid soap. Use the liquid for sprays, and the leaves for mulch on insects and other pests of the garden.

CAUTION- Overdose of tansy can lead to vomiting, fixed pupil, severe reddening of the face, cardiac arrhythmia, uterine bleeding; as well as liver and kidney damage. Death can occur in 1-3 hours. Lethal dosage of thujone rich tansy is 15-30 grams of plant material. It is a dangerous abortifacient.

TOADFLAX
BUTTER AND EGGS
(*Linaria vulgaris* Mill.)
(*Antirrhinum linaria* L.) not accepted
(*L. linaria* [L.] H. Karst) not accepted
BLUE TOADFLAX
(*L. canadensis* [L.] Dum. Cours.) not accepted
(*Nutallanthus canadensis* [L.] D. A. Sutton)
BROAD-LEAVED TOADFLAX
DALMATION TOADFLAX
(*L. dalmatica* [L.] Mill.)
SNAPDRAGON
DOG'S MOUTH
RABBIT'S MOUTH
LION'S SNAP
(*Antirrhinum majus* L.)
DWARF SNAPDRAGON
(*Chaenorrhinum minus* [L.] Lange)
PARTS USED- leaves and flowers

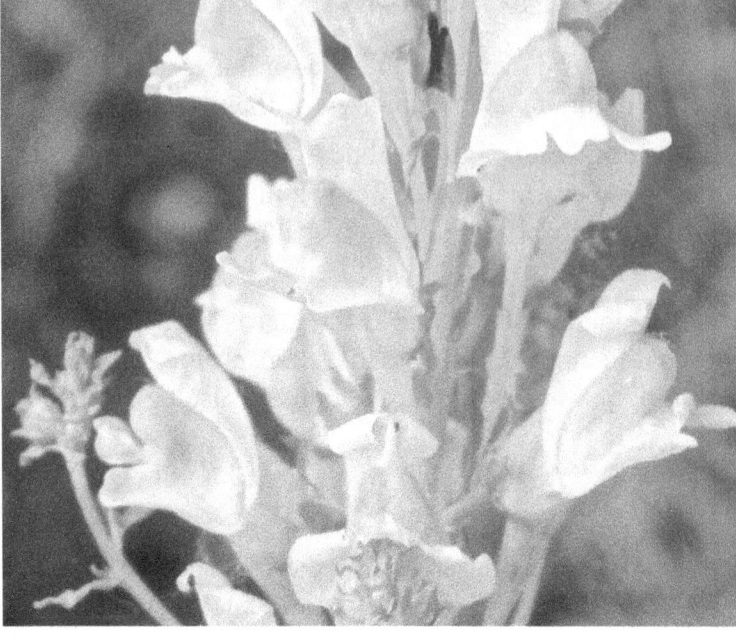

TOADFLAX

Larkspur with milk doth flow:
Toadflax without milk doth grow.

Toadflax has an interesting name. Originally it came from the Latin **BUBONIUM**, meaning the buboes, or inflamed lymph glands of the armpit and groin. A typing error changed **BUBO** to **BUFO** meaning toad.

Other scholars believe it was a misreading of **BUFONIS** from toad, and **BENEFICUS** for useful. This is a bit more of a stretch.

Linaria is from the Latin **LINUM** and Greek **LINON** meaning flax, due to the resemblance in early growth. There are some 200 species in the genus, mainly in Europe, Asia and North Africa.

Some writers believe that the Toad comes from the Old English **TOD**, a bunch or cluster, from the matted appearance. Others believe that Toad, in early English, meant "useless"; hence useless flax. This was from the German **TOT** meaning dead.

Antirrhinum refers to the snout-like form of the flowers, from the Greek **ANTI+RHIN** like a nose or snout.

Chaenorrhinum is from the Greek verb **CHAINEN** "to gape", with the noun **RHIS** "snout", as in rhinoceros. This refers to the corolla being partially open at the throat, rather than tightly closed as in Toadflax. Dalmatia is an area near Croatia.

The introduced perennial, also known as Butter and Eggs, is common throughout the prairies.

It bright yellow flowers are luminous and night, and the whole plant smells cheesy, like an un-aired dairy.

Many children know it as the closely related Snapdragon, due to the flowers opening and closing jaw-like nature. Toadflax was originally assigned to the *Antirrhinum* genus like the cultivated snapdragon.

This peculiar mouth is another example of the nature of attraction and pollination of a particular plant by a particular insect. The plants mouth remains closed and will only open when forced by bees. The conspicuous orange lip attracts bees and directs them to two orange tracks inside the flower. These in turn lead toward the nectar in the spur, and at the same time coat the bee's back with pollen.

166

Toadflax is subject to peloria, a disease which results in monstrosities, where blooms may develop from five spurs rather than one. Research shows it is induced by one-sided illumination, and scientists hope it may provide a clue as to the cause of certain human abnormalities.

In medieval times, Toadflax was worn as an amulet of protection from evil, and to break a hex. In 16th century England, three seeds were strung on a linen thread for protection. In Scotland, to this day, a spell is believed broken by walking three times around Toadflax in full bloom.

In Sussex the plant was applied to warts, and in Gloucestershire, mixed with yarrow as a poultice to ease pain, stop bleeding and induce sleep.

Among German settlers, a type of linen was woven from Toadflax that was employed by healers in casting spells. Various occult objects were kept in these toadflax bags.

The Iroquois used the introduced Toadflax infusion for removing bewitching spells. The Ojibwa made bronchial steams from the whole, dried plant called **AWACAWA' SKWUNEG**.

Older Latin scholars called the plant **URINARIA**, in reference to it's diuretic properties. Roman women incorporated the fresh juice into soaps.

The young, plant shoots may be eaten as a potherb, but I personally find them too bitter and stringy.

In Scandinavia, the plant was boiled in milk, and dishes set throughout the house or greenhouse to attract and drown flies. The fresh juice squeezed into cream is even more potent.

The Pennsylvania Dutch used fresh plant poultices for skin irritations. Johann Wolpius made a famous hemorrhoid ointment in which Toadflax was the main ingredient. He was a physician to the Landgrave of Hesse, and only divulged his secret formula to the prince after being promised one fat ox annually, to reveal the recipe.

In Bulgarian traditional medicine, Toadflax is used a laxative, and to treat inflammation of the bladder, skin rashes, and hemorrhoids. Its early use for bladder problems earned it the name *Urinalis*.

Toadflax is noted, and being further investigated for insecticide activity; with more research needed.

Dioscorides is quoted as saying Snapdragon, "being hanged about one preserveth a man from being bewitched, and that it maketh a man gracious in the sight of people."

It has come to symbolize presumption, and birth date of August 19.

In France, the flower was called Calf's head and then Calf's face, before settling as Wolf's face in the 19th century.

Snapdragon has bitter and stimulating properties; and has been used for tumors and ulcers of the skin.

Water decoctions of the whole plant are allowed to cool, and used as a wash to heal indolent ulcers. The bruised herb can be used on skin blotches or applied directly to hemorrhoids.

Dwarf Snapdragon was introduced into this country from its Mediterranean home in the last century. It has spread along the railway tracks, and earned the title of Railroad Weed.

It was originally named *Linaria minor*, and considered a diminutive toadflax, with blue flowers. But on the basis of the corolla being partially open at the yellow throat, rather than tightly closed like toadflax, it was renamed.

A seed-infesting weevil, *Gymnaetron antirrhini*, was an accidental import from Europe. The larvae appear to destroy the immature seeds, while the adults feed on the succulent stems.

An introduced perennial, Broad-leaved Toadflax has larger flowers and leaves, but otherwise looks very similar. It is quite prolific, producing up to a half million seeds per plant.

The related *L. cymbelaria* has a very interesting phototrophic system. The stalk reacts so as to turn the flower to light, but when replaced by ripening fruit, it turns from the light, in order to throw seeds towards dark walls or rock to enhance germination.

Blue Toadflax (*L. canadensis*) is used as a diuretic and laxative, and also applied to hemorrhoids as a wash or salve. This native annual looks like Common Toadflax, with light blue flowers, and is found on moist sandy soil of east central Alberta, and into Saskatchewan.

The flowers of all can be added to salads, but be warned; the aroma is strong.

An interesting note about Snapdragon. An early photosynthesizing green algae, *Chlamydomonas reinhardtii*, contains a gene involved in sensing the mineral copper. During evolution it somehow found itself into the genetic code of Snapdragon.

MEDICINAL

CONSTITUENTS- *L. vulgaris*-flavonoids including linarin, pectolarin, aurones including aureusin, and bracteatin-6-0-glucoside, quinazoline alkaloids including peganine (vasicin), antirrhinic acid, acetyl-pectolinarin (1.1% of dried flowers) neolinarin (bitter glycoside) linarascin (resin), anthokirrin (yellow colour), acacetin 7-rutinoside (flowers), choline, gamma-hydroxy-glutamic acid, scutellarein, prunin, glucosyringin, syringin, lirodendrin, 7-hydroxy vasicine, Vit C, procumbide, and antirrinoside derivatives, including 6-0-trans-p-coumaroyl antirrinoside, and 6-0-cis-p-coumaroyl antirrinoside; as well as 0-beta-D-glucopyranoside and primveroside. Also includes eight organic acids, including oxalic, aconitic, citric, ketoglutaric, ascorbic, malic, shikimic and fumaric acids.
Other constituents include antirride, 6-beta-idrossiantrride, 10-beta-glucosil-aucubina, and 4-carboxy-bornein.
The main active ingredients are the flavone glycosides linarin and pectolinarin, pectin, phytosterol, tannic acid and Vit C.
S. dalmatia- kaempferide
N. canadensis- aerial- two iridoid diesters of glycopyranose, eight flavones including apigenin, diosmetin, genkwanin, luteolin, luteolin 7-O-glucoside, luteolin-7-O-glycuronide, genkawanin 4'O-rutinoside and quercitin 7-O-rutinoside.
A. majus- leaves and flowers- choline, various alkaloids, including 4-methyl-2,6-naphthyridine, prunin, iridoids (antirrhinoside, antirrhide, 5-glucosyl-antirrhinoside, and linarioside); beta sitosterol, as well as branched chain fatty acids of the iso- and antisio-serides, along with linolenic, linoleic, oliec, trans-hexadecanoic, palmitic and other saturated fatty acids.
Sixteen amino acids have been isolated from aerial parts, as well as gamma amino butyric acid (GABA), and anthranilic acid.

Warm infusions of Toadflax help soften the stool and increase peristalsis of the intestine, as well as stimulate the liver to break down inflammatory compounds like histamine. It helps stimulate bile secretion when insufficient, but will also quickly reduce bilirubin levels when they are too high.

The leaves alone are better for diarrhea, while the flowers more so for constipation.

Michael Moore writes, "As a tonic, let's just say that Toadflax stirs things up, causing a moderate, scatter-gun stimulus of liver enzymes and fluid transport. By itself, this is just an empty increase in hepatic 'gray-noise' levels, which needs to be assisted either by other herbs that heat or stimulate liver function (for dry skin, blood-sugar reactive and allergen prone, liver deficient folks) or herbs that disperse and cool liver excitability in anabolic stress types…best combined…with such herbs as Oregon Grape and Yellow Dock (hot and stimulating) or Burdock, Dandelion or Redroot (cooling and contracting."

For liver stress from poor diet, or mal-absorption, Toadflax helps decongest and repair. Likewise in alcohol excess, or post-hepatitis exhaustion, it helps detoxify and soothe the liver. It combines well with dandelion, red root and yellow dock root; and is useful in all spleen and liver enlargements and inflammations, as well as hemorrhoids.

For lymphatic congestion, toadflax combines well with cleavers and red root.

Warm leaf infusions help break down and excrete kidney stones and gravel; as well as soothe bladder and prostate inflammation; and where there is difficulty urinating. Tinctures are reportedly better for cases of prostate inflammation.

Decoctions of the entire plant are diuretic, and were formerly given after childbirth for expelling afterbirth.

Externally, herbal fomentations or poultices relieve hemorrhoids, phlebitis, varicose veins, varicose ulcers and sciatica pain.

Warm decoctions or compresses also serve well in various skin rashes, applied to affected areas. Linarin, pectolinarin and luteolin are all active against collagenase, suggesting benefit in collagen-related disorders. Widyowati R et al, *Chem Pharm Bull* (Tokyo) 2016 64(5): 517-21.

The whole plant appears useful for those children with a tuberculin tendency.

It improves the nutrition of children with calcium deficiency, and wasting diseases, helping increase weight and strength. It should be kept in mind for obscure blood disorders in children.

Rademacher recommended the herb for knotted bunches of hemorrhoids, phlebitis and inflammation of the optical vessels. The latter indication was a decoction made into a compress and applied over the eyes in headstrong, willful children with inflamed eyes.

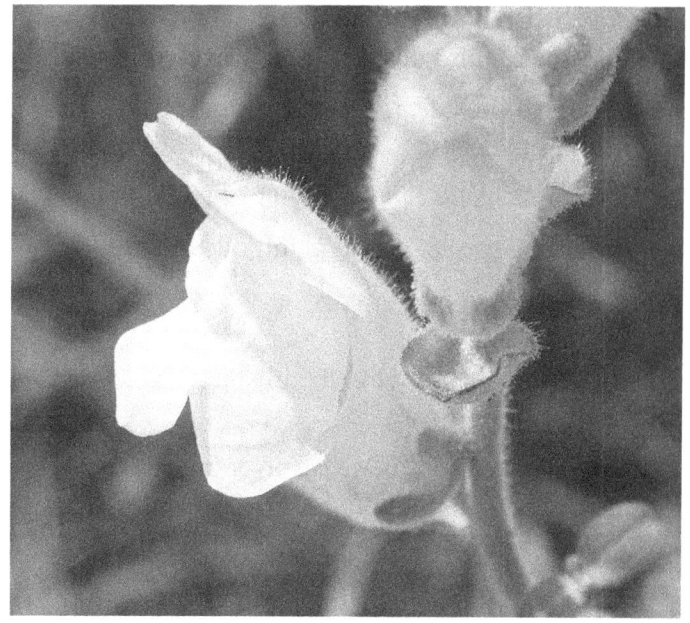

SNAPDRAGON

In TCM, the liver and eyes are closely related organs in terms of energetics.

Toadflax can be combined with yarrow, artemisia and/or false solomon seal root for making a good sweat bath. Simply decoct the plants and add the liquid to the hot rocks, inhaling the fumes.

Pectolinarin is strongly cytotoxic on large cell lung, hepatocellular, renal, amelanotic melanoma C32, colorectal carcinomas. Linarin, isolinarin A & B show similar activity. Tundis R et al, *Bioorg Med Chem Lett* 2005 15(21): 4757-60.

The same compounds show remarkable anti-diabetic activity, greater than the drug glybenclamide, in rats. Cheriet T et al, *Nat Prod Res* 2016 Dec 29: 1-7.

Scutellarein is found in Scullcap species, and has a wide range of activity.

Snapdragon ethanol extracts show activity against two candida species, in tests conducted by Jawad et al in Iraq (1988). Flower extracts alone show mycobacterium activity.

Peganine (vasicine) also found in Peganum species, is a powerful uterine stimulant, oxytocin in activity, as well as strong bronchodilator, antitussive and expectorant.

Vasicine shows potential activity against *Mycobacterium tuberculosis*. Chaliha AK et al, *Comb Chem High Throughput Screen* 2016 19(1): 14-24.

Vasicine is also a potent inhibitor of acetylcholinesterase and butyrylcholinesterase, suggestive of benefit in Alzheimer's disease and related senile dementia conditions. Liu W et al, *PLoS One* 2015 10(6).

Prunin, present in Snapdragon and Toadflax, as well as *Matthiola incana*, is strongly anti-fungal. Work by Rzadkowska-Bodalska et al, *Bull Pol Acad* 1995 43 found Toadflax active against *Candida albicans, Rhodotorula rubra* and *Aspergillus fumigatus*.

Earlier research by Damtoft at the University of Denmark, showed the iridoid antirrinoside was produced from 8-epi-deoxyloganic acid.

Work by Hobedal et al, also from Denmark, showed seasonal variation in plant iridoid content. Antirrhinoside is highest before flowering, and antirrhide during flower.

Infusions of the plant have been shown to possess cardiotoxic, hypotensive and sedative action.

Linarin has been found to inhibit acetyl-cholinesterase, suggestive of application in Alzheimer's disease and various other neuronal conditions. Fan et al, *Pharm Bio* 46:9.

Acacetin 7-rutinoside, found in the flowers is an inhibitor of lens aldose reductase, iodothyronine deiodinase, and histamine release.

Urchovska et al, *Nat Prod Res* 2008 22:9 identified anti-oxidant activity.

Kaempferide, from *L. dalmatia* inhibits inflammatory conditions. It is also found in willow and birch buds.

HOMEOPATHY

Linaria (Toadflax) acts prominently on the vagus nerve, and will calm nausea vomiting, and feelings of pressure on the stomach.

In jaundice, hepatitis, as well as liver and spleen enlargement, Toadflax will give quick relief. Along with the intestinal feelings, there can be great drowsiness, and feelings of faintness, sleepiness, and confusion.

Involuntary bedwetting is sometimes relieved. Copious urination or high colored like dark beer.

The tongue is rough and dry, and the throat may feel constricted. The symptoms are made worse by walking in the open air.

Stupid feeling of indifference, ill-humor and dull frontal headache. Confused feeling in head, and irresistible sleepiness.

Fainting spells occurring, three to four times a day. Sensation of fainting.

DOSE- Third to 30th potency. Muller, Jenicek, Raidl and unnamed woman self experimented with 5-30 drops of tincture. MacFarlan used 30x and lower potencies on patients.

FLOWER/LEAF OIL

Cover one part of fresh bruised Toadflax flowers and leaves with ten parts of hot canola oil, and let sit for twenty four hours in a loosely sealed thermos, or warm spot. Strain and use in hemorrhoid ointments, skin problems, etc. It combines well with fireweed oil for anal fissures; in the form of suppositories.

An ointment, or better yet, lotion or water made from the flowers was at one time, an ophthalmic remedy for eye irritations.

SEED OIL

The fatty acid content of toadflax seeds is two-thirds linoleic acid, with traces of linolenic, and about 22% oleic acid. The seeds contain up to 37.5% oil, with a specific gravity of 0.9217. The iodine value is 140, indicating a very drying oil. It is an edible and delicious oil that is produced in Russia to this day.

Snapdragon seeds yield an edible oil, similar to olive oil in texture and taste.

HYDROSOL

The distilled water of toadflax is excellent for treating dropsy, for it forceably expels trapped urine, is also helpful in treating jaundice, and will open blockages of the liver and spleen, when taken in three ounce doses in the morning before breakfast.
                                                                                                    SAUER

The distilled water of the herb and flowers ...doth somewhat move the belly downwards, opens obstructions of the liver, and helps the yellow jaundice; expels poison, provokes women's courses, drive forth the dead child and afterbirth.

The distilled water, dropped into the eyes, is a certain remedy for all heat, inflammation and redness in them. The water put into foul ulcers, whether they be cancerous or fistulous, with tents rolled therein, or parts washed and injected therewith, cleanses them thoroughly from the bottom, and heals them up safely. The same water also cleanses the skin wonderfully of all sorts of deformity, as leprosy, morphew, scurf, wheals, pimples, or spots, applied of itself, or used with some powder of Lupines. **CULPEPPER**

FLOWER ESSENCES

Yellow Toadflax flower essence is useful where pride and arrogance lead us to shut others out. It is for those feeling bitter, lonely, angry and in pain. It is for accepting oneself, seeing one's behaviour and opening the door to others, and returning to joy and love. **CANADIAN**

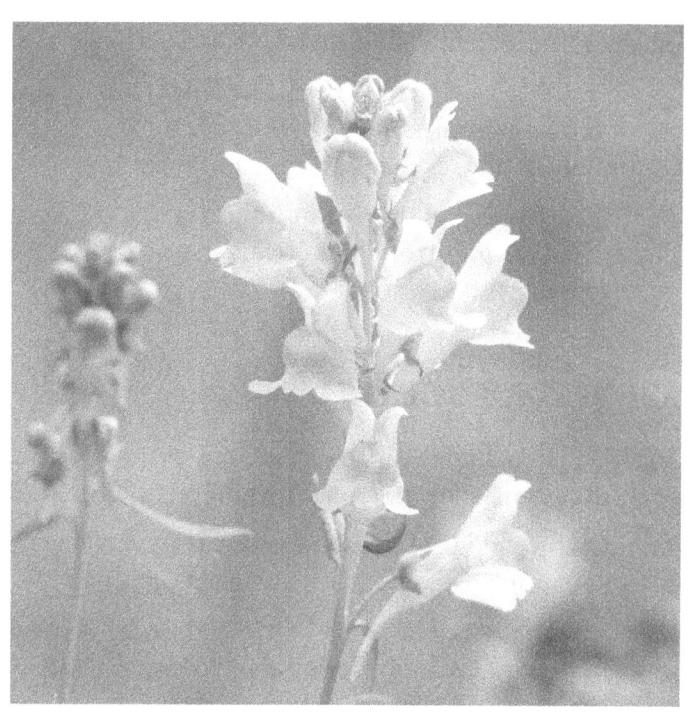

TOADFLAX FLOWERS

Toadflax flower essence is helpful to those individuals that catch themselves saying " I should have.....". By stuffing down what they were feeling or experiencing at the moment, out of fear, or embarrassment; they deprive themselves of the opportunity to grow and expand. Toadflax helps bring individuals out of their mental and emotional shells. The essence is useful for those who have difficulty with quiet, in either a social or one- on-one situation. They may feel the need to fill the "void" with constant chatter; which is a type of avoidance. An indigenous elder said, "Much silence has a mighty roar". Toadflax essence is indicated for those who have difficulty with meditation, or activities that require silencing the conscious mind for focus and inner attention. The essence may be of special importance to children with Attention Deficit Hyperactivity Disorder (ADHD) or autism. Toadflax may help create focus and attention, by filtering out disruptive, or secondary stimuli. For ADHD, consider combining toadflax with Algae Maze mushroom essence. Rogers (2016). Algae Maze is useful, as well, for obsessive-compulsive disorder (OCD) and various related behavior and neuroses. For OCD, try Algae Maze for a lunar cycle or more, combined with Alum root flower essence. For autism spectrum disorder, a good combination may be Toadflax combined with Wood Ear mushroom essence. This combination may be helpful by creating more opportunity for listening and expression. **PRAIRIE DEVA**

Butter and Eggs essence supports and stabilizes the Central Nervous System in times of stress. **EASTERN**

Snapdragon flower essence is useful to those who experience difficulties in speaking or expressing their feelings. It allows one to free repressed emotions through verbal expression. **DEVA**

Toadflax essence helps recognize our own values so that we do not need to constantly prove something to others. **MIRIANA**

The name and shape of Snapdragon's flowers show that it is predominately associated with treating the vocal cords, lips, jaw, and facial tissues, and muscles.

All the cranial plates are aligned. It treats tetanus, Bell's Palsy, lip cancer, some forms of arthritis, especially of the jaw, TMJ, and imbalances of the throat region, including laryngitis, and strep infections.

The essence also treats allergies that have a tendency to cause spots on the skin. Along with meditation, kelp and silver it may help alleviate tic douloureux.

On the cellular level, it strengthens the enamel of the teeth, and the connective tissues and joint structures are also enhanced.

Damage to the brain's speech centre could be treated with snapdragon. Stuttering is an example tissue. This can be associated with a problem with one's parents. While it is not associated with acts of violence, there can be a real release of suppressed emotions, which can include rage and screaming.

The budding of fruit will be slightly enhanced by using this essence. The fruit will appear sooner and be stronger.

GURUDAS

There can be extreme tension in the jaw and mouth, grinding of the teeth, or the need to eat foods that provide continuous biting, crunching and chewing activity.

At the deepest level, the Snapdragon helps the soul to distinguish its use of creative forces—especially those that radiate from the lower energy centres, and those which are used for the spoken word. By harmonizing the relationship between these energy centres, the soul evolves in its use of creative power.

FLOWER ESSENCE SOCIETY

SPIRITUAL PROPERTIES

Toadflax has a double capacity from the spiritual point of view. Orange is the colour of knighthood in the ranks of spiritual work, for it denotes the ability to "know" the truth which goes beyond that normally found.

Yellow is the colour of the sun, whose love for all creation is so vast as to be unimaginable to mankind. Yellow is also the universal or Christ-love in action.

This combination of love and knowledge is very potent, and the seeker may move more quickly by eating one of these flowers each day during the blooming season.

The flowers may be soaked in olive oil for three days in a light proof container. This oil may be dabbed on the third eye, and left for twenty minutes. During this time, attention should be directed to this spot. Then remove the oil. In two weeks, infra red light may be directed at the spot while the oil is in place. **HILARION**

Baby Snapdragon (*L. maroccana*) is symbolic of expressive silence. This means that certain silences are revelations and are more expressive than words can ever be. **THE MOTHER**

MYTHS AND LEGENDS

In European superstition, the Toad was an attribute of death and was often shown in arts with a skull or skeleton, or eating the genitals of a naked woman as a symbol of lust. The toad was a loathsome familiar of witches, suggestive of the torments of the damned – a demonic symbolism that stems from the ancient Near East, based perhaps on the toad's toxic secretions. These were used medicinally in China where the toad was a lunar, yin and humid symbol, a rain bringer, and therefore associated with luck and riches.

In folklore, a three-legged toad lived in the moon: it was said that a lunar eclipse was the act of the toad's swallowing the moon. Rain and fertility symbolism appear in Mexico and in parts of Africa where the toad is sometimes given the status of culture hero. Alchemy associated the toad with the primal elements of earth and water. **JACK TRESIDDER**

RECIPES

DECOCTION- Take one to two teaspoons of dried plant to one pint of water. Simmer for twenty minutes. Drink one-half cup up to three times daily.

INFUSION- two tsp of herb in one cup of hot water. Steep 18 minutes. Drink throughout day.

TINCTURE- 20-40 drop three times daily. Take fresh leaves and flowers, and make a 1:5 tincture at 60% alcohol.

COMPRESS- Take 20 grams of dried herb to 500 ml of milk and make a mushy compress.

BATH- Two tablespoons of herb per pint of water are infused and added hot to baths.

CAUTION- Do not use during pregnancy or breastfeeding. Do not use with barbituates or ACE inhibitors, or any prescription drug for that matter.

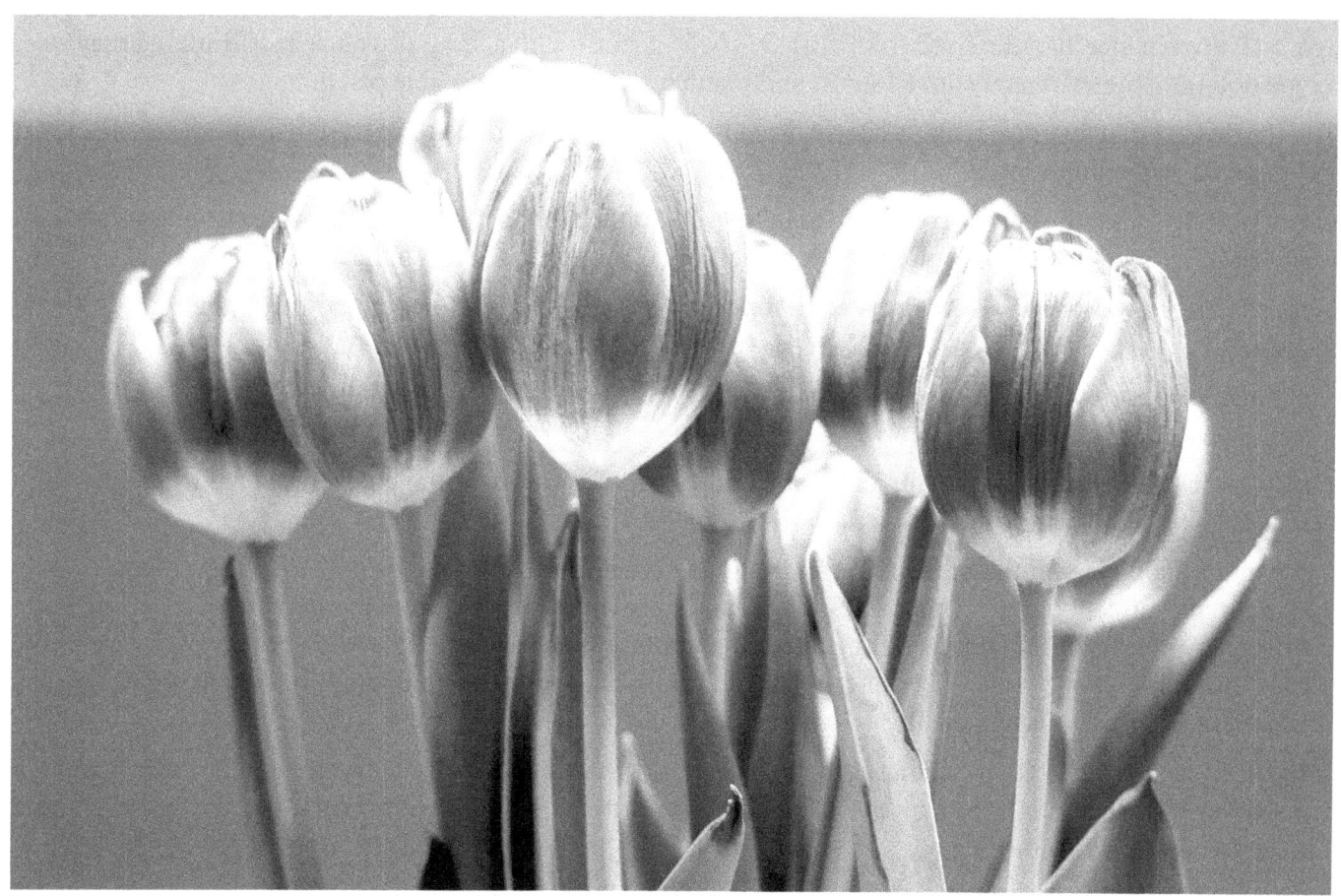

TULIPS

TULIP
(***Tulipa edulis*** [Miq.] Baker)
(***Amana edulis*** [Miq.] Honda)
(***Tulipa gesneriana*** L.)

Then comes the tulip race, where beauty plays her idle freaks: from family diffused to family, as flies the father dust
The varied colours run: and while they break on the charmed eye, the exulting
Florist marks with secret pride
The wonders of his hand.
                                                                                        J THOMSON 1730

She has the color of violet, and the curved form of the new moon…her shape is like the almond, needle like, and ornamented with pleasant rays. Her inner petals are like a well, as they should be; her outer petals a little open, this too as it should be…she is the chosen of the chosen.   **WILFRED BLUNT**

Perhaps the tulip knows the fickleness
Of Fortune's smile, for on her stalk's green shaft,
She bears a wine cup through the wilderness.
                                                                                        HAFIZ SUFI POET

Tulip is from the Arabic **TULBAND,** or **DULBEND,** meaning a turban. The Turks would show their gardens to European merchants and diplomats, and then point out the resemblance of the flower to their turban. The visitors took the name and corrupted it to **TULIPAN,** and later abbreviated to tulip.

The wild progenitor was known as **LALE,** in the area formerly known as Persia. In Arabic script it is composed of the same letters as Allah, the name of God. Tulips were planted in order to help their souls ascend to heaven.

Turkey is considered the native land for many of the species. When first introduced to Holland, over 400 years ago, an Antwerp merchant received from Turkey, a bale of cloth, with a few bulbs enclosed. Thinking they were a type of onion, the merchant cooked some, and planted some in his vegetable patch.

The red flowers that sprang up, made him realized that the tulips had traveled to him in disguise, and the great Tulip mania was soon to begin.

Other stories suggest the bulbs were imported in the 16th century by the Austrian ambassador to Constantinople, Busbequius. He acquired some bulbs at a dear price and sent them back to Vienna.

Conrad Gesner was a Swiss botanist who first described tulips as 'red lilies' after seeing them in flower in Augsburg in 1559.

Tulip mania appeared in the Netherlands in the mid-17th century.

Tulips take seven years from seed to flower, so bulbs are used to create true offspring. Tulip trade made some men wealthy, with buyers purchasing in bloom, and taking possession of the bulbs in the fall when lifted and cleaned.

Middlemen soon entered the fracas, and this progressed to florists selling tulips not yet in their possession, in a manner reminiscent of today's futures market. This paper trade was robust with everything depending upon ever higher prices. Sound familiar? They were all gambling on a living thing and someone else's care of the plants. The tulip frenzy reached fever pitch in 1636-37, with houses offered for a single bulb. Still standing today in Haarlem, Holland, it is named The Tulip House.

It all ended on April 27, 1637 when not a single buyer could be found for bulbs at any price, after the government issued restrictive legislation to bring speculations to a halt. It was reminiscent of Black Tuesday in 1929, when the stock market came crashing down.

Today, the tulip still symbolizes Holland, with some two million bulbs exported annually.

Tulip bulbs are very high in estrogenic activity. During World War II, women in Holland, who ate large quantities showed uterine bleeding and other menstrual abnormalities.

MEDICINAL

In China, bulbs of *A. edulis* are used medicinally for ulcers, abscesses and tubercular cervical nodes. Known as **SHAN T'ZU KU,** or **SHAN CI GU,** or **GUANG CI GU** (stem stolon), the bulbs are cold and sweet, and at the same time peppery in taste.

The name is derived from the likeness of the bulb to a merciful nun. I have also seen the name **LA YA BAN** for the stem tuber. The bulb is used for sore throat, scrofula, ulcers and postpartum blood stasis.

Presently it is widely cultivated and used in the treatment of tumors, such as esophageal, lymphoma and breast cancer. Yeh S, *Am J Chin Med* 2009 1: 271-4; Miao Y et al, *Ind Crop Prod* 2015 66: 81-88.

They help lower fever and detoxify, resolving sputum and easing constipation. A poultice of the mashed bulb is used for tubercular cervical nodes.

One constituent of the bulb has been shown to inhibit the influenza virus.

Ethanol extracts of *T. edulis* help eliminate stagnation and treat swelling and abscess.

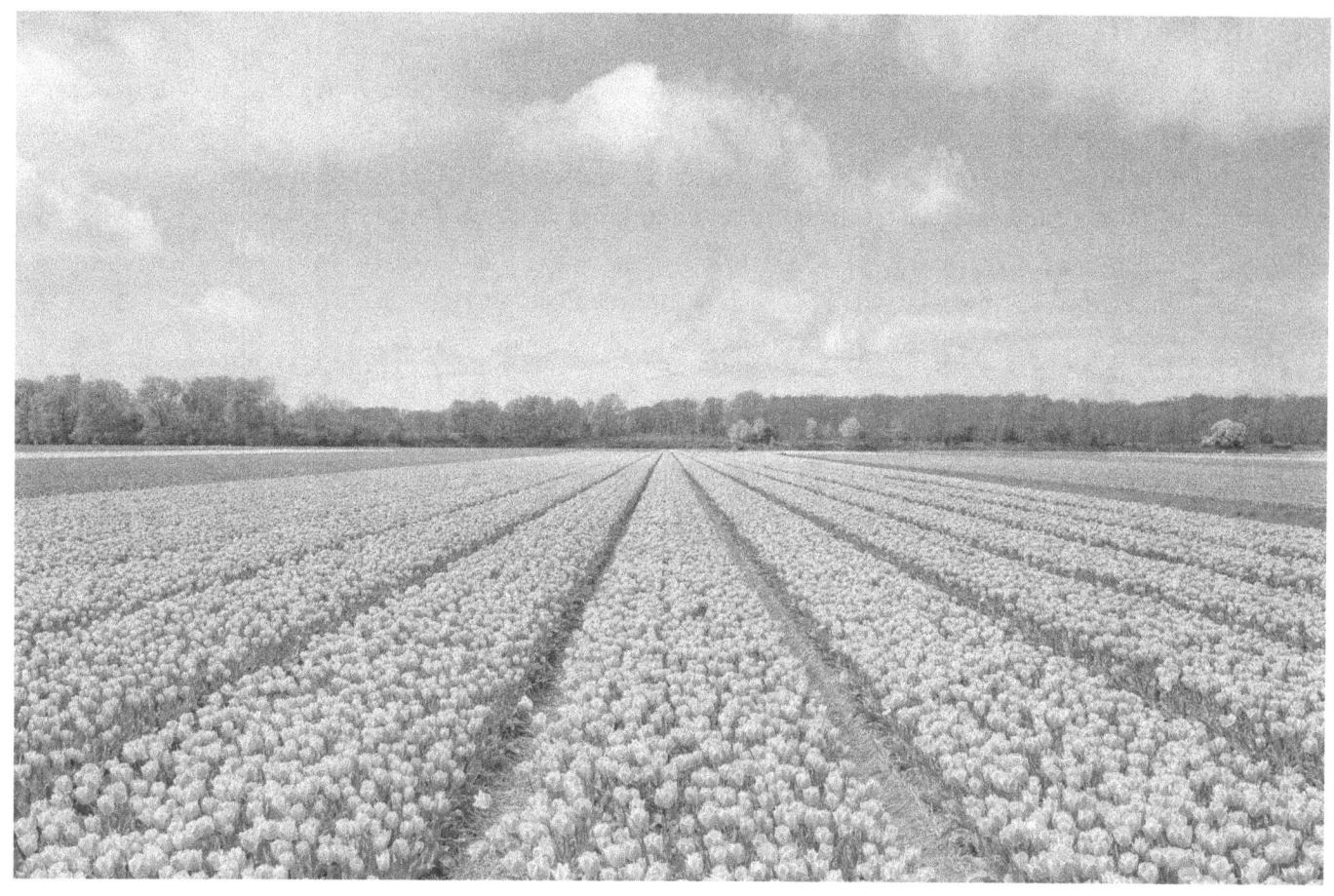

TULIP FIELD

They also inhibit the growth of human gastric carcinoma cells, due to mitochondria-mediated apoptosis. Lin R et al, *Oncol Lett* 2015 10(4): 2371-77. It is widely used in TCM for treatment of breast cancer, either singly as an edible or in various formulas.

Tulipine is cardiotonic in nature, but tulipine A is the major allergen.

Tulip bulbs contain glycoproteins, and glycosidic esters, namely tuliposide A and B. Through hydrolysis they produce carboxylic acids which lactonize spontaneously to form methylene lactones, tulipalins A and B. These compounds are powerful fungicides.

A mixture of flavonoid glucuronoides isolated from the perianth of *T. gesneriana* shows protective activity against skin vascular permeability in rabbits.

Compounds from this tulip show antibiotic activity. Tschesche R et al, *Tetrahedron Lett* 1968 6:701-6. Tulip sap shows anti-microbial activity. Dansi A et al, *Ric Sci* 1967 37(6): 524-8.

Other work shows tulip lectins exhibiting mitogenic activity on both mouse and human lymphocytes.

The people of Kurdistan use *Tulipa systola* for pain relief and as anti-inflammatory agent.

The only other reference I have found to medicinal properties is from the poet, Abraham Crowley. He wrote:

I am a flower for sight, a drug for use,
By secret virtue and resistless power
Those whom the jaundice seizes I restore;
The dropsie headlong makes away
As soon as I my arms display.

HOMEOPATHY

Tulip (*Tulipa gesneriana*) is a remedy for crossing borders, or growing in general. It is the archetype of orgasm, growing process blasting away borders.

Pure, un-inhibited sex, extremely fast remedy. Craziness, aimless activity, lazy pleasure seekers addicted to sex and kicks. Distant and numb, as if the spiritual energy has descended into the genitals. The thrill lies in forbidden things.

DOSE- 4C. First clinical proving by Olaf Posdzech with three males in 1999

FLOWER ESSENCE

Black Tulip clears the third eye. It brings clarity, perception, vision and originality.   **HABUNDIA**

Red tulip is used to provide grounding and centering to those who are too intensely seeking their spiritual path. Brings us out of our head and helps us to enjoy the journey rather than solely focusing on the end result.
RAVENWORKS

Wild Yellow Tulip (*Tulipa sylvestris*) is the native European wild tulip. I did not plan to make that essence, until I saw these flowers.

Dainty yet expressive, they are the only wild tulip that does not simply come up straight and unfolds, but that snakes around and moves almost like an animal while growing, unfolding, blooming and waning. Wild Yellow Tulip essence touches upon the principal of how we express ourselves in motion, as well as in emotion. E-motivity should here be understood as inner movement. Wild Yellow Tulip essence forces us to express that which has been held inside for too long, helping us to speak emotional truth. Despite of being yellow (orange typically goes to the sexual chakra), it seems to strongly act on the uterus, in the sense of acting on cramping or strong emotions held there. Looking much like the Fallopian Tubes in its movement, or like the dancing devotees of Bacchus, god of wine, Wild Yellow Tulip flower essence acts on wild, upwelling, and instable emotions. "It really settles them", says a young woman in emotional upheaval from a painful relationship breakup. Bringing light–"sunshine"–into the pelvis, this essence inspires our energy and body to move, in ways such as belly dance or bending backwards into a bridge. It is helpful for hysteria, a condition in which the ancient Greeks thought the uterus was wandering freely within the abdominal cavity, and adjusts both, hyper-emotionality and lack of emotions, a wandering as well as a rigid uterus. A typical MAM use would be an external application to adjust a prolapsed uterus that refuses to return to its original position, especially if the prolapse was asymmetrical. Wild Yellow Tulip is the most sensitive lily in the circle with Madonna Lily; the blossom dances in the sunlight as it unfolds. It inspires kundalini energy, as well as loosens and mobilizes stiff parts, such as the shoulders or pelvic area.
JULIA GRAVES

SPIRITUAL PROPERTIES

The message of the Tulip flower spirit is one of growth and regeneration…It is an evocative representation of all that is new, fertile and fresh. Its paper-thin petals appear almost as if by magic on a long elegant stem, but although delicate in appearance, this growth from a tight, hard bulb displays its powerful life force.
ECLARE

Tulip's alignment with the heart can help us notice and feel grateful for all our many blessings. And because like attracts like, the more grateful we feel, the more we have to be grateful for. With that in mind, tulips can help us develop our prosperity conscious-ness and attract abundance and blessings of all forms.
TESS WHITEHURST

PERSONALITY TRAITS

Tulipa, half flower and half woman, was the favourite of the Sultan Shahabaan. She was the daughter of a Dutch sea captain, and had been captured by pirates.

Tulipa is depicted surrounded by courtiers and eunuchs in tulip-shaped turbans.

Beautiful, but rather a bore, and not nearly animated for her pleasure-loving husband, Tulipa was no good at all at singing or dancing or making calembourgs. Shahabaan soon tired of her, had her sown up in a leather sack, and dropped into the Bosphorus.

COATS

Solid, reliable and conservative, patients who need Tulipa focus their attention primarily on people close by, the family, the household. It is as if they live under a glass cover, their picture of the world limited.

Very religious but in their own way; have religious feelings yet do not go to church. Find it difficult to digest new information, especially when there are many new or strange ideas. When the source of a new idea is unknown it is more difficult for them to accept.

Tend to become restless and frustrated if they do not succeed according to their own views and high standards… very perfectionistic. Strength is brought to light by preparing themselves for the worst. Might become workaholics. Reluctant in showing themselves emotionally, similar with *Natrium muriaticum*. Tend to be very mental.

Sadness can be salted away [like money], but when the tears come out, they can really break through and the person can weep long and intensely…Like the flower that is a bit haughty, the Tulipa-patient can have an inner pride that can be observed when you look for it.

GIO MEIJER MD

MYTHS AND LEGENDS

Near a pixie field there lived an old woman who…cultivated a most beautiful bed of tulips. The pixies so delighted in this spot that they carried their elfin babies there, put them inside the tulips, and sang them to sleep. The delicate music would float in the air and the beautiful tulips waved their heads to the evening breezes…As soon as the elfin babies were lulled asleep, the pixies…began their dancing. They danced all night in the fairy ring, but at first light of dawn they returned to the tulips.

The old woman tended the bed…and never let even one of the blooms be plucked. The pixies surrounded the tulips with a perfume more fragrant than roses. But at length the old woman died. The new owner removed the bed of tulips and planted parsley instead. But the parsley withered and nothing ever grew well.

And so the people of Devon say: Before you remove a bed of tulips, check to see if they have a fragrance, and watch to see if they last longer than the other flowers. If they do, then it is better to leave them be, for they might be pixie cradles.

PALLOWSKI

RECIPES

DECOCTION- 3-9 grams in decoction internally. External poultice as needed.

TUMBLEWEED
RUSSIAN THISTLE
(***Salsola kali*** L.)
(***S. australis*** [L.] Br.)
PRICKLY RUSSIAN THISTLE
(***S. kali* ssp. *tragus*** [L.] Celak) not accepted
(***S. tragus*** L.)
KARELIN
(***S. richteri***)
PARTS USED- aerial

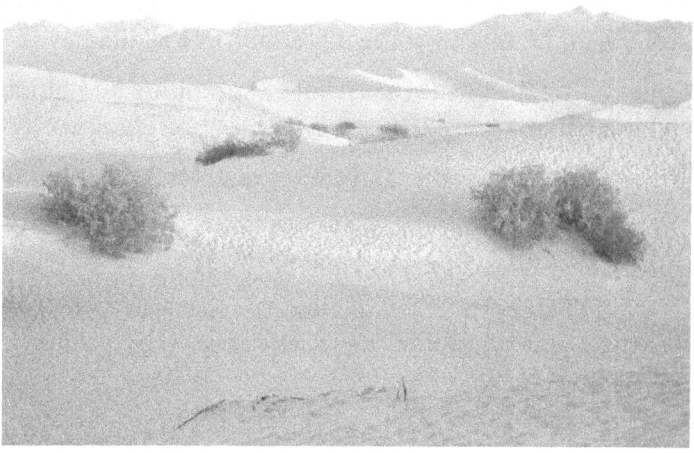

TUMBLEWEED

For though thou wash thee with nitre, and take thee much sope. **JEREMIAH 2**

The legendary tumbleweed is really a nurse crop that protects the growth of prairie grasses under its shade, and then it sacrifices itself and blows away. **ANTOINE PREDOCK**

The airy balls of tumbleweed resembled rolling brains and were another of the Southwest's emblematic organisms, like the saquaro and sagebrush, the roadrunner, the coyote and the sidewinder. **ALEX SHOUMATOFF**

Salsola is from the Persian word for "carpet". **SALSUS** is Latin for salt. Kali is from the Arabic **ALQALIY** meaning the ashes of saltwort, another common name.

Tumbleweed conjures up images of prairie storms, with tumbling balls of fire spreading grass fires. It became known as witch grass, the destroying angel of the early pioneer.

In Russia it is known as **PERIKATI POLYE** meaning, "roll-across-the-field".

It arrived in North America in the early 1870s with a group of Russian emigrants who settled in South Dakota. In their baskets of flaxseed, was the stowaway which over the next twenty years moved northward through every state and province.

A later group of Mennonites, with tumbleweed seed mixed amongst their wheat seeds sewn into their clothing, brought more into Kansas, and the assault was on.

The typical tumbleweed is a globe of wiry branches with over 12,000 small spiny leaves and minute greenish-pink flowers. It is well adapted for the prairies, flourishing in the sun, resistant to salty, alkaline soils. When seeds are ripe, a strong wind breaks the weak stem, and away it goes, sowing over 20,000 tiny, black glossy seeds over a ten-mile radius. The pollen is prolific, and has been found on the Shroud of Turin, enshrined in an Italian cathedral since 1538.

Unrestricted, tumbleweed sows itself so thickly it looks like a green carpet in spring. The seed can germinate in 36 minutes. The Apache quickly learned to eat the young green shoots, when about two inches tall.

The pretty seedpods can be used in fall dried flower arrangements, as the pink colour will stay for several months.

The herb was used in traditional European folk medicine as a laxative, diuretic and vermifuge.

The alkaline salts used in soap manufacture during Biblical times were from burning tumbleweed. The soap was made, by mixing the ash with olive oil.

In the former Dutch East Indies, the same ashes were used as a therapeutic dressing, antiseptic and cleansing agent.

Various leaf and stem boring moths (*Coleophora sp.*) have been introduced in attempts to control the spread of Russian Thistle with limited success.

New reports out of eastern Oregon find glyphosate resistance in *S. tragus*.

The amino acid content of the seeds and stem leaves has been analyzed. The plant contains 55% digestible protein, and has 80% of the digestibility of alfalfa hay.

Considering it was the first plant to sprout life and bloom after atomic testing on Utah deserts, it may be with us for a while.

The pollen is allergenic, and causes distress in a high number of people.

MEDICINAL

CONSTITUENTS- *S. kali-* alkaloids D-salsolidine (80%); and L- salsolidine (14%), as well as salsoline; estrone (3 ppm), cholesterol, beta sitosterol, nitrates, soluble oxalates and oxalic acid, isorhamnetin-3-0-glucoside, methyl carbamate and rutinoside. Ash residue is 22.64%.
S. richteri- salsoline

Russian Thistle has been suggested as a cathartic, diuretic, emmenagogue, stimulant and vermifuge.

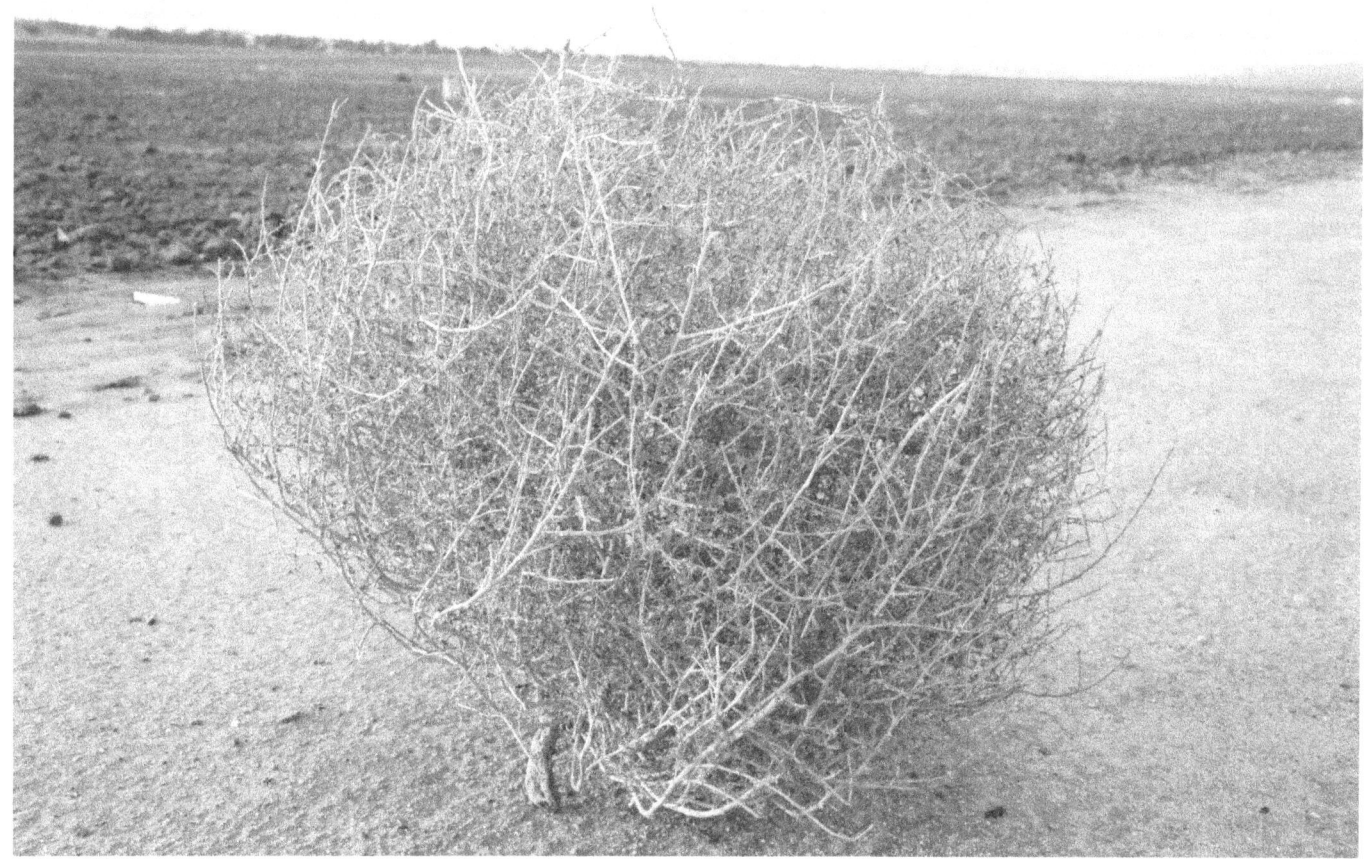

TUMBLEWEED

In Hartwell's book on cancer and plants, he lists Russian Thistle as a folk remedy for the cancerous condition known as superfluous flesh.

It has been used in cases of dropsy, or edemas.

Studies conducted by Sabahi et al at Karman University in Iran in 1987 found *S. kali* was a highly inhibitory plant against microorganisms.

In laboratory studies, the plant has been shown to exhibit hypotensive and smooth muscle relaxing activity.

Work by Turdis et al, *Pharmazie* 62:6 found aerial parts of *S. kali* contain alpha amylase inhibitors and exhibit hypoglycemic activity.

Karelin (*S. richteri*) contains salsoline and is used in Russia for the treatment of hypertension.

Salsolidine, and salsoline have been found cardioactive in nature. Salsoline is both hypotensive and anti-histaminic. It is said to resemble papaverine in its effect on vasoconstriction and hydrastine in its effect on smooth muscles of the uterus.

Tumbleweed decoction lowers oxidative stress and prevents cardiac toxicity against adriamycin, in male Swiss albino mice. Aniss HA et al, *Redox Rep* 2014 19(4): 170-8.

The closely related *S. collina* (*S. ruthenica*) is used in Traditional Chinese Medicine as a hypotensive with analgesic properties. It is known as Zha Peng Ke in Mandarin and is comprised of both the root and herb. It is called Zhumaocal, or Ci Peng, and has sweet, bland, and cool properties that relieve headaches. The anti-hypertensive effect lasts from 7-30 days after administration is stopped, with direct vaso-dilating and indirect CNS inhibition.

It contains succinic acid, betaine and a variety of polysaccharides, as well as salsoline, salsolidine, and a variety of organic acids and sugars. Normal dose is 30-60 grams in decoction.

The related *S. opposifolium* has been found to inhibit growth of hormone dependant prostate carcinoma. Tundis et al, *Z Naturforsch* 2008 63:5-6.

The plant inhibits butyrl-cholinesterase, suggestive of benefit in Alzheimer's and other neurological disease. Tundis et al, *J Enz Inhib Med Chem* 2009 24:3.

Another related fruit-bearing herb, *S. komarovvi* shows hypotensive effect, while the tiny seedlings exhibit significant pressor effect, but no hypotensive effect.

HOMEOPATHY

Salsola tragus has been proved at C4 and 30C.

The former C4 dilution, given to four females and two males in 2005, and summarized by Judy Schriebman, reported disjointed, almost chaotic kind of energy. Conversations erupted spontaneously, and people broke into song and laughter with much absolutely silly joking and wordplay.

The issue of abundance occurred and appetite was ravenous. Symptoms associated with sidedness, primarily left but mainly head, eye and ear symptoms. Eyes sensitive to light, tired. Hearing extremely acute, or muddled, and the sensation of being underwater. Frequent urination was noted.

In the latter 30C trial conducted by Todd Rowe on 15 females and two males in 2005, symptoms were different. Eurphoria, high spirits, were observed but dirt and dusty feelings were present in dreams, sensitivity to light and odour, with dusty, musty tobacco imagined.

Dryness of nose, face, mouth, throat and legs was noted with right side more affected. Headaches made worse from light noise and odor, and better from pressure.

SEED OIL

The seeds contain 22% oil with a fatty acid composition of 10% saturated, 30% monoenes, and 50% dienes.

PERSONALITY TRAITS

The tumbleweed stood for everything a cowboy was; a little ugly, lanky, and a foot loose rambler.

TODD ROWE

TURTLEHEAD
BALMONY
CHELONE
SALT- RHEUM
FISH MOUTH
SNAKE HEAD
(**Chelone glabra** L.)
PARTS USED- aerial parts

The turtlehead's a tightlipped plant-
It keeps its secrets sealed
And, unlike the banana, can't
Reward you as it's peeled.
Yet, what's so great inside that shell
That makes the bee elate?
And when it blooms each day, pray tell,
Does it "open"- or "inflate"?

JACK SANDERS

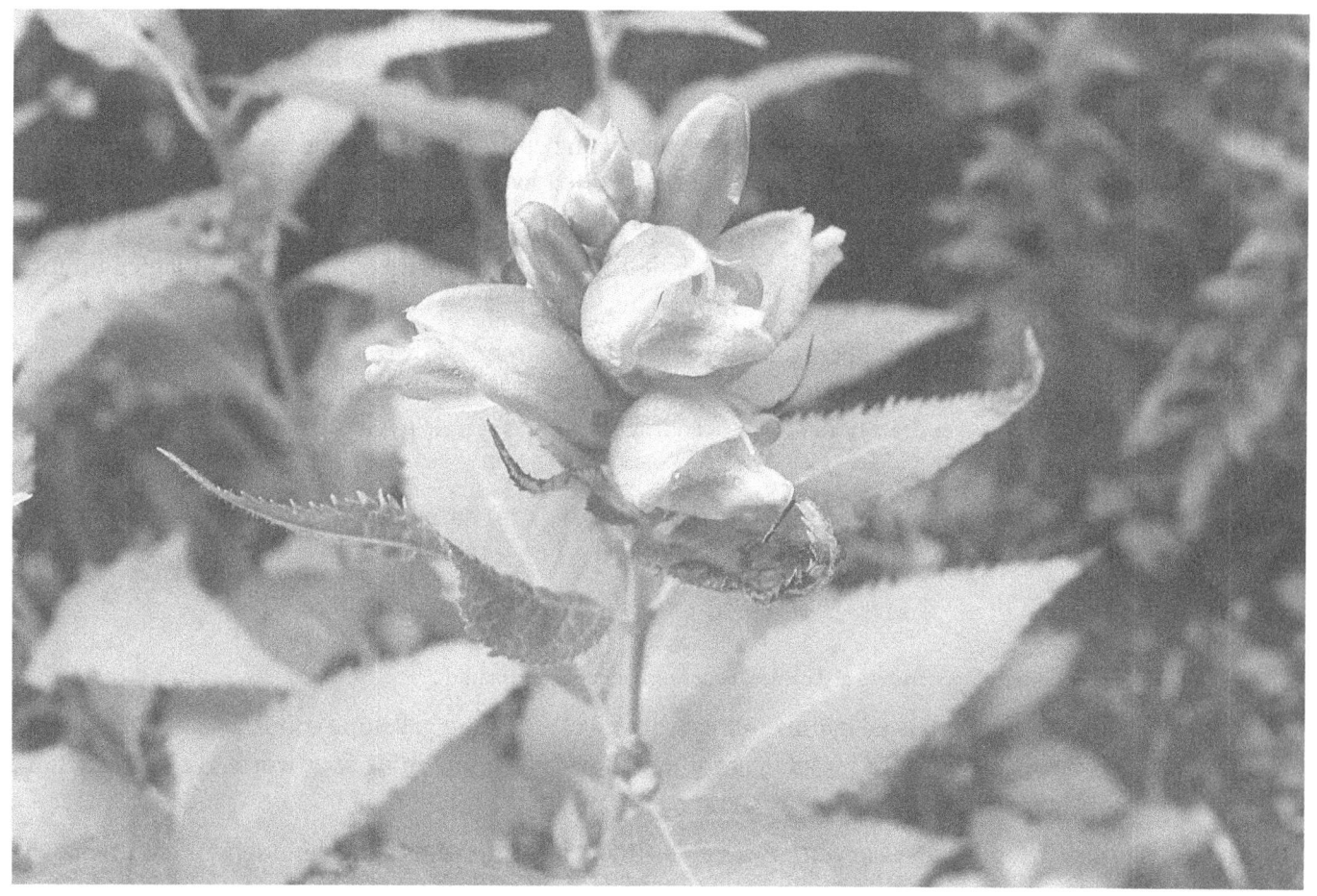

TURTLEHEAD (*C. obliqua*)

Chelone is Greek meaning turtle, referring to the flower head's resemblance to the tortoise head. Chelone is a Greek nymph. Glabra means smooth, describing the stems and leaves.

Balmony is a derivation of Baldmoney, an early name for some gentians, also called Bitterworts. Balmony is more likely related to the use of leaf salves for skin tumours, and ulcers.

Salt Rheum is from the Greek word for flux or flow, and thus a remedy for rheumatism, bursitis or gout.

Turtlehead is a perennial that thrives in wet woodlands and on riverbanks in Manitoba. It transplants easily, and one plant can become a colony very quickly if kept evenly moist. It will do best in moist, wet soil that is slightly acidic. It is a favorite browse plant of deer.

Chelone glabra is a diploid species, and *C. obliqua* occurs as a tetraploid and hexaploid.

The Cherokee infused the flower heads as laxative, as well as worms and fevers. Externally, the flowers were used for sores and skin eruptions; but internally to increase appetite.

The Iroquois used the root as part of a compound decoction for excessive bile secretion. They infused the roots in anti-witchcraft medicine. The Algonquin combined the root with cedar bark (*Thuja occidentalis*) as an unspecified medicinal tea. The Mik'maq used the plant to prevent pregnancy.

Several of the Eclectic physicians of the 19th century praised Balmony for its digestive influence.

The work of Rafinesque began with information passed on by Dr. Lawrence. "They are powerful, tonic, cathartic, hepatic, and anti-herpetic. The whole plant is used, but strictly the leaves; they are extensively bitter, one of the strongest of our bitters, without any aromatic smell and very little astringency.

Their tincture becomes black, and the use of dyes the urine the same colour...in small doses it is laxative, but in full doses it purges the bile and cleans the system of the morbid or superfluous bile, removing the yellowness of the skin in jaundice and liver diseases."

Dr. Felter saw it a "useful remedy for gastro-intestinal debility with hepatic torpor or jaundice. Dyspeptic conditions attending convalescence from prostrating fevers are often aided by it, and should be studied particularly for vague and shifting pain in the region of the ascending colon".

Dr. King agreed with all the above, and also recommended ointments of the herb for painful, inflamed tumors, irritable, painful ulcers, inflamed breasts, and hemorrhoids.

Dr. Cook added his astute opinion. "Few tonics are equal to Balmony in cases of enfeebled stomach, with accompanying indigestion, biliousness, costiveness and general languor. It arouses the gastric and salivary secretion, and decidely improves digestion... It is not so intense as the American Gentian, but is more stimulating than boneset (as a laxative tonic)."

He suggested it combines well with goldenseal and dogwood for the treatment of intermittent fevers, and with dogbane and poplar to treat intestinal worms.

MEDICINAL

CONSTITUENTS- resins, bitters, iridoid glycosides including catalpol and aucubin.

Balmony is a strongly bitter herb used mainly to treat the gall bladder and gallstone conditions. By stimulating bile flow, it has some laxative properties that combine well with its anthelmintic, or worm-removing action. The energy is cool and dry.

The herb is useful in cases of nausea and vomiting, intestinal colic, and yet is gentle enough for children.

People with poor fat metabolism, accompanied by gas, belching and chronic constipation, may find this a very useful herb.

Skin problems, such as acne, psoriasis, or eczema, related to poor digestion and elimination may benefit.

It has some minor anti-depressant properties; especially if associated with anorexia.

Catalpol shows in animal studies it might be of value for global cerebral ischemia. The highest levels are found in *Verbascum Thapsus, Plantago major, and Euphrasia officinalis*.

Catapol is neuro-protective and anti-inflammatory. Brain inflammation is believed to be important factor in cognitive dysfunction, including progressive memory loss, and impairment of spatial and perceptual recognition. Catapol has demonstrated improvement in cognitive function. See Speedwell for more information.

Aucubin has a wide range of medicinal benefit, including prevention of liver fibrosis. Lv PY et al, *Environ Toxicol Pharmacol* 2017 50: 234-9. The compound enhances lysosomal activity, resulting in hepatic dyslipidemia. Lee HY et al, *PloS One* 2013 8(12).

However, none of the isolated compounds fully explain its amazing benefits.

Rafinesque reported, "the Indians use a strong decoction of the whole plant in eruptive diseases, bile, hemorrhoids, sores, etc. Few plant promise to become more useful in skillful hands: it ought to be tried in yellow fever and bilious fever, the tropical liver complaint."

Dr. Porcher wrote, "It is administered by the vegetable practitioners as an anthelmintic; also in jaundice, in hepatic disorders generally, and in constipation."

It is rare to find a digestive tonic that is from the aerial parts of a plant, most being from perennial roots. It combines well with Oregon grape root, purple fall leaves of bunchberry (*Cornus canadensis*) and aspen poplar bark in cases of anorexia, or general appetite stimulant. For jaundice, combine with milk thistle and Oregon grape root. It combines well with elecampane and pineapple weed in treating pinworms and with Oregon grape root for *Giardia*. It is very safe for children, but just pay attention to dosage.

Blackwood's Manual is most specific. "This agent through its action upon the liver is cathartic with tonic effects. It is also an anthelmintic. It is indicated in cases of debility from loss of tone of the digestive organs, liver or from exhausting diseases. There is hepatic torpor with pain and soreness in the left lobe of the liver and jaundice. The pain extends downwards in a line from the hilus of the liver and fundus of the uterus.

The feeble digestion is dependent upon lack of tone of the stomach; with the jaundice there is loss of appetite, constipation and debility. It is of service in dumb ague and in the quinine cachexia, when it starts the secretions and removes the malaria cachexia. It is indicated in dumb ague when there is an ill-defined chill, aching, with fever and general distress. In the form of an infusion it is employed as an enema in the relief of pinworms."

Do not use Balmony, however, in cases of diabetes, or enlarged spleen.

Potter's New Cyclopaedia of Botanical Drugs and Preparations, mentions an anti-depressant quality to the herb. This makes sense, as all bitters have this quality.

When collected in the wild, the tops can be cut in flower, to ensure a constant supply. The fresh leaves make the best ointment or balm for hemorrhoids, tumours and skin ulcers.

Bergeron et al, *Int Journal of Pharmacognosy* 1996 34:4 found dichloromethane extracts of the whole plant active against Gram negative bacteria such as *E. coli*. Early work by Bishop and MacDonald, *Canadian Journal Botany* 29 found water extracts active against *Staphylococcus aureus*.

The Baltimore Checker Spot butterfly lays its eggs on the leaves, from which hatch orange and black caterpillars.

They munch on the leaves and spend the winter in thick woven webs. The next spring they feed again and construct their chrysalis. Observing the butterfly will help you find the herb; and vice versa.

It is interesting to note, that Turtlehead is much more popular amongst English-trained herbalists, than their North American colleagues. It is one more example of looking on the other side of the fence for the more exotic, when what you seek is right in front of you.

HOMEOPATHY

Turtlehead (*Chelone*) is a remedy in liver affections with pain or soreness of the left lobe of the liver, extending downwards.

It can be useful in intermittent fevers, followed by malaise and debility. There is soreness to external parts, as if the skin were off.

Dyspepsia with liver torpor is also a symptom leading to this remedy, as well as jaundice.

It is specific to round and thread worms, and is an enemy to every kind of worm in the human body.

DOSE- Tincture in one to five drops. The mother tincture is made from aerial parts during flower.

LEAF OIL

Sun infuse one part of day-wilted, fresh leaves to five parts of canola or olive oil for 10-14 days. Strain and use as part of hemorrhoid ointments, combining well with fireweed; or combined with cleavers or plantain oil for mastitis.

On its own, it can be useful for skin tumours and painful ulcers that refuse to heal. Use crock pot for four hours as alternative.

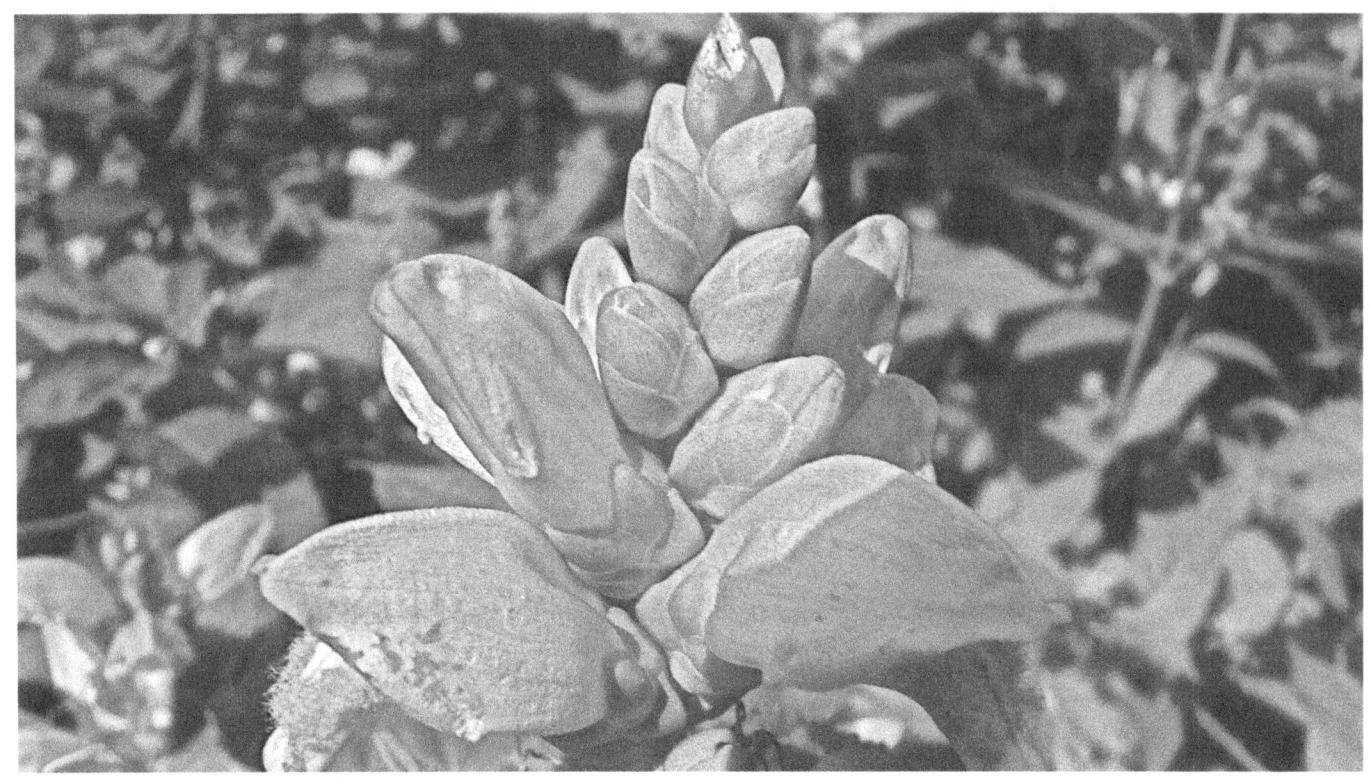

TURTLEHEAD

FLOWER ESSENCE

Turtlehead flower essence is for those who feel they have waited too long to say or do what they really want. They are finally ready to stick their necks out and speak their truth. **PRAIRIE DEVA**

SPIRITUAL PROPERTIES

Herbs like Chelone and Joe Pye Weed are considered Turtle Medicine. Matthew Wood puts it well in his description of Turtle Medicine, from *The Book of Herbal Wisdom*.

"Turtle is thus a symbol of the doorway to the Underworld. The dark eyes of Grandfather Turtle are filled with the wisdom of the ages. All things, which have ever been true, are registered in the soul of Grandfather Turtle, from the beginning of time down to the present.

The impression of the eternal upon the temporal is also stored here, so that the interface of the Great Mystery with time and space is not forgotten, but recorded indelibly. Grandfather Turtle says, "Everything you always knew to be true, is true".

The Indian people have an inalienable genetic access to the inner secrets of Mother Earth. They have long been famed and known as the bearers of some wonderful secret, from the time they were first "discovered" by outsiders.

And yet, this depth of knowledge is for them a terrible burden to carry under the present regime. We live in an age when Mother Nature is ruthlessly exploited to yield her treasures.

Grandfather Turtle is the root of wisdom, the philosopher's stone, in which the mysteries of Mother Nature are revealed. We are able to understand the plants, minerals and animals in their true nature from this source only. This is the true medical school where the true physician obtains his or her degree. With this knowledge it is possible to see the inner essence of the sick person, the disease and the medicine. Nature is also the true pharmacy, from which we obtain our store of medicine. **WOOD**

PERSONALITY TRAITS

Chelone is a Greek nymph who ridiculed the marriage of Zeus and Hera. She was metamorphosed into a silent turtle (chelonia) as punishment.

Many scholars believe that the marriage of Zeus and Hera was a forced joining of the indigenous pre-Hellenic goddess religions, with the patriarchal theology of the Indo-European tribes.

Viewed in this manner, the story is a slightly veiled threat to anyone objecting to the enforced religious change, and may be viewed as a memorial to the silenced priestesses during this social upheaval.   **ANON**

Chelone, the Turtle Goddess, is the spirit of silence. She may be invoked by those who need silence, as well as by those, who have been silenced. Chelone is the matron of political prisoners and the homeless.
JUDIKA ILLES

The turtle is a shore creature using the land and the water. All shore areas are associated with doorways to the Faerie realm. The turtle is sometimes known as the keeper of the doors. Turtles thus were often seen as signs of fairy contact and the promise of fairy rewards.

In Nigeria, the turtle was a symbol of the female sex organs and sexuality. To the Native Americans, it was associated with the lunar cycle, menstruation, and the power of the female energies. The markings and sections on some turtles total thirteen (13). In the lunar calendar, there are either 13 full moons or 13 new moons alternating each year. Many believe this is where the association with female energies originated. Turtle is the symbol of the primal mother.   **ANDREWS**

MYTHS AND LEGENDS

The Seneca consider Turtle, or Hahnowa to be a warrior. One day, while travelling in his canoe, he meets an elk that asks to join him. He asks him to run, and says that the elk is not swift enough to join him. Turtle then meets Skunk, and grants his request to join him. He also invites Porcupine. Buffalo fails the speed trial, but Rattlesnake is invited to join.

This band of warriors decides to attack the seven sisters. The Skunk sits next to a fire, ready to attack with odour; Porcupine in the woodpile ready to attack when they come for wood; Rattlesnake in the corn bucket when they come for food; and Turtle hides near a spring when they come for water. The first three attack and are beaten to death by the sisters. When one sister goes for water, Turtle attacks and bites her on the toe and won't let go. She limps back to camp, carrying Turtle. Her mother tells her to throw Turtle in the fire, but he laughs and says he cannot be destroyed by fire because he came from fire and enjoys a good fire. The mother then takes him to the creek to drown him, and Turtle pleads not to be thrown in the water, but they do anyways. He sinks to the bottom, but then rises, holds out his claws and laughs, for water is his home.   **SENECA**

In Chinese myth, the turtle guards the north quadrant of the world and serves as an emblem of earth, one of the four primal elements of nature. The phoenix represents fire, the dragon represents water, and the unicorn represents air. Of these four animals, only the turtle exists outside the mythological realm.
TAMRA ANDREWS

Turtles have a special meaning to indigenous people. The pattern of scutes on the shell define the lunar calendar cycle. Around the edge you will find twenty-eight individual scales that represent the lunar cycle. And in the centre of the shell are thirteen larger scales, representing the year's lunar calendar. It is traditional to use thirteen poles when setting up a tipi. Within the following chapters will be found my writings on twenty-eight medicinal plants. Turtle Island is the name given to North America by various native peoples. The "original" legend was passed on from the Lenape (Delaware) people, but has been embraced, with slight variation, throughout the continent.

Sky Woman fell to earth and was carrying child. The whole planet was water with nowhere to stand or sit. A giant turtle was swimming in the great abyss and was a refuge for various animals. In order to create a land base, various creatures dove deep into the water, attempting to retrieve some soil.

After many tried and failed, muskrat made the journey. He was gone a long time and when he floated to the surface he was dead. But between his paws was a small piece of mud. Sky Woman was so grateful she breathed life back into the little hero. The soil was spread over turtle's back and became Turtle Island, now called the continent of North America. **PRAIRIE DEVA**

RECIPES

INFUSION- One tablespoon of dried aerial parts per cup of boiling water. Take four ounces several times daily as needed, before meals. Cold infusion is better- 1-3 ounces three times daily.

POWDER- 0.5 to 1 gram daily.

TINCTURE- 30-60 drops twice daily for adults for vermifuge action. Half dosage for children, or for adults seeking digestive stimulating properties. Take 60 drops one half hour before meals. Dried tincture is prepared at 1:5 and 50% alcohol.

The fresh herb tincture is prepared at 1:2 and 50% alcohol. Only take 10-20 drops three times daily of this superior preparation. It should have a spicy, peppery taste if well prepared.

CAUTION- Do not use in acute inflammation or liver disease.

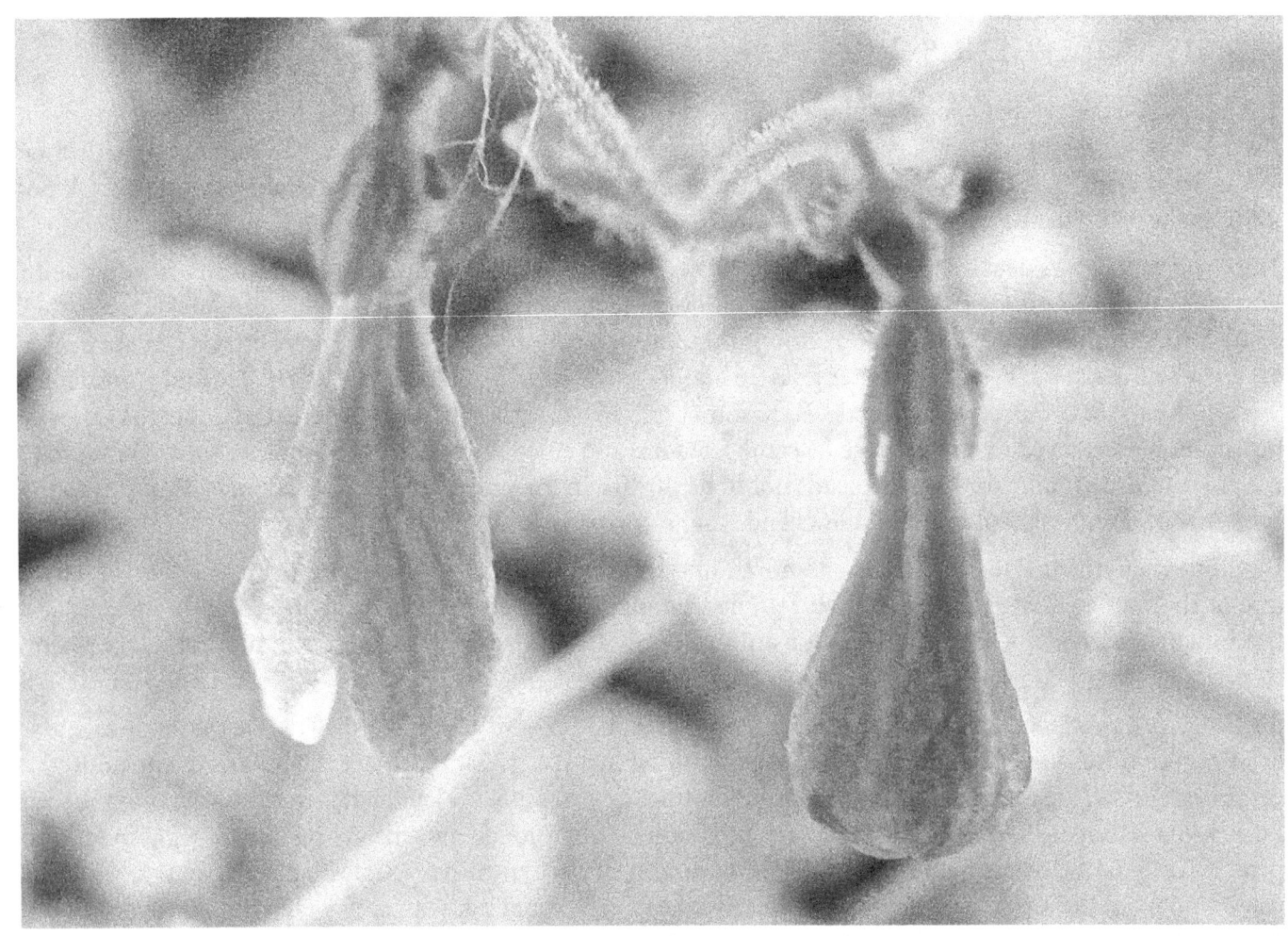

TWINFLOWER FLOWER BUDS

TWINFLOWER
(***Linnaea borealis* var. *borealis*** L.)
LONG TUBE TWINFLOWER
(***L. borealis* var. *longiflora*** Torr.)
PARTS USED- aerial parts

He saw beneath dim aisles, in odorous beds,
The slight Linnaea hang its twin-born heads;
And blessed the monument of the man of flowers,
Which breathes his sweet fame through the northern bowers.

R W EMERSON

Linnaea is named in honor of Carolus Linnaeus, who founded the modern botanical system of taxonomy, or plant identification. The small flower, abundant in his native Sweden, was a personal favorite, and he chose to name it after himself. Borealis means northern, after the Greek God of the North Wind, Boreas.

The plant is circumpolar, with three recognized varieties. Long tube twinflower is more common in the Pacific Northwest.

Linnaeus said it is " a little northern plant, long-overlooked, depressed, abject, flowering early." It has a very pleasant honeysuckle-like perfume at dusk. In 1740, he introduced the plant as Lapp tea, in an attempt to urge others to cultivate or utilize medicinal herbs of Lapland's tundra. Thirty years later, the aging naturalist still expected his namesake would be widely cultivated as the national beverage of Sweden.

Linnaeus was appointed professor of medicine in 1741 at Uppsala. Twenty years later, he was granted a title by Gustavus III of Sweden, and thereafter called himself Carl von Linne.

Linnaeus Day is still celebrated each year, in his country of birth, on May 23rd. The flower is the "unofficial" national flower of Sweden.

Indeed Twinflower is often overlooked in the boreal and mixed forests. It is often missed in the mishmash of entanglements of uva ursi, and bog cranberry, with all three spreading together in some spots.

The Iroquois decocted the stems and gave the tea to children with cramps, fever or crying spells.

The Montagnais mashed the plant and used it as a poultice for inflammation of the limbs. Other indigenous healers used leaf tea for treating insomnia.

It was used as a cold and flu remedy by the Snohomish, while the Potawatomi used the whole plant for unspecified female trouble during pregnancy or menstruation. The Algonquin women drank infusions of the whole plant during pregnancy.

The Dena'ina call it **K'ELA TL'LIA** meaning, "mouse's rope".

The Ojibwa call the flower, **NEEZHODAEYUN**, meaning " twins".

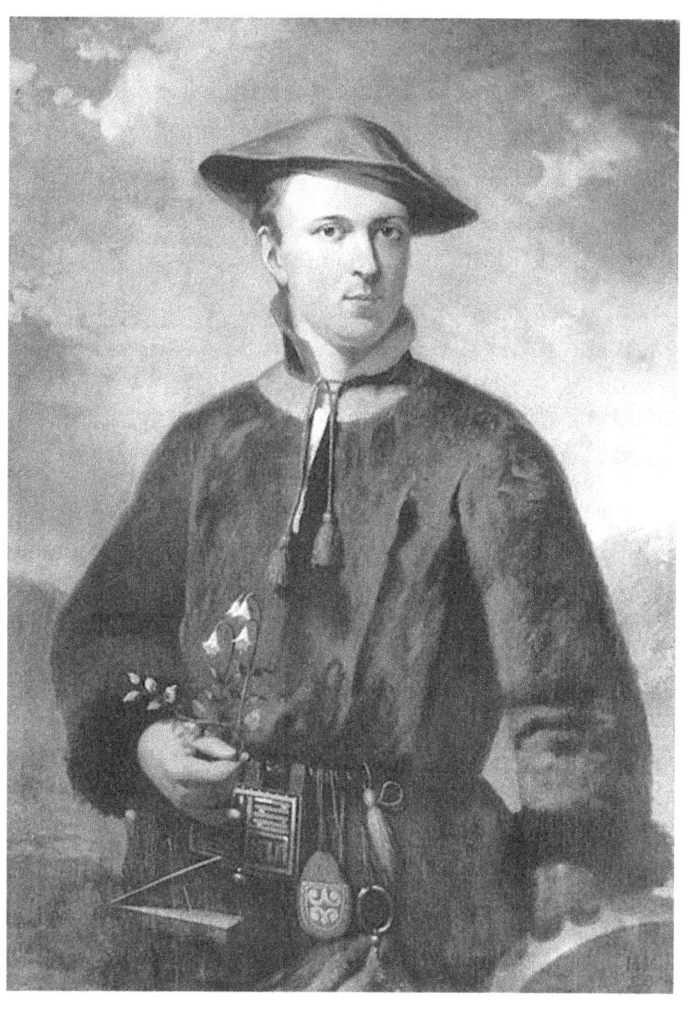

LINNAEUS WITH TWINFLOWER

187

Water and acetone extracts from the plant show activity against *Staphylococcus aureus*. Bishop and MacDonald, *Can J Botany* 29.

The flower contains a cyanidin glycoside that has not been positively identified.

Twinflower is the floral emblem of the Botanical Garden at Memorial University in Newfoundland. I have had the wonderful pleasure to visit this beautiful spot, years ago.

In parts of Norway, the plant is used to treat shingles (*herpes zoster*) pain. Alm et al, *Bot J Linnean Soc* 2006 151:3.

A pathogenic fungi is sometimes found on the stems and leaves, called *Kohninia linnaeicola*.

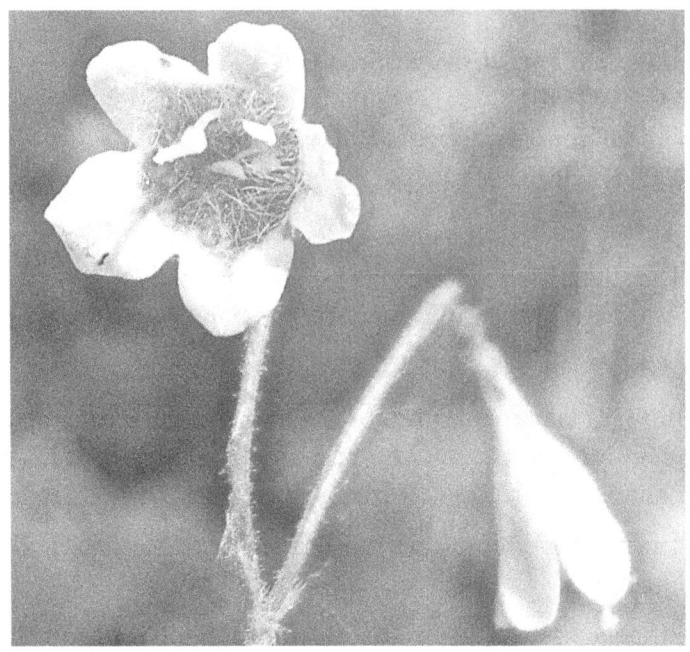

TWINFLOWER

FLOWER ESSENCE

Twin Flower (*L. borealis*) flower essence is primarily a mental remedy that promotes an awareness that it is all much bigger than we are able to perceive and understand. Twin Flower fosters optimism and humility.

Making judgment leads to rigidity and resistance. We can only release judgment when we are peaceful with ourselves. Then we can greet every situation with a breath of release and with the deep knowing that what we put out we will get back. It is with this mental framework that we are able to be in the process of our lives without getting stuck on fixed positions. **PACIFIC**

Twin Flower essence is for development of our ability that we may understand the subtle messages we receive. It brings wonderful insights into life. **CANADIAN FOREST**

Twinflower essence is for balance in communication, listening and speaking to others from a place of inner calm and focused neutrality. **ALASKA**

SPIRITUAL PROPERTIES

Cultures the world over have always been fascinated with the idea of twins, giving them prominence in their lore, from the Greek Gemini to Dylan and Lleu, personifying the powers of light and darkness in Celtic mythology. Similarly, Iroquois cosmology has Mother Earth giving birth to the primal twins of good and evil, named Sky Holder and Flint respectively. Ojibwa tradition says that the Earth was created on the back of a turtle, amid a great flood, so that Sky Woman, **GEEZHIGO-QUAE**, could give birth to twins, who subsequently spawned the human race. **BENNET**

PERSONALITY TRAITS

Did Linnaeus note a resemblance between this humble plant and himself.

He, like the flower, unfolded "in a remote northern region...unknown and overlooked, without the advantages of fortune or place. The world thought not of him, while in poverty and obscurity he pursued his scientific researches: few knew or valued this solitary wanderer...who explored the recesses of nature, and culled the treasures of the mountain and glen, the forest and the moor...which in due time, he presented, arranged...to the delight and astonishment of kindred mind in every region." **C.L. BRIGHTWELL**

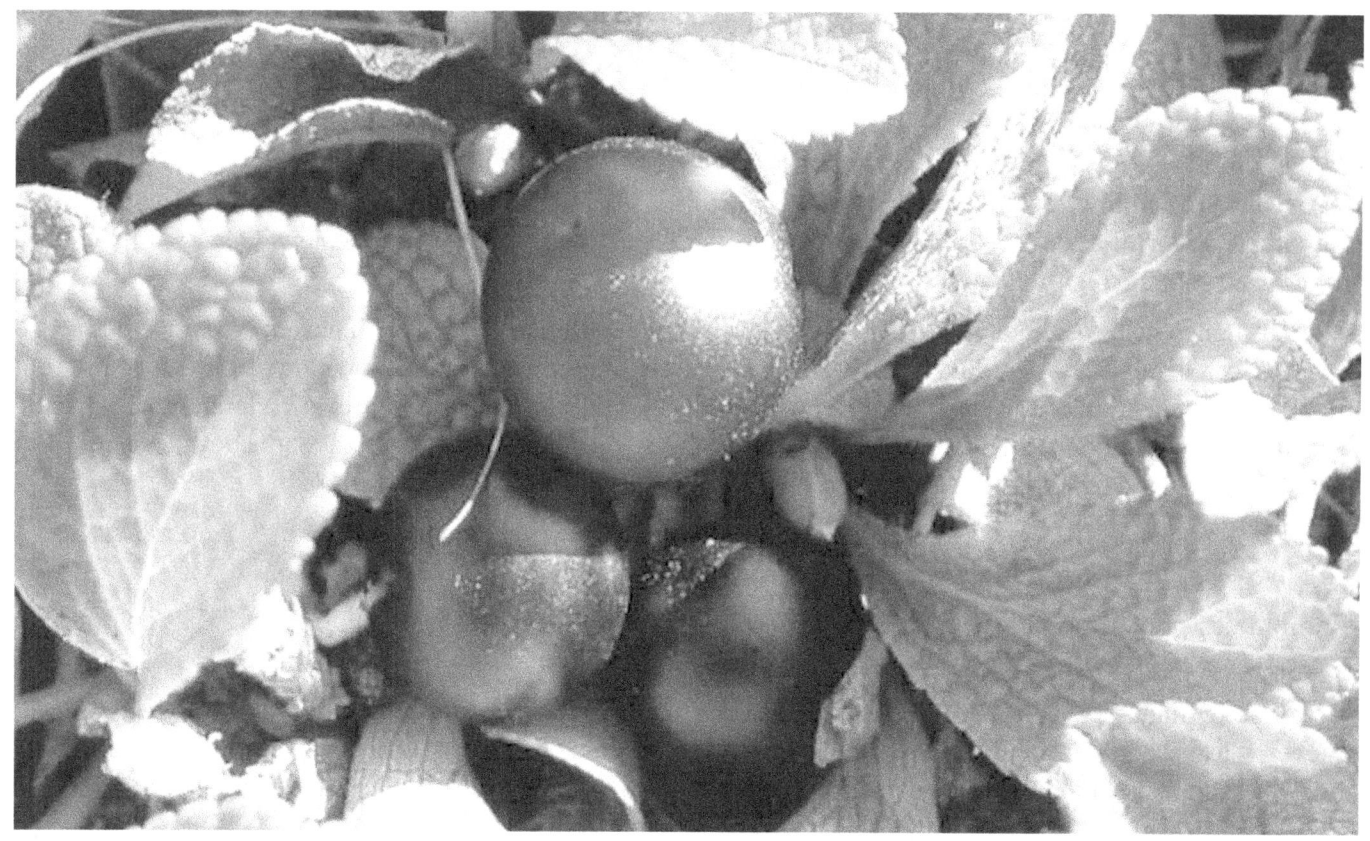

ALPINE BEARBERRY

UVA-URSI
BEARBERRY
(*Arctostaphylos uva-ursi* [L.] Spreng.)
(*A. uva ursi ssp. adrenotricha* [Fern & Macbr]
         Calder & Taylor) not accepted
(*Arbutus uva-ursi* L.) not accepted
RED BEARBERRY
(*A. rubra* [Rehder & Wils.] Fern) not accepted
(*Arctous rubra* [Rehd. & Wilson] Nakai)

ALPINE BEARBERRY
BLACK BEARBERRY
(*Arctous alpina* [L.] Nied)
ARBUTUS
PACIFIC MADRONE
(*Arbutus menziesii* Pursh.)
PARTS USED-leaves, root, berries and flowers

The tawny hill bends off its snow
Under the west wind's palmy tongue
How succulent curls the bearberry then
Its gleaming wintergreen, its blushing fruit
(a tonic for bears, eaten in spring)
tinges this chiaroscuro.
Sanguine the warp
and weft, padding a dream bed
Deer and hunter rest at the foot of the dawn
Spill, clouds, over Livingstone
Sacrifice! Conjure, like Brings-Down-The-Sun.

SID MARTY

189

ARCTOS means bear, and **STAPHYLE** a bunch of grapes. Uva ursi means grape of bear or bear's berries. This derives from the belief of the 17th century French botanist Michel Adanson, the fruits were eaten by bears. He was right!

In fall, bears will ingest massive amounts of the berries, creating a numbing/paralyzing action on the intestine.

Bears will often follow this meal with *Carex*, a rough-edged sedge that will go right through the intestine, dragging tapeworms and other parasites, previously paralyzed. This is important, as parasites can drain energy from the animal during their winter "sleep".

Another name given to this plant is kinnickinnick or kinnikinnik "that which is mixed" in reference to the use of leaves as a ceremonial or smoking mixture. It arrived with early fur traders and came to mean a smoking mixture containing tobacco, uva ursi, red osier dogwood, and other herbs. Kinnikinnik is the longest palindromic word in the English language, meaning an anagram that is spelled and pronounced the same both forwards and back. Palindrome is from the Greek **PALIN DROMO**, meaning running back again.

One famous palindrome was written, by Leigh Mercer. "A man, a plan, a canal; Panama!" Another is "Lewd did I live, evil I did dwel."

Kinnikinnik is not always burned and can be simply a blend of pleasant scented herbs carried as an offering, or used to ward off evil spirits.

Some native plants used in kinnikinnik include angelica leaves, various asters, wild bergamot, birch bark, blueberry leaves, goldenrod, fleabane, lobelia, licorice root, meadowsweet, mints, mullein, various artemisia and everlasting, sweet clover, sweet coltsfoot, tamarack, wild lettuce, willow bark and leaves, and yarrow.

Each kinnikinnik mixture was regionally unique, to the extent that certain mixtures were valued trade items. They were based on medicinal uses for physical, mental, emotional and spiritual issues.

In a funny turn around, indigenous people named it "**SACACOMIS**", after the smoking pouches worn by Hudson Bay clerks. This is from **SAC** meaning bag, and **COMMIS** meaning clerk, or commissioner.

Today, the herb is used in ceremonial pipes as part of spiritual ritual. The Cree call it **PITHIKOMIN**, mealy berry, or **MUSKOMINANATIK**, meaning Berry Bush. Another name, **OCHIKASIPAKWA** refers to the lack of flavour in the berries.

The berries are cooked and combined with raw fish eggs, or made into a cider drink.

The root is decocted as a tea for persistent coughs, or combined with other herbs for slowing excessive menstrual bleeding.

The Thompson of British Columbia prepared root decoctions for spitting up of blood. When dried and smudged, or smoked the scent of burning root is said to be irresistible to deer, and used as an attractant. If a large enough central root can be found, a pipe bowl can be carved from the heartwood. You can then use this to smoke your own kinnikinnik!

Stem decoctions were drunk to prevent miscarriage, to bring on menstruation, or to speed a new mothers recovery after childbirth.

A sitz bath containing leaf decoctions helps sooth uterine and vaginal inflammation after birth, and lessens chance of infection. The leaf and stem were sometimes mixed with blueberry leaf for the latter condition.

The fruit, combined with grease, was given to children for diarrhea, and when fried until they split open, are much tastier, like dried apple, than in raw form. Several groups, including the Thompson, rubbed the berries inside of cedar root baskets to seal and make them watertight.

The Blackfoot call it **KA-SIXIE**, **KAKAHSLIN** or **JACKASHIPUCK**. They used the dried berries in rattles; preferring them to stones as they were lighter and didn't make dust. They were strung on necklaces; as well as eaten fresh, or dried and then soaked later with sugar. The presence of numerous berries during the summer, was believed to foretell of a hard winter.

The whole plant was boiled with grease and applied to cradle cap, itching scalp and other skin disorders. A mouthwash for canker sores is prepared from the leaves.

According to Matthew Wood, an Indian name for the uvula is "bearberry", so the plant is credited with a relationship to the throat.

The Chipewyan call the plant **DE(LH)NI**, meaning crane food, and the leaves, **'INT'ANE**. Today, in Fort Chipewyan, the local residents call it Chicken Berry.

The Gitksan of northern British Columbia preserve the berries of **T'MII'IT**, in grease for winter. Sophie Thomas, a Sai'Kuz healer, calls the plant **DUNH T'AN**. It is known as the women's medicine due to its use during menopause. The whole plant with root and berries is boiled to give relief from menstrual cramps and used with wild raspberry or Oregon grape stems for easier delivery of babies.

The leaves are mixed with juniper berry for diabetes and with wild raspberry leaves for high blood pressure. Ritch-Krc et al, *J Ethnopharm* 1996 52 85-94.

Further north, the Slave call it **NETENE**, while the Gwich'in on the Mackenzie delta call the fruit Stoneberry, or **DÀN DAIH**.

They mix Stoneberry with pounded dry fish as a dessert, or combine with fish liver or roe as a meal. The sweet flowers were eaten in spring as a treat.

Further northeast, the Inuit of Baffin Island know the plant as **KALLAT**. The leaves are used to make a strong and tasty tea.

The Crow of Montana pulverized the dried leaves and applied the powder to canker sores in the mouth. The neighboring Flathead predicted the severity of the upcoming winter; few berries meaning a mild season, and many berries suggesting a long cold one. When someone had an earache, they would smoke the leaves until the stem of the pipe was quite warm. They then removed the bowl and blew the hot smoke directly into the affected ear.

The Cheyenne moved into Montana and brought their medicines with them. They boiled the stems, leaves and berries for persistent back pain.

They combined the leaves in a mixture burned on coals to drive evil spirits out of people going crazy. A combination of berries from this plant, saskatoon and chokecherry were used in an unknown manner.

The berries are a good laxative. They are edible but not what I would call tasty. The seeds from the berries have a somewhat paralyzing effect on the human intestinal tract, as well as bears mentioned above.

Some tribes fried the berries in a pan of grease until they swell like popcorn. Others mixed the berries with fruit juices to make a fermented "cider" said to help control allergies.

The Chippewa, Ojibwa and others smoked bearberry in their pipes as part of the attraction of game. They recognized the clinging activity of the berry seeds, and called the plant Berry with Spikes, or **SAGA'KOMINAGUNJ**.

The berries were rubbed on the inside of coiled cedar root baskets to make them waterproof, and used for cooking and whipping buffalo berries to froth.

The Anishinabe know the plant as **MUKWA MISKOMIN**, which roughly translates as Bear-His Red Berries. They traditionally used the leaf tea as a douche for urethritis.

The high tannin content of the leaves has, in the past, made it a favorite of Russian leather tanners.

There, the leaves were made into a bitter tea called **KOUTAI**, used to treat various stomach problems.

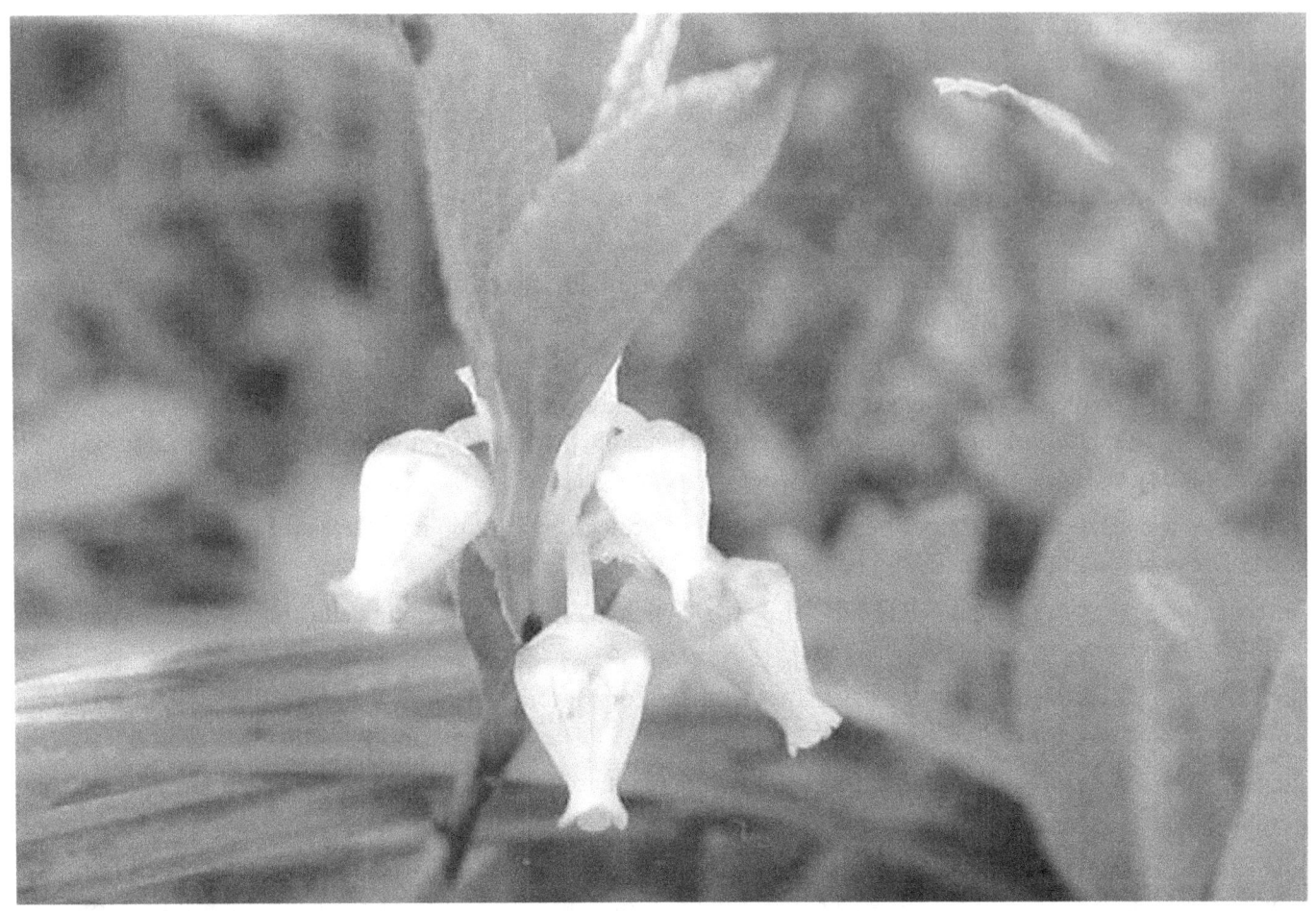

RED BEARBERRY FLOWERS

The plant is ruled by Mars and Pluto, and often added to sachets for increasing psychic powers.

Several patents exist; one for a plant growth promoter containing inositol hexaphosphate; and another as part of an astringent composition for improving the form and appearance of the female breast.

Hydroquinone and arbutin derivatives are inhibitors of melanin synthesis. They can be used as skin bleaching agents, and recommended for local treatment of scar tissue, hyper-pigmentation, pregnancy mask (cholasma), and freckles.

In France, the incorporation of 2% hydroquinone (arbutin) is allowed into cosmetic products. Use it to treat small areas as in large areas the skin can develop a marble effect. Excessive light exposure will increase re-pigmentation. Hydroquinones inhibit tyrosinase, the enzyme responsible for L-tyrosine oxidation in the pathway to melanin.

Bearberry extracts reduce melanoderma. Piechota-Urbanska et al, *Polim Med* 2010 40:3. Make a sun infusion of fresh bearberry leaves, 1:2 in rosehip seed oil, shaking daily for two weeks.

Applied twice daily this will lighten the pigmentation of pregnancy mask.

An extract of bearberry containing flavonoids and tannins mixed with a non-reducing marine polysaccharide possesses anti-free radical and anti-inflammatory properties, and anti-glycation properties. The product, called *Aglycal*, is marketed by Laboratoires Serobiologiques.

Ursolic acid inhibits elastase and exerts anti-inflammatory activity on skin.

A patent from Japan by Nanba et al, 1986 is a novel agent for dental caries, with the active ingredient derived from bearberry leaves.

Recent work by Dr. Ron Pegg with University of Saskatchewan Food Product Innovative Program looked at bearberry leaves as a food preservative.

Studies showed anti-oxidant potential in both the beta-carotene linoleate system, as well as for processing in a meat system probably due in part to polyphenolics.

Red Bearberry has bright red, and juicier berries than its cousin. As it name suggests, it is found on montane slopes and heaths. The Slave call it **O"KA DZHI**.

The leaves turn brilliant red in late summer and fall off before winter.

The Gwich'in of the Mackenzie delta call the berry Bird's Eye, or **DZHII NDEE'**. It was sometimes added to pemmican, or eaten fresh to quench thirst.

Alpine, or Black Bearberry, has similar leaves, but more spoon-shaped, wrinkly and leathery; and stay on the plant for several years.

The flowers are more yellow, while Red Bearberry flowers are white. The leaves are medicinally interchangeable with uva ursi.

Alpine Bearberry is known as **TCHAKO-SHE-PUKK**, to the Cree.

The fruit is shiny black and known to the Slave as **DZHTA DE**. The Chipewyan eat the fresh berries, which have little flavour, and call them Whiskey Jack's Eye, or **JIZE NAGHE**. Another common Chipewyan name is **KLEH**.

According to Mors Kochanski, the berries may be rubbed on burns to alleviate pain.

In one dialect of the Inuit, Inuktitut, the alpine bearberry is known as **ATUNGAWIAT**. The Dena'ina of Alaska name is **GIZHA NAGHA**, meaning "gray jay's eye".

Early French voyageurs called it Caribou Herb, or Herbe à Caribou.

Uva ursi leaves can take from 2-3 weeks to dry thoroughly after harvest. When shredded and put through screens 0.3-0.7 cm, the material takes half the space and less drying time, with no adverse effect on arbutin content. The *British Pharmacopoeia* recommends collecting the leaves in September and October from sterile branches.

I suggest picking the in early summer before flowering, or berry formation.

Bearberry that is ethically wild-crafted will regenerate to its original health in 3-5 years. Fall harvest optimizes arbutin content, especially from south facing slopes. Take no more than 25% biomass at time and it will completely regenerate in 3-4 years. Recasens et al, *J Herb Spice Med Plant* 2008 14:1-2.

Studies out of Russia indicate that seeding Bearberry is difficult, once it has been eradicated. Regeneration from seed is poor, due to poor germination, high seedling mortality up to the age of 5 years, and stunted growth until year 40.

Root cuttings can be propagated in sand, with an 80% survival rate, if treated with a solution of indole butyric acid at 100 milligrams per liter of water.

Bearberry often grows in the same habitat as bog cranberry. However, the uva ursi leaf is cross-veined on the underside, while the latter is dotted.

Methanol extracts of the leaf produce anti-algae results when tested on ponds, probably due to the tannins precipitating the algal proteins.

They inhibit *Arcobacter butzleri* and related pathogenic microbes in chicken and turkey operations. Cervenka et al, *Curr Microbio* 2006 53:5.

Pacific Madrone is a beautiful, monoecious, evergreen of western North America. The thin, multi-layered bark is red to orange brown, and later green, red, orange and brown as it peels with age. The white to pink flowers are sweet and fragrant, and fruit is round orange-red drupe with warty skin that takes a year to mature.

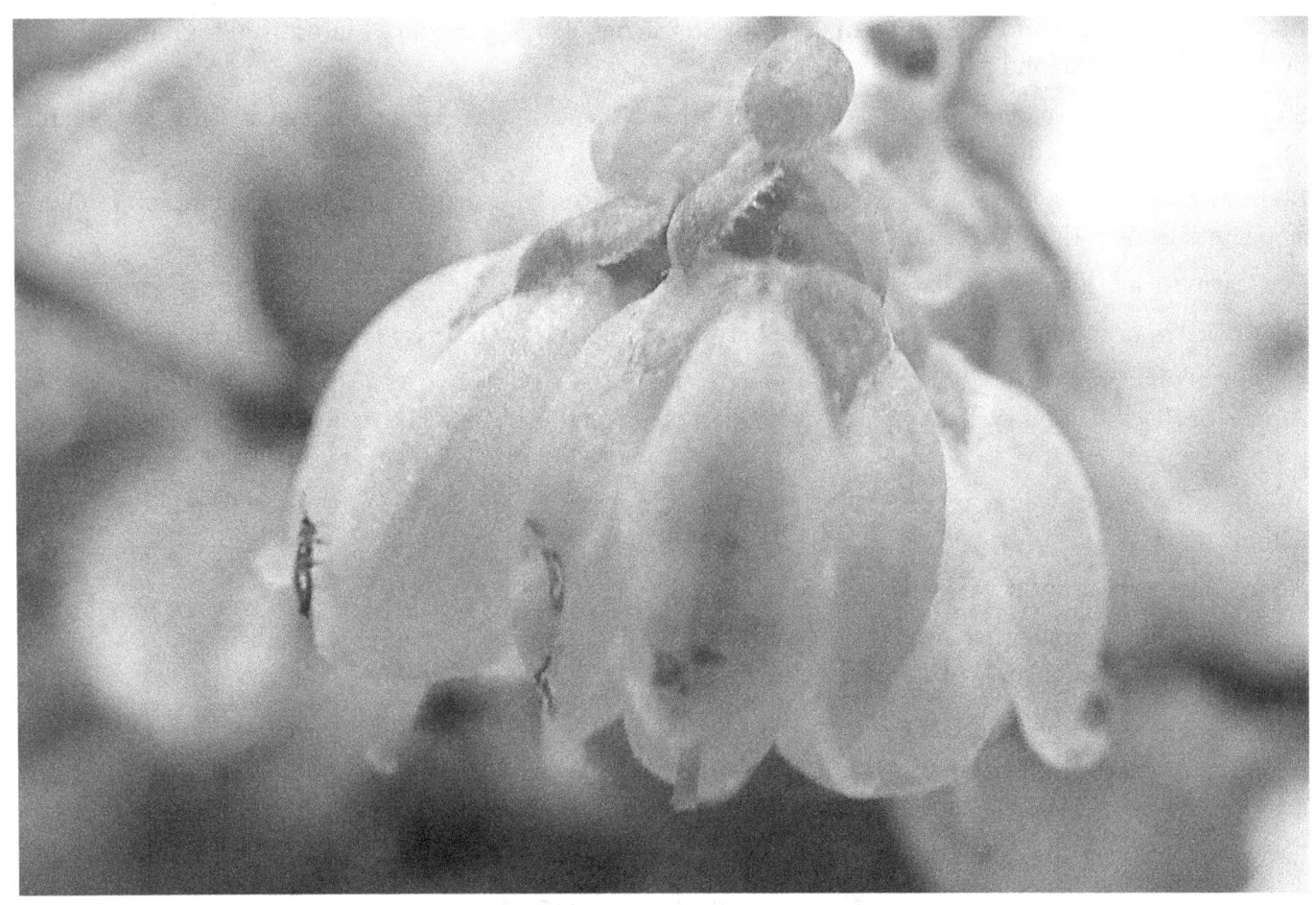

UVA URSI FLOWERS

Arbutus is a major hub of mycorrhizal fungi diversity and connectivity in a mixed evergreen forest. It helps enhance below ground resilience to disturbance. Kennedy PG et al, *Am J Botany* 2012 99(10):1691-1701.

Various coastal tribes used the bark for stomach ailments, peptic ulcers, burns, cuts, sores and impetigo, bad colds and for puberty ceremonies. Bark decoctions were generally used, including for strep and sore throats. The leaves were rubbed on rheumatic pain.

Indigenous people of the Saanich Peninsula on Vancouver Island know the tree as **KEKEILC** (*qweqwey-ilhch*).

MEDICINAL

CONSTITUENTS- leaves- various glycosides including, arbutin (12%), methyl-arbutin (4%), ericolin, various gallotannins (6-20%), hydroquinone glycosides (up to 18%), phenolic acids including caffeic, ellagic, salicylic 16mg/100g, p-hydroxybenzoic, vanillic, gentisic, homo-protocatechuic, protocatechuic, syringic 16.8 mg/100g, p-coumaric 18 mg/100g, ferulic, sinapic and ascorbic acid (191 ppm), phenolics (300 mg/g), essential oils, ursone, ursolic acid (4000-7500 ppm), uvaol, lupeol, alpha and beta amyrin, erythrodiol, ursolic and oleanolic acid, myricetin glycosides, corilagin pyroside, isoquercitin, cyandin and delphinidin, and other anthocyanin flavonoids; as well as iridoids such as monotropein, piceosides, ursone, allantoin and various minerals, including calcium (10,000 ppm), iron (1,050 ppm), magnesium (1,200 ppm), potassium (3,830 ppm).
The arbutin content is highest in the leaves (up to 14%), lowest in flowering and highest when fruit is ripe.
The roots contain various triterpenoids including ursolic acid, uvaol, alpha-amyrin, beta-amyrin, oleanolic acid, lupeol, unedoside, and betulinic acid; as well as unedoside (iridoid glucoside).
fruit- 36% sugars, vitamin C (40.3 mg/100 grams fresh) vitamin A (885 IU's per 100 grams dry weight), fat (15%).
seeds- 25% protein, 50% fat
A. alpina fruit- 52.5 mg vit C and 30 RE of vitamin A per 100 grams fresh.
A. rubra fruit- 82.3 mg vit C, 0.5 g protein per 100 grams fresh.

Bearberry's major disinfecting and anti-inflammatory agent is arbutin. Since it requires an alkaline environment to transform into P-dihydroxybenzene, or hydroquinone, an alkalizing diet helps accentuate its action.

Ericolin breaks down to the volatile ericinol, which is also antiseptic.

Like many herbal medicines, healthy intestinal flora is necessary for proper conversion and activity.

Arbutin is hydrolyzed by intestinal flora to the aglycone, hydroquinone. This in turn is metabolized and conjugated by the liver to glucuronate and sulphate esters and then excreted in the urine. It is believed that in an alkaline environment, the glucuronate and sulphate esters release small amounts of hydroquinone.

The anti-microbial activity is directly dependent on the beta-glucosidase activity of the infective organism, according to work by Jahodar et al, *Ceskoslov Farm* 1985 34.

The presence of *E. coli*, for example, in an infected urinary tract may enhance hydroquinone levels, by reversing the conjugation process and metabolizing hydroquinone glucuronide and hydroquinone sulphate back into free, active hydroquinone. Work by Siegers C et al, *Phytomed* 2003 10 (Suppl 4) 58-90 suggests alkalizing urine does not appear necessary to improve antiseptic properties of arbutin or hydroquinone.

Early work by Frohne et al, *Planta Med* 1970 18 found "the crude extract of uva ursi to be of more benefit as an antimicrobial than arbutin".

It is both a soothing and restorative agent to the urinary tract. It's cold, astringent properties make it well suited to acute urinary and intestinal infections. The antiseptic effect takes place 3-4 hours after oral ingestion.

Escherichia coli, a common Gram negative bacterial source of urinary tract infection, especially in women, thrives in alkaline urine. Normal, slightly acidic urine does not allow it to thrive and adhere to bladder wall. *Proteus mirabilis* another bacteria that causes infections, also loves alkaline urine.

In a clinical trial with 302 women with irritable bladders, a mixture of 23 parts pumpkin seed oil, 8 parts sweet sumach, 5 parts uva ursi, 2 parts hops and 1 part of peppermint, was used. The blend produced good and lasting control of the symptoms where many previous measures had failed, and with no side effects. Mohr et al, 1970.

Another study of 915 patients suffering strangury, enuresis and painful micturition, involved a mixture of uva ursi, peppermint and hops. After six weeks, success was reported in 70% of patients. Lenau et al, *Therapiewoche* 1984 34.

One double-blind, placebo-controlled randomized clinical trial with uva ursi and dandelion showed effectiveness in recurrent cystitis. Larsson et al, *Curr Ther Res Clin Exp* 1993 53:4.

After one month of treatment, there were no further cystitis episodes in the following year, while the placebo group had at least one episode in 23% of women.

It is not the powerful diuretic often insinuated in older herbals. Larger amounts will only further irritate a tender urinary tract. It does, however, combine well with plantain, yarrow, usnea and couch grass for various urinary problems.

It combines well with dandelion leaf, horsetail, and nettles where an active diuretic is needed for more chronic problems, and with marshmallow root or couch grass in cases of stone and gravel.

For prostatitis combine with thuja, juniper berry, hydrangea root and horsetail.

For bedwetting in children, try two parts uva-ursi with one part each of sumach berries and yarrow.

If used, be prepared to see your urine turn brownish-green, due to oxidation of hydroquinone.

It removes uric acid and has a well-deserved reputation for preventing uric acid stone formation, hence usefulness in gout.

Intestinally, it is effective against fungal infections like *Candida albicans*, as well other microorganisms such as *E. coli, Proteus vulgaris, Staphylococcus aureus, Streptococcus faecalis, Bacillus subtilis, Mycobacterium smegmatis, Shigella sonnei, S. flexneri* and *Salmonella typhi*.

In fact, over 70 urinary tract bacteria show reactivity to uva ursi extracts.

Highest enzymatic activity was found against *Enterobacter, Klebsiella* and *Streptococcus* genera, and the lowest by *E. coli* in work by Jahodar cited above. *In vitro* studies of 30% ethanol leaf extracts show inhibition of *Bacillus subtilis, E. coli, Pseudomonas aeruginosa, Salmonella typhimurium, Serratia marcesens* and *Staphylococcus aureus.* Extracts from 95% ethanol showed no activity.

It was found effective against *S. aureus* in work by Snowden R et al, *J Altern Complement Med* 2014 March 17. Both uva ursi and garlic were slightly less effective than goldthread or sage, interestingly enough.

The anti-microbial effect may be due to influence on cell surface characteristics.

In one study of 40 *E. coli* strains from urine of patients with pyelo-nephritis, the herb increased the hydrophobocity of the microbial cell surface, decreasing the ability of the microbe to adhere to cell wall. Turi et al, *APMIS* 1997 105.

Water extracts inhibit the growth of *Streptococcus mutans* associated with dental caries.

Work by McCutcheon et al, found branches and roots active against 9 of 11 bacteria species tested. *Journal of Ethnopharm* 1992 37. Of note is inhibition of *E. coli* equal to gentomycin, and strong inhibition of *Pseudomonas aeruginosa* from leaf and branch extracts.

Vaginally, it makes an effective douche to prevent post-partum infection or correct an ulcerative cervix; or add a decoction to a sitz bath after birthing to reduce inflammation and prevent infection. Combine it with the tincture internally to help restore the uterus to normal size.

It works well for atonic, boggy bladder and ulcerative cystitis, as well as bacterial venereal infections like blennorrhagia.

It is contraindicated in large amounts during pregnancy because it can cause mild vasoconstriction to the endometrium of the uterus.

This same property, however, makes it useful for painful and heavy menstruation, or in promoting strong labour contractions with its oxytocic activity.

And this same property can help incontinence by contracting the sphincter muscle.

The dried berries can be powdered and put in capsules for cardiac edema, or dropsy as the old herbals call it.

Tincture of bearberry leaf is taken internally to prevent post-partum hemorrhage.

Ursolic acid and other components are a strong antibiotic against *Staphylococcus aureus, S. mutans, E. coli, Pseudomonas aeruginosa,* and 70 other urinary tract bacteria.

Some bacteria, such as *Proteus* and *Klebsiella* species, associated with urinary tract infections, produce, and enjoy a urine pH of higher than 7; due to degradation of urea with release of ammonia. This assists the anti-microbial activity of uva ursi.

Other bacteria do not, and thus the need for sodium bicarbonate in some cases.

Work by Shimizu et al, identified a compound in bearberry, corilagin, that combines synergistically with oxacillin in the treatment antibiotic resistant *Staphylococcus aureus. Antimicro Agents Chemotherapy* 2001 45:11.

Paraplegic patients are prone to cystitis and will find bearberry or pipsissewa a healthier alternative to antibiotics. Ursolic acid exhibits cytotoxic and anti-leukemic activity; as well as anti-diabetic, anti-hepatotoxic, and anti-edema activity.

Arbutin from bearberry inhibits human bladder carcinoma cell proliferation via up-regulation of p21. Li H et al, *Pharmazie* 2011 66:4. It combines well with *Rhodiola rosea* in the treatment of bladder cancer.

Bearberry inhibits growth of micro-organisms like Klebsiella and Proteus, believed by some scientists to be involved in auto-immune response in some rheumatic disease. It combines well with juniper berry in treating cystitis and recurring rheumatic or arthritic pain.

For vaginitis or leucorrhea, combine with *Rumex* species root both internally, and as a douche or vaginal bolus.

Drug-resistant gonorrheal organisms are susceptible to alcohol extracts of uva ursi leaves. Roseroot (*Rhodiola rosea*) was even more active in this study by Cybulska et al, *Sex Trans Dis* 2011 38:7.

Annuk et al, University of Tartu, Estonia tested bearberry on *Helicobacter pylori*, and found it possessed marked bacteriostatic activity, and enhanced cell aggregation. By contrast, Pineapple Weed blocked aggregation of *H. pylori*, and did not reveal any anti-microbial activity. A full report is available in *FEMS-Microbiology Letters* 1999 172:1.

Leaf extracts inhibit viruses such as herpes simplex type 2, influenza virus A2, and vaccinia virus at 10% solutions.

In cancers, where the onset is attributed to viral infection, remember to use uva ursi in herbal combinations. The shriveling anti-protein effects on the cell wall of viruses, bacteria and fungi is due to the many tannins and pseudo-tannins such as oxalic, malic, tartaric and ursolic acids.

Hydroquinone, but not arbutin, has been found cytotoxic against hepatic cell lines. Assaf et al, *Planta Medica* 1987 53. The compound showed activity against L1210 and sarcoma 180 tumor cell lines.

Tetragalloylglucose (TgG) extracted from bearberry, has been found to induce apoptosis in human colon and stomach cancer cell lines; as well as human histiocystic lymphoma U937 cells. *Planta Medica* 2000 66:2.

Saeki et al, *Planta Medica* 65:3 found TgG inhibited Lewis lung carcinoma cells, which are highly metastatic, probably by preventing cell adhesion of the tumor cells.

Carpenter et al, *J Med Food* 9:2 found bearberry leaf reduces oxidative stress induced by etoposide treatment, suggesting a possible adjunct therapy for some cancers.

Beta-carotene is present in useable form to help regenerate new epithelial cells, combining well with allantoin (corn silk or comfrey) for both bladder and lung issues. The numerous flavonoids contain various anti-spasmodics that work well on soothing the smooth muscles, including relief of painful menstruation.

Oral doses of arbutin have been shown to suppress the cough reflex, in a manner stronger than dropropizine, and comparable to codeine.

The leaves have hypoglycemic effect, and combine well with blueberry (bilberry) leaves to treat diabetes. This is mainly due to arbutin, which has been found to inhibit insulin degradation.

Alcohol extracts (50%) inhibit the effect of tyrosinase activity. It appears that the melanin formed from DOPA using tyrosinase, as well as from Dopa-Chrom through auto-oxidation, are both inhibited by uva ursi extracts.

Further studies reveal the de-pigmenting mechanism of arbutin in humans involves inhibition of melanosomal tryrosinase activity, rather than a suppression of tyrosinase. Bearberry extracts could have a bleaching effect on freckles and other hyper-pigmented skin disorders. Age spots, resulting from a buildup of lipofuscin, can be reduced in darkness in 3-4 weeks with hydroquinone compounds.

Synthetic hydroquinone is used for skin whitening creams and has been shown to lead to increases in bladder cancer. The European Union banned its use in cosmetics in 2001.

A double-blind, randomized study by Larrson et al, *Curr Ther Res Clin Exp* 1993 53 of 57 women with recurrent cystitis supports the benefit of bearberry leaf. In the year-long study, none of the thirty patients taking uva ursi for first month had a recurrence; while 5 out of 27 in placebo group suffered at least one episode.

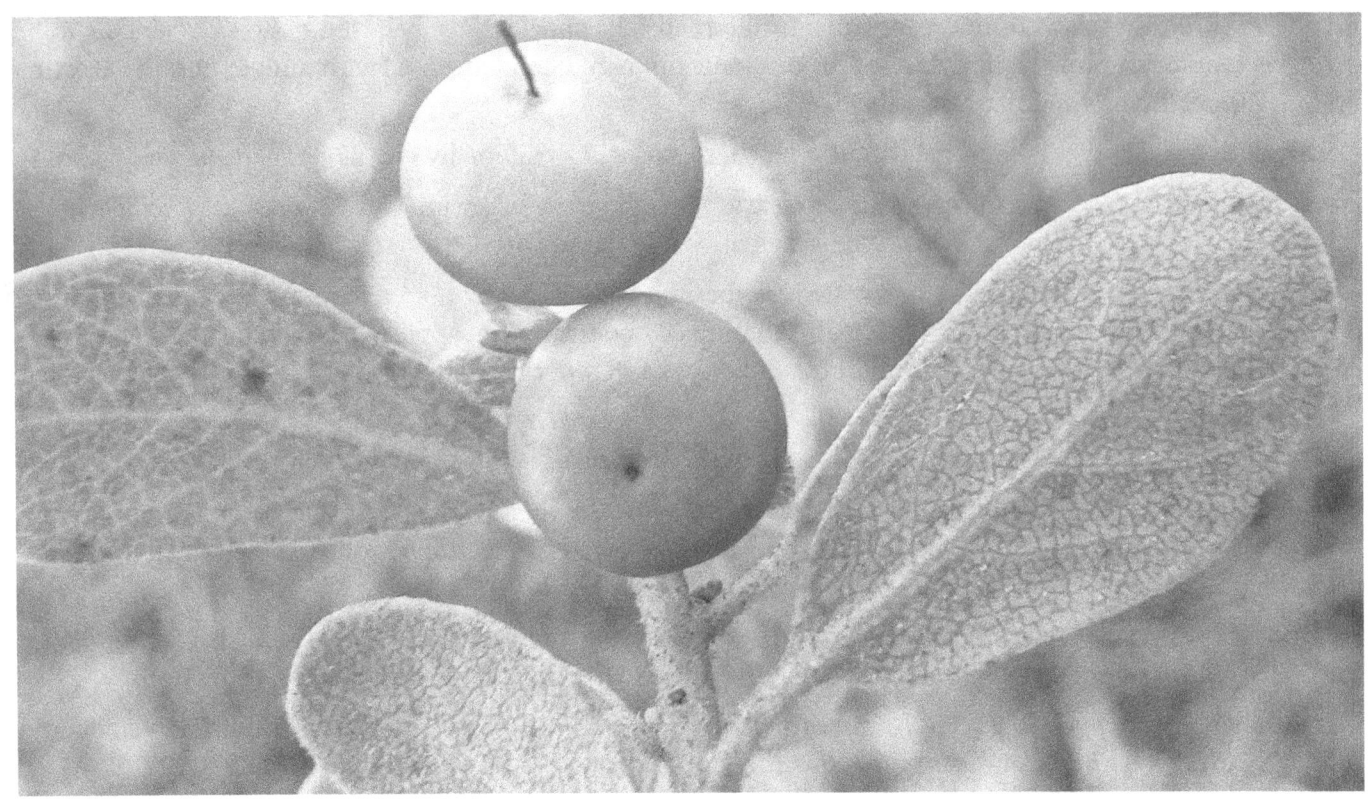

BEARBERRY LEAF AND BERRY

Work by Matsuda et al, found bearberry water extracts at 1-2% helped increase the anti-inflammatory action of synthetic cortisone ointment dexa-methasone. *Journal Pharm Society Japan* 1992 112. The same author found similar effect with indomethacin.

A 50% methanol extract of leaves enhanced the anti-inflammatory effect of subcutaneous prednisolone. Kubo et al, *Yakugaku Zasshi* 1990 110:1.

Corilagin is an ellagitannin that found to exhibit activity against MRSA, or methicillin resistant *Staphylococcus aureus*. This "superbug" evades antibiotics by making a more slippery version of a protein that the antibiotic would normally bind to. Penicillin binding proteins are enzymes that help bacterium create cell walls, and corilagin prevents these wall-building enzymes from forming. This suggests a new, or novel approach to this emerging problem. Shiota et al, *Microbiol Immunol* 2004 48:1; Shimizu et al, *Anti-microbial Agents Chemother* 2001 45:11.

Corilagin inhibits liver carcinoma cell growth by inducing G2/M phase arrest. Ming Y et al, *Cell Biol Int* 2013 37(10): 1046-54. The compound inhibits ovarian cancer by blocking the TGF-beta signaling pathways, a route not observed in paciltaxel. Jia L et al, *BMC Complement Altern Med* 2013 Feb 15:13:33.

Bearberry prevents LPS induced up-regulation of nitric oxide production and down regulation of induced TNF, or tumor necrosis factor production, in a manner similar to grape seed extract. Shanmugan et al, *Mol Nutr Food Res* 2008 Jan 9.

The leaf inhibits active pancreatic lipase suggesting application in weight loss and hyperlipidemia formulas. Stane et al, *Phytother Res* 2009 23:6. Work by Slanc et al, *Phytother Res* 2008 Dec 23 found leaves inhibit lipase production associated with fat digestion.

Ursolic acid, also present in cranberry, is a terpene that exhibits cytotoxic and anti-leukemic activity.

Avicularin is found as well in bilberry, labrador tea and *Dryas* species. Quaijaverin is present in fennel seed and knotweed (*Polygonum aviculare*).

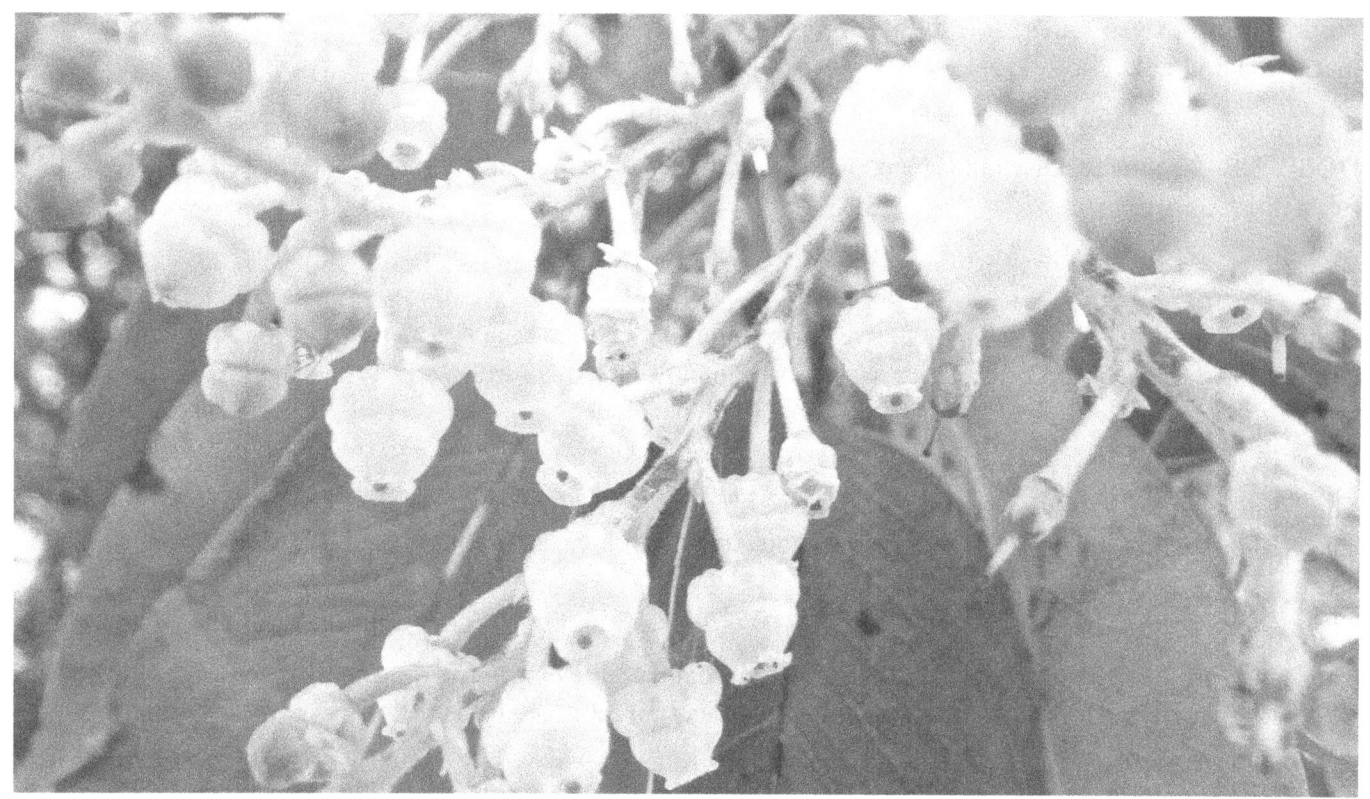

ARBUTUS FLOWERS

Uva ursi combines the best of the astringent and demulcent worlds- a rare combination in the herbal repertory.

Arbutus or Pacific Madrone trees are so beautiful, and make the coast of British Columbia a treasure to walk.

Russell Willier, noted Cree healer, uses the bark in a combination for heart and liver problems, as well as lowering blood pressure and controlling sugar diabetes. He shared this knowledge in *A Cree Healer and his Medicine Bundle*, co-authored by David Young, Russell and myself in 2016.

HOMEOPATHY

UVA URSI

The urinary symptoms are the most important indication with uva ursi. Bladder infections with bloody urine, or uterine hemorrhage call for its use. If there is burning after urination with frequent urging and severe spasms of the bladder, it is recommended.

Excess mucus in throat. Cystitis with blood.

DOSE-Mother tincture. Use 5-30 drops up to four times daily as needed. The mother tincture is prepared from the fresh leaves. Clinical observations in Boericke and effects of 10M by Macfarlan in 1892.

ARBUTIN

The active principle of uva ursi is used as a urinary antiseptic and diuretic.

DOSE- 3-8 grains on sugar cube three times daily.

ARBUTUS MENZIESII

There is loss of ambition, adversion to company, withdrawal from reality and lack of confidence.

Dullness as if in fog, mind and body as if separated [Thuja]. Want to sit and do nothing, no ambition, slow to answer, want help from others, mental confusion. Separation from reality.

Thirsty, cannot sleep on left side, desire to be near water, aversion to meat and vegetables, bad effects from marijuana and LSD.

Sensation that hands are not attached to arms, very dry mouth and yet sticky, ropy saliva. Inflammation of bladder.

DOSE- 30c. Proving by Olsen in Canada with two female and two male provers at 30c, as well as three clinical cases in 1995.

LEAF OIL

Gently heat one part uva ursi leaves to five parts canola oil in a crock pot at low setting for eight hours. Strain and use for skin sores, cradle cap and assorted skin conditions, including age spots.

ESSENTIAL OIL

The fresh leaves of uva ursi contain 0.01% essential oil that contains 7.8% alpha terpineol, 7.3% linalool, 4.1% (E) geranyl acetone, and 4.5% hexadecanoic acid. Radulovic et al, *Molecules* 2010 15 6168-85.

HYDROSOL

The leaves, and flowers of bearberry are good for sick and feeble eyes, according to Brunschwig in his *Book of Distillation* written in 1530. "And in the summer to look upon the green fields and places comforeth also the eyes."

WAX

A wax is extractable from the leaves of uva ursi. It has a melting point of 285° C and is thought to be a derivative of ursolic acid.

FLOWER ESSENCES

Bearberry flower essence helps to strengthen and increase psychic abilities. Often this ability is present, and it is simply a matter of "re-awakening" the stored energy. When first accessed, this may result in many unpleasant physical, mental and emotional sensations, as kundalini energy begins to move up through the spine and re-shape the energetics of the body and mind. Resistance at this stage can exhibit all the symptoms of psychosis as a transmutation, on the various planes, manifests. Bearberry flower essence helps reveal some of the underlying patterns that are part of a smooth transition of energy and matter. It will help individuals who occasionally have intuitive flashes, but are frustrated by their inability to access this ability on a regular basis.

During the movement of Kundalini energy, there is desire, on the personality level, to return to previous experience, or to deny the process that is manifest. Bearberry flower essence helps assist one in recognizing that the path is straight ahead and that all their past experiences have led them to this moment of possibility. Bearberry flower essence calms the individual and allows them to see themselves in this new place of awareness. In beginners, the essence reminds one that the journey toward self-awareness has begun, with the first few steps just underway. The use of yoga, tai chi, and Qigong assists the process and helps move the energy through the various chakras more efficiently and quietly. Blockage or resistance at any level will manifest in feelings of constriction, including heart palpitations, restricted breathing, sore throat, or headaches.

An excellent book by Sannella (1987) examines the issue of kundalini and psychosis. A few drops may be applied to affected areas to alleviate burning and heat associated with this process. Putting a few drops of Bearberry essence by your bedside, to use in the middle of the night, may help relieve some of the unpleasant hot and cold sensations, including the hot flashes associated with menopause and andropause.

A Japanese female in her 40s related her experience. "Although Bearberry is the essence of 'intuition power' I was talking on the phone with my friend one day and asked her, 'what were you doing this morning?' and she answered, 'I was sleeping most of the time at home'. Right after the phone was hung up, I felt immediately that she told a lie to me. So, I asked her the same question next day. In fact, she told me she had gone out that morning! I was so surprised because it happened to me right after drinking Bearberry essence."

PRAIRIE DEVA

Kinnickinnick flower essence allows people to create networks more easily in a conscious fashion, and to break these connections when they are no longer necessary. It assists people in moving in a freer and easier fashion, and alleviates unwanted past life connections.

PEGASUS

Uva Ursi flower essence nurtures the feminine, the vessel of creativity, the deep dark void from which all life flows. It helps one access the healing and creative powers of the deeper resources within. Physically, it is for healing the ovaries.

WOODLAND

Kinnickinnick flower essence encourages you to gentle snuggle into open-hearted love for yourself.

TREE FROG

SPIRITUAL PROPERTIES

Uva ursi's keyword is empowerment. Uva-ursi gives one power after walking into life and into the wisdom of self-discovery. It supports those that are ready to embrace their power and to fully express themselves and live out their true potential. It helps to integrate the fruits of life's experiences and gives certainty to direction and action to be taken.

MULDERS

Uva ursi's Bear Medicine is not only reflected in the power animal for which it is named, but also in the deep reservoir of the kidneys and urinary tract system…The Medicine Bear Lodge…is a place of deep introspection during the winter months.

The shadow cave, or the darkness of the void, is where we enter the dreamtime. The feminine mysteries represented by water, emotion, darkness and intuition speak of this metaphorically. It is from the dark womb of the Great Mother that we take our watery birth.

While uva ursi's medicine may help to heal a urinary tract infection, it is important to use it energetically by journeying inward with the spirit of this plant as an ally. Within the cave of our inner knowing is the answer to the question of how to take better care of our health.

THEA SUMMER DEER

MYTHS AND LEGENDS

The Trickster came upon a clump of bearberry. Hungry as usual, and cunning as ever, he decided to capture the berry. By dint of flattery he addressed it. "You remind me of tears on the cheeks of my favourite and most celebrated uncle." But the berry was not fooled. "Who doesn't know you, Weget?" it said, and rolled off the bush and hid in the safety of the woods. The little brown lines that may form on the berry are said to be the marks of Weget's uncle's tears.

GITKSAN MYTH

Pitch used to go fishing before the sun rose, and retire to the shade before it became strong. One day he was late and had just reached the beach when he melted. Other people rushed to share him. Fir [Douglas Fir] arrived first and secured most of the pitch, which he poured over his head and body. Balsam [Grand Fir] obtained only a little; and by the time Arbutus arrived there was none left.

Arbutus said, "I shall have to peel my skin every year and have a good wash to keep me clean." But just then XELS appeared and said, "You shall all be trees and Fir shall be your boss." So now the Arbutus sheds its bark every year, and [Douglas] for has more pitch than any other tree. **JENESS** recorded by Nancy Turner in *Saanich Ethnobotany*.

Bear related phytonyms are common throughout the botanical world. Kolosova V et al, J *Ethnobiol Ethnomed* 2017 13(1):14 is a great summary of European origin plant names.

PERSONALITY TRAITS

Uva ursi people smolder with age-long resentment about being underdogs. A "chip on the shoulder" may also indicate a stone in the kidney or bladder.

Always on the defensive, the Uva ursi person assumes that everyone is out to get them. They are never neutral—they love or hate you!

While fiercely loyal to friends, relatives and others, they stand united against the outside world and what it is doing to them. They remember all past humiliations and are ruthless when they become the BOSS! They harbour grudges and enjoy getting their own back.

The negative uva ursi has difficulty leaving the past and living in the present. It is with reluctance they will smile. Their instinctive reason seems to be to hurt someone else. They can be very selfish and self-centred. They refuse to believe that anyone else has troubles.

Those around often live in fear of their tempers, especially after alcohol starts affecting their liver and kidneys. They may suffer lower back pain or griping indigestion.

When positive, uva ursi people manage to bury the past and leave revenge to fate, or karma. They know that while there is an effect of the past; it halts humanity and deposits calcium. They choose not to dwell there too often, or let it restrict their view of life today.   **DOROTHY HALL**

BOTANICA POETICA

BEARBERRY
(*Arctostaphylos uva-ursi*)

If urination causes pain
Your bladder, you cannot contain
It's acid fire when you pee
Something's off about the stream
Infection in the urine's path
Has made you wriggle round in wrath
It's Uva Ursi you might need
To stave off germs, your pain to ease
This little shrub of Evergreen
Has got some healing in its leaf
Known to be a diuretic
Urinary antiseptic
A strong astringent quality
That has a complex chemistry
But tannins aren't for daily feed
So do not use too regularly
It's an herb for inflammation
Works to rid you of infection
Bearberry leaf, in my tea
Bladder health restore to me!

SYLVIA CHATROUX MD

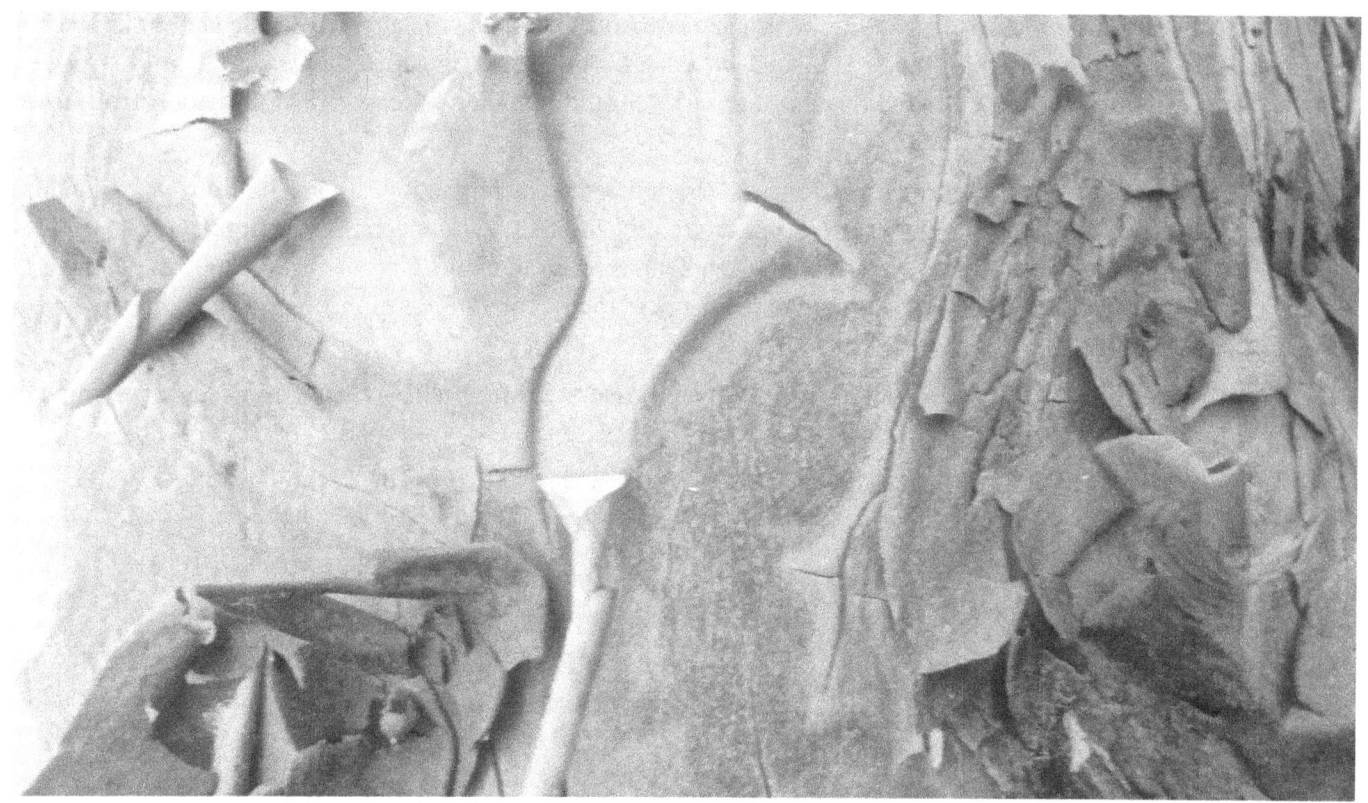

ARBUTUS BARK

RECIPES

COLD INFUSION- Leaves are crushed and steeped overnight in cool water. In the morning, warm up the drink, but do not boil. This decreases tannin irritation, and gives better levels of arbutin.

DOSE- Take three to five ounces at a time. This is an effective urinary disinfectant if the urine is alkaline. If not, use a small amount of sodium bicarbonate in water to alkalize urine. Vitamin C (ascorbic acid) and fruit juice should be avoided, due to their acidifying nature, but calcium and potassium citrates will help. Do not use for more than two weeks.

Doses up to 20 grams have not caused harm in human studies.

TINCTURE- 60 drops up to five times daily. This is best made with a 60% alcohol/water and fresh leaves in 1:2 ratio.

When combined with pipsissewa and usnea, use up to 90 drops 4x daily. Combining uva ursi with mullein leaf, which has a moderate alkalizing effect on urine, may be useful.

FREEZE-DRIED- 500 mg three times daily in capsule form.

SOLID EXTRACT- The ideal arbutin content is 10%. Take 250-500 mg or one quarter teaspoon three times daily.

SITZ BATH- One-quarter cup of leaves are simmered in four litres of water for twenty minutes and then cooled to body temperature. This can be splashed vaginally for three to five days after birthing. Whole body baths are useful for chronic conditions of rheumatism and tuberculosis.

BEARBERRY BUTTER- Cook cleaned berries with water to cover until they open up. Strain and throw seeds away. Add sweetener of choice and return to stove. Use one package of pectin for 6 quarts of pulp. Pour into sterilized jars. Use like apple butter.   **SNELL**

CAUTION- Do not use uva ursi in patients with kidney disorders, or during pregnancy, or lactation. Do not use sodium bicarbonate with high blood pressure patients. Large doses can cause nausea and tinnitus; as well as aggravate constipation, and stomach ulcers. Bearberry should be taken at least two hours apart from iron, or alkaloid containing herbs.

A patient ingesting uva ursi tea for three years for a recurrent urinary tract infection showed bull's eye maculopathy in one case reported by Wang and Del Priore, *Am J Opthamol* 2004 137. The mechanism is unclear but suggests caution in chronic use with retinal concerns. Work by Chauhan et al, *Can J Physiol Pharm* 2007 85:9 suggests both water and methanol extracts of uva ursi possess high cytochrome P450 inhibition and may interfere with drug absorption or kinetics.

Bearberry may increase the effect of NSAIDs. An isolated case of lithium toxicity was reported, involving uva ursi, parsley and other herbal diuretics.

Work by de Arriba SG et al, *Int J Toxicol* 2013 32:6 442-53 suggests uva ursi is safe for humans, based on a wide variety of human cell assays.

WESTERN CANADA VIOLET
TALL WHITE VIOLET
(*Viola canadensis* L.)
(*V. rugulosa* Greene) not accepted
HEARTSEASE
JOHNNY JUMP UP
LOVE-IN-IDLENESS
(*V. tricolor* L.)
FIELD VIOLET
WILD PANSY
(*V. arvensis* Murray)
YELLOW PRAIRIE VIOLET
(*V. nuttallii* Pursh)
SAGEBRUSH VIOLET
VALLEY VIOLET
(*V. vallicola* A. Nelson)
YELLOW WOOD VIOLET
PIONEER VIOLET
(*V. glabella* Nutt.)

EARLY BLUE VIOLET
WESTERN DOG VIOLET
HOOKED SPUR VIOLET
(*V. adunca* Sm.)
(*V. aduncoides*) not accepted
BOG VIOLET
(*V. nephrophylla* Greene) not accepted
(*V. sororia* var. *affinis* [Leconte] L. E. McKinney)
(*V. maccabeana* M.S. Baker) not accepted
(*V. pratincola* Greene) not accepted
DOWNY YELLOW VIOLET
(*V. pubescens* Ait.)
SWEET VIOLET
(*V. odorata* L.)
(*V. odorata* var. *konigin* **Charlott and others**)
PARTS USED- flowers, leaves, seeds

Who bends a knee where violets grow
A hundred secret things shall know.   **ANON**

The garden's gem
Heart's ease, like a gallant bold,
In his cloth of purple and gold.   **LEIGH HUNT**

A violet by a mossy stone
Half hidden from the eye!
Fair as a star when only one
Is shining in the sky.   **WILLIAM WORDSWORTH**

I [violet] am hidden and stooped and shun conversation.   **GOETHE**

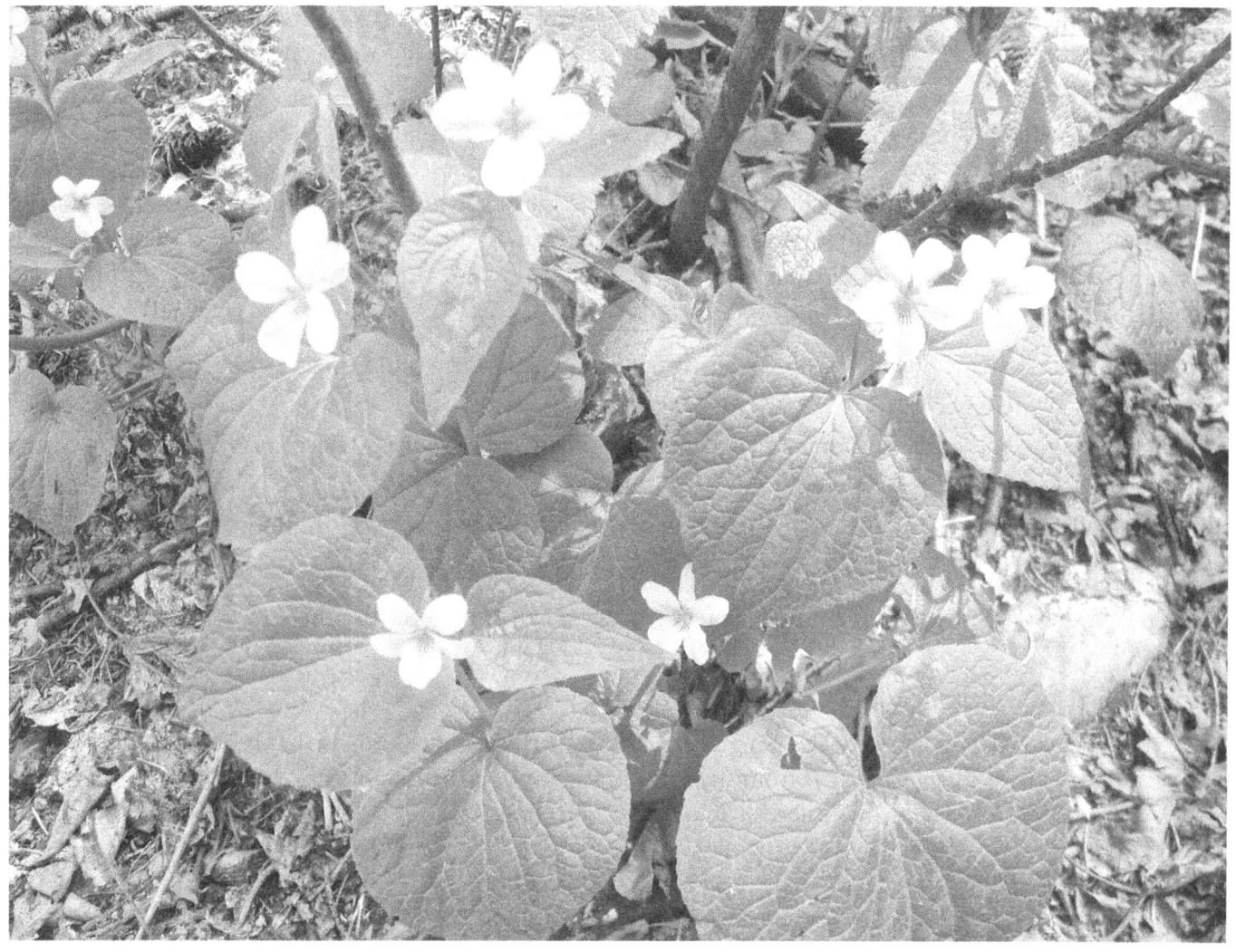

TALL WHITE VIOLET

When beechen buds begin to swell,
And woods the bluebird's warble know,
The yellow violet's modest bell
Peeps from the last year's leaves below.

WILLIAM CULLEN BRYANT

Come, Oh gods of Olympus, come and receive the springtime tribute of these violets plaited in rings; for a brilliant feast awaits the poet when the purple-veiled seasons reopen their dwelling and fragrant spring revives the divine freshness of the plants.

PINDAR

Yet mark'd I where the bolt of Cupid fell:

It fell upon a little western flower,

Before milk-white, now purple with love's wound, and maidens call it love-in-idleness.

Fetch me that flower; the herb I shew'd thee once: the juice of it on sleeping eye-lids laid will make a man or woman madly dote upon the next living creature that it sees.

SHAKESPEARE A MIDSUMMER NIGHT'S DREAM

He…set himself to discover…what there was in frankincense that made one mystical; and in ambergris that stirred one's passions; and in violets that woke the memory of dead romances…

OSCAR WILDE

Viola is from the ancient Latin name for the flower. It probably comes from the diminutive of **VIA**, meaning love. Other authors believe it is from the Latin **VIA**, meaning road or wayside, as in Via Rail, the Canadian passenger train.

The verbal root is prehistoric, probably back to the Greek **ION**, for a purple violet. The Latin **IO** is the daughter of the river god Inarchus. According to legend, Zeus, after casting his affections of Io, her priestess, turned her into a white cow to save her from his significant other, Hera, the queen of Heaven. As a consolation, he created violets (ions) to provide sweet fodder for his beloved cow goddess.

Ion was the legendary founder of Athens, and hence the violet became a symbol of the city. Athenians used the flowers to moderate anger, produce sleep and comfort and strengthen the heart.

The ancient Greeks made crowns of violets for their feasts, particularly those honoring Dionysus, associated with drinking and debauchery.

The Romans, on the other hand, thought violets were flowers of mourning, and decorated tombs with wreaths on the Day of the Dead, also known as *Violaris Dies*.

Romans also wore wreaths to cool the brow, or relieve headaches from over-consumption of wine.

This translated into medieval times where violet necklaces were said to protect from deception and inebriation.

Io is a moon that circles Jupiter, the Roman version of Zeus. Ionosphere is from the same source and likewise iodine.

Celtic mythology associated it with the Unicorn, youth and virginity.

The Greek root was later adapted to Old French giving the chemical name iodine. That is because both the gas and various salts were purple. Pansy is from the French, **PENSEE**, for "thought", or "remembrance". A famous Shakespeare quote from Hamlet is "There's pansies, that's for thoughts".

Pansy is closely related to the Greek Gods, Pan and Pandora. The latter was a companion of Hecate in the underworld, and responsible for letting loose the ills that afflict mankind. Pan was a nature god, known for his pipes, dances and sexuality.

In Germany, the pansy is known as **STIEFMUTTERCHEN**, meaning Little Stepmother.

Heartsease was a name from Elizabethan times, and associated with innocent, unspoiled love. In the language of flowers, the three colors of pansy, purple white and yellow, stand for memories, loving thoughts and souvenirs, to ease the hearts of separated lovers. The sweet, glutinous taste of violet suggests a plant signature related to soothing and emollient properties. The plant has a birth date of March 29th. The 7th Norse Rune, Gyfu, is associated with *Viola tricolor*.

Canadensis means "from Canada". This is the tallest of the violets in our region, usually found in mixed woodlands and some shade, whitish with purple and yellow spotting. Arvensis means, "of the field". Tricolor is for the three-colored flowers, purple, white and yellow. Adunca means hooked, due to a hook on the flower spur.

Violets have played a role in art, poetry and folklore.

The Greeks used them "to moderate anger, procure sleep, and comfort and strengthen the heart".

Courtesans of ancient Greece used violet to perfume their erogenous zones as it blends with the natural odor of feminine secretion and was believe to alleviate the melancholia of the oldest man, and torment youth beyond endurance. No doubt!

Earlier, the ancient Egyptian Ebers Papyrus, spoke of the medicinal benefits of violets over two thousand years ago. The Koran says "the superiority of the extract of violets above all other extracts is as the superiority (of Mohamet) over the rest of men."

Scented violets have three petals above and one below, while pansies and other violas have four petals above and one below.

In the 1700s a lozenge made from violet conserve called **PLATE**, was used medicinally for bronchitis.

Napoleon was the Corporal Violet leader, the dainty flowers serving as a secret emblem for his followers. On their wedding anniversary, he gave Josephine a bouquet of violets; and when he died, a locket around his neck contained her hair and a dried violet flower.

Because of this seditious association, French law prohibited public display of art featuring these flowers for over a half century. The flower is thus associated with modesty, chastity, loyalty and love.

On the other hand, a shrinking violet is someone shy, unassertive, or retiring; in the shadow like the flower itself.

Shrinking Violet was a member of the Legion of Super-Heroes in Action Comics. She was brought into being, by Jerry Siegel, the co-creator of Superman.

The ancient Celts steeped violets in goat's milk, to increase female beauty. Queen Victoria had three thousand violet plants grown at Windsor, so much did she love the flowers. In Scotland, the petals were soaked in white wine to make shrub, a popular drink.

The Irish herbalist K'Eogh wrote heartsease flowers, "cure convulsions in children, cleanse the lungs and breast and are very good for fevers, internal inflammations and wounds."

Hildegard of Bingen recommended a violet salve for ulcerated tumors and other skin cancers, as well as connective tissue cysts, lumps, precancerous growths, muscles sores, etc. She recommended, "one suffering tertian fevers should take violet and a third as much plantain and two-thirds as much savory. He should frequently eat these herbs with vinegar or roasted salt."

Anthony Askham, in his *Little Herbal* of 1550, wrote "For them that may not sleep for sickness, seethe the violets in water, and even let him soak well his feet in the water to the ankles: and when he get to bed bind of this herb to his temples, and he shall sleep well, by the grace of God."

The first whitish flowers of spring don't generally produce seed. Later in the season, small greenish flowers, or "cleistogamous buds", that remain underground, or right at the soil surface, don't open and self-fertilize, ensuring seed production.

Violet seeds have attached, special oily bodies called elaiosomes, that attract ants. They carry the seeds away to their nests, eat the oils, and toss the seeds, helping disperse them further.

Violets display, appropriately, ultra-violet patterns visible to bees, and other pollinators, but not to humans.

The qualities of color, structure and sweet scent are why they flourished in the gardens of Greece, and served as a symbol for Athens.

The dried leaves have been burned as part of incense blends for protection from illness.

All violet leaves and flowers are edible and delicious additions to salads, soups and omelets. The leaves, specifically, help thicken soups and stews, due to their mucilaginous nature.

The leaves of some species have five times more Vitamin C than oranges, and twice the Vitamin A of spinach. The steamed leaves retain some violet flavor and even fragrance, are slightly astringent, and similar to spinach.

The roots and seeds of *V. odorata* are considered toxic, however.

The Ojibwa tribe used decoctions of Western Wood Violet root for back pains and concerns of the bladder.

The root contains a wintergreen-flavored pepsin. A weak root tea can be used for prolapsed bladder or uterus.

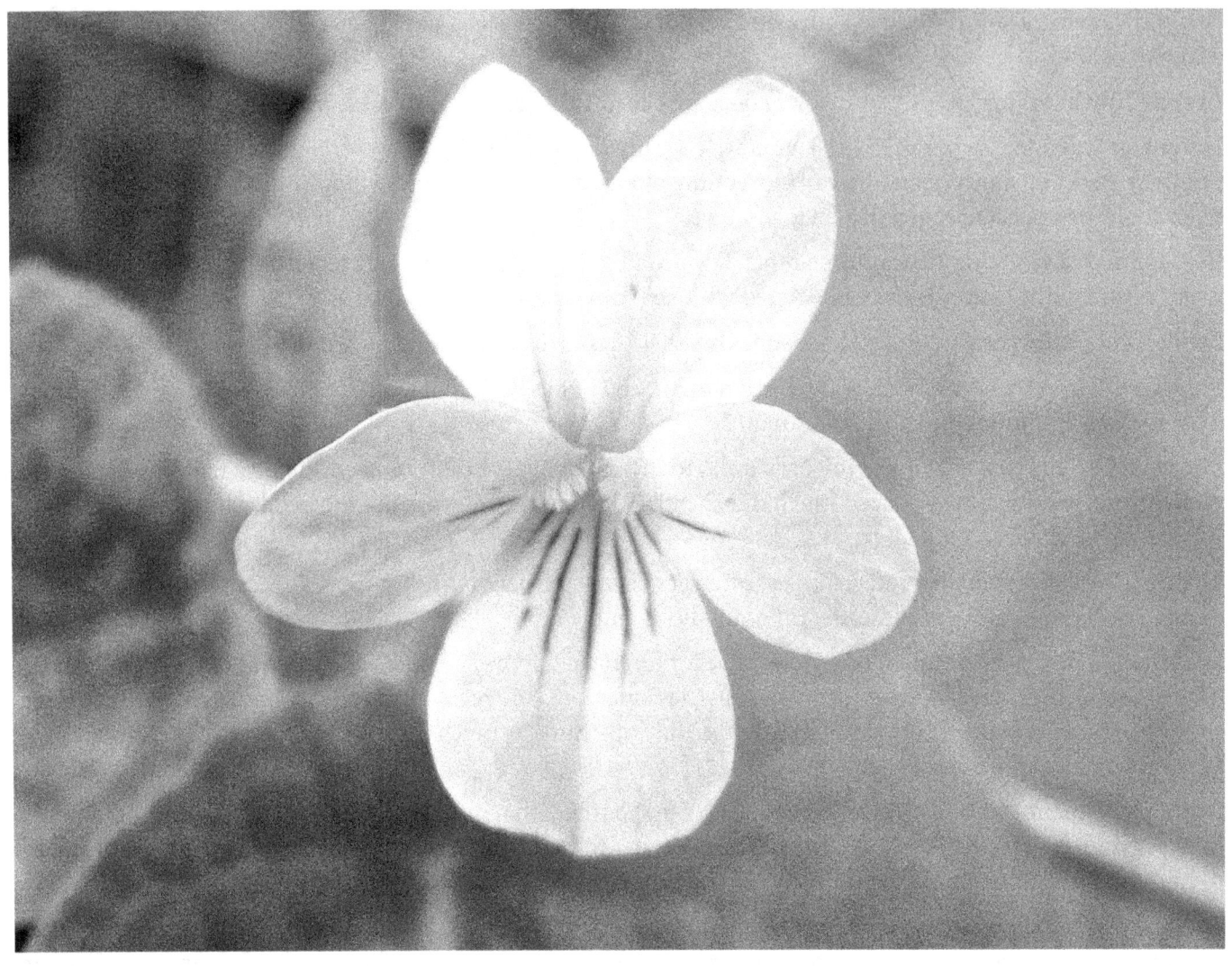

WESTERN WOOD VIOLET

The Early Blue Violet was poulticed as an analgesic by the Klallam, applied to the chest or sides for pain. The Makah women chewed on the roots and leaves during labor. The Blackfoot of southern Alberta used a blue dye from the flowers on their hunting arrows.

They called it Blue Mouth, and brewed a tea from the leaves for children with respiratory difficulty. The Cree name **MEHKWAKANASKOS** means, "little face plant".

Other groups used the plant wash on sores and swollen joints, stomach pain, and childhood asthma.

The Blackfoot call this species **KOMONO** as well as Red Mouth or Blue Mouth. The blue dye was used to dye arrows. The leaves and roots were decocted for tea to relieve asthma, or applied externally to painful joints.

The blue flowers give up their color quite easily to hot water. When acid is added the color turns purple to red; while alkali such as baking soda turns green and then yellow, suggesting use for determining pH of any substance.

Yellow Prairie Violet is widespread in the southern prairies.

The roots of *V. glabella* were boiled, by indigenous healers of Alaska, as a purgative.

Downy Yellow Violet is more common to the eastern prairies. The Ojibwa decocted the root and used it as a gargle for sore throat, while the Potawatomi considered the root a heart medicine.

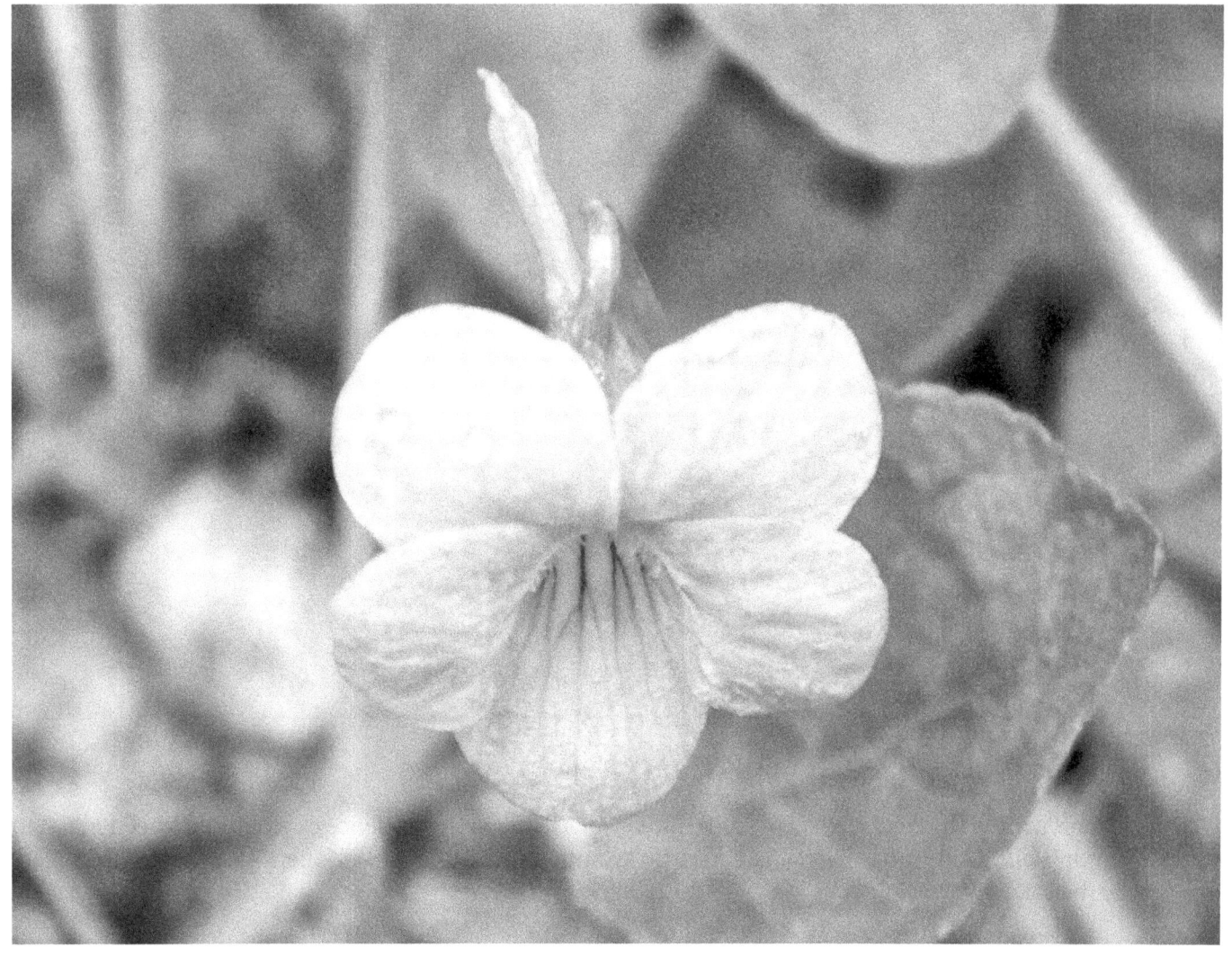

EARLY BLUE VIOLET

The Cherokee soaked their corn in root infusions to prevent insect invasion. Medicinally, the leaves were used for headaches, and a nasal spray for catarrh. The crushed root was applied to boils.

The cultivated *V. tricolor hortensis* has the same medicinal value, a quality not always shared by wild and tame cousins. It was the result of a cross between *V. lutea* and *V. altaica* in 1810.

Tall White Violet has purple tinged petals, and is, what some scientists including Sir John Lubbock, call a violet in the process of evolving from white to purple, the most advanced flower color.

The introduced violet or pansy from Europe looks very similar, with some taxonomists using size to differentiate between Pansy and Johnny Jump Ups.

Field Pansy is very similar, but the flowers are smaller and mainly creamy or white.

They both possess the same properties. Johnny Jump Up is from England and derived from the phrase, Johnny Jump Up and Kiss Me.

In one Romanian tale, the pansy was once a beautiful servant in the royal court. She was transformed by a jealous queen, when her son, the prince, fell in love with her. The Queen wished to make her a toad, but she was so lovely that she could only make her into a pansy.

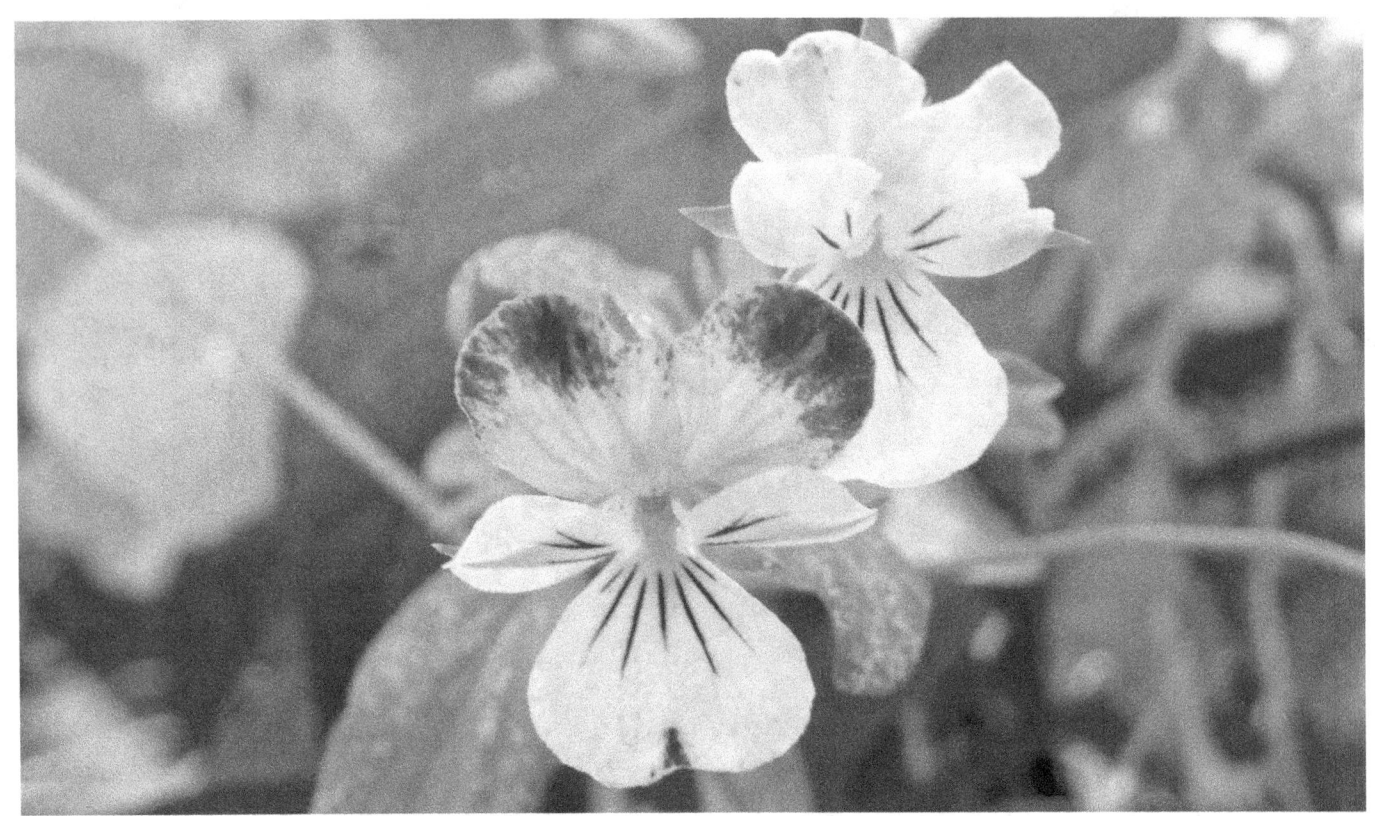

JOHNNY JUMP UP

Dr. Millsbaugh wrote, "the emetic effect of some of the violets, due to the presence of violine, has been noted to some extent in (wild pansy). The most characteristic symptom of its action is an offensive odour of the urine, like that of the cat."

Sweet Violet (*V. odorata*) is famous for its perfume, from both flower and leaf. It is considered hardy only to zone 5, but many scented hybrids do very well in zone 2-3, if protected and planted close to house foundations.

Violet flower tea can be used for determining acid and alkaline direction, in the manner of litmus paper. Simple prepare an infusion that is blue. Add an alkali and it turns yellow green; but add acid and it turns red.

The flowers of *V. odorata* are used in India medicinally as an anti-pyretic, diaphoretic and febrifuge; and known as **BANAFSHA**.

Traditionally, a syrup was made from the flowers and called **IOSACCAR**.

A famous French liqueur, **PARFAIT AMOUR** traditionally contained distilled flower oil. Probably not today!

Purple Violet (*V. cucullata*) is the provincial floral emblem of New Brunswick. This variety was suggested for use by Jethro Kloss, in combination with red clover and vervain, for the treatment of cancer and cancerous skin growths.

For nervousness and general debility, he suggested combining violet, scullcap and black cohosh, equal parts. This will relieve severe headaches and congestion in the head.

Various violets are the state flowers of Wisconsin, Rhode Island, New Jersey, and Illinois. Violets are the national floral symbol of Poland and Northern Portugal.

Mrs. Grieve wrote "they seldom do well near a town, because the undersides of the leaves are covered with hairs, which catch the grit, thus blocking the breathing pores."

Geo-botanical prospecting, or the observation of which plants grow near which minerals is an interesting field. The same plants also lend themselves to land remediation, especially with regards to heavy metals, and the concentration of organic metals for human and animal health.

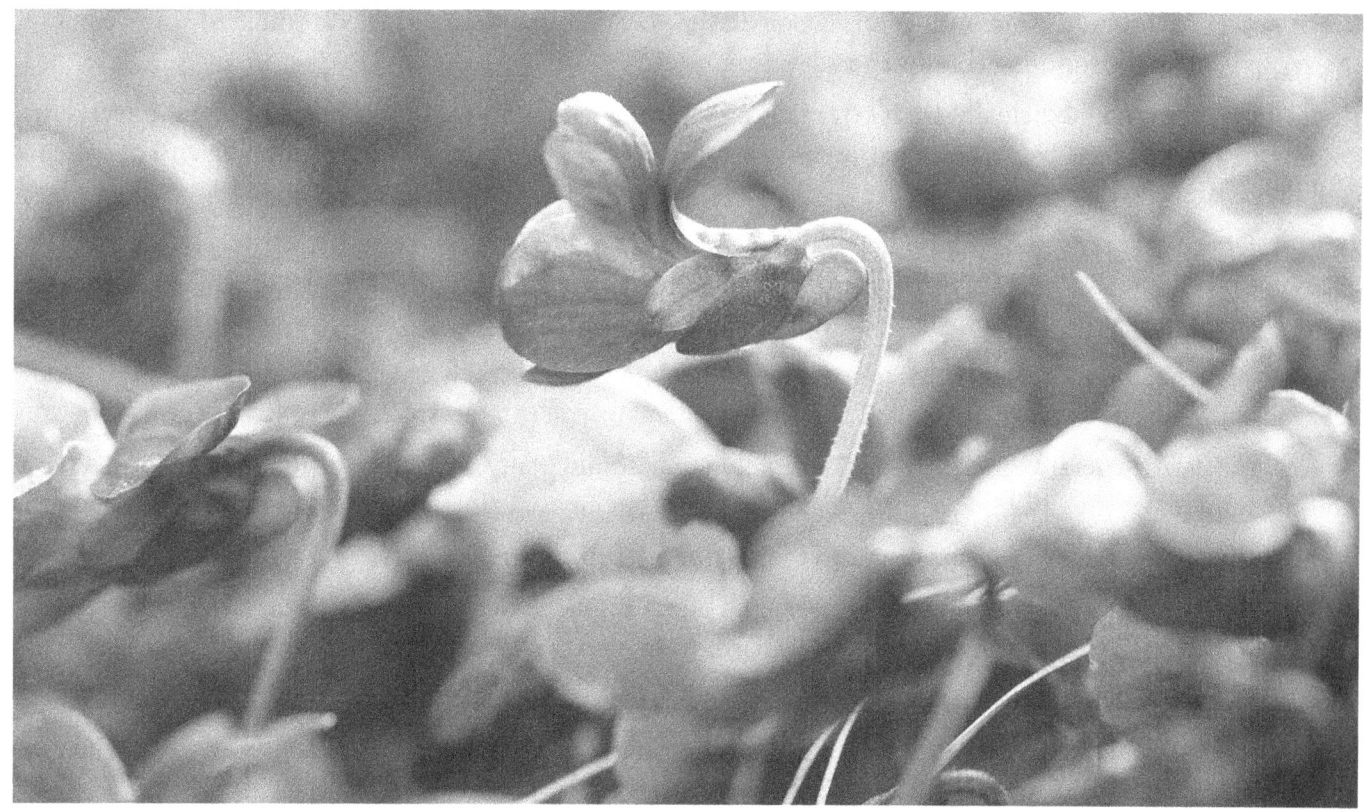

SCENTED VIOLET

The wild pansy (*V. calaminaria*) of China, is a zinc loving plants, with 1% of its ash composed of this mineral. Various violet species hyper-accumulate cadmium, suggesting use in phyto-remediation.

MEDICINAL

CONSTITUENTS- *V. tricolor* aerial parts- salicylic acid, methyl salicylate (0.43-1.3%), alkaloids, flavonoids including violarvensin- a di-C-glycoside flavonoid, glycosides like violanthin; scoparin, saponarine, delphinidin triglycoside, vicenin-2, vitexin-phenol carboxylic acid; violutoside, vitri A-F, cycloviolacin-O2 violaquercitin, and anthocyane (violanin); gums, mucilage (10%), coumarins, umbelliferone, cyclotides, flavonoids including rutin (violaquercitin), violanthin, scoparin, saponarin, and the C-glycosides vitexin, saponaretin, orientin, and iso-orientin; patulin, tannins, essential oils, calcium and magnesium salts, and seven novel macrocylic polypeptides or cyclotides (vavpeptides A-H), with 29-30 amino acid residues.
The flowers have carotenoids including auroxanthin and violaxanthin. The rutin content at the start of flowering is 0.15% at the start of flowering, tripling to 0.45% at fruit set. Also contain flavonxanthin, myricetin, myrosine, quercitin, rutin (2-23% dried), salicylic acid, tocopherol, violanine, violanthin, zeaxanthin.
seed-myrosin, and a glucoside.
V. arvensis- cyclotides similar to *V. tricolor* and *V. odorata*; violarvesin (flavonoid di-C-glycoside); salicylic acid, arbutin, catechol, caffeic, ferulic and p-coumaric acid, hesperidin, scopoletin, umbelliferone, rhamnose, arabinose, galactose, glucuronic acid, apigenin, luteolin, kaempferol, quercitin, vitexin, dicoumarin, ellagic acid.
V. odorata- aerial parts- saponins, myrosin, violamin, viola-quercetin, gaultherin, viola-emetin, salicylic acid methyl ester (0.04%) volatile oil; beta-nitropropionic acid, friedelin, odoratine (alkaloid).
Flowers- violin, volatile oil, rutin 2%, cyanin 5.3%, chromogen, a glycoside of methyl salicylate, sugar, tocopherols, anthocyanins 4% including violanin, melatonin, nicotiflorin, minerals 8.5% and mucilage 18%.
Leaves- above and triterpene friedelin, beta sitosterol, alkaloids, essential oil, alcohol. Cycloviolacin 02 and cyclotides consisting of "cyclic cystine knots", salicylates, ferulic and sinapic acids.
Root- saponins (0.1-2.5%), essential oil similar to flowers, 2-nitropropionic acid, alkaloid with hypertensive activity, triacetonamine (odoratine). Leaves, roots and flowers all contain cyclotides.
V. yedoensis- cerotic acid, alkaloids, flavonoids.

Violet flower tea and syrup are both gentle laxatives, the yellow ones more so. When combined with coltsfoot, the syrup is good for soothing coughs and sore throats.

Violet leaves are used medicinally, both externally and internally for various skin conditions including eczema, cradle cap, impetigo, psoriasis, acne, nettle rash and scabies. Cradle cap is helped by softening and decreasing of skin oils and waxes.

Wild violet leaves are covered with boiling water and allowed to stand for twelve hours. This is gargled and used as a compress in the treatment of throat cancer. Tea of fresh or dried wild violet leaves is a specific for cancerous growths of the throat. A cold infusion is best.

Salicylic acid, one of the constituents, promotes skin healing by generating a more rapid turnover of new skin cells. Some violets have up to 4000 ppm of salicylic acid, mainly in the roots, stems and leaves.

As well, it relieves general skin itching, and chronic rheumatic and gouty conditions, through a dredging action. This is useful for scanty dribbling urination, bedwetting, difficulty in urination and excessive mucous in urine.

Some people complain of a cat-like odour to their urine after drinking violet tea.

Heartsease activates immunity, reduces infection and promotes tissue repair. It can be used in chronic infections such as herpes or in treating infantile eczema caused by drinking cow's milk, being both gentle and efficient.

It is a useful addition to lymphatic decongestant formulas that include, cleavers, blue flag and red root.

Violets help restore and relax the nerves, useful in exhaustion, and nervous heart palpitation as well as twitching, spasms, and cramping of muscles.

The various violets are non-sedating calmatives, useful for cranky, overheated congested emotions and lymphatic systems. For the latter, combine with cleavers.

Tis Mal Crow, a Native American Root Doctor/Herbalist uses violet as an activator or accelerator herb in plant combinations. He believes that violet potentiates the activity of green medicinals in a ratio of 1:32.

Field Pansy (*V. arvensis*) has been found to show cytotoxicity against ten human tumor cell lines, in work by Lindholm et al, in Sweden.

Johnny Jump Up has been used in treating skin cancer, bronchitis, rheumatism, and whooping cough. Water extracts of the leaves have shown activity against both gram positive and myco-bacteria. Witkowska-Banaszczak et al, *Fitoterapia* 76:5.

Research by Papay et al, *Acta Pharma Hung* 1987 157 indicates chemical substances useful for preventing heart spasms and anti-inflammatory effect. Recent work by Tolu et al, *Rev Med Chir Soc Med Nat Iasi* 2007 111:2 found *V. tricolor* tincture to possess anti-inflammatory activity.

For angina pain, hypertension or a slow, sluggish heartbeat, use the flower tincture in the same dosage. Extracts show anti-thrombin and anti-cancer activity. Goun EA et al, *J Ethnopharm* 2002 81 337-342.

It is worth noting Heartsease and Johnny Jump Up growing in rye fields are believed to be therapeutically superior, to those growing elsewhere. There appears to be a symbiotic relationship between the two, and in the past, skin eruptions caused by excessive rye in the diet, were cured with Heartsease tea.

Other skin conditions such as cradle cap, impetigo, psoriasis, acne, hives, herpes and allergic/atopic eczema all may be treated with the herb infusion or tincture. This indicates, in the example of infantile eczema, an immune-regulating and anti-histamine response. Asthma, particularly allergy related, also responds well to the activity of Heartsease. This may be due, in part to the content of cyclotides, which inhibit proliferation of activated lymphocytes in an IL-2 dependent manner. Overly active immune system response is calmed down. Hellinger et al, *J Ethnopharmacol* 2014 151(1): 299-306.

Cyclotides are plant-derived mini proteins, genetically encoded as precursor proteins that become post-translationally modified to yield circular cystine-knotted molecules. Because of this, they resist enzymatic degradation in biological fluids. As of 2015, over 164 cyclotides have been discover in *V. tricolor*. It is estimated as many as 150,000 individual cyclotides may be eventually found in Viola species. Hellinger R et al, *J Proteome Res* 2015 14(11): 4851-62.

Vicenin-2, one constituent of *V. tricolor*, possesses hypotensive activity.

Vigno cyclopetides induce apoptosis in cervical cancer cells. Esmaeili MA et al, *Fitoterapia* 2016 109: 162-8.

A tincture of the aerial parts exhibits an anti-inflammatory effect on bone marrow acute phase response. Toiu et al, *Rev Med Chir Soc Med Nat Iasi* 2007 111:2.

When treating babies, you can use pansy tea instead of water in preparing their food. It can also be added to milk. Note however, that dairy allergies are one of the leading causes of eczema in young children.

Pansy flowers contain up to 23% rutin, which contributes to lowering of intraocular pressure of glaucoma. Three fresh flowers daily give the recommended daily dose of 60 milligrams of rutin.

V. tricolor has been shown to reduce glucose transport from the intestine into the bloodstream, in a manner similar to fenugreek seeds.

The plant contains utero-active peptides, as well as possessing anti-microbial activity (Kalala-peptide B1), that is being researched as a starting point for the design of new peptide antibiotics.

Work in Sweden suggests cyclotides responsible for anti-cancer activity are 14 times higher in mid summer.

Work by Hermann et al, *Phytochem* 2008 69:4 found Viola cyclotides active against lymphoma cell lines.

Viola tricolor induces apoptosis in cancer cells and exhibits anti-angiogenic activity, thus promoting cell death and preventing blood vessels from feeding tumors. Sadeghnia HR et al, *Biomed Res Int* 2014: 625792.

Tang et al, *Peptides* 2010 31:8 identified vitri A, vitri F and cycloviolacin O2 as most cytotoxic against five cancer cell lines, including ovarian, breast and prostate.

Crude extracts of V. tricolor were analyzed for cytotoxic activity against lymphoma and myeloma cell lines. Three small proteins, virti A, varv A and varv E, cyclotides, were shown to be potent anti-cancer compounds. Svangard E et al, *J Nat Prod* 2004 67(2): 144-7.

This is not surprising, and in fact, more research will probably discover both immune stimulating and regulating properties in the plant.

Cyclotides, particularly cycloviolacin O2, disrupt human lymphoma cell line U-937 GTB and disintegrates cell lipid membranes within five minutes. Svangard E et al, *J Nat Prod* 2007 70(4): 643-7.

Like our native Violets, the flowering plant soothes scanty and difficult urination, or bedwetting as the case may be.

The flowering tops are one of our most important sunscreen protectants. Work by Khazaeli et al, *Iranian J Pharm Res* 2008 7:1 reported an SPF of 25.69.

Leaf extracts of *Dracocephalum moldavica* were close second at 24.79.

Students at Northern Star College steam-distilled the latter plant at Gordon Steinrath's farm a few years ago. The oil is distinctly lemony, and more in the direction of lemon balm than lemongrass or any citrus oil.

A gel, containing *Viola tricolor* extracts, was tested on ultraviolet B induced burns. Piana M et al, *J Ethnopharm* 2013 150(2):458-65. Results were positive.

As a hot infusion, it relieves cold and flu, or even chronic bronchitis, croups and respiratory infection in general.

Be careful where it grows, as *V. tricolor* is a high accumulator of cadmium.

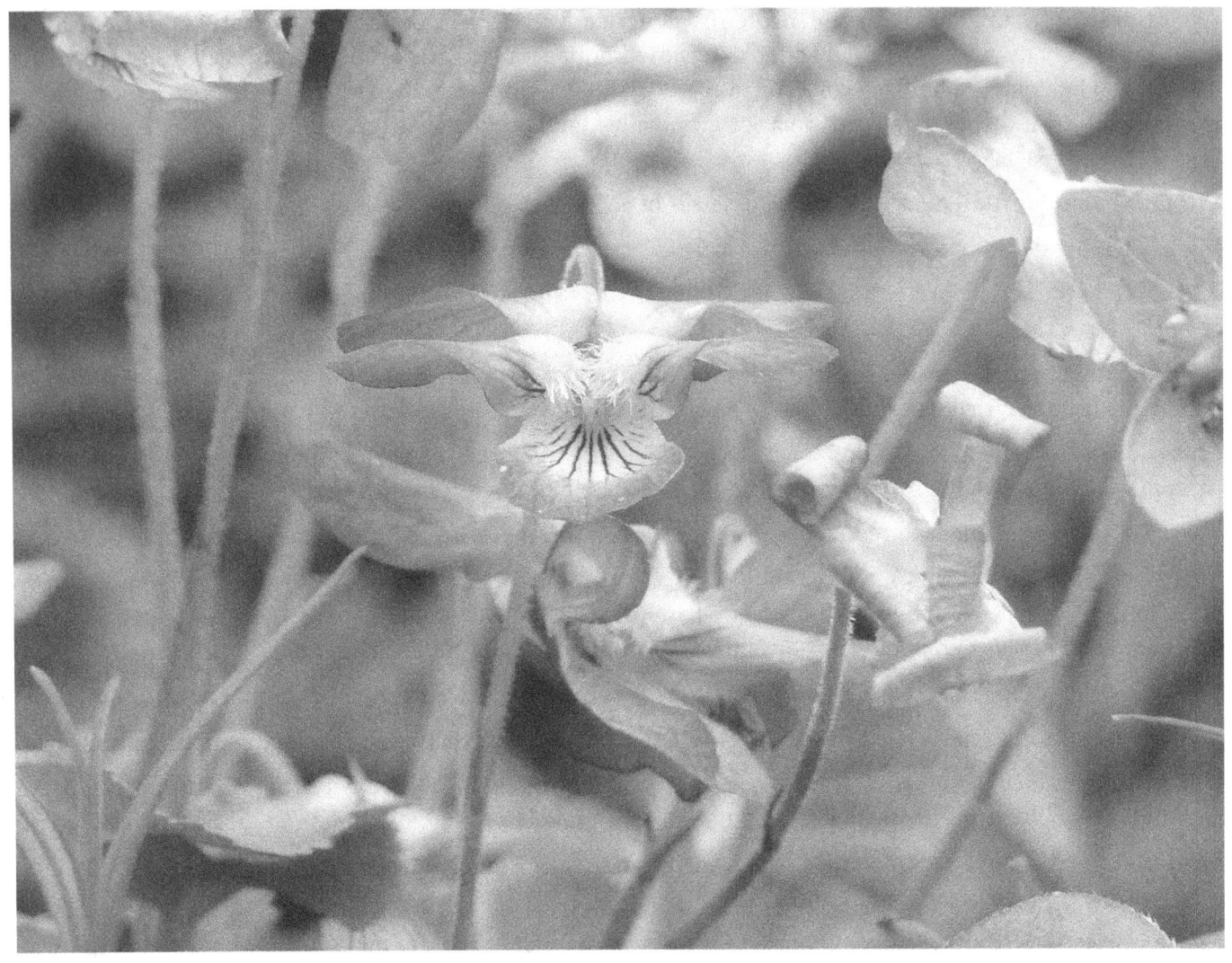

VIOLA ODORATA

Both *V. tricolor* and *V. odorata* extracts protect neuronal cells from serum/glucose deprived cell death, in part due to antioxidant activity. Mousavi SH et al, *Avicenna J Phytomed* 2016 6(4): 434-41.

Sweet Violet leaf and root is similar with two exceptions. It has better mucolytic and anti-tussive activity than Heartsease, and is therefore a better choice in hot, damp inflamed lung conditions such as whooping cough.

Sweet Violet leaves, flowers and roots all possess anti-tumor activity, especially in the treatment of lung, breast, stomach, intestinal and throat cancers. It appears that the tincture discourages growth of new blood vessels that feed cancer cells, thus starving them of nutrients. It can be used after cancer surgery to help prevent metastasis.

Note the roots and seeds of this species are semi-toxic, and should not be used long term.

Unique cyclotides isolated from aerial parts exhibit strong cytotoxic activity against a whole range of human tumor cell lines. The IC50 against chronic lymphocytic leukemia cells was 0.1 microM compared to 0.87 microM against healthy human lymphocytes. A different mode of action from anti-tumor drugs is at work. Lindholm et al, *Mol Cancer Ther* 2002 1.

Friedelin inhibits breast cancer MCF-7 cell growth. Subash-Babu P et al, *Exp Toxicol Pathol* 2017 June 12.

It also shows strong activity against *Mycobacterium tuberculosis* strains. Chinsembu KC et al, *Acta Trop* 2016 53: 46-56.

Violet leaf tea helps alleviate menopausal hot flashes; as well as offering hormone sensitive cancer prevention.

Sweet Violet leaf extracts have been found comparable with aspirin in reducing fevers. Khattak et al, *J Ethnopharm* 1985 14.

Decoctions and syrups have been used traditionally for coughs and insomnia, or applied topically for anti-inflammatory agents. Kroustil et al, *Chem Abstract* 1969 71 significant anti-inflammatory activity was found in herb decoctions.

Sweet Violet flowers contain measurable amounts of melatonin, especially in tincture form. Ansari M et al, *DARU* 2010 18(3): 173-8.

Sweet Violet is frequently used in skin disorders such as juvenile acne, herpes, urticaria, eczematous varicose ulcers, chronic psoriasis and eczema. It is a tonic to the venous system, and effective for treating hemorrhoids, phlebitis and constipation. A strong tea, or diluted tincture of the leaves and flowers can be used in the form of a compress or a liniment rub on affected limbs. In season use the fresh leaf poultice for even better effect.

The leaves and flowers contain anti-allergic and anti-inflammatory properties useful for treating arthritis and rheumatism.

In British herbal medicine, the leaves and flowers are used for treating stomach and breast cancers. In India, the fresh leaves are infused to relieve the pain of cancerous growths, especially of the throat. To cancerous growths of the skin, a fomentation or poultice of fresh leaves is applied.

The dried root is used for constipation, and as an emetic in larger doses. It contains violine. The stems can be used as an ipecac substitute to induce vomiting, in doses of 40-50 grains; or an infusion of two ounces of the stem.

The root saponins are useful as a tea for dry catarrh, chronic bronchitis and rheumatic conditions; and as well for sore throats in the form of a gargle.

The leaf is useful for various throat and lung inflammations, as well as nervous strain, insomnia and hysteria. The flowers are emollient, demulcent, astringent, diaphoretic, diuretic and laxative. They can be used in bilious conditions, nervous disorders, including epilepsy, uterine and rectal prolapse, and inflammatory swellings.

Sweet violet and rue (*Ruta graveolens*) water extracts exhibit synergy in the treatment of *Trichomonas vaginalis*. Al Heali FM et al, *Turkiye Parazitol* Derg 2006 30(4): 272-4.

The leaf extract showed anti-hypertensive and anti-dyslipidemic activity in both *in vivo* and *in vitro* studies. Work by Siddiqi HS et al, *Lipids Health Dis* 2012 Jan 10;11:6 suggests the vasodilating effect is mediated through inhibition of Ca(++), and NO pathways. This may explain the fall in blood pressure observed.

As a hot tea, the flowers are diaphoretic, and useful for coughs, sore throats, as well as kidney and liver complaints. The flowers are used in the form of syrup, or as an infusion in one part to 100 parts water.

Combine violet flowers and hops in a 1:6 ratio to increase milk production in nursing mothers.

A 50% alcohol tincture of the flowers turns pale green-yellow color. It is said to be very calming to the nerves and emotions, especially when one is over-stimulated or constipated due to stress. A few drops in water can bring a content and relaxed feeling.

Extracts of flowers possess significant antioxidant activity. Stojkovic et al, *J Herb Spice Medicinal Plants* 17:3.

Of course, the flowers and leaves are used in perfumery and aromatherapy. Ionine, the chief interesting component of violet flowers, dulls the sense of smell, so that continual exposure dulls not only the scent of violets, but everything else as well. Try it!

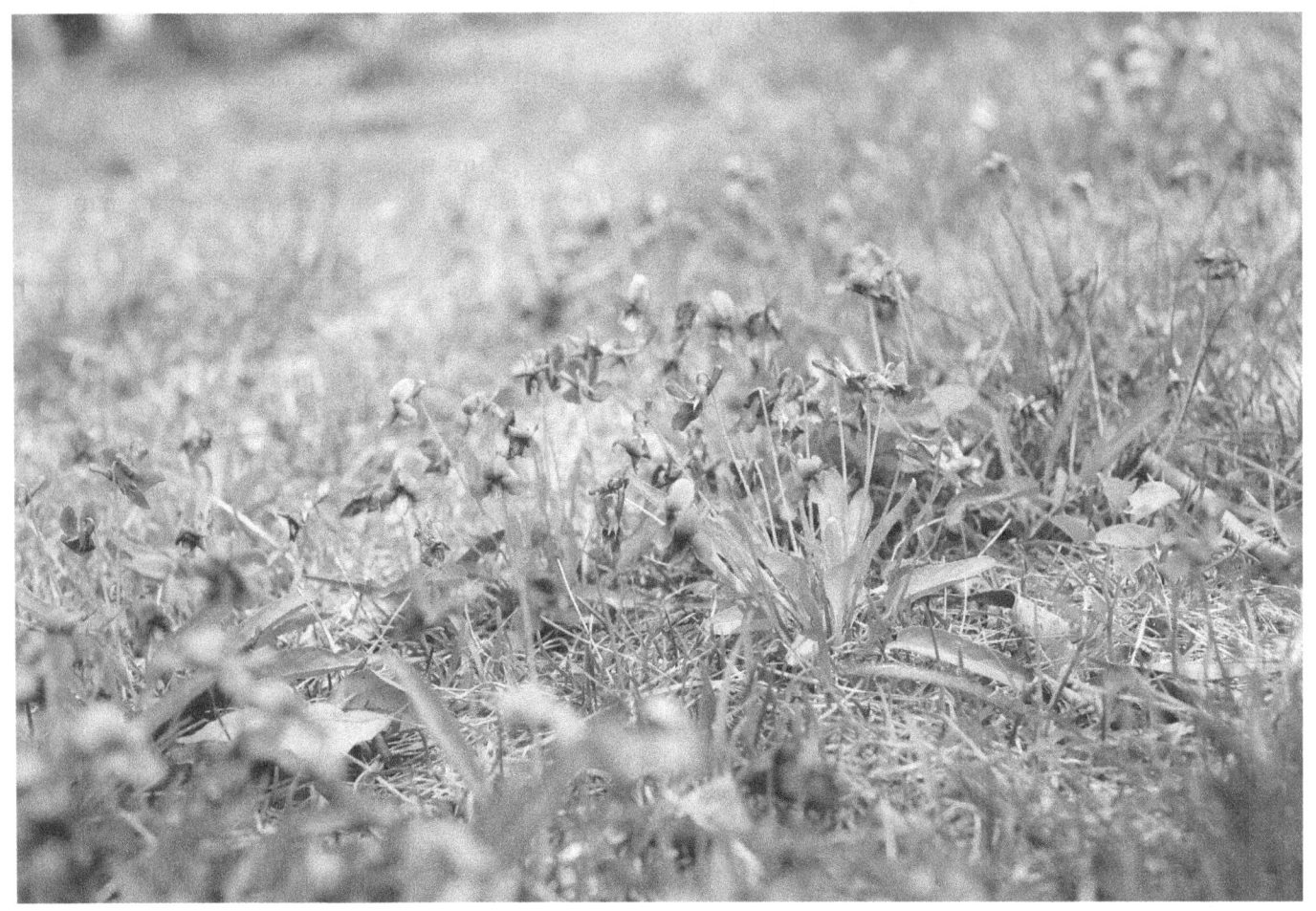

VIOLA YEDOENSIS

Yedeon's violet (*V. yedoensis*) is native to China and Japan, and used for many of the same skin related diseases as their western cousins.

In Traditional Chinese Medicine, it is known as **ZI HUA DI DING**, and in Kampo medicine of Japan as **SHIKAJICHO**.

Kampo herbalists use the whole plant when flowering, or in fall when the fruit has ripened, including root for hot swellings and tumors, mumps and abscesses. It is especially indicated in lymphagitis, and lymphadenitis, where abscesses of the head, back, breast and intestine are prevalent, and where boils, furuncles and various sores and wounds require detoxification. The herb has been shown to clear the body of chlorides but not sodium or potassium for increasing water excretion.

This same species of violet is used in the Great Ormond Street Children's Hospital in London for treating childhood eczema.

Chang et al, *Antiviral Research* April 1998 found this violet keeps HIV from "erupting from infected cells. It contains compounds that inhibit the reproduction of bacteria responsible for tuberculosis, a common complication of AIDS."

Cycloviolacin Y5 is the most active cyclotide, against HIV and is most hydrophobic. Wang CK et al, *J Nat Prod* 2008 71(1): 47-52.

This is only true of *V. yedoensis*, not our North American species. It contains various saponins and cerotic acid; and is bacteriostatic to *Streptococcus species* and *Pseudomonas aeruginosa*.

Moon et al, *Bioorg Med Chem* 2006 14:22 found *V. hondoensis* inhibits aldose reductase, suggestive of diabetic support for eye health.

Creeping Violet (*V. diffusa*) another annual Violet from China, is known as **P'U-FU CHING** or **DI BAI CAO**. The whole plant has cooling properties with a somewhat bitter and acid taste. It is often used in Traditional Chinese Medicine for aplastic anemia, and other leukemias, as well as mastitis, mumps, boils and abscess.

One to two ounces of the whole plant is decocted at a time.

Another violet, *V. collina*, or **TI HO TAO**, is used in China, with properties similar to our own species.

All of these violets can be easily cultivated on the prairies. They appear to hyper-accumulate zinc, which is involved in skin health.

HOMEOPATHY

Pansy (*V. tricolor*) is indicated for cradle cap and other kinds of skin eruptions such as eczema, dermatitis, acne vulgaris, impetigo and dermatitis *exfoliativa neonatorum*.

It is useful in alternation and support with Sulphur for bronchial asthma. The throat may be swollen, causing difficult swallowing, and constant hawking of mucous and phlegm.

The face may be hot and sweating after eating, with swollen glands.

It Germany, it is indicated for eczema and inflammation of the urinary passages, in the *Bundesanzeiger*, or Federal Gazette. The urine may be copious, disagreeable with a cat-like odour. The symptoms are worse in winter and around 11 a.m.

DOSE- lower potencies. The mother tincture is prepared from the fresh plant in flower. Proving by Franz on self and four others with tincture.

Violet (*V. odorata*) is indicated for violent earaches with discharge. Or, myopia with pains in the eyes.

Rheumatism of the right wrist as well as inflammations of the joints of the right wrist and hand also point to its indication.

Locally, it is used for pain due to uterine fibroids.

Respiratory inflammation is also eased, as is dyspnea during pregnancy.

It assists bedwetting in nervous children. Milky urine that smells strong is also helped.

DOSE- The mother tincture is prepared from the whole fresh plant in flower. Self experimentation by Hahnemann, Stapf and Gross with tincture, as well as clinical observations by Hering, Clarke, Cooper, Mangialavori.

ESSENTIAL OIL

No essential oil is produced from Violet, but both a flower and leaf absolute are made from *V. odorata*.

The volatile oil component is very small, at 0.003%, and is composed mainly of trans alpha ionone (parmone), with the chief constituents being (-)zingiberene, (+)-curcumene, dihydro-beta-ionone, 2,6-nonadien-1-al, undecan-2-one, and isoborneol.

The flower absolute is made by washing of petroleum extracted concrete, but is becoming more and more uneconomical and rare.

It is greenish-olive colored or creamy green with a very delicate sweet floral note, reminiscent only when diluted down to 1% or less.

The price is prohibitive-one kilo of absolute was worth over $15,000 Canadian before World War II! Be wary if offered this product from France. A small production out of China is sometimes available. Ionone, the main aromatic element in violet flowers was synthesized in 1893.

Violet leaf absolute, on the other hand, is still widely available, and extensively cultivated in the south of France, and north of Italy for this purpose. It is pricey.

It is produced by ether extraction from the fresh leaves, alcohol washing, chilling, filtration, evaporation in vacuum, etc.

The absolute is intensely green and possesses a powerful and peculiar odour, green yes, but with an indisputable floral note. It is used extensively in perfume blending as unique cucumber green note.

It is sedative and cooling, with particular affinity for the liver as a detoxifier. On a psychological level, it relieves fear, and is used to treat anxiety, insomnia, nightmares, restlessness and over excitement.

A new *V. odorata* cultivar, Vesna, developed in Russia, produces 21% more raw material and 29% more production and better quality concrete, than standard cultivars.

The distinct violet leaf odor is related to content of 2-trans-6-cis-nonadienal.

The absolute is composed of 40-58% octaceda-9, 12-dienoic acid, 8-17% hexadecanoic acid, 5-18% nona-2, 6-dienal, 4% cis-hex-3-enol and other compounds.

Hexane extracts contain 16% pentadec-3-enal, 13% non-2, 6-dienal, 13% hexadec-1-ene, 11% octadec-1-ene, 5% nona-2, 6-dienol.

Viola tricolor, when steam distilled fresh, yields 35 compounds, with 60% sesquiterpenes, including 29% bisabolone oxide. The dried plant yields just 24 compounds, mainly aliphatics and 1% beta ionone.

V. arvensis, when dried and distilled yields 59% aliphatics, with beta-ionone at 2% (the distinct violet odor), and 5.4% pentyl-furan.

HYDROSOL

CONSTITUENTS- *V. tricolor* ssp. *arvensis*- camphor 30%, linalool 24%, eucalyptol 20%, cis thujone 4%, endo borneol 4%, and minor components.

Crisp cluster plunged in shadow.
Drops of violet water and raw sunlight
Floated up with your scent.
A fresh subterranean beauty climbed up from your buds, thrilling my eyes and my life...
Fragile cluster of starry violets, tiny, mysterious planet of marine phosphorescence, nocturnal bouquet
nestled in green leaves; the truth is
There is no blue word to express you.
Better than any word is the pulse of your scent.   **PABLO NERUDA**

The water of Violet flowers, cools the blood, the heart, liver and lungs, overheated, and quenches an insatiable desire of drinking.   **CULPEPPER**

The water of Blue Violets is good for the heat of pestilence, and it cools the heart, liver and stomach. **BRUNSCHWIG**

The water of Yellow Violets is for comforting those that have lost their wits. It comforts the liver and causes women to be fruitful. It purifies after childbirth, warms the heart, and is good for palsy or paralysis associated with trembling and loss of speech. It causes to be merry the heart and mind of man and purifies destroyed blood.   **BRUNSCHWIG**

The distilled water of the herbe or floures (*V. tricolor*) given to drinke for ten or more daies together, three ounces in the morning, and the like quantitie at night, doth wonderfully ease the paines of the French disease, and cureth the same, if the patient be caused to sweat sundry times. **GERARD**

Costaeus in his booke of the nature of all plants saith, that the distilled water of Harts ease, is commended in the French disease, to be profitable, being taken for nine days or more, and sweating upon it, which how true it is, I know not, and wish some better experiences were made of it, before we put any great confidence in that assertion. **PARKINSON 1629**

FLOWER ESSENCES

Violet (*V. odorata*) flower essence is for patterns of profound shyness, reserve, aloofness, and fear of being submerged or lost in groups.

On the positive side, it will helps instill sensitivity, elevated spiritual perspective and a sharing with other while remaining true to oneself.
FLOWER ESSENCE SOCIETY

Bog Violet essence is for dealing with secrets, self-preserving or self-satisfying.
ROCKY MOUNTAIN

Yellow Evergreen Violet essence deals with those who want other to do it for them even if it cost the others great effort.
ROCKY MOUNTAIN

Pansy essence allows us to look at nostalgia for what it often is: painful memories that we can't let go of. Nostalgia can keep us bound to the past, bound to tradition, bound to our families' co-dependent patterns. Pansy can allow us to let go of outworn family baggage that no longer serves us. **JADE**

Blue Violet essence helps increase awareness of signs/symbols/omens; to perceive evolving patterns and their relationship to the Whole. It promotes silent observation, adaptability, swiftness and sureness of thought and action.
LIGHT MOUNTAIN

Heartsease helps to fill energy holes, rather like the way it grows in a garden wall. It is very healing and helps repair damage to the aura, especially from long standing emotional hurts. **OLIVE**

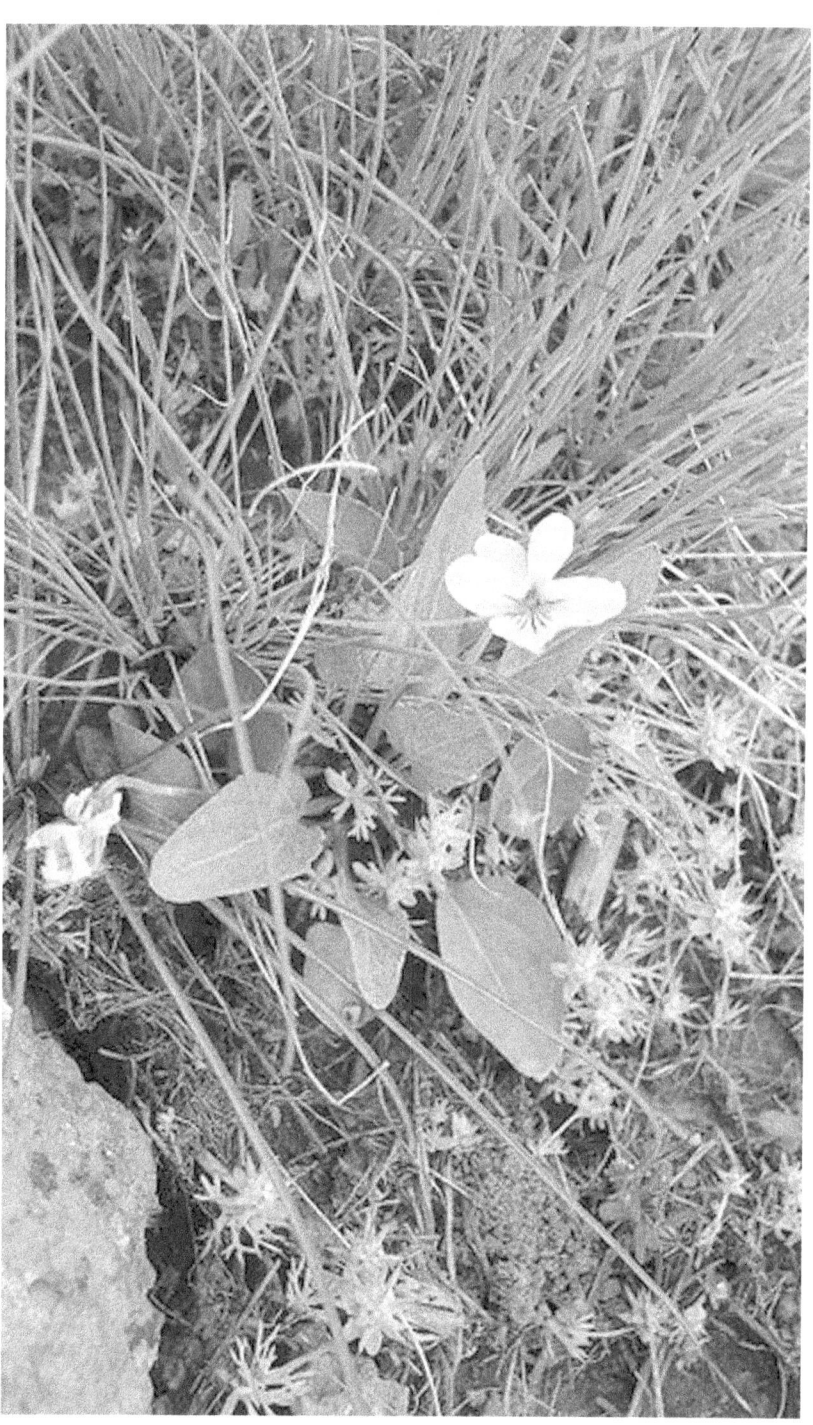

YELLOW PRAIRIE VIOLET

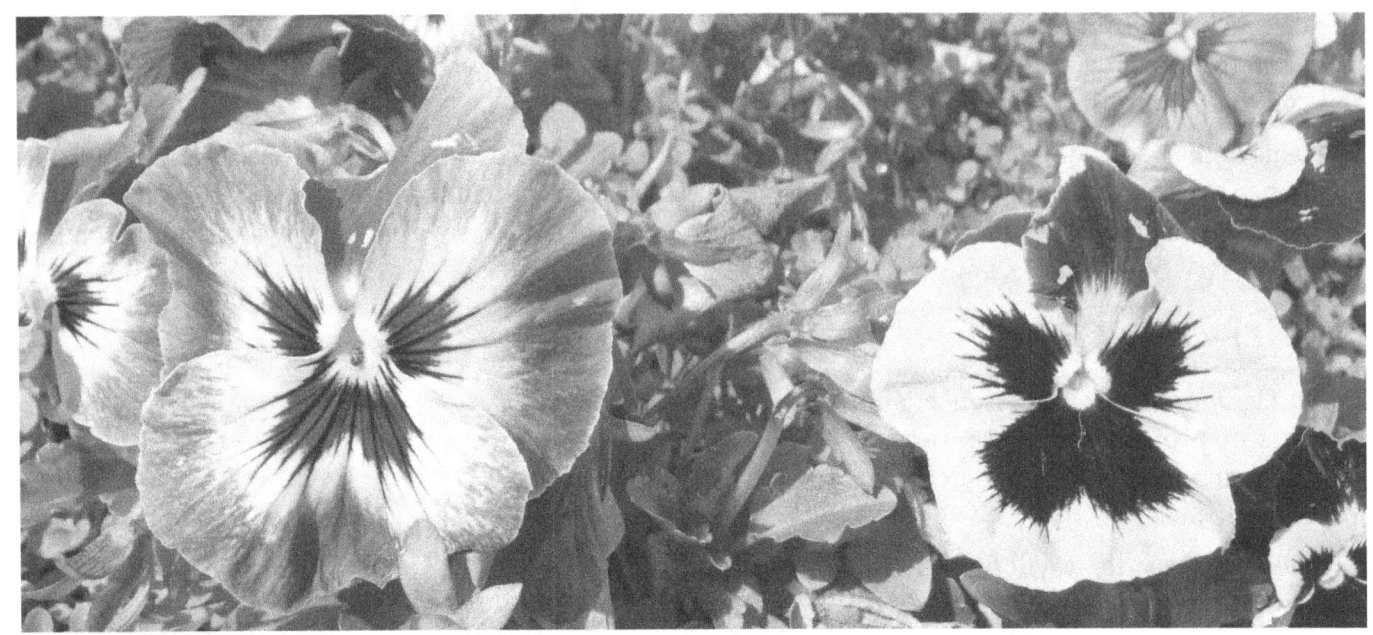

PANSIES

Pansy is an exceptional remedy to prescribe against most forms of viruses, from the common cold or AIDS to herpes or hepatitis.

Since orthodox medicine has generally not overcome most viruses, you have many volunteers for this flower essence without too much interference from chemical drugs, and the clinical results should be fairly easy to measure.

Pansy is also effective against the radiation and psora miasms.

Homeopathic potencies of pansy are recommended because the virus thought form is not fully conscious, assimilative, or understandable to animals.

Pansy is quite useful in treating bovine leukemia and the new forms of AIDS, characterized as HTLV II as well as HTLV I, which also affects bovine leukemia.

This is a mutating form that will likely, become a common inflammation difficulty and experience for the cattle kingdom.

New mutations of viruses may result form the overuse of herbicides, particularly those deriving form nay other substances that have derived from dioxin or Agent Orange, and from many other substances that have derived from this. The tobacco mosaic may be one that will shift in time, and pansy is excellent to treat this.

GURUDAS

PERSONALITY TRAITS

The growth pattern of violets is strange. The original patch may die, but the creeping stolons travel away, relocating and sending down roots elsewhere. In Europe, the Violet has symbolized death of one kind and rebirth in a different dimension.

Some years ago, while preparing a lecture on the lymphatic system, I was struck by the pattern of resemblance between the creeping linked-beads of this system with its root nodes and runners, and its patches at points of major collection under arms, at the groin, etc. Suddenly some of the ancient texts made sense: the medicinal uses of the Violet flowers and leaves, and creeping roots had previously been obscure to me, but if the plant cleared lymphatic blockages, and renew normal lymph flow, then the ancient writer's observations made sense.

ANON

When I discovered that an alkaloid similar to Emetine (also in Ipecachuana) had been extracted from the plant, the relationship was complete. Even as recently as 1931, Violet leaf tea, for lymphatic cancer of the throat, was listed in the British Pharmacopoeia!

Ancient herbalists practiced empirical medicine: if something worked it was tried again, and again, and with variations. **HALL**

Johnny Jump Ups keep popping up in my yard. They seed and re-seed, spreading from flower garden to vegetable patch, lawn and rockery.

The thing that amazes me about these flowers is how well they seem to keep other plants away. Even weeds are intimidated by their presence. They seem harmless enough, but something about them deters neighbouring plants from getting too close. Other kinds of plants are like that too, producing toxins, hogging the light, or crowding out the roots of other plants.

Johnny Jump Ups remind me of some people- those individuals who have a way of keeping others at arm's length, even alienating them.

It may be through gossip that poisons, an overbearing manner that suffocates, or a self-centeredness that covets the spotlight. They crowd out everyone else and eventually end up with only themselves for company. **G. MOHAMMED**

At first glance, you could easily mistake the blue violet for a weak, tender perennial. But if you take a closer look you might see the young, eater spirit within the plant that can hardly wait to emerge form frozen lawns and snowy hillsides. No matter how old or deeply rooted a particular stand of violets may be, they seem to exude a child-like exuberance as their blue and purple flower heads burst open. To me, spring violets radiate a beautiful vitality that teaches us we all have the potential to begin again and see the future with renewed hope. **DEWEY**

As I researched and reflected on the Twelve Windows of Perception, I have come to know Violet in a different way. I noticed that it really makes a connection with the Violet individual where they are at. This makes it easier for these people to trust and take the first step. You can't push or intimidate the Violet type or they won't partake. Viola at a deep level must know this. Violet gently lowers its head in invitation and patiently awaits your readiness to enter. The flower slowly brings you in and offers you safety in its compact, protective center. The lateral and upper petals are paired and they will give you support on your journey. It offers you gifts of transformation. **MARY, STUDENT AT NORTHERN STAR COLLEGE 2010.**

Let's compare Dandelion to Violet. Dandelion loves the sun and people's lawns whereas Violet loves the shade and the seclusion of the woods. Each plant has its own personality…so that Violet is soothing, cooling and contains mucilage whereas Dandelion stimulates digestion, tones the liver, and aids the gall bladder. Violet is shy and unassuming while Dandelion is bold verging on aggressive. **MONTGOMERY**

The pansies and violets are cheerful appearing flowers, with the characteristic quaint little faces, bobbing up to face the sky. They seem to be smiling and one can't help but smile in return. They are know as great ornaments because of their perky colourful prettiness and the mute eloquence of their fragrances…Their appeal gives them the self-assertion to expand and occupy all areas with a loyal, devoted and vigorous entrenchment…On the contrary, one flower is the emblematic shy 'shrinking violet'. Small, sweet, sensitive, subdued as well as retiring, reserved and unassertive, they display intrinsic meekness and modesty. There is the overall feeling of being humble, lowly, diminutive and insignificant. They dislike conversation and remain elusive, aloof and secretive…

Herein lies the dilemma for Violaceae. On one hand their innocent attractiveness, cherry disposition and sweet shyness creates the popularity that gives them universal appeal…Without their pleasing humble nature, there is a risk of losing the very loyalty on which they depend for their popularity. It is time to return to being the meek, shrinking violet again. It is true that it is the meek which inherit the earth. **VERMEULEN**

MYTHS AND LEGENDS

There are several legends about the flower from Greek and Roman mythology. In one, Jupiter turned his lover, Io, into a white heifer, to disguise her from his jealous wife, Juno. Then, he created violets for her to eat as she was too delicate to eat grass.

In another, the violet flower is hidden under its leaves. This represents a beautiful, young girl who is hiding from the unwelcome advances of the god, Apollo.

In another version, the violet is dedicated to Orpheus, the god of music, because the flower grew where he dropped his lyre.

In yet another Greek myth, Attis is driven mad with love, castrates himself and dies; with violets springing up from the blood.

The legend of the Violet originated in Rome, where Venus and Cupid eyed a group of beautiful, dancing Earth maidens. Envious, Venus turned to Cupid and asked if he found them more pleasing in form than she. As he indicated a preference towards the maidens, she became outraged and beat them all until they were blue and purple. When Cupid saw them, he turned them into flowers. We see from this legend where the words violent and violate are derived. Perhaps too, this also is the reason why the music of the violin is so said.

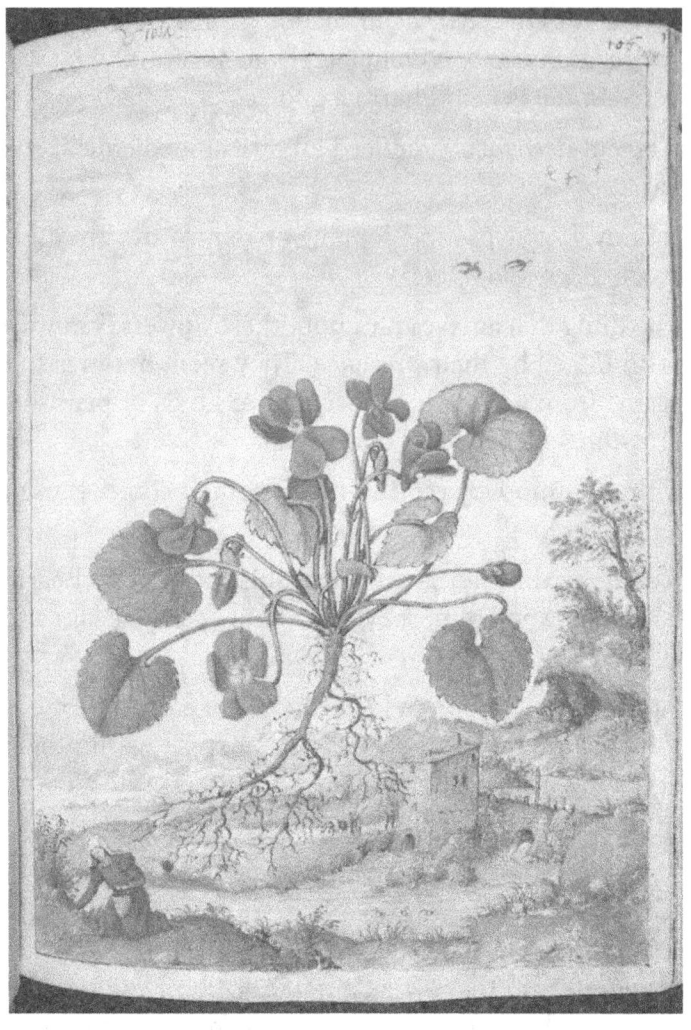

OLD HERBAL MANUSCRIPT

Knowing the legend, one can understand the gentle un-obstructive beauty of the flower. Not wanting to draw attention to itself for fear its beauty may not be appreciated, Violet has remained small and modest throughout our history. Its purple colour arouses idealism, spiritual development and love.   **RUDGINSKY**

The curious construction of the pansy gives the imagination an opportunity to indulge in several quaint conceptions. In the centre of every blossom lives a little old man, who, for punishment, must feel cold and be always wrapped up in a yellow blanket. He sits in the middle of the flower, with his feet in a foot tub, a queer little long narrow tub, so narrow that one wonders how he can get into it. If you will pick a pansy carefully apart you will see the little man, the little feet and the little tub.   **BEALS**

Long ago…a grateful nymph wished to reward a poor farmer and his wife. The nymph noticed that they took great pleasure in the few violets that grew by the doorstep of their cottage. Each time, upon entering or leaving their home, they sniffed the blossoms to catch the most fragrance that wafted up into the air.

"I shall give you a field full of the loveliest smelling violets that I can find," said the nymph. "But take care that you keep the flowers to yourselves".

Overnight, the meadow in back of the poor cottage was filled with a new kind of violet, with larger petals of velvety smoothness. Best of all, the flowers had a perfume unlike anything that existed before. The couple named the new flower "pansy", and took great delight in it.

But they could not resist showing it to their neighbors and friends. Everyone rushed to exclaim over the beautiful flowers and to smell the enticing smell. They stamped down the grasses and…soon there was nothing but bare earth. The couple called on the nymph. "I cannot take away a flower once it is growing, but I can take away the smell". And she did. Since that time, the pansy remains a lovely, velvety flower, but it has no fragrance at all.

PELLOWSKI

One night, just before Midsummer eve, the fairies had gathered to make preparations for their annual revel and were discussing what they could do to make the world brighter for their being here. One little one timidly made a suggestion that they make a new flower. The rest were greatly pleased and the very next night they went to work. Getting out their paint boxes they blue from the sky, different shades of red from the sunset clouds, yellow from the sunbeams and a warm brown colour from mother earth. These colours they mixed in a corn cup with their brushes made of dandelion down. All night they worked and when morning came there were the flowers gorgeously coloured. Some of the fairies had sketched in portraits of their fellows, so that the bed of pansies looked like a bed of cheerful little faces. The earth has been brighter and better, ever since, for that night's work.

BEALS

The prevailing cause for a Viola tricolor-pathology lies in a "step-mother-situation". The patient suffers from neglect or unjust treatment by someone he is depending on so much that he can neither escape the situation nor stand up for his right.

There is a close similarity to the situation of the Magnesiums, but the resulting state of mind of *Viola tricolor* is a much deeper emotional imbalance than in the Magnesiums, who lack the syphilitic element. *Viola tricolor* patients usually have a difficult character and they are unlikely to be among those you feel most at ease with.

WOLFGANG SPRINGER

PANSY- THE LITTLE STEPMOTHER

The stepmother is number 1. You will note that she is wearing the most beautiful dress. Numbers 2 and 3 are her own daughters. They, too have lovely dresses, although not as beautiful as her own.

Numbers 4 and 5 are her step-daughters. They wear plain, unadorned dresses.

If you turn the flower over, you will see the sepals which represent chairs. The stepmother has two chairs while her daughters, numbers 2 and 3, each have a chair to sit on. But sadly, her stepdaughters, numbers 4 and 5, must share one chair.

LOVEJOY

SPIRITUAL PROPERTIES

Pansy (*V. tricolor hortensis*) represents thoughts turned towards the Divine- a certitude of beauty.

THE MOTHER

Sweet Violet (*V. odorata*) is related to modesty that is satisfied with its own charm and does not draw attention to itself.

THE MOTHER

The open-armed flower spirit of the pretty Violet is calling on us to become more companionable with one another. Begin to reconnect with friends, neighbours, family, and community members. Create your own extended family with the people you love and enjoy.

ECLARE

In calling the spirit of the plant, a female essence appears to me. She is a luminescent one, bearing somewhat androgynous features. Ensconced in a flowing white robe, her hair drops down her back and nestles against her face. She is surrounded by beams of violet blue light, that cradle her every shadow…She is the plant spirit of harmony.

AVENSARO

BOTANICA POETICA

Viola odorata
Helps to soothe your cough
Rids you of catarrh
Try it as a broth
Some say it can fight cancer
Lumps and bumps can soften
A mild sedative as well
Okay to use it often
Soothe your rheumatism
Ease a UTI
Lots of Vitamin C in it
For eczema apply
The flower of Aphrodite
'Twas sexy even then
It's fragrance oh so fleety
And then it pulls you in.
Eat the flower, steam the leaves
Violets for a snack
These gentle benefits
To keep your health on track!

SYLVIA CHATROUX MD

BOTANICAL POETICA

Frollick Virgins once these were,
Over-loving, (living here)
Being here theirs ends deny'd
Ranne for Sweet-hearts made, and dy'd.
Love in pitie of their teares,
And their losse in blooming yeares;
For their restlesse here-spent houres,
Gave them Hearts-ease turn'd to Flow'rs.

ROBERT HERRICK

RECIPES

INFUSION- 8 hour cold water maceration, followed by a slow warming is best to retain all of the benefit of the plant. Use distilled water for babies. Dr. Madaus suggests using *V. tricolor* as an antidote for those allergic to rye. Use 1:20 ratio.

FLUID EXTRACT- 1:1 ratio of 20% alcohol. Ten drops as needed.

TINCTURE- FRESH PLANT- 1:4 at 40%. 25-40 drops as needed. A standardized extract should contain not less than 0.2% flavonoids calculated as hyperoside.

Viola odorata root and seeds are emetic, and should be avoided, or at least limited when used for medicinal purpose.

VIOLET SALVE- Press the juice from fresh violets, and strain through cheesecloth. Add one part olive oil to three parts juice and three parts billy goat fat. Boil in a pot.

Either violet flowers only or flowers and leaves may be used. Another option is to take five parts coconut oil to one part fresh wild violet leaves and simmer in low temperature crockpot for four hours. Strain.

SYRUP OF VIOLETS- Take one pound of fresh sweet violet flowers and leaves (2:1) to two and half pints of boiling water. Infuse for 24 hours, pour and strain. Add double the weight of sugar and make into syrup without boiling. It can be combined with almond oil for constipated children, or used straight for irritating coughs, or sore throats.

CRYSTALLIZED VIOLETS- Pick the fresh flower head, wash and drain, and then wash with a solution of arabic gum and rose water; or foamy egg white. Then dust them with fine fruit sugar, and dry in a very low oven.

Store in an airtight container, or up to a year in a freezer.

CAUTION- *Viola tricolor* should be avoided by people with favaism or G6PD deficiency. This is an inherited disorder making people susceptible to haemolytic anemia in presence of faba beans, morel mushrooms and other triggers.

A nine-month oil infant given a half cup of heartsease tea became ill with moderate haemolysis and recovered in 24 hours. Behmanesh et al, *WHO Drug Information* 2002 16 15-16.

VIPER'S BUGLOSS
BLUE DEVIL
BLUE CAT'S TAIL
(***Echium vulgare*** L.)
VIPER'S BUGLOSS
PATERSON'S CURSE
(***E. lycopsis*** L.) not accepted
(***E. plantagineum*** L.)
SMALL BUGLOSS
(***Lycopsis arvensis*** L.) not accepted
(***Anchusa arvensis*** [L.] M. Bieb.)
PARTS USED- leaf, flowers

A spiny stem of bugloss flowers,
Deep blue upon the outer towers.

N. HOPPER

There thistles stretch their prickly arms afar,
And to the ragged infant threaten war;
There poppies, nodding, much the hope of toil;
There the blue bugloss paints the sterile soil,
Hardy and high, above the slender sheaf,
The slimy mallow waves her silky leaf.

GEORGE CRABBE

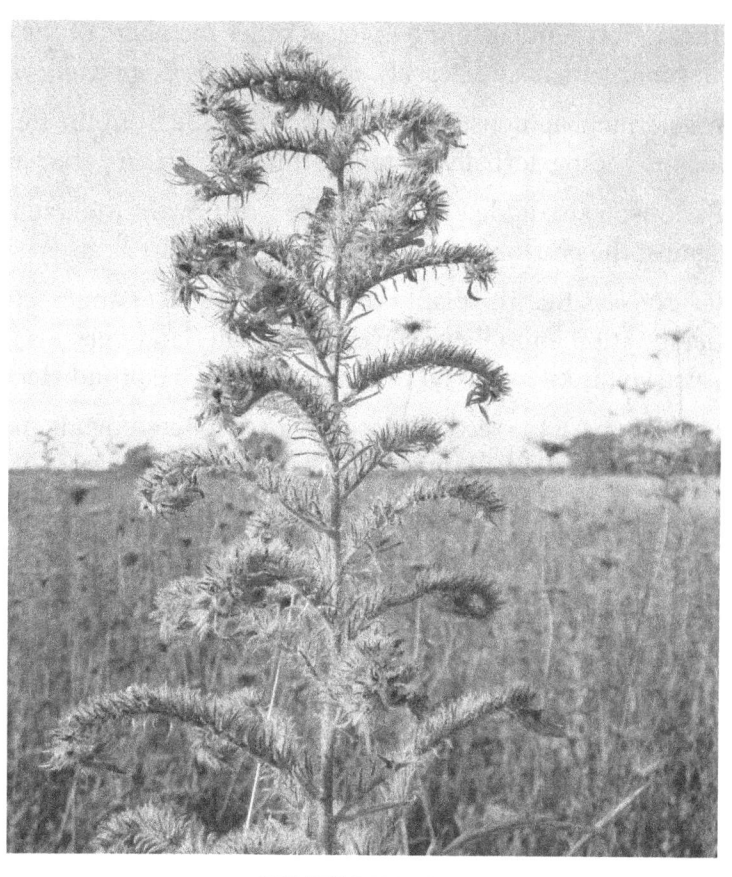

VIPER'S BUGLOSS

Echium is from the Greek **EKHION** or Ekhis, meaning a viper. The Greek **ECHIS** is derived from a genus of carpet vipers, while **ECHINO** means hedgehog or spiny.

The common name was given to the plant, according to Lyte (1578) "because it is very good against the bitings of serpents and adders, and because also his seed is like the head of an adder or viper." The latter indication dates to Dioscorides who observed the nutlet shape and its similarity to a viper's head. Giambattista Della Porta wrote that the herbs "bear seeds like a viper's head, and these are good to heal their venomous bitings."

It was thought that the red spots on the prickly stem resembled a snake's skin, and the viper-headed seeds help round out the doctrine of signatures.

Bugloss is derived from the Greek **BOUGLOSSUS** meaning cow or ox-tongue. This was for the broad rough, tongue shaped leaves. The German name **OCHSENZUNGE** means ox tongue.

Lycopsis means "wolf-like", vulgare means common, and arvensis, of the field.

Viper's Bugloss is an introduced biennial/perennial with a long, black taproot that has bright blue, purple and red flowers in the second year. This tri-colour variation led to the rustic, and biblical name Abraham, Isaac and Jacob.

It is considered, a hateful, invasive weed by some farmers. The hairs on the stem and leaf can produce painful dermatitis.

In England, the plant was praised by John Evelyn, who found the flowers "greatly restorative, being conserved."

Culpepper recommended the root or seed syrup for comforting the heart, and expelling sadness and melancholy. "The seeds being drunk in wine procureth abundance of milk in women's breasts. The same also being taken easeth the pains in the loins, back and kidneys".

This is very similar to the usage of other members of the borage family, including borage itself. In fact, early German settlers and herbals, such as Sauer's *Compendius Herbal*, recommend substituting one for the other.

A soft, mucilaginous and saline juice is made from the fresh plant. This was used traditionally as a demulcent for the chest externally; or for soothing the urinary tract and bowel as a laxative when taken internally.

Parkinson also added his two pence worth with "the water distilled in glasses, or the roote itself taken is good against the passions and tremblings of the heart as also against swoonings, sadness and melancholy."

Grieve says that the plant is diuretic, demulcent and pectoral. The leaves make a good infusion that induces perspiration and relieves fevers, headaches and nervous complaints; as well as inflammatory complaints. In Austria it is known as **STOLZER HEINRICH**, proud Henry, or **HIMMELBRAND**, sky fire.

Decoctions of the seed in wine were used for comforting the heart and driving away melancholy, increase breast milk flow, and treat lumbago.

In China, it is known as *IAN JI* meaning blue luck.

After its introduction to North America, it spread wildly. Indigenous tribes like the Cherokee began to utilize the plant as part of a decoction for milky urine.

The Iroquois used the root as part of an infusion for ensuring the complete removal of the placental after birth. The Mohegan used root and leaf infusions for various kidney disorders.

The root yields a red fabric dye.

Dr. King noted its diuretic and pectoral properties. He noted that the root, when properly burned, was used as a fine grade charcoal by artists.

One of the insects that rendezvous at feeding sites are solitary bees of the genus Hoplitis. The females, and the males as well, eat the nectar and pollen of viper's bugloss. Males seek out these plants and remain by them for long periods of time as they fly from blossom to blossom searching for sexually receptive females that come to feed.

Work by Giasson and Jaouich, *Vecteur Environ* 1998 31 found the plant removed heavy metals from contaminated soil in Quebec. A follow up study by Tamas et al, *Z Naturforsch* 2005 60:3-4 found the plant accumulates lead, copper and zinc in the new shoots, and could be used for bioremediation.

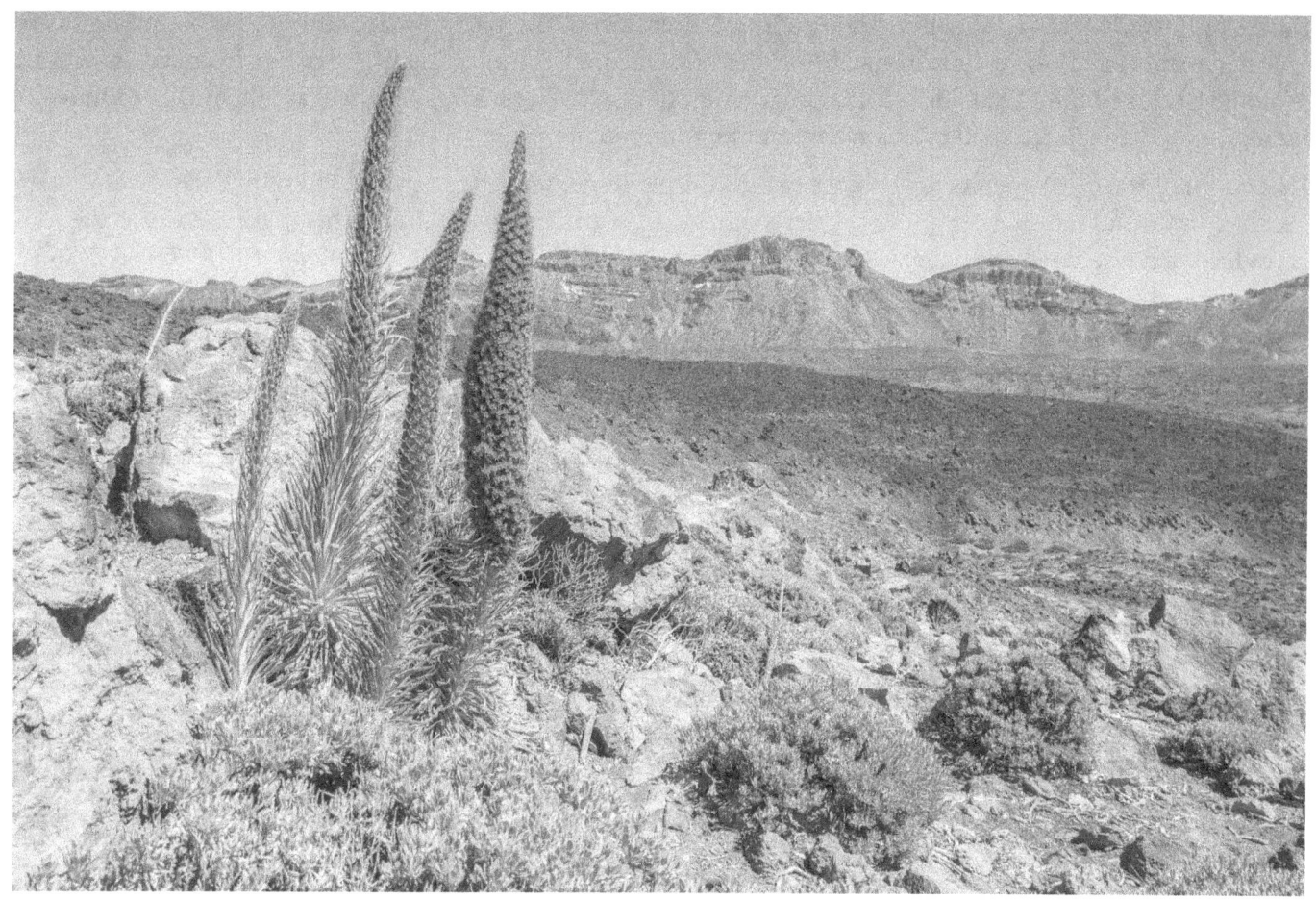

ECHIUM PININANA GROWING ON TENERIFE

Viper's Bugloss growing on copper and zinc soils increased the allantion content ten fold in root and four fold in shoots. It also increased shikonin by three fold compared to plants grown on uncontaminated soil. Dresler S et al, *Phytochemistry* 2017 133: 4-14.

Pyrrolizidine alkaloid rich plants, eaten long term by livestock, have been found to lead to low, acute toxicity, but elevated liver copper accumulation, and depressed levels of vitamin A. Horses, cattle, rabbits, sheep and rats all exhibit similar effects.

The species, *L. lycopsis* is often offered by seed companies as *L. vulgare*. It will grow as a true annual.

Small Bugloss (*L. arvensis*) is an introduced annual found on dry fields and waste ground throughout the prairies.

While vacationing on the Canary Islands, I noted the giant *E. pininana*. It takes several years to flower, but then produces a twelve-foot tall flower with thousands of pink and blue buds. A common name is Tower of Jewels.

MEDICINAL

CONSTITUENTS- 18 pyrrolizidine alkaloids (0.055% fresh; 0.25% dried) including echimidine (49.8%), 3'-acetylechimidine (10.2%), echimidine isomer (20.9%), retronecine, 7&9-angel-oylretronecine, 7&9-tigloyl-retronecine, 9-senecio-nyl-retronecine, heliosupine, asperumine, echihumiline, consolidina, equiina; allantion, lithospermic acid, naphthoquinone pigments alkannin, shikonin, stigmast-4-ene-3,6-dione; mucilage
Pollen- echivulgarine, vulgarine, 7-O-acetylvulgarine

In many respects, Viper's bugloss is similar to borage. Both are diuretic and diaphoretic, when taken as tea internally. For the latter effect, drink the tea when hot.

227

Pyrrolizidine alkaloids (PAs) have drawn a lot of attention in the past few decades. These compounds are found in plants like Borage, Comfrey and *Petasites*, with rat studies indicating liver damage from excessive, and prolonged intake of the alkaloids. Mucilaginous compounds, in Viper's bugloss, help soothe inflamed mucous membranes in a manner similar to comfrey and hound's tongue.

Like comfrey and other members of borage family, the plants contain allantoin and shikonin derivatives. A 41% increase in wound tensile strength was observed from a 1% ethanol root extract. This makes sense, as the root is traditionally used in Turkey for ulcers, burns and wounds. Eruygur N et al, *J Ethnopharm* 2016 185: 370-6.

Much has centered on the liver toxicity, as well as the mutagenic and carcinogenic activities of these alkaloids. Viper's Bugloss also contains the toxic naphthaquinone pigments, shikonin and alkannin.

These plants are a source of anti-mitotic, anti-tumor, anti-spasmodic and eye-pupil dilation activity. They should not be used for extended periods of time.

Some of the pyrrolizidine alkaloids have been found to exhibit anti-tumor activity. Pukhalskaya et al, 1959. As well, they possess diuretic, hypotensive and CNS inhibiting activity.

Work by Atanasova-Shopova et al, *Izv Instit Fiziol Bulg Akad Nauk* 1969 12 found *E. vulgare* extracts possess anti-convulsive activity.

The herb contains organic acids that exhibit contraceptive and anti-gonadotropic activity. Man'ko et al, *Farm Zh* 1971 26; Kozhina et al, *I Rast Resursy* 1970 6.

The more concentrated stem is used for baths to treat hemorrhoids. When decocted, the plant is a weak diuretic and sudorific, appropriate for the treatment of colds and bronchitis. The allantoin content, in mucilage, makes the plant useful in soothing all kinds of skin conditions. *Gibbs* 1974.

The tea makes a mild tonic for nervous headaches.

As a poultice or plaster, it can be used for boils and carbuncles. Studies by Wang et al, 1988, have shown shikonin to be useful clinically in treating phlebitis, vascular purpurea and other skin conditions.

Laboratory studies confirm activity against *Enterococci* and *Staphylococcus* bacteria. Peter et al, 1968 & 1970.

It is, however, toxic to cold-blooded animals, and paralyzes the nervous system. Over 50 kilograms of the plant will produce just one gram of the toxin.

Lithospermic acid, also present in comfrey, gromwell and bugleweed, is a known anti-contraceptive. Work by Manko et al (1977) showed various organic acids responsible for contraceptive activity. Kozhina et al (1970) found the plant to possess anti-gonadotropic activity. See Gromwell (volume 2).

Alkannin and shikonin are red pigments found in the root cortex, with anti-microbial activity against *Bacillus subtilis, Staphylococcus aureus, S. epidermis,* and *Sarcina lutea,* as well as lactic acid bacteria. Tabata et al 1975; Papageorgiou 1980; Shervanivs'kii 1971. The pigments may possess anti-tumor activity, according to the last named researcher.

Shikonin has been used clinically to treat skin conditions such as vascular purpurea, and circulatory concerns such as phlebitis.

Shikonins are 2.5 times higher in Viper's Bugloss than the annual *E. plantagineum*.

Polysaccharides from the flowers of the former show activity against two *Listeria* bacterium, *L. ivanovii* and *L. monocytogenes*. Tahmouzi S, *Int J Biol Macromol* 2014 69: 523-31.

Rosmarinic acid is found in self heal, rosemary and a number of plants with anti-oxidant capability. Tandogan B et al, *Pharm Biol* 2011 49(6): 587-94.

Extracts from aerial parts of Small Bugloss have been shown to be unique anti-coagulants. In studies by Chiryat and Rusakova in 1994, the plant extract showed 90% inhibition of the transformation of fibrogen to fibrin.

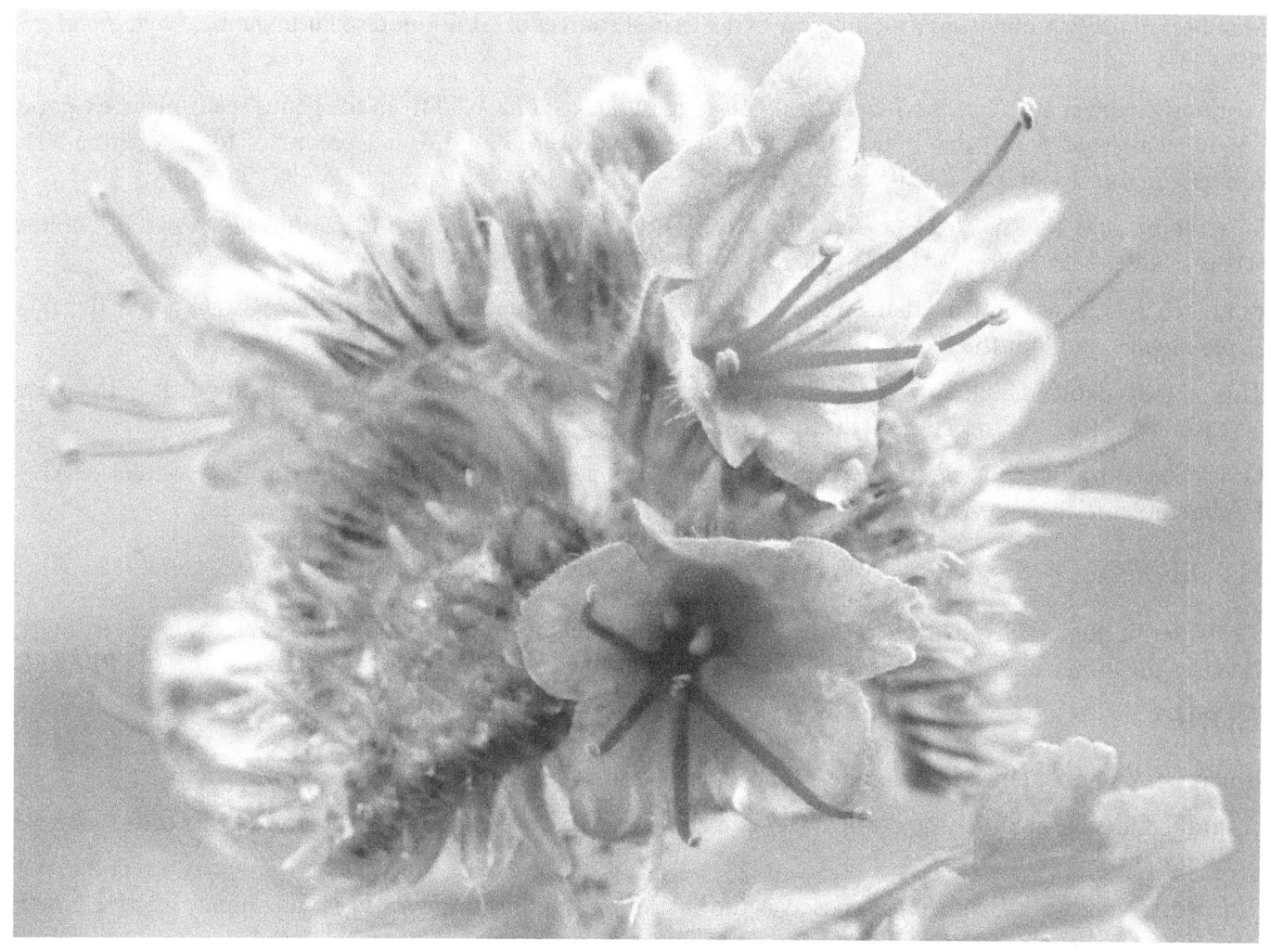

VIPER'S BUGLOSS FLOWERS- CLOSE UP

When intravenous preparations were given to rats, the extract resulting in persistent dose-dependent hypo-coagulaemia. Common Comfrey showed similar results. More information is available in *Rastitel'nye-Resursy* 30:4.

Some of the citations above, listing only year were originally found in hardcover copies of this Russian journal. Unfortunately, I no longer have access to it. Sorry.

Echinone, from the callus of closely related *E. lycopsis*, shows activity against Gram positive bacteria.

The related *E. amoenum* shows relief of mild to moderate depression significantly better than placebo, in studies by Sayyah et al, *Prog Neuropsychopharm Biol Psychiatry* 2006 30:1. The plant shows appreciable anti-inflammatory and immune modulating effects, including inhibition of lymphocyte activation, suppression of cellular and humoral immunity and induction of apoptosis. Amirghofran Z et al, *Iran J Immunol* 2010 7(2): 65-73.

SEED OIL

Members of the Echium genus, from Micronesia, were investigated for content of GLA, or gamma linolenic acid. Of 19 species studied by Guil-Guerrero et al at the University of Almeria, Spain, all contained high numbers ranging from 9.5% Paterson's Curse (*E. plantagineum*) to 26.31% (*E. callithrysum*) of the total seed fatty acids.

GLA related to total seed weight was also significant, ranging from 1.77% (*E. sventenii*) to 5.02% (*E. nervosum*). The seed oil of *E. italicum* contains 9.7% GLA. Abbaszadeh et al, *J Med Plants Res* 2011 5:19. Seed oil content of *E. amoenum* is nearly 34%.

Members of the Echium genus contain some of the richest sources of GLA found so far in nature. *Phytochemistry* 2000 53:4.

Work by Zhang et al, *J Nutr Biochem* 2008 19:10 suggests stearidonic acid from the genus seeds may be a good botanical alternative to fish oil for reducing triglyceride levels in blood. It is a precursor to EPA with a 30% conversion rate as compared to flax seed oil at 10%.

Stearidonic acid 18:4 n3 (SDA) metabolizes to EPA and is comparable in mice studies for lowering lipids, atherosclerosis, etc. Forrest LM et al, *Atherosclerosis* 2012 220:1 118-21.

Botaneco, a Calgary company that specializes in safflower oleosomes partnered in 2008 with Croda to develop *E. plantagineum* oil for the EPA/Omega 3 market.

This oil is available in bulk for various skin and cosmetic purposes from Jedwards International, Inc. The price is reasonable. The PAs are removed during extraction.

Our local, introduced *E. vulgare* seed oil contains 9.2% GLA, significant amounts. The seed content of ALA (alpha linolenic acids) reaches 39.3% by 20th day after flowering.

HYDROSOL

The water of Bugloss distilled when their flowers are upon them, strengthens the heart and brain exceedingly, cleanses the blood, and takes away sadness, grief and melancholy. **CULPEPPER**

HONEY

It may be of some interest to beekeepers that Viper's Bugloss could prove of economic importance.

A study conducted at the University of Waikato in New Zealand assessed the anti-bacterial activity of 345 samples of unpasteurized honey.

This work by Allen et al, in 1991 was used as the basis for a significant move of Manuka honey into the North American market for treating *Helicobacter pylori* bacteria responsible for stomach ulcers.

What was overlooked in the study was the high anti-bacterial activity of viper's bugloss honey. More information can be obtained from the *Journal of Pharmaceutical Pharmacology* Dec 1991.

Work by Beales et al, *J Ag Food Chem* 2004 52, looked at the pyrrolizidine alkaloids in honey from the related annual *E. plantagineum*. Up to 2000 ppb, compared to commercial retail samples of honey from multiple floral sources of approximately 250 ppb. The PAs (pyrrolizidine alkaloids) in Viper's Bugloss honey come mainly from the nectar, in form of echimidine (N$^+$oxide).

FLOWER ESSENCES

Viper's Bugloss essence helps you develop your warmhearted side and teaches you that a smile can often open doors; it enables you to recognize that humor and friendliness take you farther than a grim sense of duty or discipline. **OLIVE**

Viper's Bugloss helps to realign how love flows in the system. When this is out of balance, people may become the perpetrator or victim of manipulative patterns in an effort to get their needs met. **SUN**

Viper's Bugloss essence is for those who suffer abuse, whether of a physical, mental, emotional or sexual nature. **CHOMING**

Viper's Bugloss essence helps one become more aware that humor and friendliness make it easier to solve problems. **MARIANA**

SPIRITUAL PROPERTIES

The Bugloss was made the emblem of falsehood because of its use in many kinds of dyes.

In early days, it was used to colour women's faces before more delicate means were discovered The tint lasted for some days without renewal, and washing the face with water actually revived the colour rather than taking it off.

So Bugloss, with all other constituents of make-up, was dutifully defined as falsehood. Many ladies did not care a jot, as long as they achieved the desired effect.

Matthew Arnold declared:

I must not say that thou wert true,
Yet let me say that thou wert fair;
And they that lovely face who view,
They will not ask if truth be there.

But Keats had met and conquered this dispute long before:

"Beauty is truth, truth beauty"- that is all Ye know on earth, and all ye need to know.

Anatole France had the last word, however: "If I were called upon to choose between beauty and truth, I should not hesitate: I should hold to beauty, being confident that it bears within it a truth both higher and deeper than truth itself. I will go so far as to say there is nothing true in the world save beauty."   **POWELL**

WATER ARUM
CALLA LILY
(*Calla palustris*)
PART USED- root, flower, leaves

Calla is from the Latin and Greek **KALLOS** meaning beautiful. Palustris means marsh loving. Arum is an ancient name, believed derived from the biblical Aaron Rod. More likely, it is from **AUR**, meaning fire, in reference to its acrid juice, or from the Hebrew **JARON**, a dart, in allusion to the spear-like leaf shape.

Calla Lily is a member of the Arum family, and closely related to Skunk Cabbage. Taxonomists are having a difficult time classifying its placement within Aroideae. We will leave this problem (?) to them.

Because of its suggestive shape, and fancied sexual connotations, the Arum was often touted as an aphrodisiac. In the 1st century AD, Dioscorides praised its erotic properties. And in 1601, John Lyly wrote again of its supposed virtue of stimulating the passions.

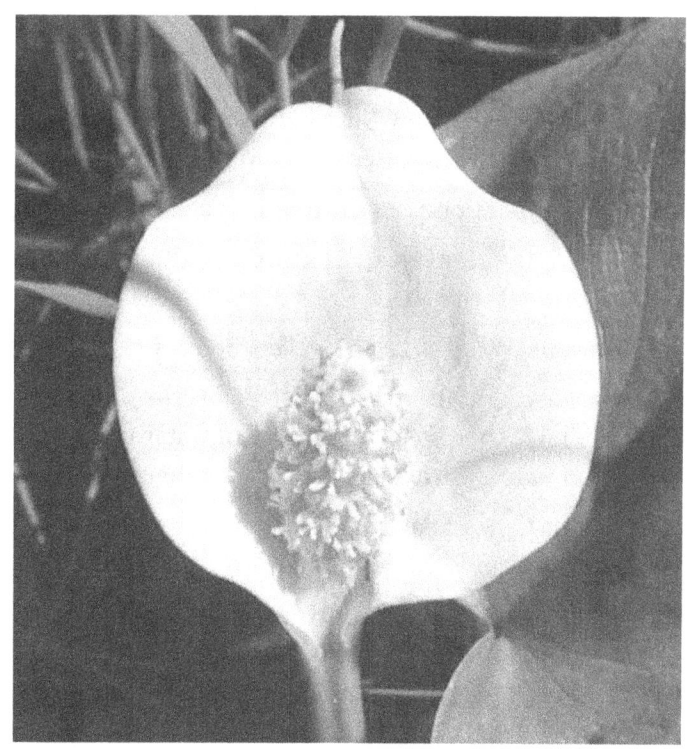

WATER ARUM FLOWER

Water Arum, similar to Skunk Cabbage and Calamus root, thermo-regulates the temperature of their flowering parts to spread their odour far and wide. This heat is generated by the spadix and is mediated, in the Arum family at least, by salicylic acid, which acts as a hormone that influences both scent and heat.

In order to attract carrion seeking flies and other insects, the compounds contain skatole and indoles.

One Brazilian philodendron raises the temperature of its spadix to 46° C. Oxygen consumption during this time is similar to that used by a hummingbird.

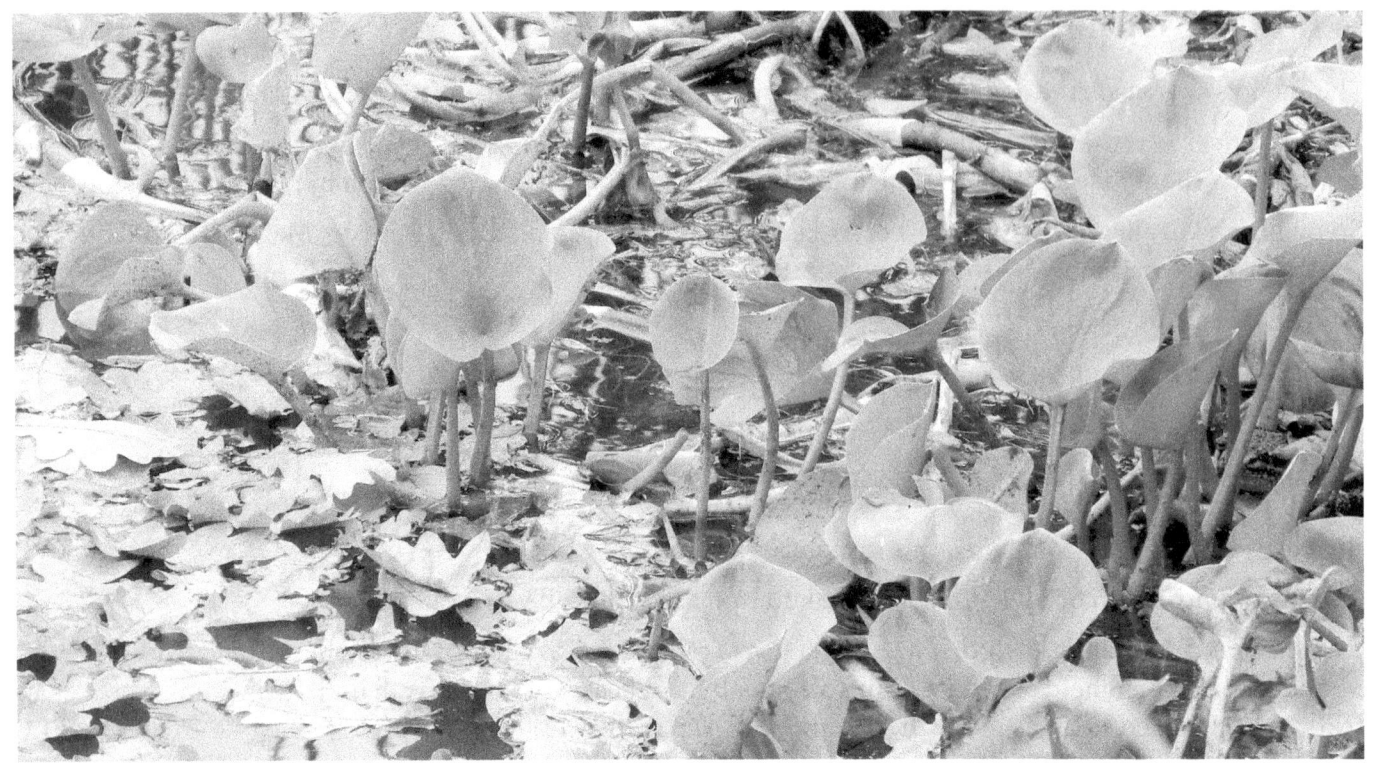

WATER ARUM

The Gitksan of British Columbia used root decoctions for hemorrhages, influenza, and shortness of breath. They also used the root decoction for "cleaning out the eyes of the blind".

The Potawatomi pounded the root into a poultice, and applied it to various parts of the body to reduce swellings.

So too, did the Chipewyan of northern Alberta, who know the plant as **TLH' OGH CHENE SLINI** meaning, "Grass stem which is bad".

In *Discovering Wild Plants*, an excellent book by herbalist Janice Schofield, the medicinal uses of Calla Lily are discussed.

An Athabascan elder in Alaska, collects the wild calla leaves in spring, before the flowers develop and dries them well. He then steeps them in hot water for colds, flu and arthritis. He used them as a steam bath for sore aches and pains, as well as arthritis and rheumatism.

The Woods Cree of Saskatchewan call the plant **OCICAKOKATASK**. It was believed poisonous to touch and eat, but bears could eat it without problem. The aerial stem was used to treat a sore leg.

Elders consider the rhizome to be poisonous. The Algonquin, for example, call it **EHAWSHOGA**, or "plant that bites back at the mouth". The Slave near Greater Slave Lake chewed the dried rhizome and swallowed the juice only for sore mouth and throat. The pulp was spit out.

Some natives believed rubbing the white root juice on hands protects one when handling rattlesnakes.

While the plant is acrid and burning when fresh, the dried roots have been used in Lapland to make a kind of bread called **MISSEBROED**. The dried root is ground, and then boiled and macerated, and this powder mixed with other flours, including fir bark.

It was used in Finland as an emergency food, and baking the sliced rhizomes at 180-200°C for hour or more, most of the toxicity is removed.

Pigs are less sensitive to acrid substances and in part of Germany the plant is called **SCHWEINEKRAUT** or swine herb. The red berries contain minor amounts of calcium oxalate.

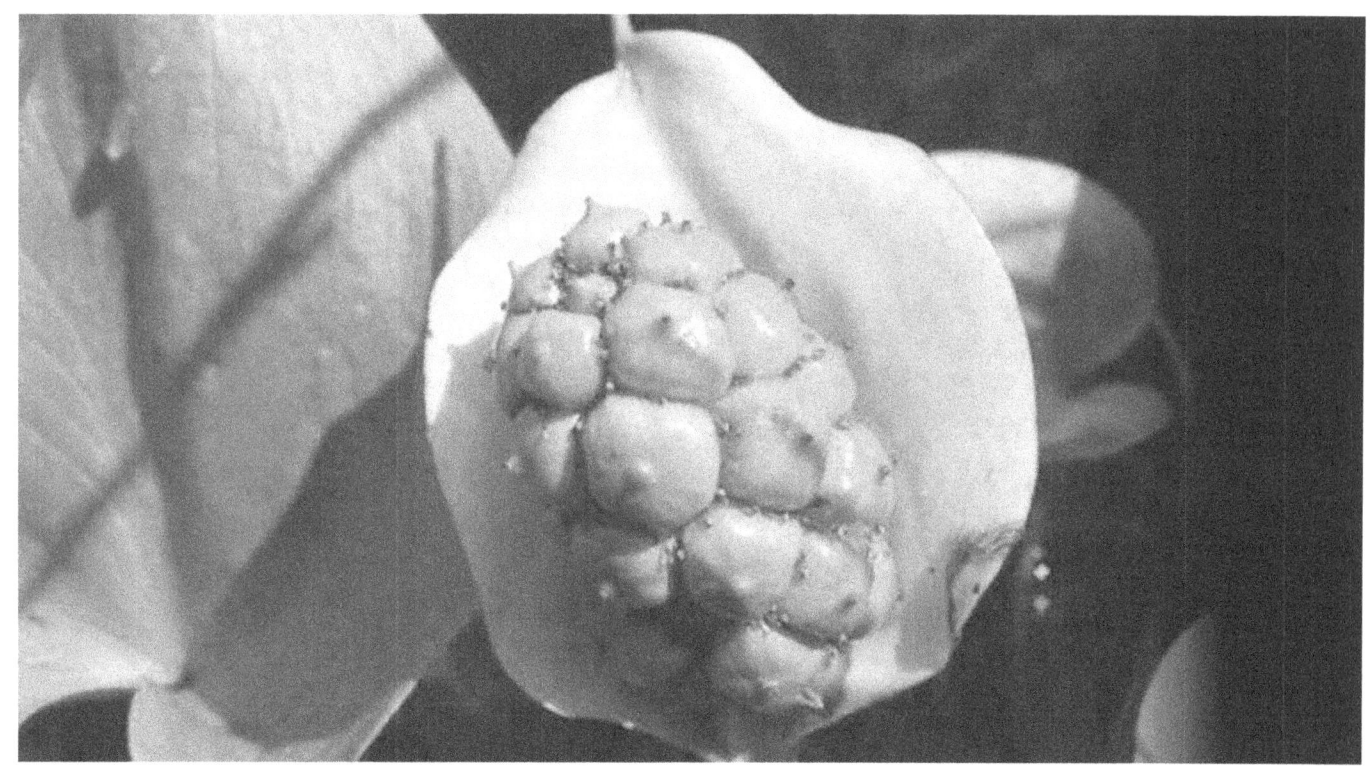

WATER ARUM GOING TO SEED

SPIRITUAL PROPERTIES

The Arum plant has many European names that identify it as a lingam-yoni symbol more than anything else. It is known as Adam and Eve, Bulls and Cows, Ladies and Gentlemen, Stallions and Mares, Kings and Queens, Lords and Ladies, Dog's Dibber, Bull's Pintle, Priest's Pintle, or Parson's Billycock.

Geoffrey Grigson wrote of it, "Here's the penis of the lecherous cuckoo, who cuckolds the birds, and here's the penis inside a hood, or in a cowl-that is to say, the penis of a priest, or monk, or friar, who goes round cuckolding husbands".

Cuckoopint comes from the Anglo Saxon root **CUCU**, meaning lively, and **PINTLE**, one of many words for penis.

PERSONALITY TRAITS

By contrast, water arums, transitional now between flowering and fruiting, seem derelict- the immaculate hooded spathes sullied by decay; the massed yellow stamens on the clubbed flower heads shriveled, and the young seed capsules an indeterminate green.

Their glory will not be regained until the transfiguration of their ripe capsules to a deep, glistening blood red is complete.   **GRIFFITHS**

MYTHS AND LEGENDS

The ancient Germans believed that where the arum prospered the wood spirits were happiest. It was also said that when Aaron's rod was planted in the ground the first Arum sprouted from the soil as a symbol of abundance. The plant has a strange sexual symbolism, for in many parts of the world superstitious farmers assess the fertility of the forthcoming year from the size of the Arum's spadix. Should it be large they rejoice; if otherwise they prepare to mourn.   **MAPLE**

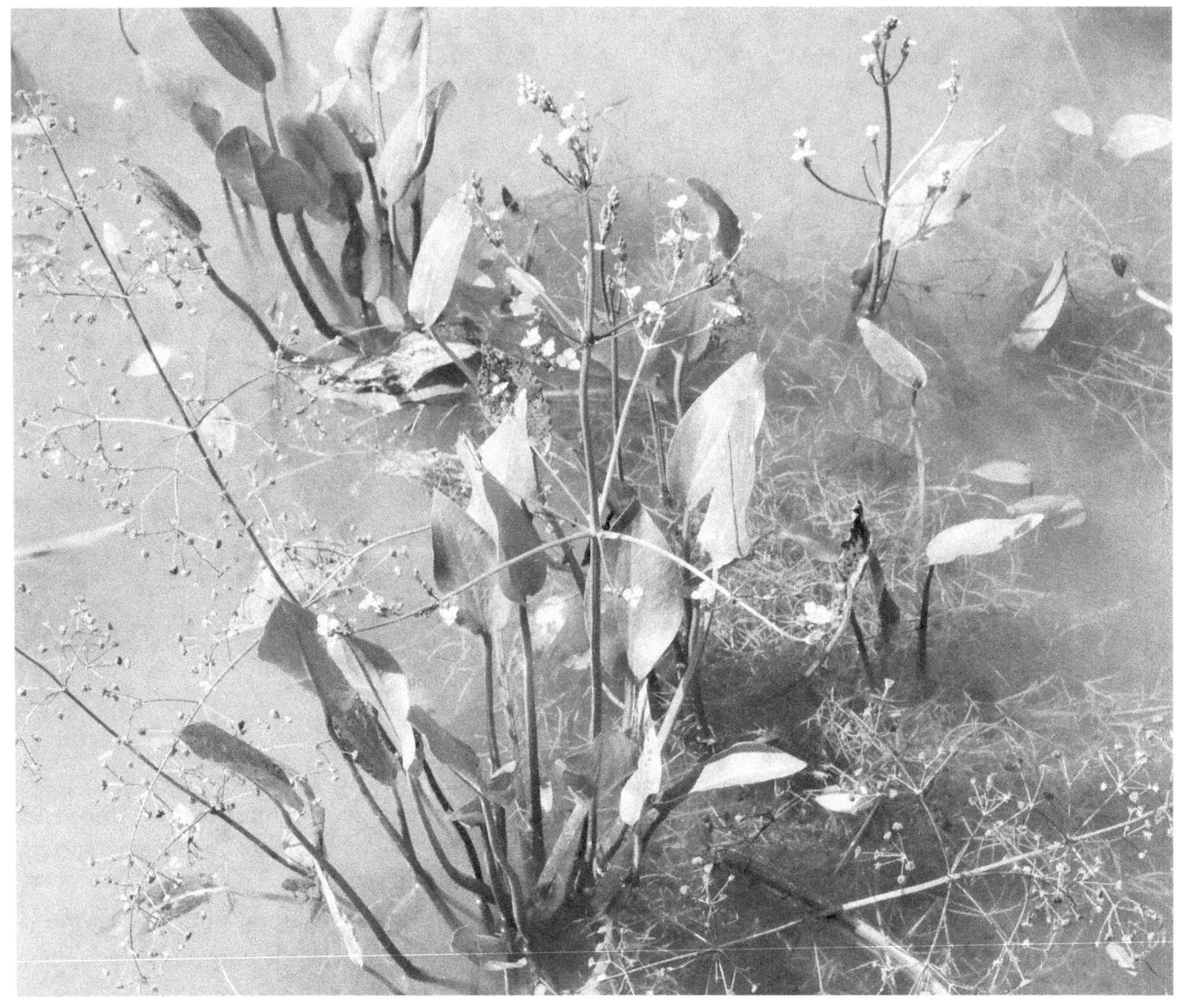

WATER PLANTAIN

AMERICAN WATER PLANTAIN
EUROPEAN WATER PLANTAIN
(*Alisma triviale* Pursh.)
(*A. plantagoaquatica* L.)
(*A. plantago-aquatica var. americanum* J.A. Schultes) not accepted
(*A. brevipes* Greene) not accepted
(*A. parviflorum* Pursh.)
ASIAN WATER PLANTAIN
(*A. plantago-aquatica* **subsp.** *orientale* [Sam.] Sam.)
(*A. orientale* [Sam.] Juz.)
NARROW-LEAVED WATER PLANTAIN
(*A. gramineum* Lej.)
(*A. geyeri* Torr.)
PARTS USED- whole plant, root

Alisma is from the Celtic **ALIS** meaning water. Plantain was name given by early botanists/taxonomists who noted the similarity of leaves with *Plantago* species, but ignored the flowers and other dissimilar traits. Water plantain is plentiful throughout Alberta, certainly a common perennial near the shores of Lesser Slave Lake, and up into the Peace Country. It likes water, so is plentiful in central Manitoba and north.

It has numerous pale lilac blooms that stay closed all morning, open for the afternoon and close again in early evening.

The Cree of Northern Saskatchewan call it **MITIHIMASKIHKIA**, meaning heart medicine. The dried stem was eaten directly or grated and taken in water for heart "troubles", including heartburn. The stem base was used for stomachache, cramps, constipation and flu. The stem base was given to a mother during childbirth to prevent fainting.

The Iroquois used infusions of the whole plant for "womb trouble", while the split roots were used for lame back or kidneys; probably applied externally.

The leaf infusion was used as a runner's liniment, and the raw root chewed to strengthen varicose veins. The whole plant including root was decocted for treating tuberculosis.

Early German settlers swabbed a woman's nipples with water plantain juice to stop breast milk production.

In 1899, Dr. Laws wrote in the California Medical Journal about a valuable local remedy for nasal catarrh. He applied equal parts of the tincture of the roots of water plantain, water and glycerin on cotton balls placed in the nasal passage with excellent results.

TSE-HSIEH the name given in Traditional Chinese medicine means literally "a flood unleashed from a marsh" implying it's rapid de-humidifying and diuretic action.

It is known as **ZE XIE** in Mandarin, and **JAAK SE** in Cantonese; and was first mentioned in Chinese Medical texts around 200 AD.

Other names include **HU XIE**, meaning Swan Drain, and **MANG YU**, Awned Yam.

They consider the root the most important part for medicine, believing it stimulates the female genitalia. Extracts are used for increasing urination; and removing dampness caused by stagnation and urinary difficulty.

In Kampo, the Japanese herbal tradition, Water plantain is used in the treatment of diseases related to fluid imbalances in the ear, such as dizziness and tinnitus, or ringing in the ears. It is known as **TAKUSHA**, and in Korean, the very similar **T'AEKSA**.

It is not recommended in Traditional Chinese medicine for men prior to attempts to conceive a child, as it is thought to lead to loss of JING, or essence being passed to the child.

Herbalists use the plant rhizome for various uro-genital complaints; as well as dysentery.

The roots are eaten as a cooked vegetable in Russia. They are rich in starch, and are eaten after drying to reduce acridity. The rhizomes are best in late fall, or early spring when starch content is highest. They are best steamed or roasted and are extremely dry texture.

At one time in Russia, the herb was considered "a capital remedy" for treating hydrophobia, and called Mad Dog Weed.

Winter harvested roots are the most potent diuretic, spring harvested roots the least diuretic. The root will easily pick up toxins, so don't pick in water you are not sure about.

In South America, it is known as *Platano Aqua*, and prized for its ability to cure snakebites. In Londonderry, the juice was used to stop spitting of blood.

Narrow-leaved Water Plantain flowers are pinker, but use is similar.

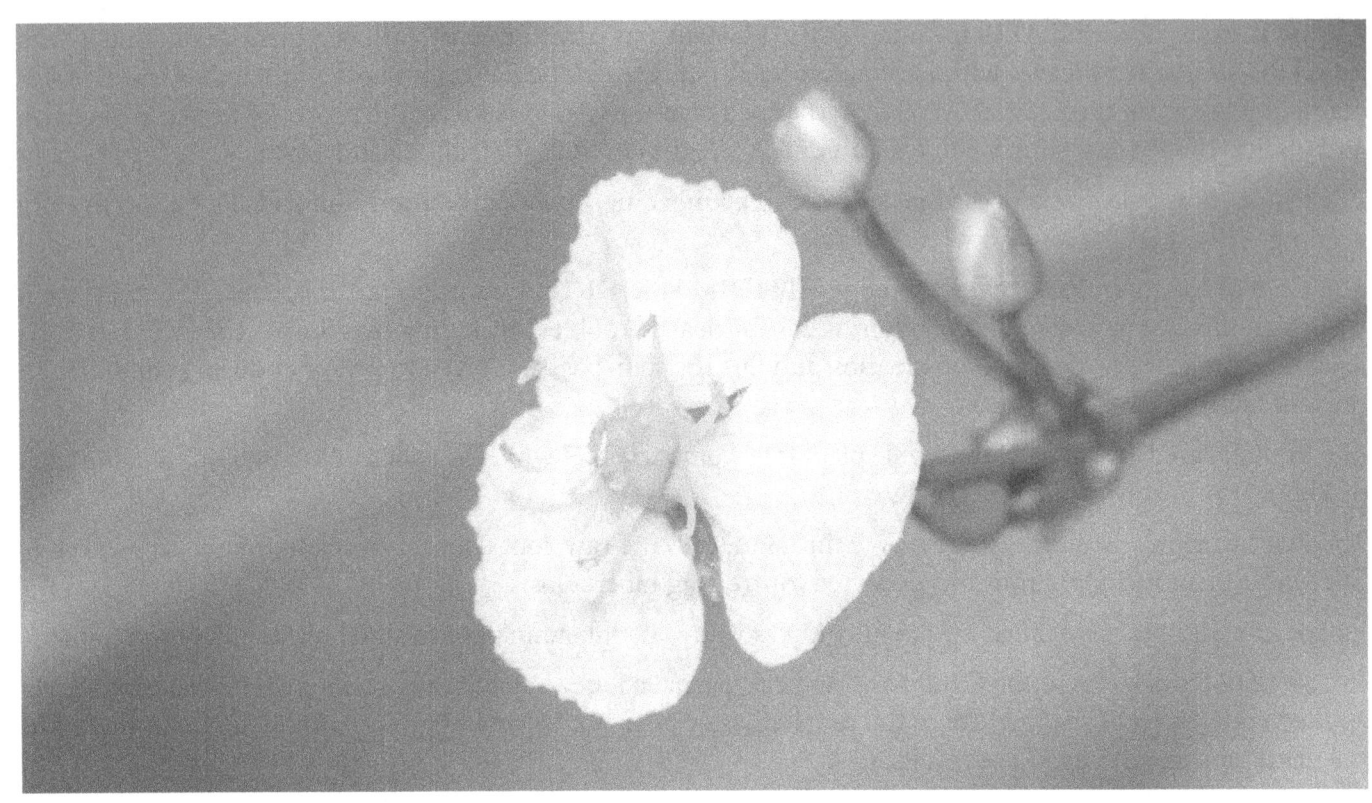

WATER PLANTAIN FLOWER

MEDICINAL

CONSTITUENTS- root- volatile oils, numerous protostane-type triterpenoids including 11-deoxyalisol C and alisols A-C and their monoacetates, epialisol; an acylated sitosterol glucoside, alismol (a sesquiterpenoid), sulfoorientalols A-D, orientalol A-C and alismol (sesquiterpenes), chlorogenic acid sulphate, luteolin, asparagine, alisman SI (a glucan), 23% starch , sugars D-glucose, D-fructose, sucrose, valine, l-asparagine and acetylvaline (amino acids), lecithin, choline, potassium 11,200 ppm, sodium, flouride, B12, biotin, furfural, lactose hexaphosphate and an acrid resin.
flower- 11-deoxy-cyclalisol
aerial parts- alismol, aps-sulfo-transferase, chrysoeriol, luteolin, nicotinic acid, pantothenic acid, proanthocyanidin, tannins, sugars
seed- 13% protein

In Japan, water plantain root is used to treat diabetes and diuretic effect, under the name **SAJI OMODAKA**. Alismol (1-hydroxyalismol), extracted from the root, is patented in Japan for use in liver disorders.

In the Kampo tradition, it is called **TAKUSHA**, and used in stimulating deficient kidneys to promote urination. In Japan, it is one of six herbs used to ameliorate neural dysfunction of the brain, such as Alzheimer's disease, senile dementia and memory loss, as well as protection against glutamate neuronal death. Liu et al, 1995.

In Quebec, the roots and leaves were employed for various urinary affections, as well as a calming effect in epilepsy.

The plant should not be used when spermatorrhea or leucorrhea (clear, thin vaginal discharge) are present due to kidney yang deficiency or any damp cold pattern. Abnormal vaginal discharge due to damp heat, however, with thick, sticky, abundant and foul smelling, yellow colour indicates use of the herb.

It can be used successfully when poor urination and accompanying edema are present; or when gravel or kidney stones are problematic.

For urinary calculi combine with moneywort, *Lycopus* and mallow seed.

It encourages urination and regulates water in the body, by increasing the excretion of sodium, chloride and urea.

For water swelling and lack of urination, the root combines well with plantain seed and the medicinal mushroom umbrella polypore, *Dendropolyporus umbellatus*. For painful urination it combines well with trifoliate akebia and amur bark.

Tinnitus, ringing in the ears, and dizziness are relieved in patients exhibiting the right constitutional picture. It is believed that taken over a period of time will sharpen the eyes and ears, and prolong life.

The root may be stir fried in bran, for more specific action on water diarrhea, or vertigo due to dampness of the middle burner. When stir-fried in salt, the root, known as **YAN ZE XIE,** is more useful for lower back pain and atony of the legs and feet, with heel pain, due to kidney vacuity.

If dry-fried, **CHAO ZE XIE**, the slightly yellow root helps harmonize stomach and spleen yang deficiency by moderating the cold property.

Numerous studies have validated the plant's use for diuretic and anti-inflammatory effect. More recently, it has been found alismol is the active principle from root that inhibits aortic contractions in laboratory studies.

Alisman SI, a glucan from the root, contains polysaccharides that exhibited significant immune stimulating effect in laboratory tests. It is considered to be both anti-tumour and interferon inducer. It is considered an immune regulator, useful in allergies such as rhinitis, asthma, and hives.

The root helps increase IgA, an antibody found in the respiratory and digestive mucosa, responsible for preventing degradation of the membranes and informing the immune system of viral or bacterial attacks.

Various complex sugars in the root stimulate the lymphatic system to consume pathogenic bacteria and fungi that infect the urinary or digestive tract.

Luteolin in the root inhibits the release of histamine from mast cells.

Ironically, the seeds are considered to promote sterility.

Isolated sulfo-orientalols inhibit contractions in isolated smooth bladder muscle.

Alisol A and B have been shown to increase sodium excretion in laboratory mice. The alisols inhibit hypercholesterolemia in rats and prevent carbon tetrachloride liver damage.

In short, laboratory studies have shown the herb to lower blood pressure, reduce blood sugar levels, and inhibit the storage of fat by the liver.

Alismol, a sesquiterpenoid, has demonstrated in vitro inhibition of noradrenaline release at adrenergic post-synaptic membranes.

In one clinical trial involving 281 patients, alisma rhizome tablets (3-4 tablets 3-4X daily of 2.5-2.8 grams each), decreased blood cholesterol and triglyceride levels by 90% and 75% of the patients. On average, blood cholesterol level was reduced by 17%, and triglycerides by 14%.

Work by Rau et al, *Pharmazie* 2006 61:11 found that of 52 herbal extracts, nearly half significantly activated perixisome proliferator-activated receptors gamma and 14 activated PPAR alpha.

The most active were extracts from *A. plantago aquatica*, as well as *Acorus calamus*, corn silk, stinging nettle and cayenne, suggesting a rationale for these herbs in anti-diabetic and anti-lipidemic formulas.

Various root compounds have been found to inhibit the hepatitis B virus, in vitro.

In vitro, the extracts inhibit the tuberculin mycobacterium.

A study by Shimizu et al 1994 found alisma contains constituents that stimulate immune system cells to kill bacteria and yeasts, in particular, *Candida albicans*.

Various compounds including Alisol A and G and other protostanes triterpenoids show 77% anti-malarial activity against K1 strain. Adams et al, *J Ethnopharmacology* 2011 135:1 43-47.

Alisma root shows synergistic growth inhibition of multiple drug resistant cancer cells, with paclitaxel, vinblastine, doxorubicin and actinoymcin D. At the same toxicity level, the herb is more effective than verapamil, due in part to its inhibition of P-glycoprotein. Fong et al, *J Phytomed* 13:9-10.

An interesting study conducted by Usuki in 1988 showed that water plantain may stimulate the corpora lutea to secrete progesterone. More study is needed, but this may explain the use in TCM for infertility, difficult labour and irregular menses. It is very valuable in late stages of labor.

Hot extracts of the root have been found to inhibit active arthus reactions in mice. *Journal of Traditional Medicines* 1998 15:4.

This is a severe local inflammation at the site of injection and a sign of hypersensitivity. It is a good thing we are not mice, nor injecting this herb.

It combines well with tree peony root for treating sensations of deep, hot pain in the bones; as well as dizziness and vertigo.

The fresh leaves are an efficient counter-irritant for swellings and contusions. Be careful that it be removed in a timely fashion, as it will irritate sensitive skin. The dried leaf is good for bruises.

Dr. Cook recommended the dry leaf tea, taken warm, to promote mild diaphoretic activity, and to quiet nervous agitation.

Infusions of the dried leaves, taken cold, are excellent for urinary problems including gravel, irritation and frequent desire to urinate.

Used warm, the infusion is diaphoretic and quiets nervous agitation.

The powdered seeds are considered hemostatic, and to act as contraceptive.

A good review of Alisma orientale has been recently published by Zhang LL et al, *Ann NY Acad Sci* 2017 June 29.

PLANT OILS

Water Plantain contains 78 mg/ 100 grams of dry weight of lipids. This in turn breaks down to 40% neutral, 40% glyco- and 20% phospholipids. The latter is of most interest, and is composed of 42.7% phosphatidyl choline, and 5.3% phosphatidyl serine.

FLOWER ESSENCES

Water plantain flower essence may help diminish excesses of the body and mind. Often these patterns develop from past trauma, where someone has felt deprived. It can also arise if our caretaker suffered deprivation, and over-compensated with our care. How it manifests will depend on the type of deprivation. If there was fear of not enough food, the result might be over-eating, or over-feeding dependents. Bulimia, anorexia, obesity or a love-hate relationship with food might develop, for example. If the past trauma was a lack of material possessions, there can be binges where buying and hoarding occur. With this pattern, a teeter-totter effect, of feast and famine might also manifest. Credit card debt or overspending could result, as could excessive saving, and difficulty enjoying spending money. Water plantain may combine well with Liberty Cap mushroom essence when dealing with addictions to shopping, consumerism, and hoarding. Rogers (2016). The excesses might also reveal themselves in emotional tones. One pattern women often manifest is being "too nice". There is often a hidden agenda behind this behavior, either wanting to be approved of and liked, or gaining power by creating a dependency. It may also be an unconscious need to submit or on some level be subservient to males; or avoid confrontation. Water Plantain can help reveal the reason behind the excessive behavior. These patterns foster inauthentic relationships and lifestyles, because they are not based on sustainable behaviors. In the case of excessive sweetness, the sweet person will eventually feel resentful and used. If they keep up the inauthentic mask of kindness the person whom they initially charmed, will eventually feel manipulated or misled. Water Plantain helps elicit clarity of intent. It may balance tension allowing clarity or laughter to intervene, allowing mountains to revert into mole hills. It helps wash away patterns of deception in interactions. The essence may reduce emotional inflation and overreaction of all types. People are freed momentarily from their usual reactions, so they have a choice. They can calmly view their patterns, and decide if and how they would like to change them. **PRAIRIE DEVA**

Water Plantain essence helps when there is trauma, bad news, shock and the individuals feels paralyzed. **MIRIANA**

PERSONALITY TRAITS

The reason why (*Alisma*) mainly treats wind, cold, damp impediment is its ability to bring up the water fluids from the lower part to irrigate the interstices of the flesh and skin through center earth. Breast milk is the fluid from the middle burner. When water fluids enrich center earth, difficult lactation is cured…Alisma can enrich center earth, so it is able to nourish the five viscera. The kidneys are organs which produce force. When water essence is upborne to supply nourishment, the qi force is boosted. When the interstices of the flesh are irrigated via the center, the person gains weight and becomes strong. **ZHANG ZHI-CONG 1610**

RECIPES

DECOCTION- 6-16 grams. Drink several cups daily.

INFUSION- One ounce of dried leaf to one pint of hot water. Steep 20 minutes. Drink 4-6 ounces 3-4 times daily.

TINCTURE- 2-4 ml. The freshly dried root tincture is prepared at 1:4 and 50% alcohol.

CAUTION- Do no use in kidney yang deficient disease such as vaginal yeast infections, and spermatorrhea. In fact, large doses, over time may lead to the latter health concerns.

"If taken for a long time, the eye and ear become acute, hunger is not felt, life is prolonged, the body becomes light, the visage radiant, and one can walk upon water". Stuart AG. *Chinese Materia Medica: Vegetable Kingdom.* Gordon Press NY 1977 (Original 1911).

The rhizome is collected in the fall, after the aerial part has withered, and dried.

When planting the seed, a depth of 5-7 cm results in over 98% germination, but at 1-2 cm the rate is still high, and results in larger corms, weight and yield.

A full study is available by Kim Jung Kon et al, from *RDA Journal of Industrial Crop Science* 1999 40:2.

WILD RICE, SOUTHERN
(***Zizania aquatica*** L.)
(***Z. aquatica ssp. brevis*** [Fassett] S. L. Chen) not accepted
NORTHERN WILD RICE
(***Z. palustris*** L.)
(***Z. aquatica*** var. ***interior*** [Fassett] Dore)
PARTS USED- seeds, hulls

Zizania is named after a Greek name for another wild grain, **ZIZANION**. The root word Zizanion, was probably the tares of scripture (see Darnel). Zizaniology was even suggested, at one time, to be the disciplinary name for the study of weeds.

Wild Rice is a tall annual grass, with long black grains that grows abundantly and dense on the edge of some northern lakes. On some lakes, it is found near inlet and outlet, but usually less abundantly. Some taxonomists distinguish between Southern Wild Rice (*Z. aquatica*) which has a thin, papery hull, and Northern Wild Rice (*Z. palustris*) whose hull is firm and leathery. In either case, the hull must be removed for edibility.

Southern Wild Rice is a non-cultivated wild rice with smaller seeds, and no longer commonly used for food. It is found around the Saint Lawrence River, in Florida and Gulf coast states.

The seed has long been gathered, as food by indigenous groups. As far back as 1828, T. Flint recommended its cultivation. John Powell, in 1900, suggested "should this natural produce come into the general use to which it seems adapted, it will add another to the many debts of Caucasian to Indian."

Today, it is a large, commercial operation, assisted by powerboats and floatplanes. Nearly 40,000 acres of wild rice lakes have been declared certified organic, as of 2003.

Native Americans called it **MANOMIN** gift of the gods. The Menominee tribe called themselves Menomin, or Wild Rice Men, to signify the importance of the plant in their lives. One lake, near Kenora, Ontario is called Zizania Lake.

In the past, it was gathered near the end of September, two to a canoe. One would carry a long hooked stick in one hand, and a straight one in the other. With the hooked stick the grains are bent over the canoe, and beaten off with the other.

When the canoe was filled, it was time to return to shore and empty.

It was then dried in the sun, and finished in an iron pot over a fire.

The grain and chaff need separation, which was done by treading it in a hide spread over a shallow pit. New moccasins or bare feet only were used!

It was then winnowed in a shallow birch bark tray, when the wind would spill the chaff away. It was then stored in baskets made from bulrush or cattail leaves.

Originally, it was boiled with meat. Sometimes it was stored with dried blueberries and cooked together in spring. Or the boiling broth of fish or meat was poured over the rice, and allowed to steam and soften.

The early voyagers called it *FOLLE AVOINE*.

It can be made into porridge, ground into flour, or soups. Today, it is a culinary delicacy that is often mixed with domestic rice.

The chaff was cooked in a similar manner to the Wild Rice kernels by the Chippewa, and considered a delicacy. Today, it is simply thrown away.

Canada produces about 5% of the world market for wild rice, with Minnesota at 30% and California a staggering 65%. In the Sacramento Valley, many farmers have switched from cultivated to wild rice, and can harvest two crops annually.

In Canada, the province of Saskatchewan produces 70%, Manitoba 21% and Ontario most of the rest, for a total value of about $3.5 million. Alberta produced nearly 80,000 kilograms in 2003, about half of Manitoba.

Seed gathered to replant or introduce the crops to other lakes is kept in burlap sacks under water until needed.

Mature seeds need to be stored for 90 days in cold water before dormancy is released.

The young edible shoots of Wild Rice are grown in Japan, northern India, China and elsewhere as a spear shaped vegetable resembling small corncobs. They are steamed, boiled, baked or sliced and stir-fried. In China, it is known as **GAAU SUN.**

In China, *Z. latifolia*, a related species develops a thickened base of the culm due to a parasitic fungi. This is eaten as a vegetable, as well as the young shoots.

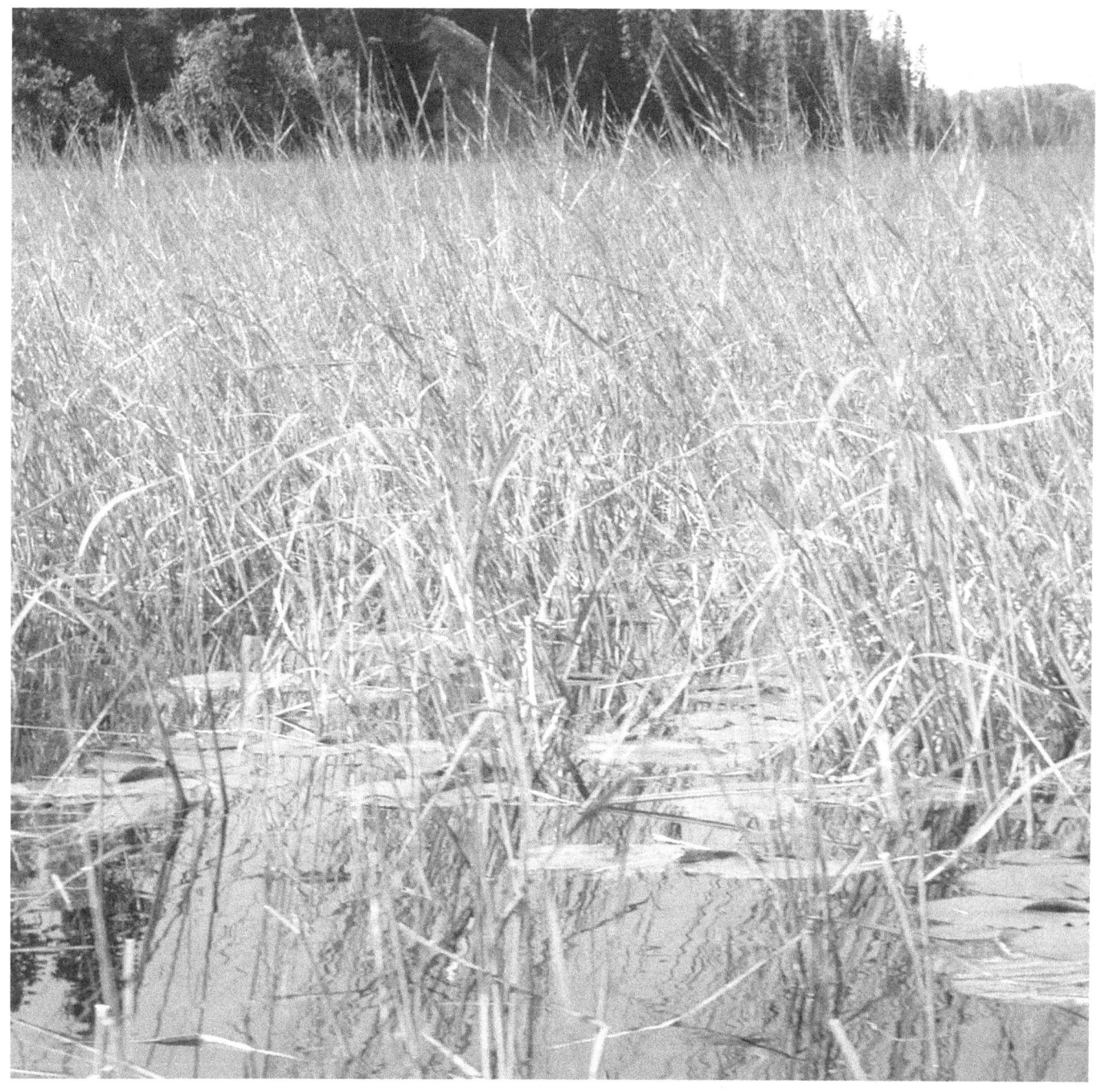

NORTHERN WILD RICE

MEDICINAL

CONSTITUENTS- *Z. palustris* grain- carbohydrates (82%), protein (12-15%), and traces of phosphorus, potassium (up to 344 mg/100g), magnesium, iron, manganese, zinc, and copper. Protein content is 15.2-17% with a protein efficacy ratio of 1.77, high for a cereal. The amino acid score is 82, with lysine the limiting factor. In all cases, levels of protein, minerals, B1 and B2, are higher than commercial rice. Niacin is 6.2 mg/100grams. Gamma oryzanol (1352 µg/g) versus only 688 for brown rice. Steryl caffeate and cinnamate also present.

The polysaccharide amylose content is nearly 24% higher than regular rice. Amylose content is 21-23%. The grain contains serotonin.

Z. aquatica- epigallocatechin, epicatechin, rutin, as well as various phenolic acids, including ferulic, vanillic, ellagic, sinapic, syringic, caffeic, gallic and cinnamic.

Wild Rice is a rich source of soluble fibre that helps normalize cholesterol and triglyceride levels. It also acts as fuel for various lactobacillus that help keep gastrointestinal health.

I have never heard of an allergy to wild rice, so that individuals with food sensitivities may have another healthful "grain" choice for their diet.

Wild Rice is indicated whenever there is a phosphorus deficiency, or when silica or organic sodium, is needed by the body. This makes it a great food for those who do excessive mental work.

It contains high levels of lysine and methionine, often lower or none existent in various grains. It contains no vitamin A but lots of B vitamin complex.

Wild Rice exhibits anti-oxidant activity that could well have commercial application. In studies by Wu et al, conducted in Minnesota in 1994, it was shown to reduce rancidity and showed appreciable anti-oxidant activity with ground beef and lard.

This may be due to the presence of polyphenol oxidase; a free radical quencher.

Wild Rice hull use was further examined by Asamarai et al in 1996, at the same University.

It has been shown wild rice hulls contain greater anti-oxidant activity than the kernels (Wu et al, 1994). This product is normally discarded at source and considering the millions of pounds of wild rice harvested annually, could potentially lead to another source of income.

The anti-oxidants extracted include anisole, m-hydroxybenzaldehyde, vanillin, and syringaldehyde.

One compound identified, 2,3-dihydroenzofuran, has been identified as a pro-oxidant.

Ramarathnam et al, *Trends in Food Science and Technology* 1995 6:3 found antioxidant activity in wild rice, and suggested the use of such foods may help prevent lipid peroxidation and the aging and disease process associated with it.

Recent work found the antioxidant activity 30 times that of white rice, no surprise, with several flavonoid glycosides believed responsible. Qui et al, *J Ag Food Chem* 2009 July 24.

Gamma oryzanol is present in levels twice that of brown rice. This compound enhances innate immune response, promoting the secretion of innate cytotkines, interleukin-8 and CCL2 which facilitate phagocytosis. Shin SY et al, *J Med Food* 2017 July 7.

It is a promising anti-obesity substance, with distinct property of being a novel epigenetic modulator. In a study on high fat diet-induced obesity in mice, gamma oryzanol modulates dopamine receptors in the brain striatum. This addiction to fat shares a common mechanism with alcohol, nicotine and narcotics. Kozuka C et al, *Diabetologia* 2017 60(8): 1502-11.

Gamma oryzanol shows protective effect against glaucoma, and can reduce optic nerve damage. Panchal SS et al, *J Ophthalmol* 2017: 1468716.

A supplementation of 600 mg/daily during nine weeks resistance training on thirty male volunteers increased muscular strength, but did not change anthropometric and body measurements. Esiami S et al, Indian *J Med Res* 2014 139(6): 857-63.

An interesting herbal compound, developed by Richard DeSylva of *Herb Works*, is called Oxygen Blend. It contains walnut leaves, chaparral and wild rice hulls in capsule form.

The grain was used at one time for burns, and ailments of the heart, lungs, liver, stomach and kidneys.

Wild Rice is contraindicated in forms of arthritis and stone formation related to phosphoric acid deposits. The more common uric acid and calcium oxalate forms are not affected.

Mice fed wild rice reduced the size and severity of atherosclerotic lesions by 61-71%. Reductions in plasma cholesterol, LDL and VLDL levels were all significantly reduced. Surendiran G et al, *Atherosclerosis* 2013 230(2): 284-92.

A good review of the nutritional constituents and health benefits of wild rice is found in *Nutrition Review* 2014 72(4), by Surendiran G et al.

The related Wild Rice (*Z. caduciflora*) or **JIAO BAI** is used in China for food and medicine. The stem is sweet and astringent, helping cool fevers, alleviate thirst and promote lactation.

The root calms fevers and is an antidote to poisons.

HOMEOPATHY

Zizania palustris patients feel flat emotionally, with aversion to interactions, and are withdrawn and desire to be left alone. There is a feeling of isolation, preoccupation with the number 2, and dreams of babies, childbirth, pregnancy, dead relatives, storms, tornados, wind and snow.

Sensitive to smell of bread, extremes of temperatures. Sensation as if falling down stairs, while lying in bed. Brain as if divided in two, with slight vertigo.

Top of head as if to explode when bending over. Lump in right side of throat. Thyroid as if swollen.

Internal vibration in legs, like touching a wire and feeling electric current.

DOSE- Twelfth to 30th potency. Proving by Jake Klakahi and Jeremy Sherr with 21 provers at 12th and 30th C potency in 2007.

FUNGI
Ustilago esculenta

A smut growing on the shoot of Wild Rice has been found to be useful as a diuretic, and laxative. It is also used medicinally for those with reddened eyes, alcohol intoxication, and for treating carbuncles.

The sori grow within the young stems, causing the stem to swell with infection. In an early stage, it can be eaten as a delicious and tasty vegetable, for easing constipation and urination.

Cut the wild rice shoot into slices and dry in the sun. To 62 grams of dried shoot add salt and vinegar and cook the mixture as a soup.

Makomotindoline, extracts from the infected shoot shows adverse effects on rat glioma cells. Suzuki T et al, *Bioog Med Chem Lett* 2012 22(13): 4246-8.

A wild rice seed ergot similar to that on rye, has been used by the native midwives of Wisconsin for hastening childbirth. *Claviceps zizaniae* is widespread, but occurs only sporadically.

ESSENTIAL OIL

Wild rice volatiles have been isolated using vacuum steam distillation, followed by solvent extraction.

One hundred and twelve compounds have been identified. Phenols contribute to the smoky character, while toasted and roasted odours are associated with pyrazines.

The alkyl pyridines identified probably contribute to the tea-like and green aromas of wild rice.

A pleasant, sweet note is 5-methylfurfrual. A strong floral aroma is due to acetophenone.

Cinnamaldehyde contributes a cinnamon like quality.

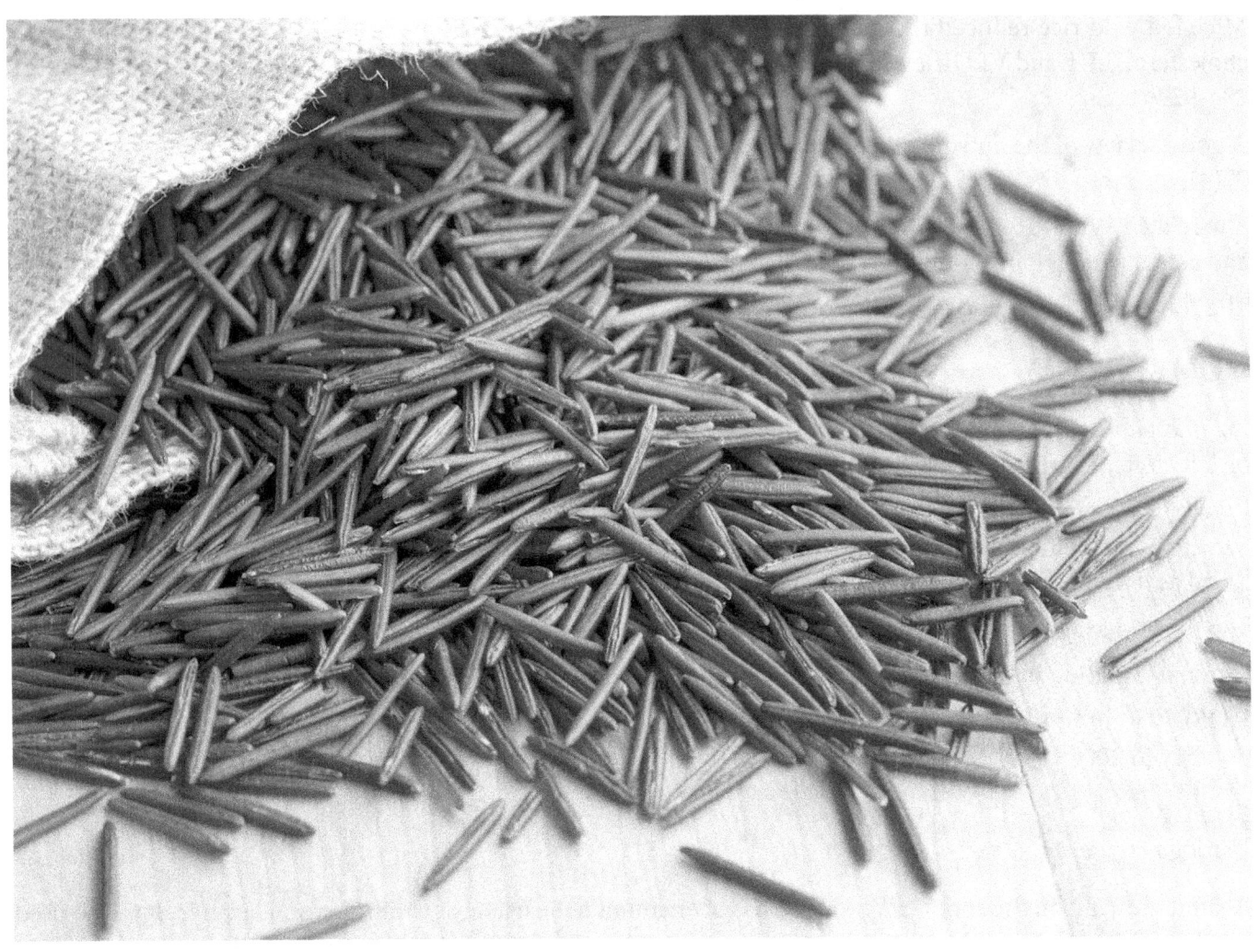

WILD RICE READY FOR COOKING

SEED OIL

Wild rice contains 0.5-0.8% lipids, composed of 30% linolenic acid, and 8% linoleic acid, 14% palmitic and 6% oleic acid.

MYTHS AND LEGENDS

Life was easy for Wenabozhoo. His indulgent grandmother, with whom he lived, demanded no work of him, and in consequence he passed through his early boyhood days.

At last, the grandmother awoke to the fact that her son lacked the initiative so essential to meet the requirements of their race and so encouraged him to go out into the world and learn for himself. He was not a skilled hunter and had to subsist on seeds, roots and tubers. One day, when he was exhausted and seeking food, he heard many plants speaking to him. Wenabozhoo gave no heed until he was attracted by the beauty of a graceful grass growing in a small lake basking in the sunshine of the open woodland. Some of these plants beckoned to him and said, "Sometimes they eat us". He was quite hungry now, and observing that the upper part of the plants was loaded with long seeds, he soon gathered some of them.

Removing the hulls, he ate the kernels and found the taste of them so pleasing and their effect upon his hunger so gratifying that he exclaimed, "Oh, you are indeed good! What are you called?" The plants replied, "We are called Manoomin".

KAHLEE KEANE

SPIRITUAL PROPERTIES

Though I speak with the tongues of men and of angels, and have not Macroneurotics, I am become as a sounding bell or a tinkling cymbal.

For though I have the gift of prophecy and can do Tarot readings, and understand all earth mysteries and oracles, but I have not Macroneurotics, then I am nothing.

And though I bestow all my goods to Oxfam or to the jumble sales of Guru Maharaji, and have not Macroneurotics, then it profiteth me nothing.

For I say unto you, Macroneurotics suffereth long, in fact is very much into suffering; Macroneurotics envieth not, and is not puffed up, unless by excessive consumption of Rice cakes.

Macroneurotics never faileth. But whether there be vegetarians, they shall fail. And whether there be vegans, they shall be wrong too. And whether there be proponents of Food Combining, yeah verily, they shall all vanish away.

But when that which is perfect comes (ie Brown Rice), then that which is in part (white rice) shall be done away. For when I was a vegetarian, I spoke as a child; and when I became a vegan, I understood as a child; but when I became Macroneurotics I put away childish things, and learned to use chopsticks.

For now we se through a Cooking Class darkly, but then face to face. Now I know Macroneurotics Studies, but then shall I know Total World Domination.

And now abideth vegetarianism, veganism and Macroneurotics, these three; but the greatest of these is Macro-neurotics.

THOMPSON

AMERICAN WINTERGREEN
SHINLEAF
(*Pyrola americana* Sweet)
(*Pyrola rotundifolia* auct. non L.) not accepted
(*P. rotundifolia* L. **var. *americana*** [Sweet] Fernald.)
not accepted
(*P. americana* **var. *rotundifolia***) not accepted
WINTERGREEN
COMMON PINK WINTERGREEN
BOG WINTERGREEN
LIVERLEAF WINTERGREEN
(*P. asarifolia* Michx.)
(*P. uliginosa* Torr. & Gray ex Torr.) not accepted
LARGE WINTERGREEN
(*P. bracteata* Hook.) not accepted
(*P. asarifolia ssp. bracteata* [Hook.] Haber)
LESSER WINTERGREEN
COMMON WINTERGREEN
(*P. minor* L.)
WHITE WINTERGREEN
(*P. elliptica* Nutt.)

ROUND LEAVED WINTERGREEN
GREEN WINTERGREEN
(*P. virens* Schweigg. & Korte) not accepted
(*P. chlorantha* Sw.)
(*P. axypetala*) not accepted
(*P. convulata* W.P.C. Barton) not accepted
ONE FLOWERED WINTERGREEN
SINGLE DELIGHT
WAXFLOWER
WOOD NYMPH
(*Moneses uniflora* [L.] A. Gray)
(*P. uniflora* L.) not accepted
SERRATED WINTERGREEN
ONE-SIDED WINTERGREEN
(*Orthilia secunda* [L.] House)
(*P. secunda* L.) not accepted
(*Ramischia elatior*) not accepted
(*R. secunda*) not accepted
PARTS USED- whole plant

All bright, and fresh, and glossy, our Wintergreens come forth as though they had been perfecting their toilet within the sheltering canopy of their snowy chambers, to do honour to the new-born year just awakening from her icy sleep.

C.P. TRAILL

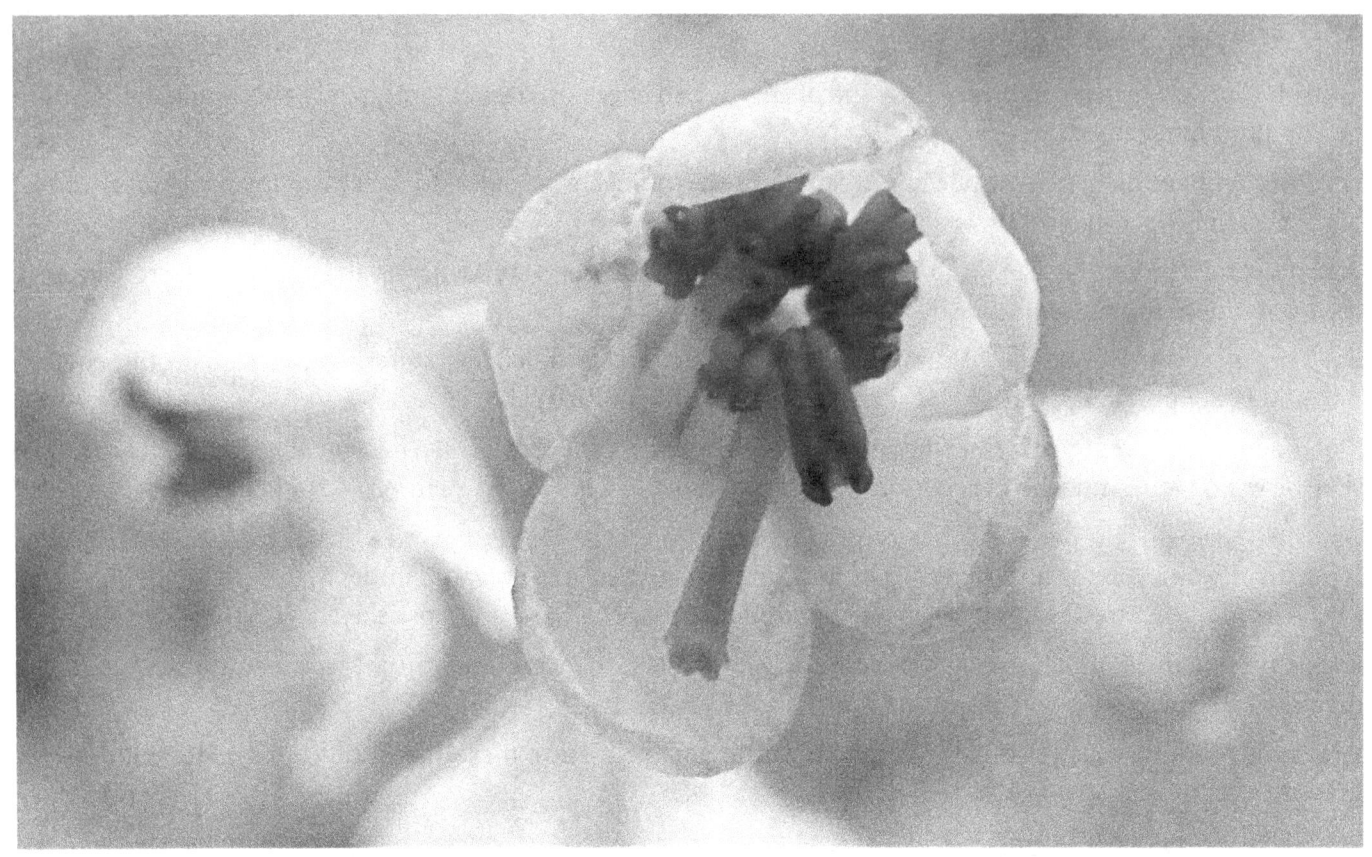

COMMON PINK WINTERGREEN

Pyrola comes from the Latin **PYRUS** meaning pear, due to the perceived leaf shape.

Moneses is derived from the Greek **MONO** meaning, one and **HESIA** meaning, delight. Orthilia is from Greek **ORTHOS**, meaning straight, and Old Norse **THILL**, meaning a stake or pole. **SECUNDA** is Latin meaning growing on one side only. Asarifolia means asarum-like leaves.

This is the true wintergreen, not the *Gaultheria*, or false wintergreen famous for essential oils. Wintergreen was a term originally applied to ivy, due to staying green all year round.

So too, does this interesting wooded plant; that in bloom has a wonderful fragrance. They are more closely related to Pipsissewa, found in the same habitat, and possess very similar medicinal value.

The number 5 prevails, with five petals, 5 parted calyx, 10 stamens, 5-rayed stigma, 5 tubercles at apex, and a 5 celled, valved seed vessel.

All the wintergreens have an herbal tradition based on their astringent action. Decoctions of the whole above ground plant have been used for skin disease, gargled for sore throat and a wash for various eye troubles.

The leaves can be simply poulticed and applied to boils, swellings, carbuncles, and painful skin tumours.

Round-leaved Wintergreen, or Shinleaf as it is also known, is widespread and common. The flowers are small, white and very fragrant reminiscent of lily of the valley. Shinleaf refers to the external application to old indolent ulcers of the leg and skin.

Culpepper placed it under Saturn, and praised its astringent qualities for, "inward ulcers in the kidneys or neck of the bladder." He suggested the herb be boiled in wine and water to stay "all fluxes as the lask, bloody fluxes, women's courses and bleeding of wounds, and takes away any inflammations rising upon pains of the heart, it is no less helpful for foul ulcers to be cured; as also for cankers or fistulas."

Common pink wintergreen (*P. asarifolia*) is infused by the Cree as a diuretic, in cases of urinary blockage. It is sometimes called **WA WIPAK**. A more common name **AMISKOWEHTAWAKEWUSKOS** or "beaver ear plant" is so-called due to the round-shaped leaves. Leaf decoctions can be used for treating coughing up blood, or to wash sore eyes.

The Chipewyan mashed the leaves with lard and apply it to cuts to stop bleeding and heal properly. For toothache the leaves were simply chewed.

Pink wintergreen is known as **SASDZAGHE**, meaning Bear's Ears.

The Slave of the boreal forest call it Beaver Berry or **TSA DZHI**, or sometimes Hoary Marmot Berry, **DEDIE DZHI**.

The latter name may relate to marmots eating the roots. The eastern Ojibwa name is **BINE'BUG**. The leaf and roots of *P. secunda* are eaten by red squirrels.

Various indigenous tribes steamed hyperactive children with the leaf tea; or simply drank it as a liver and kidney tonic.

The Nootka and Kwakiutl placed poultices of One Flowered Wintergreen (*M. uniflora*) on boils, or abscesses to draw out the pus. It was reported to be strong and caused skin blisters.

The Dena'ina call it Single Delight, Bethlehem Star, or **QUNULGGUGI** meaning, "that which ran up again". They collect the creeping stolons, soak them in water and drink this for sore throats. The chewed leaves are placed on cuts. The Chugach of the Kenai Peninsula infuse both leaves and flowers as a tea for sore throat.

The Montagnais call it **CACA'YUMNA'N** and used the steeped plant for treating paralysis.

In Germany, the plant is used in various ointments and salves. The bruised plant staunches blood, and can be used as a styptic.

The dried plant tea has a red tint and mild wintergreen with bittersweet aftertaste.

Grieve says that the leaves are decocted with a little cinnamon and red wine for curing bloody stools, ulcers of the bladder and restraining menses.

It was used as a diuretic for urinary infections; and anti-spasmodic for various nervous and epileptic concerns.

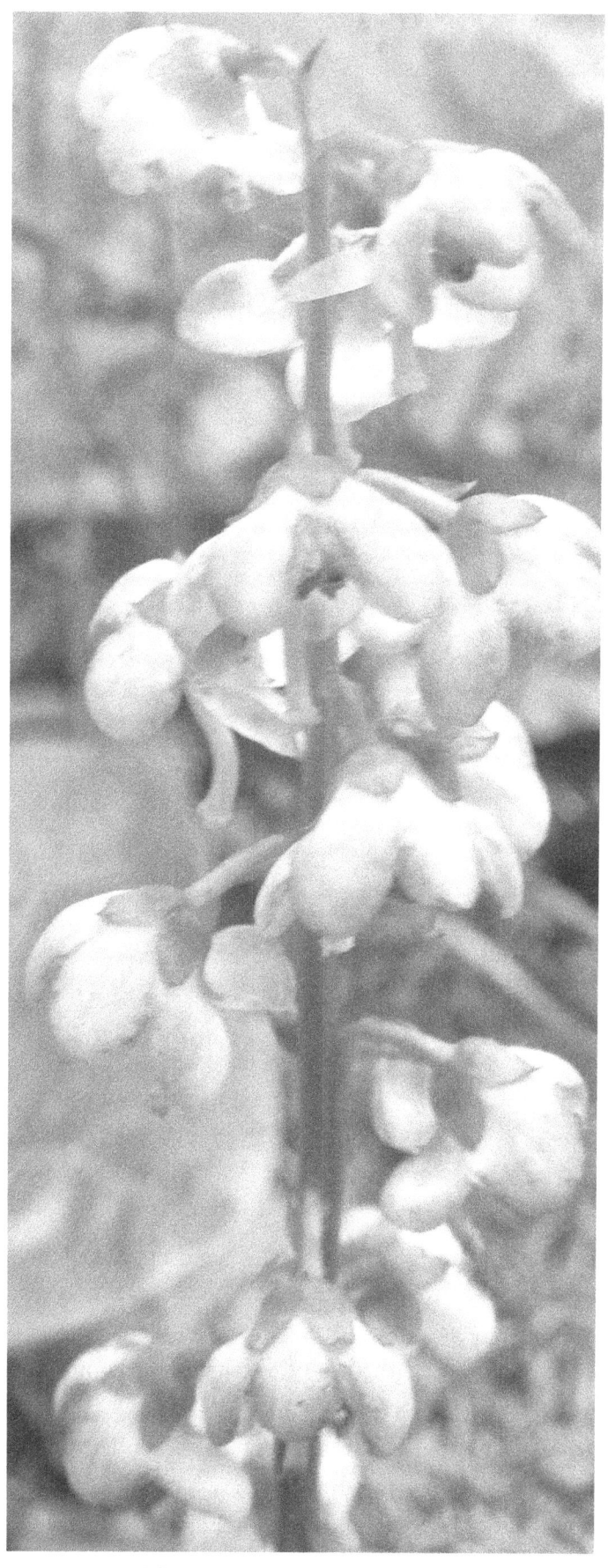

COMMON PINK WINTERGREEN

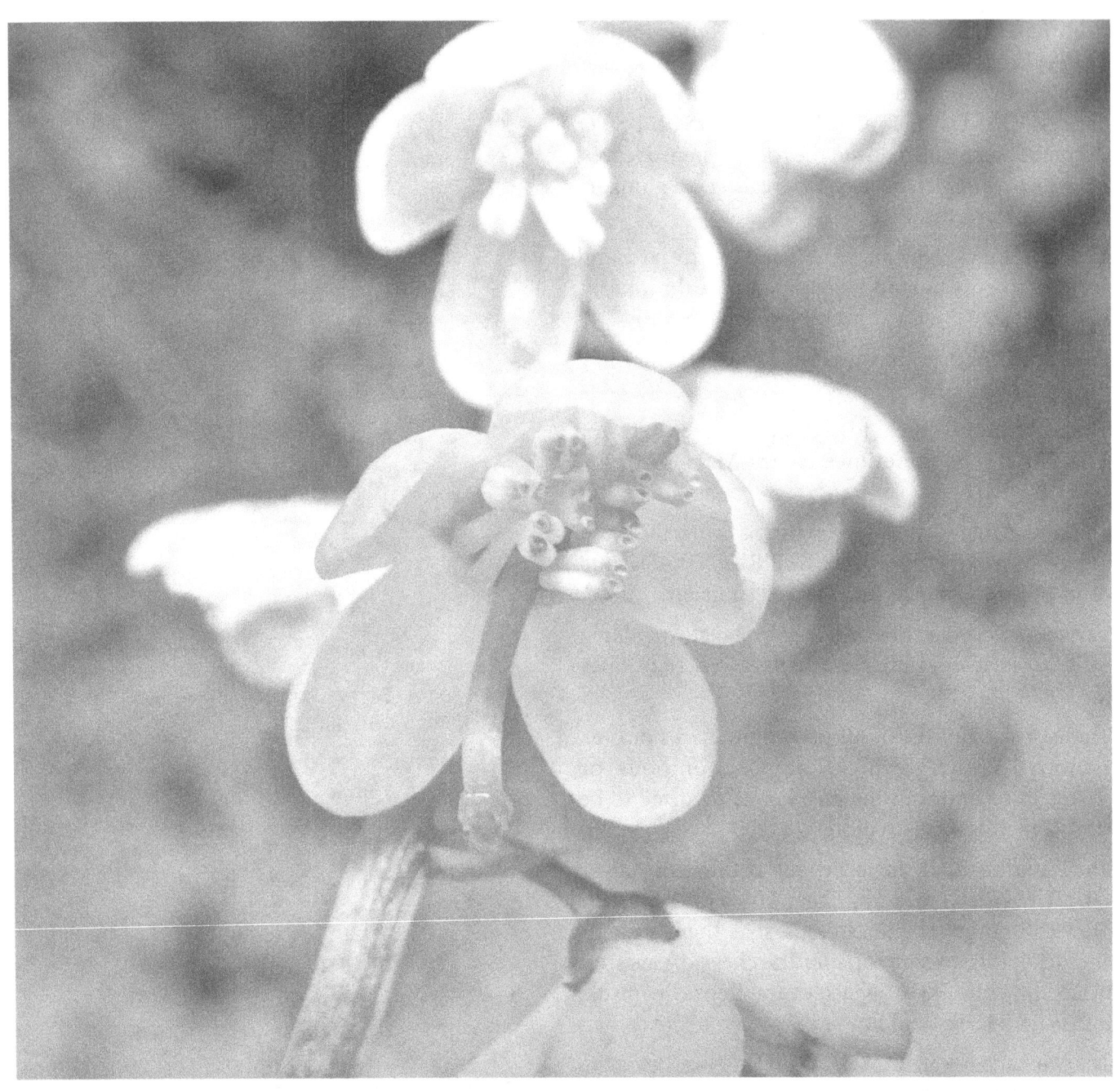

ROUND LEAF WINTERGREEN

One-flowered wintergreen is considered a powerful medicine, by the Haida. They make a weak tea from the whole plant for diarrhea, smallpox, tuberculosis, cancer, as well as for "power and good luck". They call it **XILGUUGAA**.

Writings by Swanton in 1905 record the story of a hero eating a whole mountain full of this plant to give him supernatural strength. In another journal in 1908 he wrote. "When people wanted to be chiefs, they ate bitter leaves."

The fresh, hyacinth-scented flowers have been mashed for treating rashes, bunions, and corns. In Alaska, various tribes drank the leaf tea for sore throats, gentle enough to give to children. The seeds are edible, raw or roasted.

The Kwakiutl used the plant as a poultice for swelling and pain. It was chewed or pounded on a rock, and applied to the skin where it caused blisters. They were opened, and when the loose skin was peeled off, the sore was washed with gooseberry root decoction, and then covered with plantain leaves until healed. One-sided Wintergreen was mixed, with animal fat, by Chippewa healers into a salve. The leaves were chewed for toothaches.

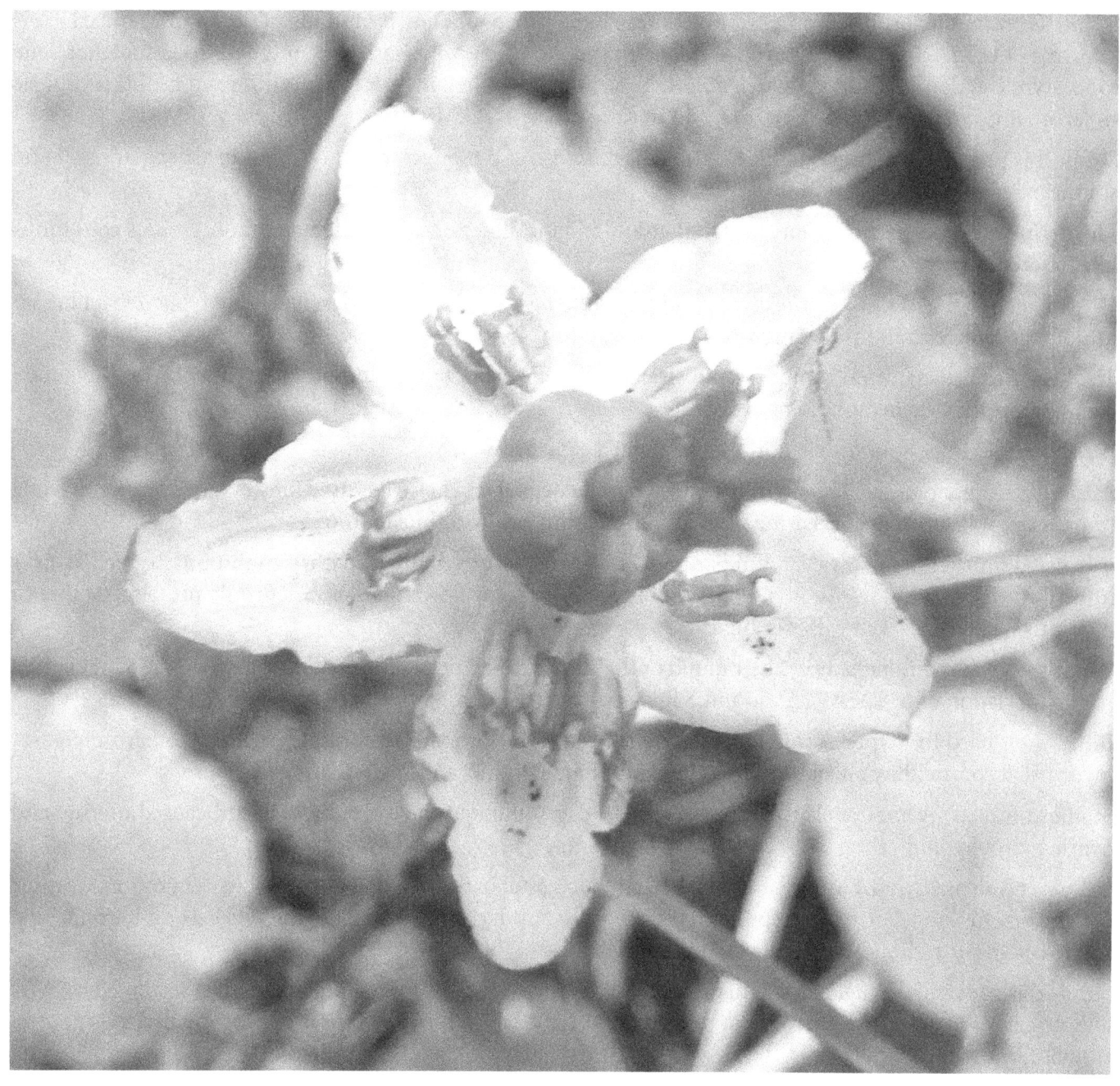

MONESES UNIFLORA

MEDICINAL

CONSTITUENTS *P. rotundifolia*- arbutin, monotropin, einulsin, isohomoarbutin, methylhydroquinone, gallic and ursolic acid, ericolin, quinone chimaphilin, ursone, tannins, bitters, invertase, renifolin, emulsin, acetovanillon, ursone, hyperin, toluhydroquinone, manno-heptulose, sedoheptulose

M. uniflora- vit C, chimaphilin, 3-hydroxychimaphilin, 2,7-dimethyl-1,3-dihydroxy-naphthyl, 4-0-alpha-L-rhamnopyranoside, 8-chlorochimaphilin, 2,7-dimethoxy-1,4,8-tri-hydroxy-naphth-alene, mannohepulose, sedoheptulosan, sedoheptulose, inositol, erythritol, mannitol, sorbitol, methyl hydroquinone.

P. virens/chlorantha- 8 flavanol glycosides based upon kaempferol, quercitin and rhamnetin; luteolin, apiginen

P. minor- mannoheptulose, sedoheptulose, sedoheltulosan, inositol, erythritol, mannitol, and sorbitol.

P. secunda- renifolin, two phenolic glycosides.

The leaves of all *Pyrola* are high in methyl salicylate.

249

Pyrola (*P. rotundifolia*) has been used in Chinese herbal medicine for thousands of years. In Mandarin it is known as **LU XIAN CAO**, or Deer's Hoof, due to the leaf shape with both root and herb used together. Due to its styptic action it is also known as Sword Tryer; the leaves helping to stop bleeding and heal insect bites. In Japan, it is known as **ROKUGANSO**, and in Korea is **NOKHAMCHO**.

Shinleaf is practically identical in herbal use to *Pipsissewa,* and more commonly found in aspen parkland and southern boreal forest.

The herb is a broad-spectrum anti-bacterial, useful in lung afflictions like cough and more serious conditions like tuberculosis.

Other bacteria including *Staphylococcus aureus, Bacillus pyrogenes* and both dysentery and typhoid bacillus are inhibited at concentrations ranging from 12.5 to 50 µg/ml.

The herb helps dispel wind dampness and strengthens sinew and bones, combining well with Water Plantain root for chronic degenerative joint disease.

It also relieves bone spurs, taking orally and applied externally.

Shinleaf is a musclo-skeletal restorative, hemostatic, and detoxifying herb. It is used for stopping internal bleeding traumas, as well as excessive uterine bleeding, combining well with Burnet root.

It is useful in rheumatic myalgia, lumbar pain, and other assorted inflammatory conditions, as well as liver infections. For painful joints, it is often combined with Fleece flower, while for chronic proteinuria due to nephritis it combines well with rosehips.

Work by Lee et al, *J Ethnopharm* 112:1 found both iNOS and NO production was lowered, as well as activating phosphorylation of p38 MAP kinase and NF-kappa B by the herb.

It has been used for hypertension where there is need for a coronary restorative. That is, the herb increases myocardial contractility and at the same time is anti-arrhythmic, and vaso-dilating in nature.

Studies of mice given 20% plant decoctions for 10 days inhibited the estrous phase and caused uterine and ovarian atrophy; indicating some contraceptive potential.

Extracts given orally, or by intravenous infusion, are successful in the treatment of pulmonary infection. Chronic coughs due to Lung deficiency respond to plant decoctions. It moistens the lungs and is best for chronic, dry, feeble coughs or asthma associated with kidney deficiency.

Shinleaf is cool and drying, and useful topically for insect bites, cuts, sores, and bruises. It is indicated in UTIs and urinary irritation. Use infusions or diluted tinctures for mouth rinse in cases of pharyngitis, canker sores, stomatitis and tonsillitis.

It is used for intestinal and urinary infections, especially pediatric diarrhea and acute dysentery.

Many of these observations may be due to the ability of the herb to activate AMPK signaling pathway. The ability to regulate glucose and lipids and increase insulin signaling as well as other parameters places shinleaf (round-leaved wintergreen) in the category of herbs like ginseng for increased metabolic rate and production of energy. Ptitsyn et al, *Fitoterapia* 82:8 1285-9.

An interesting study found a compound injection of this herb and astragalus root in guinea pigs prevented the ototoxicity and nephrotoxicity associated with aminoglycosides such as gentamicin, tobramycin and amikacin.

One-Sided Wintergreen (*P. secunda*) in ethanol extracts has shown activity against gram-positive bacteria, as did *P. rotundifolia* in both ether and acetone extracts.

Saxena et al, *Journal of Natural Products* 1995 59:1 found chlorochimaphilin, derived from one-flowered wintergreen (*Moneses uniflora*) to be active against fungi (especially *Candida albicans*), and both gram positive and negative bacteria.

Research by Bishop and MacDonald in the mid-1950s found the plant active against *Staphylococcus aureus*.

McCutcheon found the plant extract completely inhibited growth of *Mycobacterium tuberculosis* and *M. avium*; whereas earlier work by Saxena et al 1996 found no inhibition related to any isolated compounds.

McCutcheon found strong anti-bacterial activity against at least 10 of 11 bacteria tested, including MRSA.

In one study, reported in the *Journal of Ethnopharmacology* 1994 44:3 aerial parts of *Moneses uniflora* showed significant anti-fungal activity (9 of 9 tested).

In one clinical study in China, out of 18 patients suffering with pulmonary infection, sixteen were cured with methyl hydroquinone, from the plant.

In another study of 36 children with infantile and children's diarrhea, infusions were stopped after three days, due to successful cure.

The plant contains vitamin K-like activity, as well as anti-inflammatory and analgesic relief.

Chlorochimaphilin shows activity against *Staphylococcus aureus, Bacillus subtilis, Fusarium tricuictum, Candida albicans,* and *Microsporum gypseum*.

Crude plant extracts show activity against herpes simplex virus and respiratory syncytial virus. The latter is prevalent and most people have been infected by the age of three, and every year afterwards for our whole life. It can cause both respiratory bronchiolitis and urinary tract infections. A formalin-inactivated RSV vaccine produced a more severe disease when recipients became infected and has been pulled from the market.

White Wintergreen (*P. elliptica*) has shown in studies by Bergeron et al to possess biological activity against *Candida albicans* and *Bacillus subtilis* as both methanol and water extracts. Methanol extracts were effective against *E. coli* and *Cladosporium cucumerinum*.

Chimaphilin, present in pipsissewa as well, is a well-known naphthoquinone with anti-fungal, antibacterial, anti-hemorrhagic, and vitamin K-like activity. It possesses anti-inflammatory and analgesic properties.

Chimaphilin, isolated from Pyrola, was found by Kagawa et al to inhibit platelet aggregation, and may play a role in myocardial circulation. In moderate amounts, it activates phagocytose inhibition of human granulocytes, but in low doses actually stimulates phagocytosis.

Herbalist Greg Brandenburg has observed *Moneses uniflora* to possess significant pain relieving constituents. He was kind enough to share this with me many years ago.

Wintergreen (*P. asarifolia*) contains pyrolaside B that shows activity against two Gram positive bacteria, *S. aureus* and *Micrococcus luteus*.

A strong leaf infusion may help treat epilepsy and other nerve disorders.

Darcy Williamson suggests that taken as a regular tea, Pyrola strengthens cardiac muscle contraction and anti-hypoxia ability. Leaf decoctions are slow simmered.

HOMEOPATHY

Shinleaf, *Pyrola rotundifolia* helps the mind that becomes partially unconscious and patient feels like fainting, as if brain is paralyzed and mind gone. It helps melancholy and drowsiness with very weak feeling in head, or they feel like crying. Head heavy.

It seems like a stimulant running all through the blood, whole system is utterly relaxed with no strength or vigor.

Great weakness of arms, hot flushes and chilliness. Aching in vagina, labia as if inflamed, dry mouth, rose runs, pain over right eye.

DOSE- low potencies. First proving by Gatchell in USA in 1876.

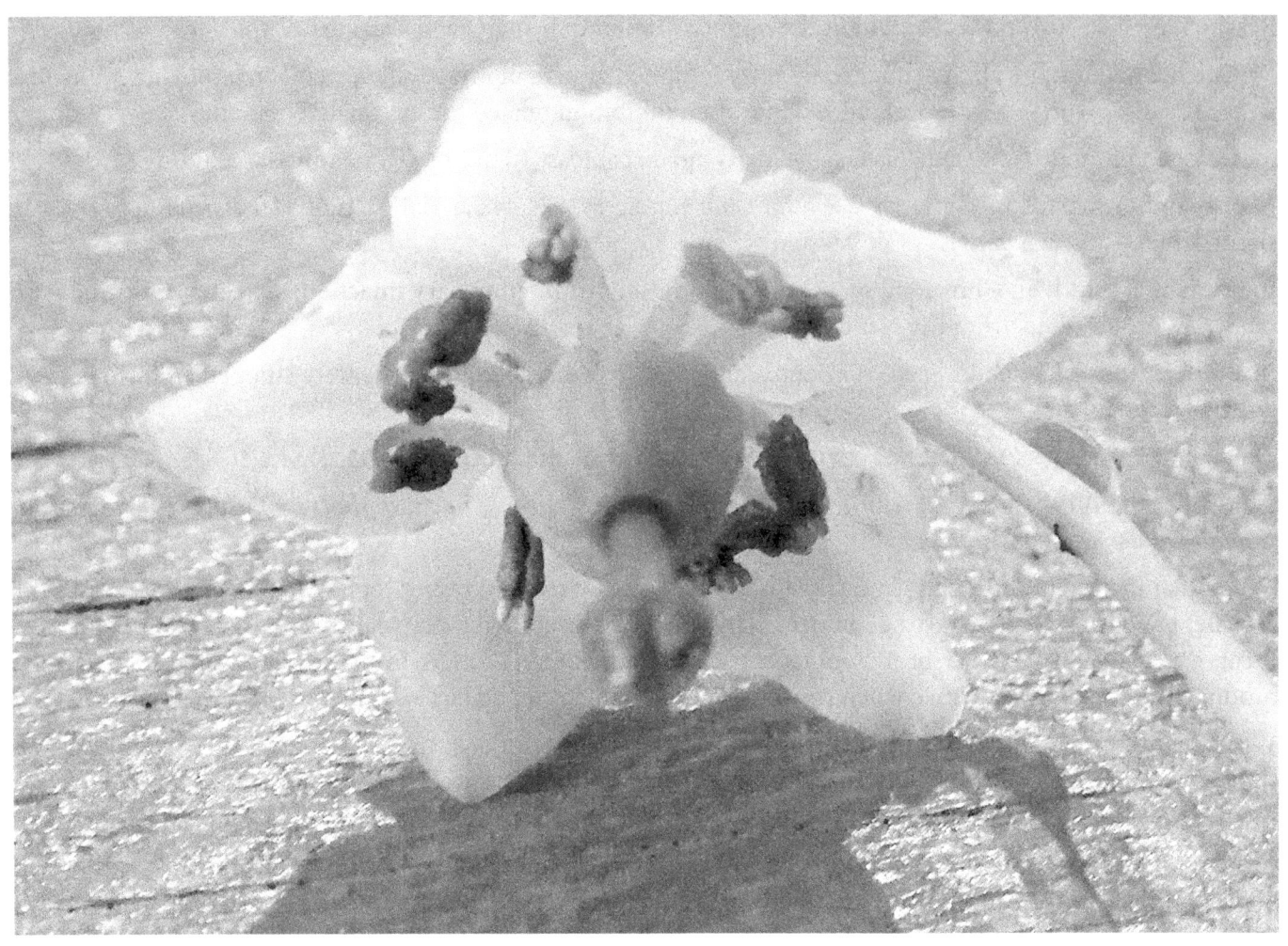

ONE-FLOWERED WINTERGREEN (*MONESES UNIFLORA*)

ESSENTIAL OILS

CONSTITUENTS- *P. grandiflora-* benzaldehydes dominant
P. rotundifolia- methoxy benzenes, and phenyl propanoids.

At the present time, there is no commercialization of essential oil extraction from Pyrola. It is due mainly to lack of demand in the marketplace. Many have an almond-like fragrance.

HYDROSOL

Pyrola water is produced from the whole plant, including root, and according to Brunschwig in *Book of Distillation*, is good for bathing fresh and old wounds and sores.

FLOWER ESSENCES

One Flowered Wintergreen flower essence is for dealing with a letdown or disappointment.
ROCKY MOUNTAIN

Wintergreen (*M. uniflora*) initiates the wakening up of consciousness by invoking aid from one's Higher Self. Particularly when we are feeling dispirited and dark, or axed by spiritual loneliness. Reconnecting to our soul ignites optimism and aspiration, whereupon we can maintain a true state of alertness and full consciousness.
FINDHORN

Bog Wintergreen (*P. asarifolia*) harkens to the instinctual nature of humanity to find its place on the planet. There's an innate sense of deserving and belonging that this plant tries to resonate and that in allowing this plant to serve you, what it will bring up…is the breaking down of the dysfunction of the generational patterns of not being in the right place at the right time.   **HIGH SIERRA**

RECIPES

DECOCTION-10-30 grams

TINCTURE-2-5ml. The tincture is prepared from the whole fresh plant including roots at 1:2 and 50% alcohol. Note: in short and long term skin eruptions, the tea may aggravate the condition temporarily. Urine will turn green but is harmless. Do not use for more than ten days at a time.

CAUTION- Pyrola is generally contraindicated during pregnancy and lactation. Due to its cool drying nature, use care if constipation is already an issue.

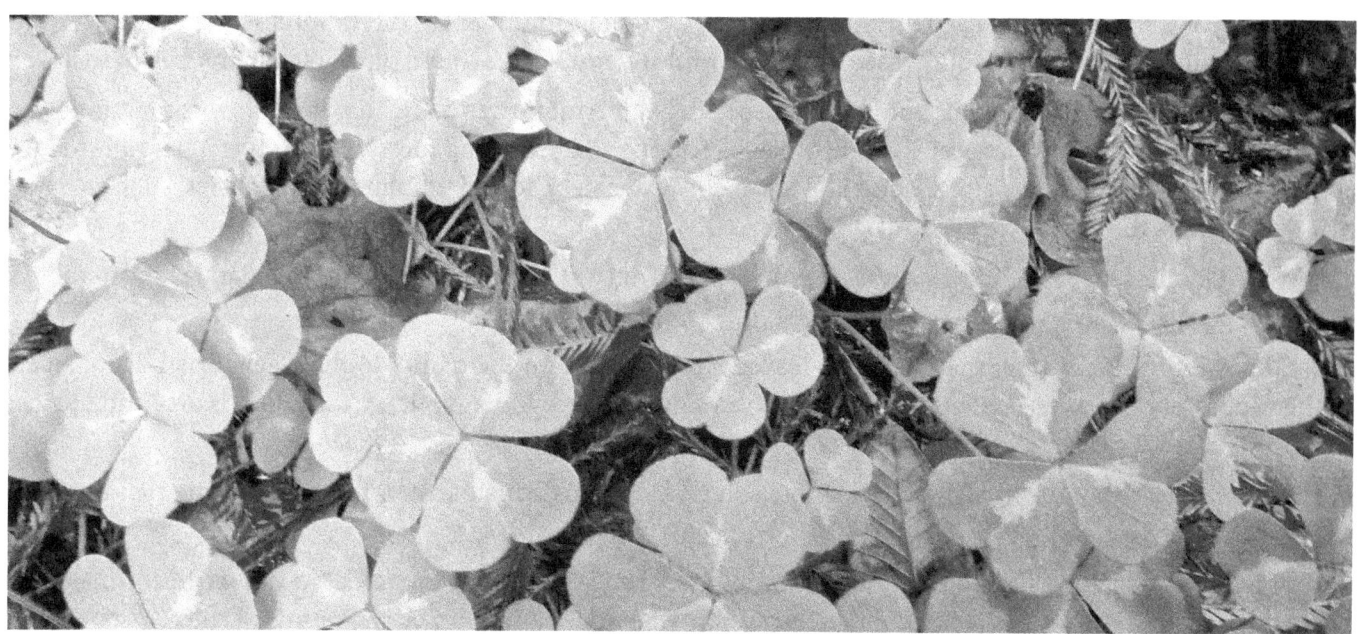

WOOD SORREL

WOOD SORREL
YELLOW WOOD SORREL
(***Oxalis stricta*** L.)
(***Xanthoxalis stricta*** [L.] Small) not accepted
(***O. europaea var. bushii*** [Small] Wiegand) not accepted
WOOD SORREL
(***O. acetosella*** auct. non L.) not accepted
(***O. montana*** Raf.)
(***O. alba*** Gilbert) not accepted
CREEPING WOOD SORREL
(***O. corniculata*** L.)
MOUNTAIN SORREL
(***Oxyria digyna*** [L.] Hill)
(***Rumex digyna*** L.)
PARTS USED- root, flower, leaf, fruit

Who from the tumps with bright green masses clad,
Plucks the Wood Sorrel with its light green leaves,
Heart shaped and triply folded; and its root
Creeping like beaded coral.

CHARLOTTE SMITH

O, the Shamrock, the green, immortal Shamrock!
Chosen leaf of Baird and Chief, Old Erin's native Shamrock.

THOMAS MOORE

Oxalis is from the Greek **OXUS**, meaning sour, or **OXYS** meaning acid. Stricta means erect. Acetosella means literally vinegar salt. Sorrel is from the Germanic **SURAZ**, meaning sour.

Digyna may be from the Greek **DI**, meaning two and **GYNE** meaning female organ system such as ovary or pistil.

Shamrock is from the Celtic or Irish **SEA MAIR** or **SEANROG**, meaning "little clover", which became Shamrog, and finally shamrock.

Creeping Wood Sorrel is an escapee from cultivation, and often found around old homesteads. Yellow Wood Sorrel is mainly confined to the southeastern prairies, while *O. europaea* is found on dry soil in the northern areas.

Wood Sorrel is a native perennial, hardy to zone 3, of North America and Eurasia. It is a low creeping flower with nodding white flowers and purple veins that prefers the shade of cool, moist woods. It is often referred to, and sold as, Shamrock, especially around St. Patrick's Day. It can be found in many old paintings, such as those by Fra Angelico, to represent the trinity.

The Triple Goddess, or Three Bridgets was common and feared by Christian authorities in Ireland who attempted to change its meaning.

Legend has it that St. Patrick used the three-leaved sorrel to explain the trinity to the Gaelic Irish. He studied in the monastery of Lerins, which was founded from Egypt, where the Egyptian trinity, Osiris, Isis and Horus, represented the father, mother and child.

Patricius was his Romanized name. He was the son of a Roman-British army officer, under the real name of Maewyn Succat.

St. Patrick's shamrock was a druidic mystic symbol associated with the ancient Celtic sun wheels. Christians created the idea of the four-leaf clover being lucky, and of course, symbolizing the points of the cross.

The plant has come to symbolize joy, and has been assigned birth date of April 21. It also goes by the name of Alleluia Flower, as it comes out at Easter and is a sign of celebration. In England, France and Italy, it was known by this name. In France, it was known as Sorrel de bois, meaning of the woods; hence wood sorrel.

It is said that if two lovers out walking should step on a wood sorrel, their marriage may be delayed.

In parts of Wales, it is called Fairy Bells, due to the belief that the swinging tiny bells made music that called elves to moonlight dance and revelry.

At night, the leaves fold in half to protect against excessive moisture.

Like many woodland plants, they have self-fertilizing, or cleistogamic flowers on curved stems at the base of the plant. It is an evergreen plant through sugar compounds with anti-freeze type ability that allow the leaves to lie dormant for winter.

The leaves have a tart, sour taste that Gerard, the English herbalist, wrote was made into a Greene Sauce that is "good for them that have sicke and feeble stomaches... and of all the Sauces, (Wood) Sorrel is the best, not only in virtue, but also in pleasantness of his taste".

Culpepper suggested the herb "to quench thirst, to strengthen a weak stomach, to stay vomiting... excellent in any contagious sickness or pestilential fever".

Grieve, in *A Modern Herbal* mentions wood sorrel "has diuretic, anti-scorbutic and refrigerant action, and a decoction made from its pleasant acid leaves is given in high fever, both to quench thirst and to allay the fever".

Francus concluded the herb of value to recruit the energies of the heart and to dispel the quinsy.

Sandro Botticelli and Fra Angelico often placed the symbolic flowers in their paintings of the crucifixion. The reddish veining of the leaves were from drops of blood shed by Christ on the cross. The Italian name Alleluia, is said to be related to Hallelujah.

The juice of the leaves turns red when clarified, and was used as a gargle for mouth ulcers, and effective when applied externally to swelling and inflammation.

Another name for the plant, Cuckoo Sorrel, originated from idea the bird used the herb to clear its voice.

Only the fresh plant juice or tincture will work well, although distilled waters and wines were used during the times of Culpepper and Gerard.

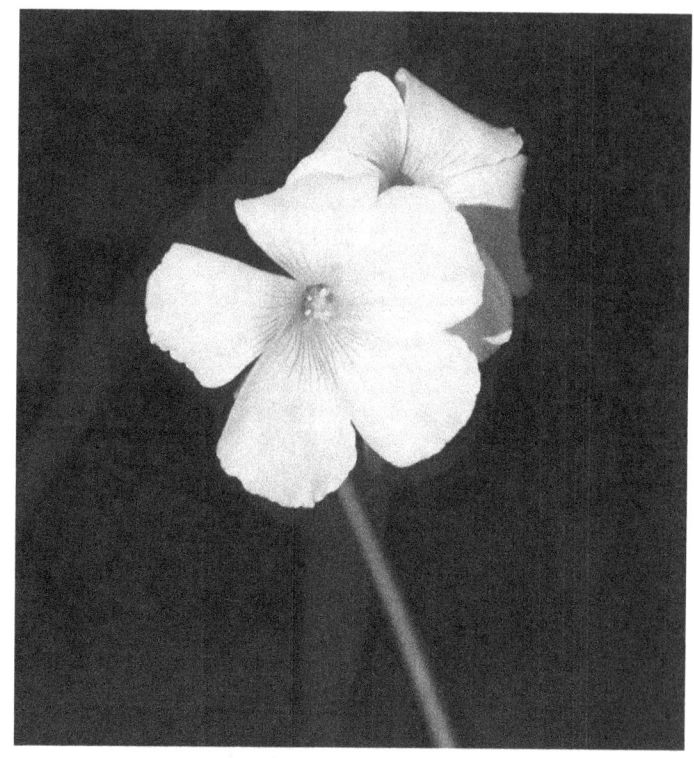

CREEPING WOOD SORREL

Apothecaries made salts of lemon from Wood Sorrel, by evaporating the juice. This was used for treating catarrh, hemorrhage and fevers. Three pounds of sap evaporated down to one ounce of the salt crystals, composed mainly of oxalic and citric acid.

The green fruit are a pleasant sour flavour, that Kindscher called "little bananas".

Indigenous healers would pound up the roots and give them to their horses to give them speed; "to put the north wind into their hoofs."

The Ojibwa call the plant **ZEEWUNUBUBUSHK**, or sour leaf. They made a bittersweet dessert of the leaves cooked with maple syrup. The Algonquin considered it an aphrodisiac, in part, because of the heart shaped leaves.

Scandinavians make a type of fermented sauerkraut from the leaves.

One Lapland recipe had the herb boiled in milk, and the coagulated mass stored underground for winter food in times of scarcity.

In *Edible Wild*, the author relates a story of traveling with Laplanders where the sauerkraut dish was served. "I liked it so much I wanted a refill but was refused- an action very uncommon among people who will share their last bit of food with you. When I asked the reason for this strange, hostile attitude, I was told that if I ate too much, the White Wolf in the sky would overtake and kill me by thirst, tied to a dwarf birch in the wilderness."

The bulbous tubers can be eaten raw or boiled. They are quite sour and probably contain oxalic acid. Small taproots, however, attached to the rhizomes are glossy and transparent looking. These are sweet and plentiful and make a good food.

The leaves can be boiled and when removed from heat, a little honey added to make a refreshing lemonade type beverage.

An unusual dish from Edible Wild mentioned above is to take a pickle of the tuberous root and a handful of red ants soaked in water overnight, in which small game is cooked the next day. Yellow Wood Sorrel was utilized by Omaha as a poultice for swellings.

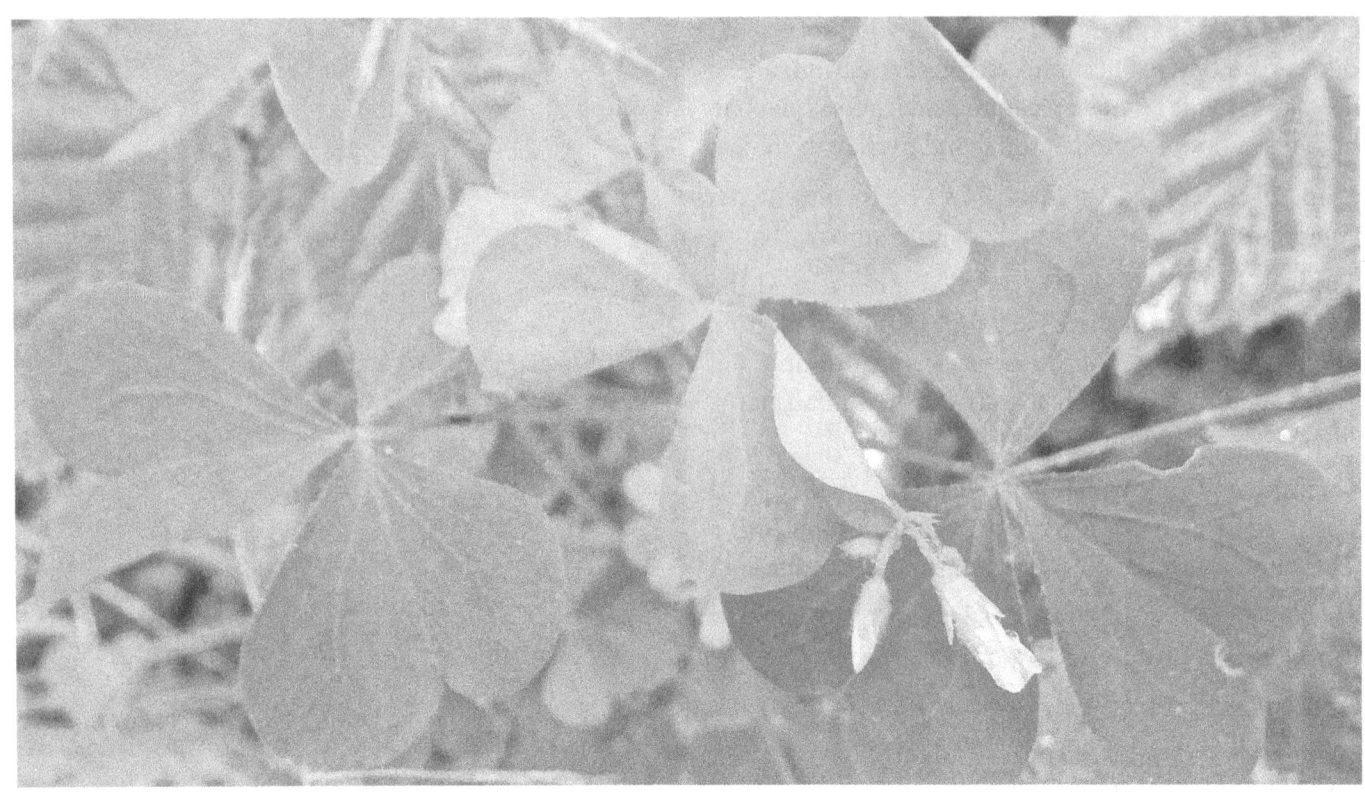

WOOD SORREL

Creeping Wood Sorrel was a favourite plant of the Cherokee who used infusions to treat hookworm in children.

A salve made from the infused leaf with sheep fat was applied to skin sores. For old sore and wounds, it was sometimes combined with Smartweed (*Polygonum hydropiper*).

Cold leaf infusions were used to stop vomiting. The leaf was chewed for sore mouth or throat, as well as problems of saliva.

They used is for cancer that has just started. The Seneca boiled Oxalis species in bear grease, for example, as part of a cancer salve.

Further north, the Iroquois decocted the roots as part of a combination for blood problems, and infusions of the plant for cramps, nausea, fever and summer complaint in children.

The Algonquin believed it to have aphrodisiac properties.

Creeping wood sorrel, as a fresh juice, is said to antidote Jimson Weed and *Datura metel* seeds as well as arsenic and mercury. The slimy mucilage was said used by magicians to eat glass.

The Sotho of Africa use plant infusions to wash snakebite, while in former Tanganyika the leaf is eaten or decocted as a cough remedy. Fresh leaf decoctions were taken twice daily in parts of Africa as an abortifacient.

For cellulitis, the steamed leaves are applied to affected area.

The fresh plant juice has been used for headache, earache and eye inflammations.

A Chinese publication from 1421, *Precious Secrets of the Realm of the Keng and Hsin* (Metals and Minerals), suggests creeping wood sorrel accumulates high levels of copper in its tissue.

The plant is used in Traditional Chinese Medicine, and has a variety of names, the most common being **TSA CHIANG TS'AO**.

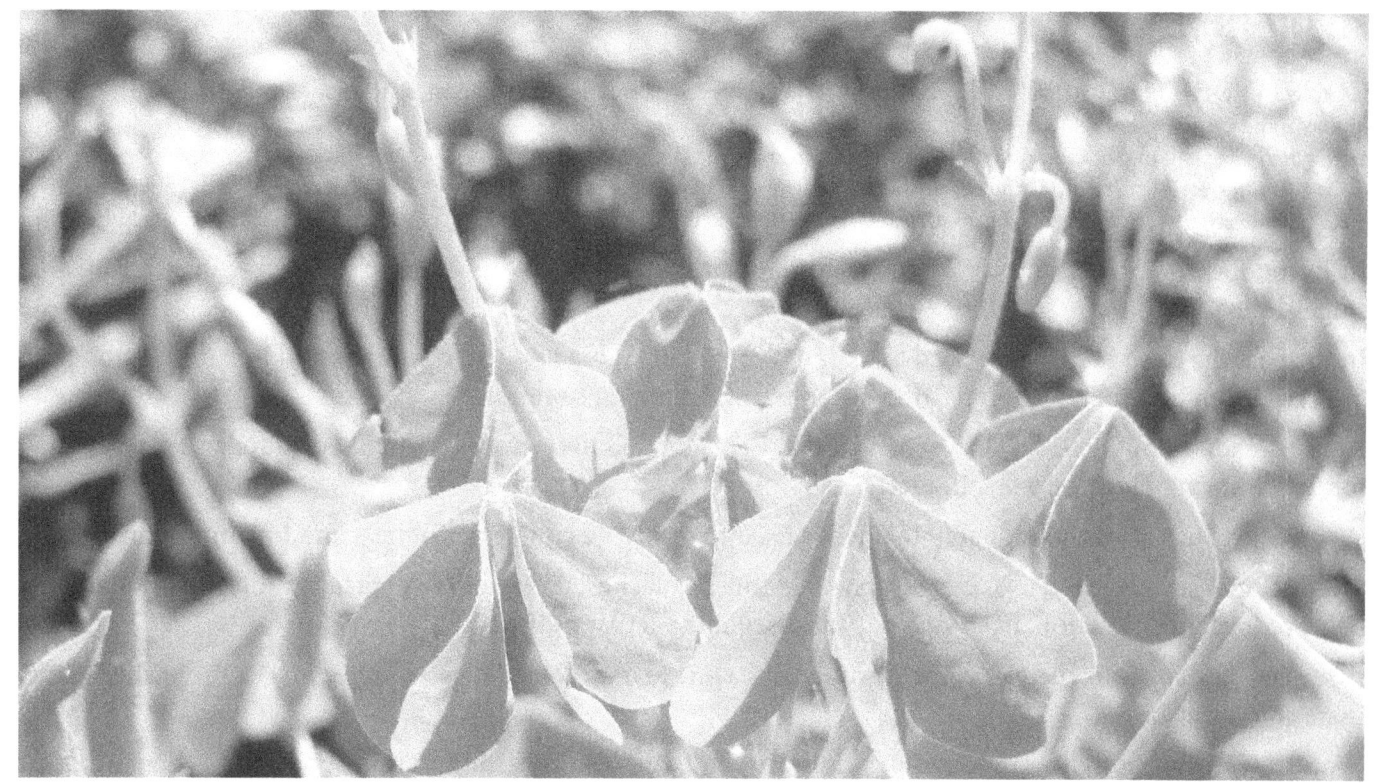

OXALIS STRICTA LEAVES

In neighboring Nepal, the plant juice is combined with butter and applied to muscular swellings, boils, pimples and other skin conditions. Taken internally, the juice is used for stomach acidity, peptic ulcer, and dyspepsia, as the leaves are good at inducing appetite.

The plant has similar usage in India, with the potherb used to treat piles and mesenteric disorders. The fresh juice is used for dyspepsia and in fevers with biliousness.

Mountain Sorrel is from a totally different genus and member the Buckwheat family. It does, however contain oxalic acid, and a sourness that reminds me of sorrel.

As the name suggests, at least in Alberta, it is confined to the foothills and montane. The plant is incredibly hardy, and thrives as far north as there is soil in which to root.

The Inuit and others fermented the leaves as a type of sauerkraut. Natives ate the hard achenes enclosed in a fleshy calyx.

The Slave call it Bear Ear, or **TSA DZI**, while the Inuit of Baffin Island call it **QUNGULIIT**. The plant is eaten to relieve stomachaches caused by too much fat intake.

Because of the sour taste, it is known as **SEERNAQ** in Greenland. As they grow larger they lose their tangy taste and become sweet, which also happens with boiling.

This is used to treat those with low energy, or to make people sweat. When chewed for a long time and the juice is gone, they are hard to swallow.

The leaves and achenes were sometimes boiled with fish roe until thick. This was then poured into small wooden frames to dry into winter cakes, or for trade.

In the early 1980s, I spent several years in Peru. On one trip to Lake Titicaca, I found the related Oca (*O. tuberosa*) growing on steep terraces alongside Maca, and Potato. Like other Sorrel, the edible tubers contain calcium oxalate. Locals dry the mature tubers in the sun for a few weeks, producing a taste similar to sweet figs.

257

MEDICINAL

CONSTITUENTS- *O. stricta*- oxalic acid (0.3-1.25%), clover acid, ascorbic acid, enzymes, hormones, beta- carotene, bioflavonoids, 4-(6'-sulfatoglucosyloxy) benzoic acid
O. digyna leaves- 40 mg vitamin C, 890 RE vitamin A, iron 3.2 mg per 100 grams
O. corniculata- aerial parts and leaves- 2"-0-(beta-D-glucopyranosyl-isovitexin), 5-hydroxy-6,7,8,4'tetramethoxyflavone; 5,7,4'trihydroxy-6,8-dimethoxyflavone, vitamin C, carotene, calcium oxalates, tartaric and citric acid, as well as malic acid in stems.

In Europe, Wood Sorrel was used to treat liver and various digestive disorders associated with overeating or sluggishness.

In the past the fresh plants were used to treat not only scurvy, but applied to wounds and inflamed gums. As a poultice it can be applied to lumps, brown spots and malignant tumors.

A paste made from the freshly bruised plant that is evaporated in the sun, is combined with dandelion extract, for the cleansing of cancerous skin ulcers.

Wood Sorrel has a cold sour quality that lends itself to resolving conditions of heat and inflammation.

This includes stomach and liver congestion including headaches, fevers and hyperacidity. Intestinally, the plant helps reduce inflammation, fight infection, and begin the repair of tissue.

It awakens the appetite, reduces vomiting and nausea due to a weakened digestive system. For simple heartburn use a cold infusion.

Wood sorrel is mainly used for acute conditions, and when skin rashes, painful boils and other inflamed conditions of the skin occur due to blood toxemia.

According to Steven Buhner, the plant has a long history of use by indigenous peoples for the treatment of cancer, particularly skin cancers.

Oxalis ointment, manufactured by Weleda, is produced from the mother tincture, and rubbed into the stomach and intestinal region for cramping, and pain.

Wood Sorrel infusions, taken at room temperature, are a good diuretic.

Like Sorrel, and other docks containing oxalic acid, the plant helps prevent depositing of calculi in the gall bladder or kidneys; and even preventing the hardening of arteries associated with mineral deposition.

It will not help an existing problem, as oxalic acid will aggravate calcium oxalate stones by stimulating their breakdown and release them too quickly. For those prone to this constitutional tendency, it can be a useful preventative. Some herbalists recommend angelica seeds, leaves, or stems be added to neutralize the acidity.

Oxalates are soluble in water as sodium oxalate or potassium oxalate and often accompanied with high concentrations of calcium.

They are normal part of diet and much ado has been written, with great ignorance, about oxalate poisoning. John Kallas in his *Edible Wild Plants* explains the issue with great intelligence, pages 375-378.

Wood Sorrel, when taken warm, will promote expectoration, remove intestinal parasites, and bring on delayed menstruation.

Peter Holmes, in his excellent book, *The Energetics of Western Herbs*, suggests that Wood Sorrel be utilized both internally and externally on the spine, to treat Parkinson's disease.

Creeping Wood Sorrel is used in Traditional Chinese Medicine for its cool and sour properties that help clear fever, reduce swelling, resolve clots and bruises, as well as treat urinary tract infections, and enteritis.

Some unusual names for the herb are **LAO YA TS'AO**, Old Crow Grass, **LEI KUNG CHIEN**, Thunder God's Scissors, and **WANG KUA SUAN** meaning, Cucumber Sour.

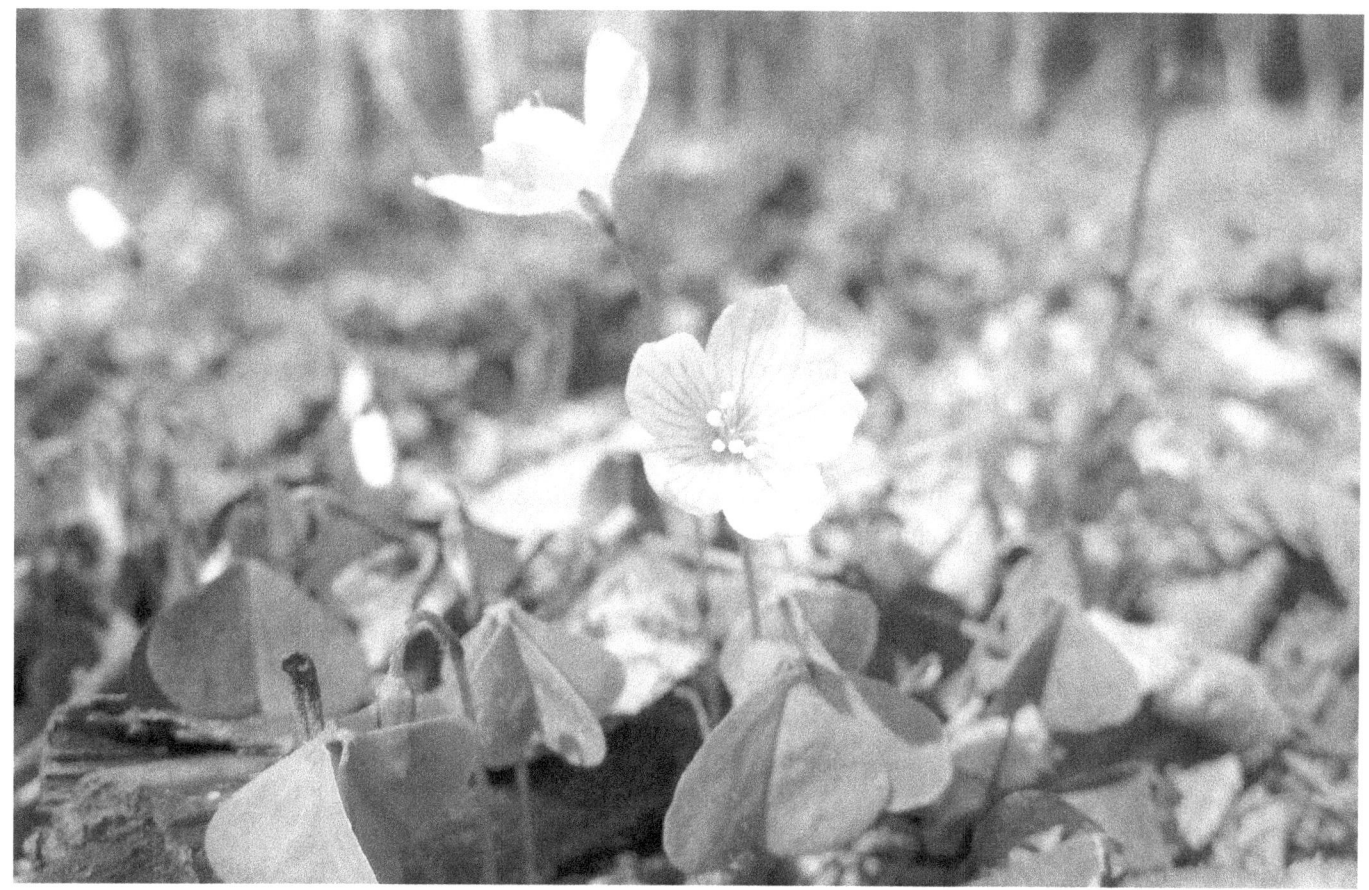

OXALIS MONTANA (formerly *O. acetosella*)

Creeping Wood Sorrel has been shown active against *Staphylococcus aureus*. The fresh juice shows activity against gram-positive bacteria, while water extracts inhibit *Micrococcus pyogenes* var. *aureus*.

Water extracts also inhibit yeast such as *Aspergillus niger* and *Pestalotiopsis theae*. Iqbal et al, *Pak J Biol Sci* 2001 4:7.

It is useful for prevention of uroliathasis. Laikangbam et al, *J Food Ag Envir* 2009 7:2.

The herb shows significant activity against *Proteus mirabilis, E. coli, Pseudomonas stutzeri* and *Klebsiella pneumoniae*, bacteria associated with promotion of stone formation via alkalization of urine. Work by Rehman A et al, *Int J Anal Chem* 2015:842468 found extracts active against *E. coli, Shigella dysenteriae, Salmonella typhi* and *Bacillus subtilis*, as well as various fungi.

Methanol extracts of *O. corniculata* show anti-cancer activity against liver (Hep2) cell lines. Salahuddin H et al, *Cell Mol Biol* (Noisy-le-grand) 2016 62(5):60-3.

The herb protects the myocardium from ischemic damage through anti-oxidant and anti-hyper-lipidemic activity. Abhilash et al, *Exp Tox Pathol* 2011 63(6):535-4.

Various studies suggests its benefit in kidney and liver toxicity.

A great review is by Badwaik et al, *Int J Phytomedicine* 2011 3:1.

Bush's Yellow Wood Sorrel has shown activity against *S. aureus* and *E. coli*.

Embelin, a benzoquinone, identified in *O. erythrorhiza* shows inhibitory effect on MRSA, methicillin resistant *Staphylococcus aureus*, as well as *E. coli*, and various fungi. It has cytotoxic effect on human lung fibroblasts.

This plant is used in Argentina to treat heart complaints related to Chagas' disease.

HOMEOPATHY

Wood Sorrel (*Oxalis acetosella*) is indicated for burning stomach pains, diarrhea, or liver problems with dyspepsia. Vomiting is sour and makes the teeth feel blunt, as in duodenal and gastric ulcer.

Angina pectoris, with sharp sticking pains in the left epigastrium and thorax, and suspicion of duodenal ulcers.

Proving by Dr. Riley in 1993 includes dizziness that is worse on waking and worse during heat.

Anxiety attacks and sweating. Tachycardia, fears of being poisoned or of impending disease. Dreams of slowly, and softly, falling.

Painful sore throat, diminished appetite, and flushes of heat in the forehead. There is increased perspiration, and swelling and stiffness of the lower extremities. Swollen feet worse at onset of menses.

He used seventeen provers at 12c potency. In one prover strange dissociative perceptions were found. "Car and driver seemed to be two distinct entities moving in separate though parallel space-time continuums. People walking in street seemed to be moving in unrelated random patterns."

DOSE- Mother tincture is prepared from the fresh plant in flower of *O. acetosella*.

Douglass in his *Characteristics of the Homeopathic Materia Medica* 1901 lists this Oxalis illusion.

"On first getting into bed, abdomen and thighs feel as though a cold, wet cloth were about them. When the eyes are shut he imagines that his abdomen and the head above the eyes are shaped like a gigantic semi-circular fungus. When the eyes are open, in a light room, the illusion vanishes, only to return the moment the eyes are closed."

HYDROSOL

Wood sorrel is more effectual in hindering putrefaction of blood, and ulcers in the mouth and body, and to quench thirst, to strengthen a weak stomach, to procure an appetite, to stay vomiting, and very excellent in any contagious sickness or pestilential fevers. The syrup made of the juice, is effectual in all the cases aforesaid, and so is the distilled water of the herb.   **CULPEPPER**

FLOWER ESSENCES

Aleluia (*Oxalis corniculata*) flower essence is for those who lost hope facing an adverse situation, as in a long, serious illness or confinement. They no longer believe they can be healed; and are generally apathetic.

Creeping Wood Sorrel can also be used in an emergency situation, when hope is lost.

FLORAIS DE MINAS

Oxalis (*O. ptychoclada*) flower essence is for things that "have you by the throat" and appear to be so overpowering that there looks like no way out.   **BAILEY**

RECIPES

FRESH PLANT TINCTURE- 10-30 drops up to three times daily for mild liver congestion. Use 90 drops three times daily as a diuretic.

COLD INFUSION- This is actually a hot infused tea, left to cool down. Drink one half cup three times daily for heartburn, and other digestive complaints.

LEMONADE- Use 30 grams of fresh leaves to one litre of water and 500 grams of sugar or honey. Let it ferment for 24 hours at 20° C, strain and refrigerate.

CAUTION- Wood Sorrel is contraindicated in cases of gout, and kidney stones. Maybe.

WESTERN YAMPA
FALSE CARAWAY
GAIRDNER'S YAMPAH
(***Perideridia gairdneri*** [Hook. & Arn.] Matthias)
COMMON YAMPAH
(***P. gairdneri* ssp. *borealis*** T. I. Chuang & Constance)
(***P. montana*** (Blank.) Dom) not accepted
(***Carum gairdneri*** Blank.) not accepted
(***Atenia gairdneri*** [Blank.] Rydb.) not accepted
PARTS USED- root, leaf, seeds

Sahcargarmeah gathered a quantity of the roots of a species of fennel (*P. gairdneri*) which we found very agreeable food, the flavor of this root is not unlike anis seed and they dispel the wind which the roots called Cows (*Lomatium* sp.) and quawmash (Camas) are apt to create particularly the latter, we also boil a small onion (*Allium geyeri*) which we find in great abundance, with other roots and find them also an antidote to the effects of the others, the mush of roots we find adds much to the comfort of our diet. **MERIWETHER LEWIS**

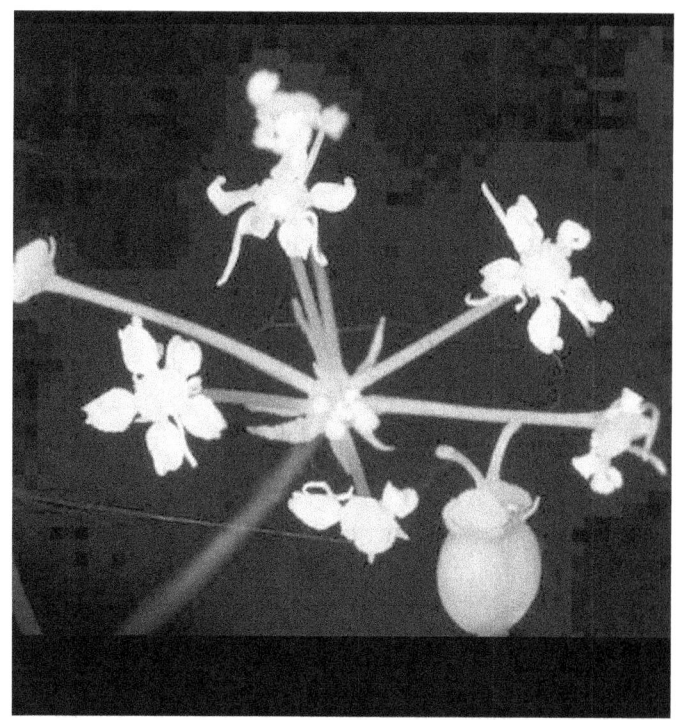

EASTERN YAMPA FLOWERS
(Courtesy southeasternflora.com)

Perideridia was name given by Heinrich Reichenbach of Dresden. It may be derived from the Greek **PERI**, meaning around, and **DERIS**, leather coat; referring to the dark, tough coated root, or around the neck bracts under umbels. Or it may be from the Latin **DERIDERE**, meaning to laugh, deride or make fun of. No one is sure.

Gairdneri is named after the surgeon and plant collector Meredith Gairdner who worked for the Hudson's Bay Company and collected many plants of the Northwest. He was born in London, and died in Hawaii.

Yampa has small white flowers borne in umbels like other members of the parsley family. The single, wiry stem is 1-3 feet tall, and often obscured by tall grass until flowering. It is a very common perennial in the dry woods and meadows of the southern prairies.

The small, oblong root is striped brown, purple and tan, and shaped like a large peanut, hence the Blackfoot name, Double Root, or disparaging Squaw Root. The Crow tribe call it split root or **BIKKA:SAHTE**.

The stem break off easily from root, so some care is needed to harvest successfully.

The roots are crunchy and sweet, resembling water chestnut in texture and taste. They can be steamed or baked, or even eaten raw. Natives dug up the roots in May and June, and sometimes dried the cooked roots, and mixed them with powdered deer meat as a special treat.

The Southern Okanagan used to boil them with Saskatoon berries, and Black Tree Lichen to make a thick pudding. On the coast it was known as Yampa, Ipo, or Sa'hweet.

They were stored raw for winter by packing them into an earth pit lined with pine needles or cottonwood bark to protect from frost and rodents.

The seeds can be gathered and used as a condiment like wild caraway, their close relative, when fresh. After parching, they were added to cooked gruels and grains. The leaves are edible.

The Blood used the fresh roots of "double turnip or double root" as a food, and also saved it for boiling in blood or broth for soups, etc. It was sometimes called wild caraway, due to the smell and resemblance to that plant.

The Blood used the roots for coughs, sore throats and trouble with the liver or urine.

The Blackfoot call it **NIITSIKAPA'S**. They chewed the raw roots, or boiled them and used the left over water for sore throats.

They poulticed the roots and applied them to the skin to draw inflammation from swellings. The children often made snacks of them while playing on the prairie.

The plant was rubbed on arrows to make them shine, and for waterproofing. The Buffalo runners chewed the root to help their endurance and keep a moist mouth.

The root was infused and given as a diuretic and mild laxative internally, or applied externally to sores and wounds.

Root infusions were used to counteract the cathartic and emetic effects of Bracted Honeysuckle berry (*Lonicera involucrata*) infusions.

Women used to treat sore breasts, often with a massage using warm stones.

The root was either chewed or infused for sore throats, or decocted as an expectorant for the lungs.

A lazy horse would be given the root to chew, for enlivening it, probably due to increased sugars. Maybe. Recent anthelmintic research suggests western yampa may be useful for controlling nematode load in animals. Acharya J et al, *Vet Parasitol* 2014 201(1-1):75-81.

Root infusions would be poured into nostrils to treat nasal gleet. The horse would snort and remove the pus.

The root was sometimes smudged and the smoke inhaled for nagging coughs. Or the powdered root was snuffed to relieve nasal congestion.

The Cheyenne call it "four grow together", or **ANO-NEVE-E?TOSE**. The roots were gathered in May or June, and eaten fresh or dried for winter. They were either scraped fine and dried, or were dried whole, or cooked, dried and later pulverized. A mush was prepared by pouring hot soup over the crushed root.

It was often combined with balsamroot, stems and leaves and boiled together as an unspecified medicine.

The tubers have a sweet, nutty, creamlike flavor; said by some people to be the best tasting wild roots in the mountains. In parts of California, the roots were at one time, sold by the tin cup full, and eaten like popcorn at rodeos and ceremonies.

The introduction of sheep and cattle to the plains has decimated the plant population.

CONSTITUENTS

Dry matter (% of fresh wt)	37.14
Total protein (% of dry wt)	8.35
Total fat (% of dry wt)	1.61
Starch (% of dry wt)	69.36
Total sugar (% of dry wt)	16.19
Fiber (% of dry wt)	5.25
Vitamin A (I.U. fresh wt)	122
Vitamin C (mg/100 g fresh)	11.22
Potassium (% of dry weight)	1.29

As can be seen, the Vitamin C content is 3 times that of apple, and a potassium content 10 times greater. Even its vitamin A content is 25% more than apples.

Yampa root is rich in methionine, cystine isoleucine, valine, alanine and proline.

Quality of protein can be expressed in a number of ways. Biological value, net protein utilization, protein efficiency ratio or protein score. Each has limitations.

When compared to the ideal egg protein, with a score of 100, the most limiting amino acid determines the protein score.

The protein score for Yampa root is 81, as compared with 58 for Jerusalem Artichoke, and 36 for Indian Breadroot covered elsewhere.

By comparison, protein scores for soybean is just 57, potato 70, corn 56, and beans, 42.

Yampah therefore, has exceptionally high quality protein.

Considering its hardiness, and exceptional food value, it would be a good choice for introduction into the natural, organic food market.

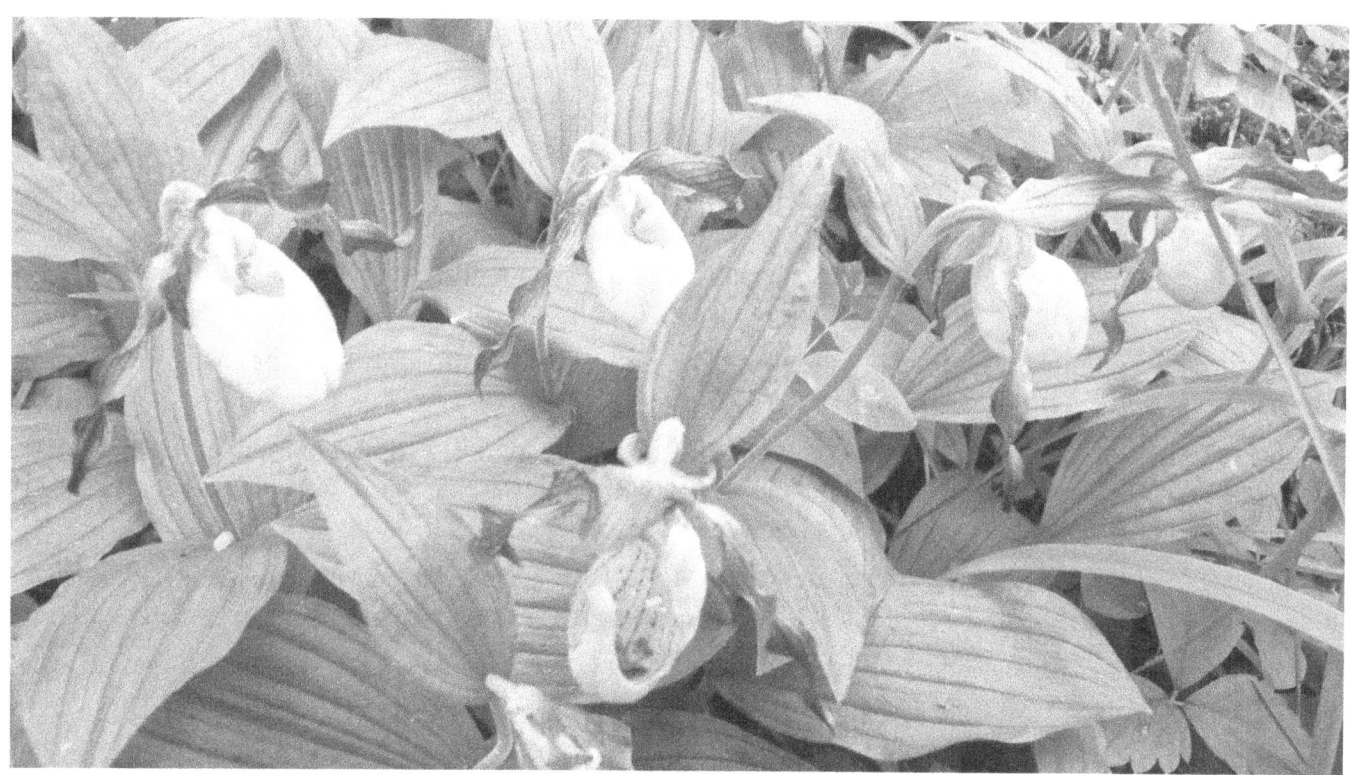

YELLOW LADY'S SLIPPER

YELLOW LADY'S SLIPPER
MOCCASIN PLANT
(*Cypripedium calceolus* L.)
LESSER LADY'S SLIPPER
(*C. parviflorum* Salisb.)
(*C. calceolus var. parviflorum* [Salisb.] Fern) not accepted
MOUNTAIN LADY'S SLIPPER
(*C. montanum* Dougl. ex Lindl.)
SPARROW'S EGG LADY'S SLIPPER
(*C. passerinum* Richards.)
PINK LADY'S SLIPPER
STEMLESS LADY'S SLIPPER
(*C. acaule* Aiton.)
(*C. humile* Salisb.) not accepted
(*C. hirsutum* Mill.) not accepted
(*Fissipes acaulis* [Aiton] Small) not accepted
PARTS USED- root

"The Cypripedium with her changeful hues
As she were doubtful which array to choose."
Where Cinderella dropped her shoe,
'Tis said in fairy tales of yore,
'Twas first the lady's slipper grew
And there its rosy blossom bore.
And ever since, in woodlands gray,
It marks where spring retreating flew,
Where speeding on her eager way,
She left behind her dainty shoe.

ELAINE G. EASTMAN

Cypripedium is from the Latin **KYPRIS**, a name for Venus, goddess of love and beauty; and **PEDILON** or **PODION** for slipper, sock, buskin or foot, referring to the shape of the flower lip. Linnaeus, the founder of today's botanical system, named it *Kupris podeion*, literally meaning Aphrodite's boot. Kupris was Aphrodite's ancient name on Cyprus, where she was created and born from foam off the seashore. Hansen gave it a twist calling it *Kypris pedion* that translates as "the genital area of Aphrodite."

Cypripedium is a grammatical error, and should be Cyripedilum. It will probably never be changed. Moccasin is corrupted from the Native American **MA'KASIN**.

Calceolus means "small shoe", referring to the pouch formed by one of the petals. Montanum means mountain, while Passerinum means "of sparrows", as the purple spots on the flower's lip reminded botanists of a bird's egg. Acaule means stem-less in reference to basal leaves.

Orchids have mesmerized humans throughout history. Marcel Proust equated them with harlots and homosexuals, and George Bernard Shaw said describing a woman as orchiaceous was to suggest that she behaved like a courtesan.

Various cultures have connected orchids with sultry sex, and the wicked female, especially in Victorian England. See personality traits below.

By contrast, the American naturalist, Henry David Thoreau believed orchids revealed the divine essence of nature. But then again, he was a life-long bachelor.

Yellow Lady's Slipper is one of the most beautiful orchids of the Northern Boreal forest. To see a whole mat of them in the wild is one of life's great joys. They are a rare and endangered plant that should not be picked.

Nor does it easily transplant to the backyard garden, due to the symbiotic nature of its environment, and various fungal and microbial contents of the soil. Leave it where you find it. Mature plants can be up to forty years of age, and it may take up to seventeen years from seed to first bloom. Take time to smell the flowers, which have a soft rose-like perfume.

Various native tribes used the root for female disorders or inducing dreams of the supernatural, including them in various love potions.

The Cree used the whole plant to treat female disorders, and the root specifically in nerve tonics. It is known as **WAPAKWANIY** (orchid), or the Blessed Virgin's shoe, **KIHCITWA-MARIE OMASKISIN**.

The Cherokee used root decoctions for spasms, fits, and hysterical affections; as well as females "weak from the rigors of childbirth".

Hot infusions were used to break flu, by inducing sweat. They call it **U TSU WODI** or Moccasin flower, or **OO KA OU LA SU LO**, meaning Nerve Root.

The Lakota call it **MAKA CANAKPA** meaning, "earth groin swelled up".

Mountain Lady's Slipper is a rare white and purple tinged orchid of the mountains and foothills. It is threatened and should not be picked. In fact, none should be picked.

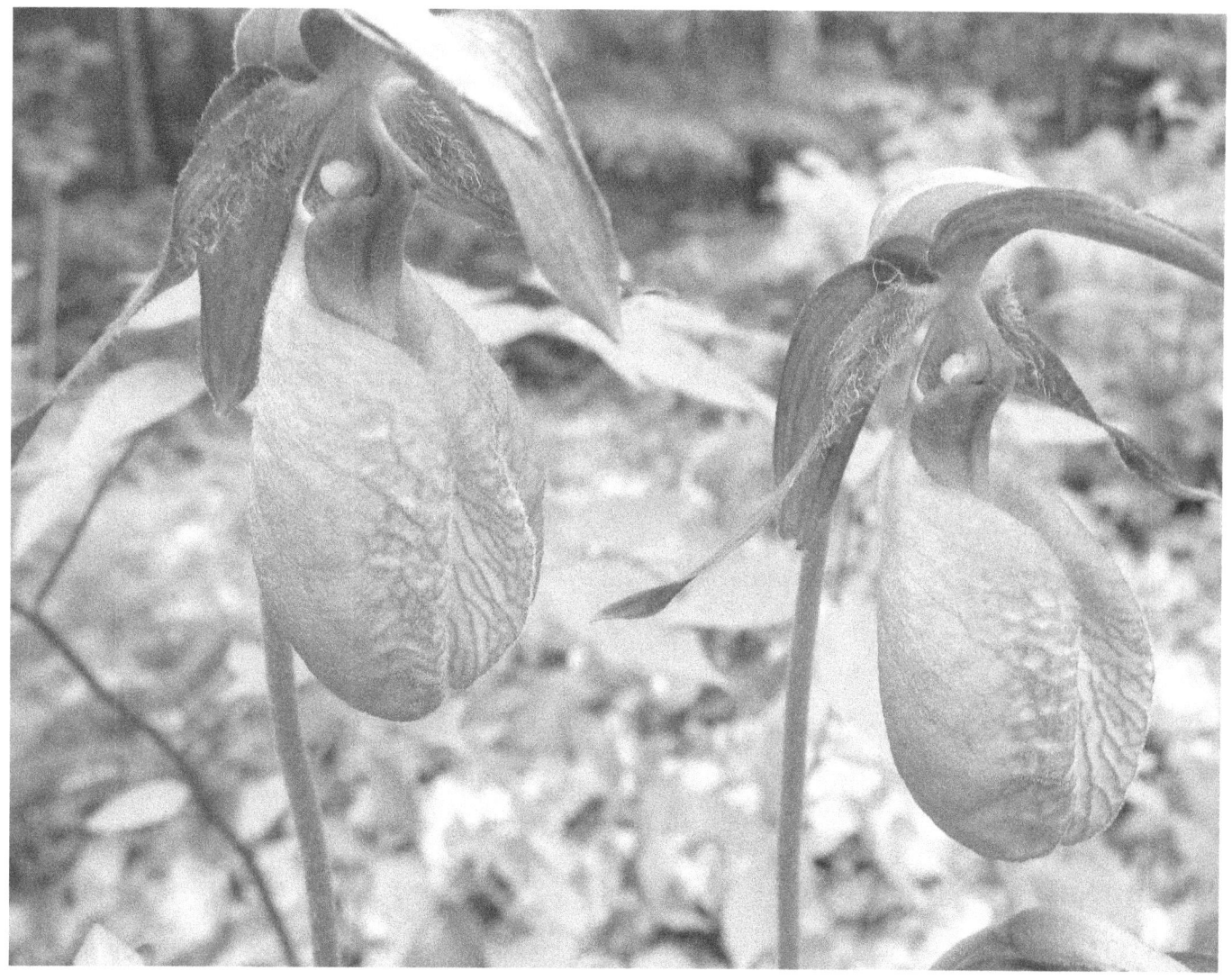

PINK LADY'S SLIPPER

Sparrow's Egg Lady's Slipper is a rare and protected species of the boreal forest.

It was prized by the Slave, of northern Canada, as a "girl medicine" love charm. A single strand of the girl's hair was tied about the stem, and was carried next to a man's heart. It is called **TSELLI NAYDI**, meaning girl, or little one medicine.

Symbolically, Lady's Slipper means Capricious Beauty. Win me and wear me.

Pink or Stemless Lady's Slipper is the only one with basal leaves, and a pink, deeply grooved pouch like lip with purple veins.

It is rare, and the provincial floral emblem of my birth province of Prince Edward Island.

The Menominee used the root for male problems associated with the urinary system, and as a love potion and sedative.

Work by Primack and Hall at Boston University have found that when Pink Lady's Slipper blooms and flowers, the leaf size is 13% smaller next year. It may take up to four years for a plant to fully recover from flowering.

Dr. Douglas Gill, U of Maryland, studied three thousand pink lady's slippers over 16 years, and found only one thousand flowered. Of these, just twenty-three plants were successfully pollinated, by bees. Once pollinated, however, a single flower can produce up to sixty thousand tiny seeds.

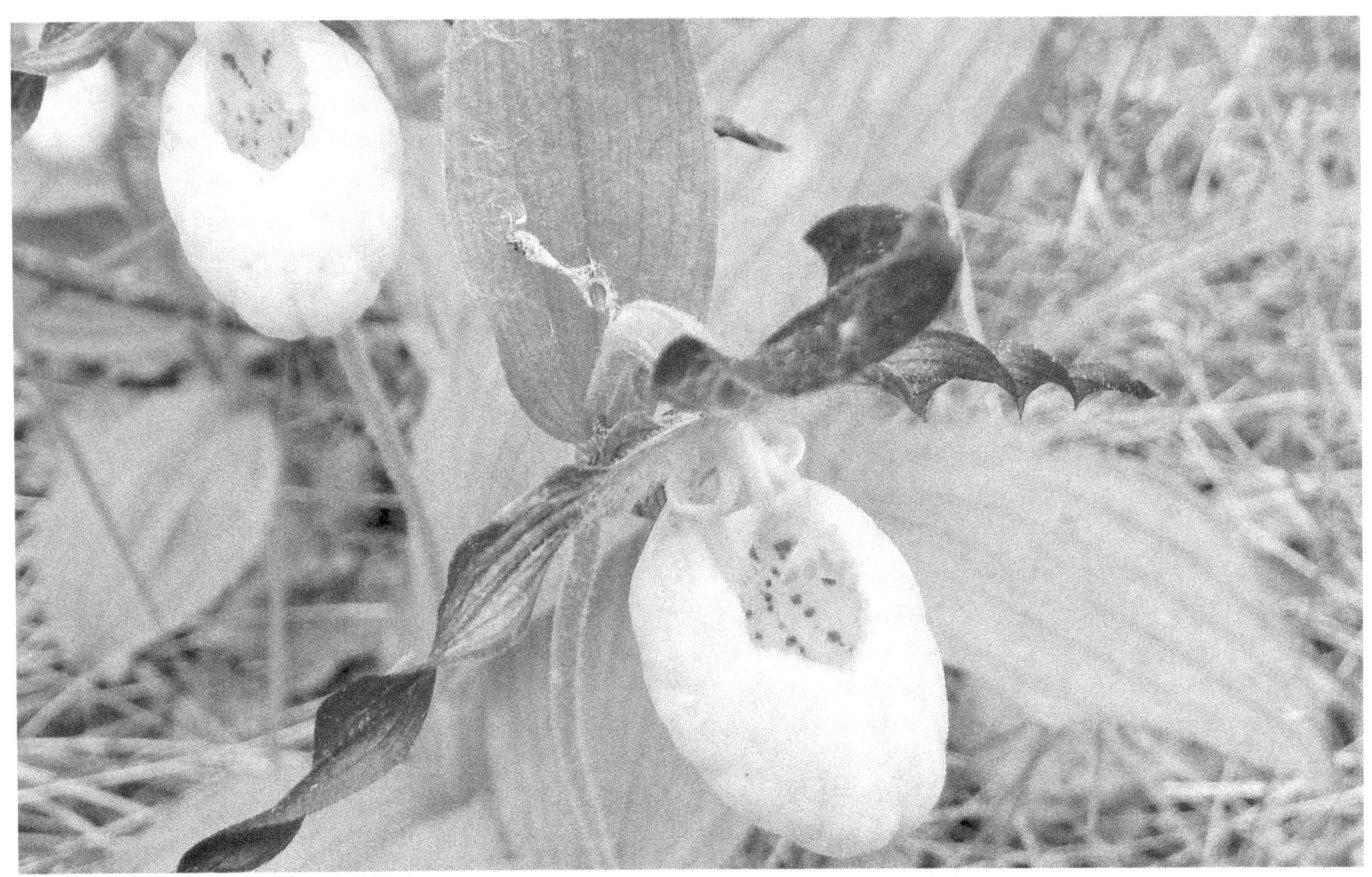

YELLOW LADY'S SLIPPER

MEDICINAL

CONSTITUENTS- root- Essential oils, resins, quinones, tannins, glycosides, Phenanthrene quinones, including cypripedin, tannins, trace minerals, gallic acid, myelin (?)
stem- raphides, quinone.

Yellow lady's slipper is almost a pure nervine that is safe and effective in large doses. The root is a nerve calmative and restorative, at the same time.

It relaxes internal spasms that are due to tension, and the internal trembling that sometimes accompanies stress, grief, anxiety and depression.

It has a bitter, cool nature that helps replenish deficient conditions of the nerves after a prolonged illness, such as post-influenza depression.

It is similar in many ways to black cohosh, scullcap and bugleweed; and yet in some patients, particularly women, it works better for lifting the spirit and ridding melancholy, like no other remedy.

Yellow lady's slipper root combines well with cramp bark for painful menstruation, relaxing the uterine spasms, and some cases of menorrhagia. It works well as a douche and wash for pruritis vulvae, or chronic vaginal itching. It works well in certain cases of nervous headache, and nervous depression that is associated with stomach disorders.

It combines well with scullcap and green-flowering oats for various nerve disorders including hysteria, headaches and low fevers. Lady's slipper is a specific antidote to caffeine poisoning. When you drink too much coffee on Sunday morning, for example.

266

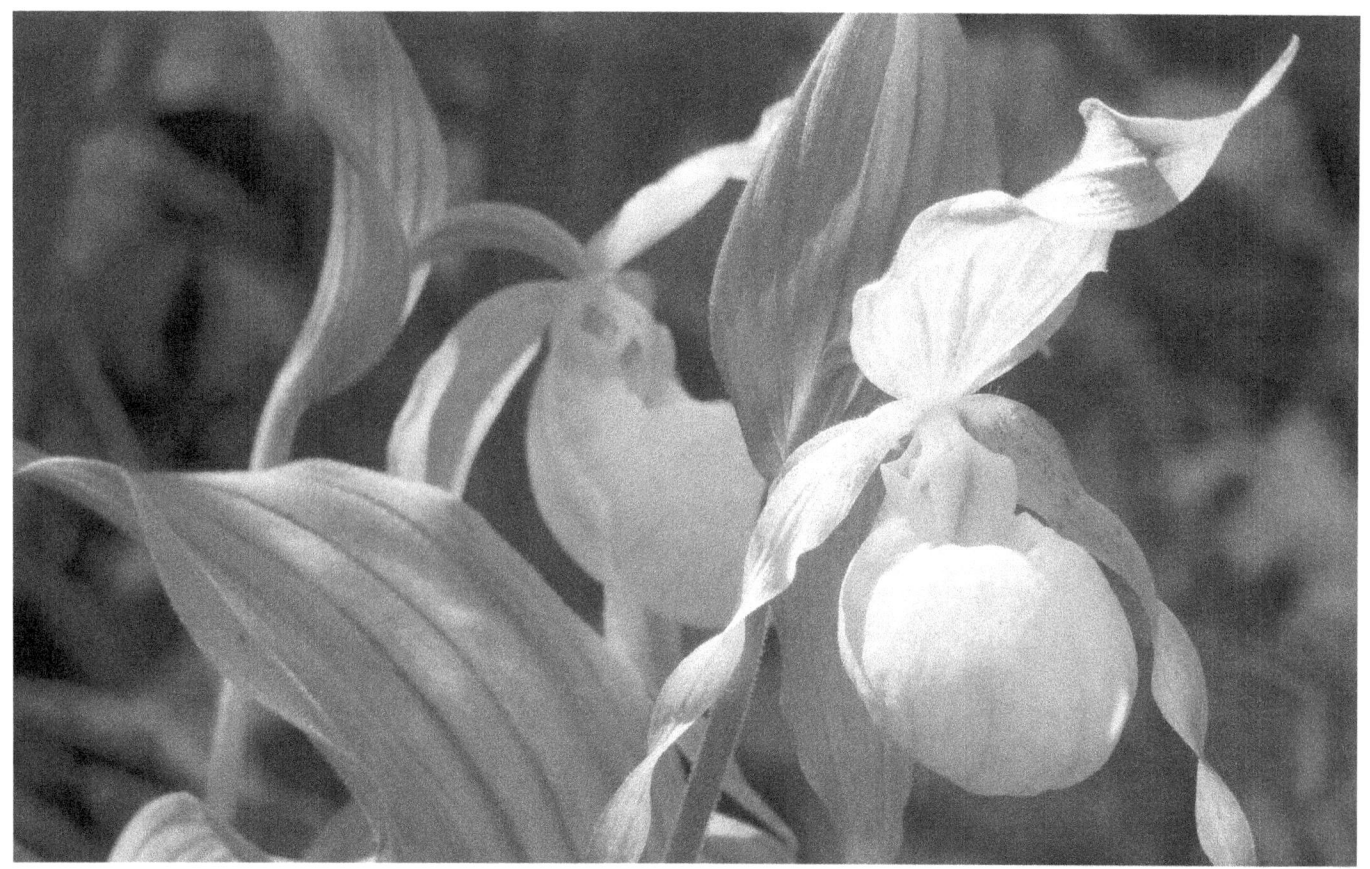

YELLOW LADY'S SLIPPER

Quinone, one of its constituents, may cause allergic reaction in some individuals, or cause contact dermatitis, according to research by Schmalle and Hausen, 1979.

In vitro studies have shown fluid extracts weakly active as a uterine relaxant.

Early work by a Dr. Nester extracted "myelin" from the plant; a compound also found in ginkgo seed and cayenne fruit. Cypripedin is anti-spasmodic and muscle relaxant.

Dr. King noted Pink Lady's Slipper is said, "to possess more narcotic properties than the others, especially when inhabiting dark swamps."

Moerman also contributes. "The roots have been used for menstrual disorders, venereal disease, stomach aches, kidney troubles of children, urinary tract problems, neuralgia and other pains, worms, spasms and fits, colds and flu, nervousness and male disorders. The Iroquois bound a poultice of smashed leaves to the bite of a mad dog."

HOMEOPATHY

Yellow Lady's Slipper infusion, in a healthy human being, causes firstly an improvement in mental function and the whole nervous activity, following which a great tranquility is observed, which finally proceeds to a considerable fatigue of the mind and body.

Cypripedium is particularly effective in nervous women, whose nerves are affected by illness or by abuse of tea and coffee. However, it is also recommended in consequences of mental over-exertion, night watching and exhaustion of the nervous system in influenza. Debility after gouty attacks is also relieved.

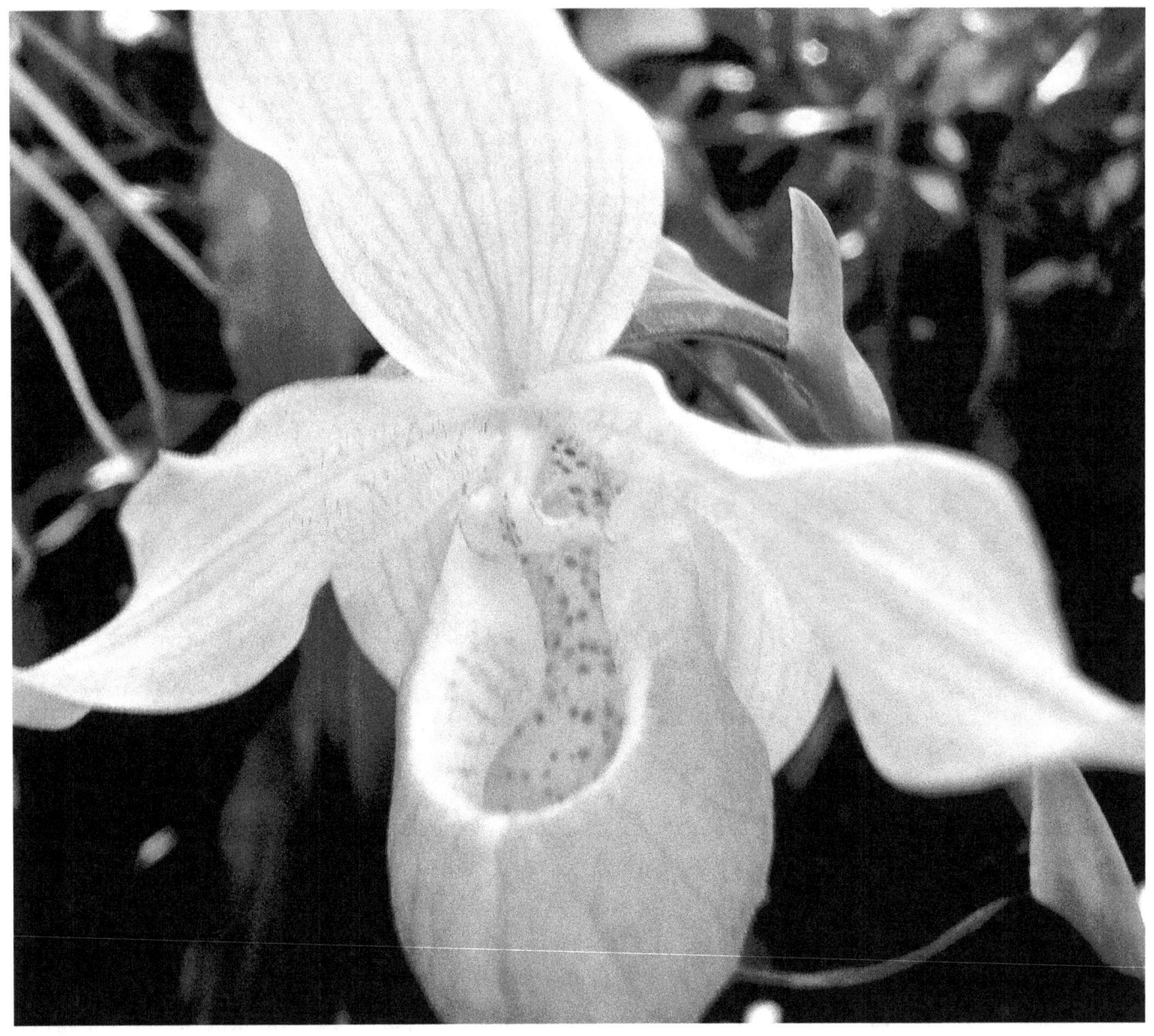

PINK LADY'S SLIPPER

It can also relieve headaches suffered both premenstrual and during the menopausal transition.

It can also be beneficial in teething complaints of children with symptoms of cerebral irritation and incipient meningitis.

The skin symptoms are similar to those of poisoning by Rhus (poison ivy), for which it has been found an efficient antidote.

DOSE- Mother tincture to sixth potency. For poison ivy, use 5 drops of tincture in water applied locally. The mother tincture is prepared from the fresh rootstock gathered in autumn. Clinical observations by Hale, Boericke, Hering and others based on use by Native Americans and Eclectics.

Pink lady slipper (*C. humile*) exhibits vertigo, has to sit down, followed by heaviness and dragging of left food. Acute stitches are in under part of toes in right foot. Severe pain in right foot, along inner margin, and an hour later, very severe in front part of left foot.

DOSE- Mother tincture. Based on fragmentary self-experimentation by Kummer of tincture. Prepared from fresh root in fall. Now known as *C. acaule*.

FLOWER ESSENCE

Pink Lady's Slipper (*C. acaule*) flower essence carries the paradox of the plant, for although this flower is one of exquisite delicateness and rare beauty, it is also one that contains a powerful vibration. It is as if the plant is able to act as a focal point for the mysterious power of the forest. Those people who feel a knowledge or wisdom within them or a deep love or joy, but feel reluctant to express this part of them will benefit from Lady's Slipper.

DALTON

SPIRITUAL PROPERTIES

But perhaps the most effective medicine of all "made" from Lady's Slippers is found simply in its company and distilled at the place of its origin- the fields, bogs and thickets that it once populated so abundantly. Here, in the quiet of its home, there emanates a deep and rewarding peace, likened to that found in the finest of nature's cathedrals, the old growth forest.

GLADSTAR

Lady's Slipper affects people on two essential levels. One of these is the level by which the feet come in contact with the Earth- the way the Earth speaks to you by motion. This enhances the ability to achieve a trance state while dancing, called trance dance.

It also makes it easier to achieve ecstatic states brought on by Sufi dancing and other similar techniques. Individuals who seek greater energy through the feet will find this accelerated and assisted by the energy of the plant.

The other spiritual effect is what happens to this energy. It is not only achieving a deeper trance state and a willingness to experience God's energy in such a state, but to utilize it in a way of fluid grace- a way the Earth is connected through your being to God, and together God and the Earth dance through you. A gentleness and grace may be achieved. There is greater ability to understand the value of dance.

The cancer and heavy metal miasms are eased. Positive aspects between the Moon and Venus are excellent indicators for using this herb.

GURUDAS

PERSONALITY TRAITS

The story of Dorothy and the Wizard of Oz illustrates some of the psychological properties of Lady's Slipper.

Dorothy grew fretful about the limiting circumstances of her life on a farm with her uncle and aunt. She wandered away from the farm. Then a tornado came and deposited her in the Land of Oz.

The first thing that happened there was that she received a pair of magical shoes, which protected her from the wicked witch. Then she set off on a path, the Yellow Brick Road. When she arrived at her destination she received the solution to her problem: " There's no place like home".

That's the message of Yellow Lady's Slipper: When the shoe fits, wear it. At times it will seem like a prison, but there is a path and we need to follow it in order to reach a destination, which will fit us.

WOOD

Another famous fairy tale illustrating the qualities of Lady's Slipper is Cinderella. Here we find the adolescent dreams of glory, the refinement of the romantic nature, the self-doubt, and the "right fit".

The young girl meets the prince at a ball, he falls in love, but in a fit of anxiety she runs away. Only her shoe is left, so the prince has to set off to find the woman who is the perfect fit for it.

WOOD

The color of the lip of (Yellow Lady's Slipper) is a lively canary yellow, dashed with deep crimson spots.

The upper petals consist of two short and two long; in texture and color resembling the sheath of some of the narcissus tribe; the short ones stand erect, like a pair of ears; the long or lateral pair are three times the length of the former, very narrow, and elegantly twisted, like the spiral horns of the Walachian ram; on raising a thick yellow fleshy sort of lid in the middle of the flower, you perceive the exact face of an Indian hound, perfect in all its parts- the eyes, nose and mouth.

C. P. TRAILL

Ladie's-slipper is an orchid…Piquant, joyful, lavish in the dispensing of an intense spicey fragrance, a fragrance that strongly resembles that of lily of the valley but with more of moss and earthiness in it; more hugging than lifting.   **EMILY CARR**

So unpleasant is the encounter [with the pink lady's slipper] that the bee will be unlikely to venture near another lady's slipper. For the orchid, the bee's wariness is dangerous, because it takes two acts of insect gullibility to complete a fertilization…Few orchid plants will breed during any given year, when one is fertilized it hits pay-dirt…[producing] ten of thousands, or hundreds of thousands of seeds…Orchids can afford to wait for the perfect pollinator. They are among the longest-lived of all flowering plants, and they have very few natural enemies. As a result, far more orchids survive from one year to the next than do most plants. Suckers may come and suckers may go, but the fakers of the world are built to last.   **N. ANGIER**

ORCHID BOOKS

The Orchid Thief: A True Story of Beauty and Obsession by Susan Orlean.
The Pretty Lady by Arnold E. Bennett.
The Flowering of the Strange Orchid by H. G. Wells.
Orchids: Strange Stories by Gustav Meyrink.

MYTHS AND LEGENDS

One day, Venus, the Roman goddess of love and beauty, was out hunting with Adonis when they were overtaken by a tremendous thunderstorm. Venus and her beloved took shelter. Naturally enough, they also took full advantage of their enforced intimacy, and this led to Venus's mislaying her slipper. When the storm had passed, the slipper was spotted by a mortal who immediately went to pick it up.

Before he could touch it, Venus's slipper was transformed into a flower whose central petal, the labellum or lip, was not only shaped like a slipper, but retained the color of the gold from which the goddess's priceless shoes had been made.   **BERLIOCCHI**

There was once a little daughter of an Indian Chieftain. One day, while she was playing far away from her camp she met a rabbit that was crying. It had hurt its feet and couldn't go home. The little girl begged the rabbit to stop crying and gave it her moccasins.

It was growing late, and the child decided to return to camp. Before long her feet were sore and bleeding. She collapsed in exhaustion and fell asleep. Before long a songbird flew by, and seeing her feet, begged the Great Spirit to help the little girl.

Upon awakening, she found a beautiful pair of moccasins hanging on two slender stems. She put them on and made her way home. And if you look inside the yellow lady's slipper orchid you will see the reddish-purple spots of blood, and some lines made by the girl's bleeding feet.   **WILLARD**

RECIPES

DECOCTION- Take four ounces of lady's slipper root and soak in one litre of distilled, cold water for two hours. Bring to a boil and simmer for 15 minutes. Strain and remove liquid. Reduce over low heat to ¾ of a pint. Remove from heat and add eight ounces of vegetable glycerine while still hot for preservation.

TINCTURE- 10-30 drops as needed. The fresh root tincture is prepared 1:2 in 45% alcohol. The resultant tincture is crimson in colour, with a nauseous fecal odour, and a taste very similar to black walnut.

POWDER- 2-4 grams three times daily. Dried powder may be put in capsules.

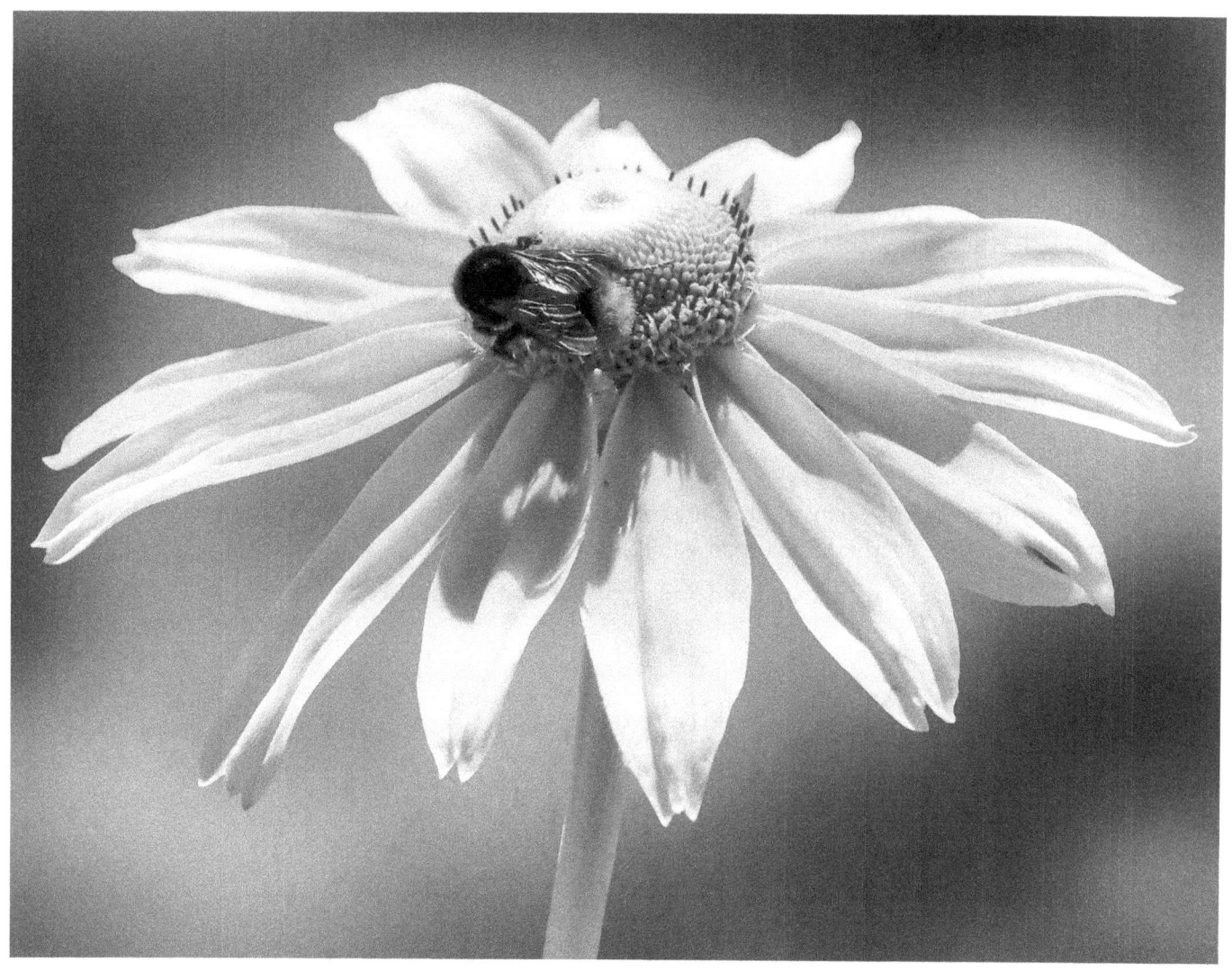

ZINNIA FLOWER

ZINNIA
(***Zinnia elegans***) not accepted
(**Z. *violacea*** Cav.)
PRAIRIE ZINNIA
(**Z. *grandiflora*** Nutt.)

Zinnia is named after Johann Gottfried Zinn, a 18th century botanist and physician, who wrote the first eye anatomy book in 1755. Elegans means youth and old age, due to how quickly it blooms, and how quickly it dies at first frost. Grandiflora means large flower.

Matilda Stevenson wrote *Ethnobotany of the Zuñi Indians* in 1915. She noted, "the entire plant is reduced to powder between stones; this is sprinkled over hot stones, beside which sits a fever patient, who inhales the fumes. This treatment is accompanied by a sweat bath, both the patient and stones with the medicine being covered with a heavy blanket."

Work by Motose et al, at the University of Tokyo reveals the presence of xylogen, an arabinogalactan protein in Zinnia. This works on some form of local intracellular communication.

The Prairie Zinnia (*Z. grandiflora*) has not been well studied. It does contain three new delta-elemanolide-type sesquiterpene lactones, zinagrandinolides A-C, as well as delta- elemanolide. All compounds exhibit strong cytotoxicity against the cancer cell lines NCI-H460 (lung), MCF-7 (breast), SF-268 (brain), and MIA PaCa-2 (pancreas). Bashyai BP et al, *J Nat Prod* 2006 69(12): 1820-2. Unfortunately, they also are cytotoxic to normal human fibroblast cell type WI-38.

When fresh, the flowers of various species can be used to give a yellow, orange or red dyestuff for wool and other natural cloth. The dried plants lose their colour, and ability to create dyes.

ESSENTIAL OILS

Zinna (*Z. elegans*) flowers have been steam distilled with germacrene D (12.4%), and p-cymene (9.1%) the major components.

FLOWER ESSENCES

Zinnia (*Z. elegans*) flower essence helps create more childlike humour and playfulness in those suffering heaviness or dullness associated with overly serious approach to life.

It also helps one experience a joyful inner child, or help bring forth a repressed inner child waiting to be heard.
FLOWER ESSENCE SOCIETY

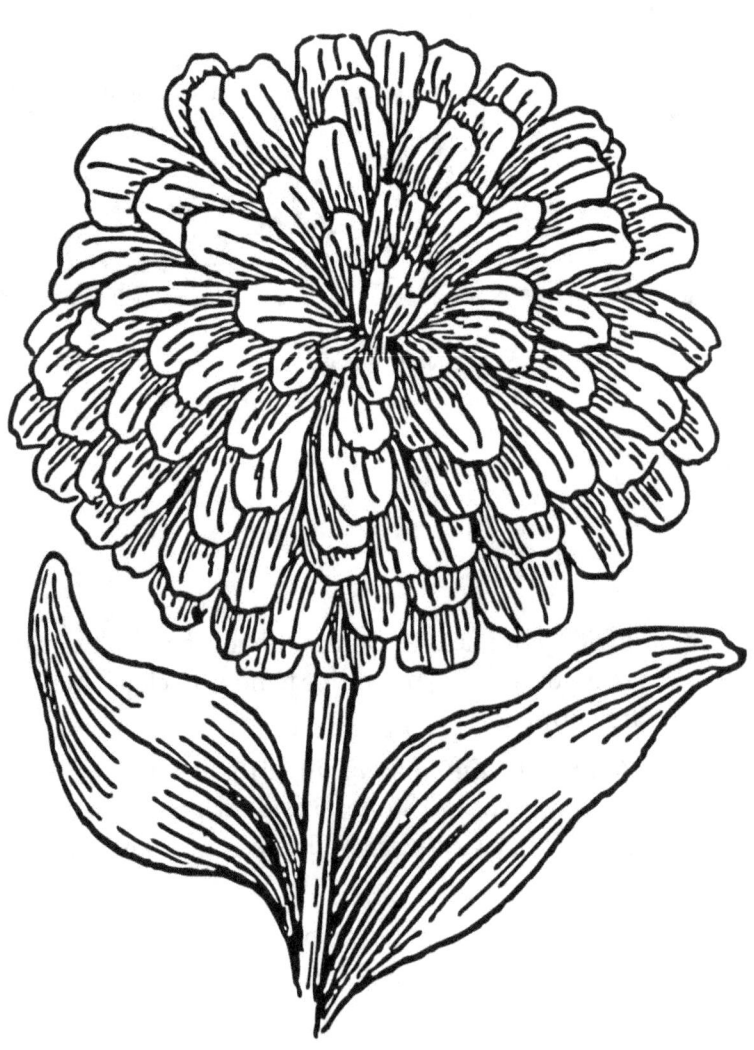

ABOUT THE AUTHOR

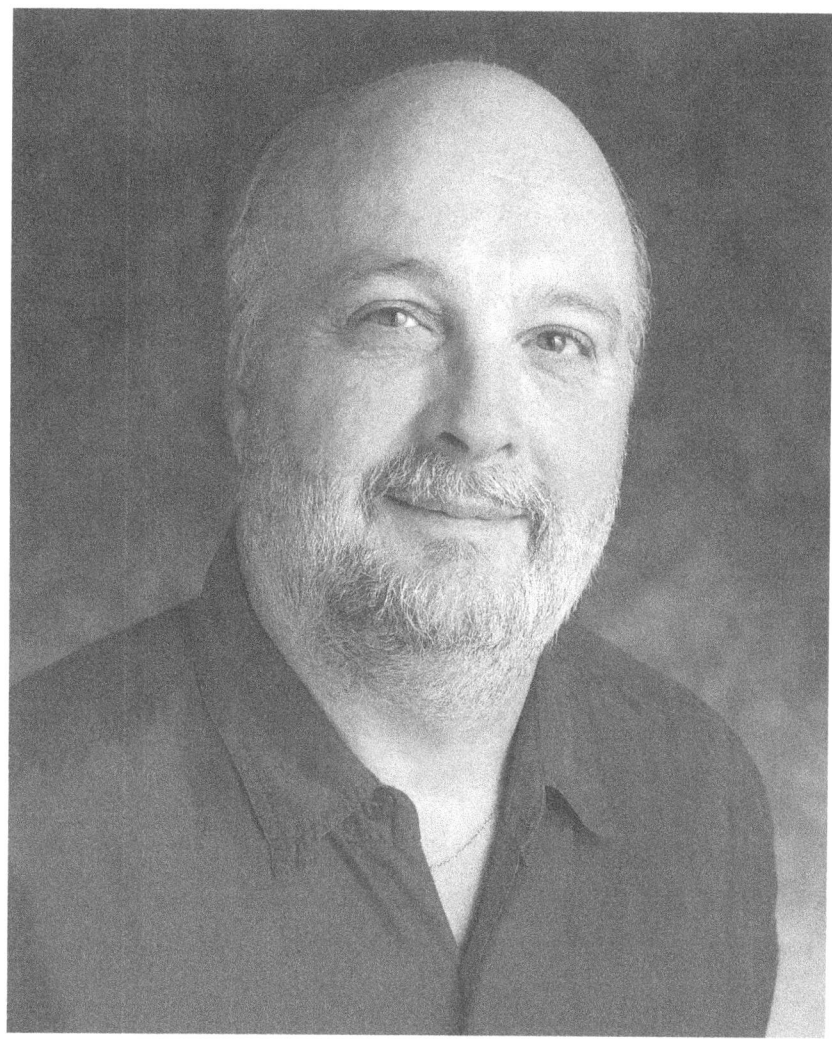

Robert Dale Rogers has been an herbalist for over forty-five years. He has a Bachelor of Science from the University of Alberta, where he is an assistant clinical professor in Family Medicine. He teaches plant medicine, including herbology and flower essences in the Earth Spirit Medicine Program at the Northern Star College of Mystical Studies in Edmonton, Alberta, Canada.

Robert is past chair of the Alberta Natural Health Agricultural Network and Community Health Council of Capital Health. He is a Fellow of the International College of Nutrition, past chair of the medicinal mushroom committee of the North American Mycological Association and on the editorial board of the International Journal of Medicinal Mushrooms. He writes occasional article for Fungi magazine.

Robert co-hosts The Alberta Herb Gathering held every second year (www.albertaherbgathering.com)

He lives on Millcreek Ravine in Edmonton with his beautiful and talented wife, Laurie Szott–Rogers and out of control cat Ceres.

You can email him at scents@telusplanet.net
or visit
www.selfhealdistributing.com

BIBLIOGRAPHY

Abbe, Elfriede, *The Fern Herbal,* Cornell University Press, Ithaca, 1981

Acorn, J. Bugs of Alberta, Lone Pine Publishing, Edmonton, AB, 2000.

Adams, J. *Les Plantes Medicinales.* Bulletin 23, Agriculture Canada. 1916

Adams, Jean. *Insect Potpourri, Adventures in Entomology.* Sandhill Crane Press, FL. 1992

Aggarwal, Bharat. Healing Spices. Sterling Pub. New York 2011.

Albert-Puleo, Michael. *Economic Botany, 32, Jan-Mar, 1978.*

Allaby, Michael. *Temperate Forests.* Facts on File. New York. 1999.

Allen, D & Hatfield, G. *Medicinal Plants in Folk Tradition.* Timber Press, Portland. 2004

Allen,E, Morrison,D, &Wallis,G. *Common Tree Diseases of B.C. Canada Forest Service,* '96

Allende, Isabel. *Aphrodite- A Memoir of the Senses.* Harper Flamingo. New York. 1998.

Alstat, Ed. *Electic Dispensatory of Botanical Therapeutics.* Ecl Med. Oregon. 1989.

Anderson, Anne, *Some Native Herbal Remedies,* Pub 8A, Devonian Botanical Gardens 1980

_____*Plants in Cree.* Duval House Pub. Edmonton AB 2000.

Anderson, C.&Tischer,T. *Poinsettias, the December Flower,* Waters Edge Press, CA, 1997

Andoh, Anthony. *The Science & Romance of Selected Herbs used in Medicine and Religious Ceremony.* North Scale Institute. San Francisco. 1986.

Andre, Alestine & Fehr, Alan. *Gwich'in Ethnobotany.* Gwich'in Social and Cultural Institute, Box 46, Tsiigehtchie, NWT, X0E 0B0, fax 1867-953-3820.

Andrews, Tamra. Nectar and Ambrosia. ABC-CLIO Box 1911 Santa Barbara CA. 2000.

Andrews, Ted. *Animal Speak- The Spiritual and Magical Powers,* Llewellyn. Minn. 1996.

_____*Animal Wise,* DragonHawk, Jackson, TN, 1999.

Antol, Marie. *The Incredible Secrets of Mustard.* Avery Pub. New York. 1999.

Aronson J K Ed. Meyler's Side Effects of Herbal Medicines. Elsevier Amsterdam. 2009.

Arrowsmith, Nancy. Essential Herbal Wisdom. Llewellyn Pub. Woodbury, Minn. 2009.

Arsdall, Anne Van. *Medieval Herbal Remedies.* Routledge, New York. 2002.

Arvigo & Balick, *Rainforest Remedies,* Lotus Press, Twin Lakes, WI. 1993

Arvigo & Epstein. *Rainforest Home Remedies,* Harper SanFrancisco, 2001.

Assiniwi, Bernard. *La Medecine des Indiens d' Amerique,* Guerin Literature, 1988

Atal C.K. & Kapur B. *Cultivation and Utilization of Medicinal Plants,* Jammu-Tawi, 1982

Attenborough, David. *The Private Life of Plants.* Princeton U Press. Princeton NJ 1995.

Ausubel, K. *Seeds of Change The Living Treasure.* HarperSanFrancisco, 1994.

Aversano, Laura. *The Divine Nature of Plants.* Swan•Raven & Co. Columbus, NC, 2002.

Ayensu, Edward,S. *Medicinal Plants of the West Indies,* Reference Publications, 1981

Baïracli Levy, Juliette *Herbal Handbook for Farm and Stable,* Faber&Faber, London, 1952

Baker, Phil. The Dedalus Book of Absinthe. Dedalus 2001.

Barl, Branka et al, *Saskatchewan Herb Database,* U. of Sask. Saskatoon, 1996.

Barlow, Max. *From the Shepherd's Purse.* 1990

Barnes J, Anderson L, &Phillipson J. *Herbal Medicines, A guide for healthcare professionals.* Pharmaceutical Press, London, 2002.

Barnett, Robert A. *Tonics,* Harper Collins, New York, N.Y. 1997

Bartram, Thomas. *Bartram's Encyl. of Herbal Medicine,* Robinson Pub. London, 1998.

Bascom, Angella. *Incorporating Herbal Medicine into Clinical Practice.* F. Davis Co. 2002

Beals, Katherine, M. *Flower Lore and Legend,* Henry Holt, 1917

Beers, Susan-Jane. *Jamu The ancient Indonesian Art of Herbal Healing,* Periplus, 2001.

Belcourt, Christi. Medicines to Help Us. Gabriel Dumont Instit. Saskatoon, SK 2007.

Béliveau, R & Gingras,D. *Foods That Fight Cancer.* McClelland & Stewart Toronto. 2006.

Belsinger S & Dille C. *Cooking with Herbs.* CBI- Van Nostrand Reinhold, N.Y. 1984.

Benjamin, D.R. *Mushrooms: Poisons and Panaceas.* WH Freeman, San Francisco, 1995.

Bennet, Doug & Tiner, Tim. *Up North.* Reed Books Canada. Markham, Ont. 1993.

_____*Up North Again.* McClelland and Stewart. Toronto, 1997.

Bennet, J & Rowley S. *Uqalurait An Oral History of Nunavut.* McGill Queens, Mont. 2004

Benyus, Janine. *Biomimicry Innovation Inspired by Nature.* William Morrow. 1997.

Berenbaum,May R. *Buzzwords, A Scientists Muses on Sex, Bugs and Rock N Roll,* Joseph Henry Press, Washington, D.C. 2000.

_____*Bugs in the System.* Helix Books, Addison-Wesley Pub. 1995.

Beresford-Kroeger, Diana. The Global Forest. Viking Penguin. 2010.

_____Arboretum Borealis. U Michigan Press. 2010.

Berliocchi,Luigi. *The Orchid in Lore and Legend.* Timber Press, Portland Oregon, 2000.

Berlund B & Bolsby C. *The Edible Wild* Pagurian Press, Toronto, Ont. 1971.

Berkowsky, Bruce. *Mount Julius Flower Remedies. Mt. Vernon Washington, 1986*

Bermejo, J & Leon,J. *Neglected Crops-1492 ...* FAO Series 26, United Nations, Rome, 1994.

Bernhardt, P. *The Rose's Kiss, A Natural History of Flowers* . Island Press, Covelo CA 1999

Bianchi, Ivo. *Geriatrics and Homotoxicology.* Aurelia-Verlag GmbH, Baden Baden, 1994.

Bianchini, F. *The Complete Book of Health Plants.* Crescent Books, New York, 1975.

Biship, Carol. *The Book of Home Remedies &Herbal Cures,* Jonathan-James, Toronto, 1979.

Bisset, Norman G. *Herbal Drugs and Phytopharmaceuticals.* 2nd Ed. CRC Press, 2001.

Blackburn, Thomas. *December's Child: A Book of Chumash Oral Narratives* , U of California Press, Berkeley, 1975.

Blanchan, Neltje. *Nature's Garden.* Doubleday, Page&Co. New York, 1900.

Bland, John. *Forests of Liliput.* Prentice Hall, Englewood Cliffs, New Jersey, 1971.

Bliss, Anne. *Rocky Mountain Dye Plants.* Juniper House, Boulder, Colorado, 1976

Blouin, Glen. *Weeds of the Woods.* Goose Lane, Fredericton, New Brunswick 1992.

_____*An Eclectic Guide to Trees, east of the Rockies.* Boston Mills, 2001.

Boas, F. *Ethnology of the Kwakiutl.* Bureau of Am. Ethnology, 35th annual report, 1921.

Boericke, Wm. *Materia Medica with Repetory.* B. Jain Publishers. 1976

Boik, John. *Natural Compunds in Cancer Therapy.* Oregon Med Press, Princeton,Minn 2001

Boland, Bridget. *Gardener's Magic &Other Old Wives' Lore.* The Bodley Head, London, 77.

Bolton, Brett L. *The Secret Powers of Plants.* Berkley Pub Co. New York. 1974.

Bolton, J.L. *Alfalfa, Botany, Cultivation &Utilization.* Interscience Pub, New York, 1962.

Bone, Kerry. *A Clinical Guide to Blending Liquid Herbs.* Churchill Livingstone. 2003

Borrel, Marie. *Healing Plants.* Cassell & Co. Wellington House, London. 2001.

Bouchardon, Patrice. *The Healing Energies of Trees.* Journey Editions, Boston, 1999.

Bossenmaier, Eugene. *Mushrooms of the Boreal Forest.* U. of Saskatchewan Press, 1997

Boulos, Loutfy. *Medicinal Plants of North Africa,* Reference Pub. Algonac, Mich. 1983

Bowles, E. Joy. *The Chemistry of Aromatherapeutic Oils.* Allen & Unwin, Crow's Nest, Australia, 2003.

Bowman, Daria. *Hydrangeas.* Friedman/Fairfax Pub. New York. 1999.

Bradley, Peter. British Herbal Compendium Vol 2 Brit Herb Med Assoc. Bournemouth 2006.

Brahmachari, Goutam Ed. Natural Products, Alpha Sci Int Ltd. Oxford UK 2009.

Brandeis, Gayle. *Fruitflesh.* Harper Collins, San Francisco. 2002.

Brennan, M. *Complete Holistic Care & Healing for Horses.* Trafalgar Sq. Pub. VT. 2001.

Bringhurst, Robert. *A Story as Sharp as a Knife.* Douglas&Mc Intyre Vancouver, 1999.

Brinker, Francis N.D. *Herb Contraindications and Drug Interactions* .Third Edition Eclectic Medical Publications, Sandy, Oregon, 2001

_____*The Toxicology of Botanical Medicines,* revised 2nd. Eclectic Med, Oregon, 1996.

_____*Eclectic Dispensatory of Botanical Therapeutics,* Vol 2, Ecl. Med . Oregon, 1995.

Brodo, Irwin & Sharnoff. *Lichens of North America.* Yale University Press, 2001.

Brown, Deni. *Encyclopedia of Herbs and Their Uses.* Reader's Digest Press, Que. 1995.

Bruneton, J *Pharmacognosy, Phtyochemistry, Medicinal Plants,* Lavoisier Pub. Paris, 1995

_____*Toxic Plants Dangerous to Humans and Animals.* Editions TEC&Doc, Paris, '99.

Brunschwig, Hieronymus. *Book of Distillation.* Johnson Reprint Co No. 79. New York, 1971.

Brynaherb Essences 29, Kells Meend Berry Hill, Gloucestershire GL16 7AD

Bubar, Carol et al. *Weeds of the Prairies.* Alberta Agriculture Pub. Edmonton, 2000.

Buchanan, Carol. *Brothers Crow, Sister Corn.* Ten Speed Press, Berkeley, 1997.

Buckle, Jane. *Clinical Aromatherapy. 2nd ed.* Churchill Livingstone, Toronto, 2003.

Buhner, Stephen H. *Sacred and Herbal Healing Beers,* Siris Books, Boulder, Co, 1998

_____*Sacred Plant Medicine.* Robert Rinehart, Boulder, Co. 1996.

_____Herbal Antibiotics. Storey Books, Vermont, 1999.

_____*The Lost Language of Plants.* Chelsea Green Pub. White River, Vt. 2002

_____Secret Teachings of Plants. Bear & Co. Rochester, Vt. 2004.

_____The Natural Testosterone Plan. Healing Arts Press, Rochester VT. 2007

Burbridge, Joan. *Wildflowers of the Southern Interior of B.C.* U. of B.C. Press, 1989.

Burger, W. Flowers- *How they changed the world. Prometheus Books.* Amherst NY 2006.

Burgess, Isla. *Weeds Heal.* Viriditas Pub Group. Cambridge NZ 1998.

Burlando, Bruno et al, Herbal Principles in Cosmetics. CRC Press Boca Raton 2010.

Caius, Rev. Fr. Jean F., *The Medicinal and Poisonous Plants of India,* Scientific Pub, 1986.

Cameron, Elizabeth. *A Floral ABC.* John Wiley and Sons. Toronto. 1980.

Carpenter D. Snr Pub. *Nursing Herbal Medicine Handbook,* Springhouse Corp. 2001.

Carpinella, Maria et al. Novel Therapeutic Agents from Plants. Sci Pub. Enfield NJ 2009.

Carr, Emily. *Wild Flowers.* Royal BC Museum, Victoria, B.C, 2006

Carroll, Roisin. *The Crane Bag Celtic Tree Ogam Oils* , Feasibility Pub. Dublin

Carter, Bernard F. *The Floral Birthday Book.* Bloomsbury Books, London. 1990.

Casselman, Bill. *Canadian Garden Words.* Little, Brown & Co. Toronto, 1997.

Castleman, Michael. *The Healing Herbs.* Bantam Books. 1995.

Castro, Miranda. *The Complete Homeopathy Handbook.* MacMillan, 1990

Catty, Suzanne. *Hydrosols the next Aromatherapy,* Healing Arts Press, Vermont, 2001.

Cavers, Paul ed, *The* Biology *of Canadian Weeds* 62-83,Ag Institute of Canada, Ottawa, 1995

_____84-102 Ag Inst. of Canada, Ottawa, 2000.

_____103-129 Ag Inst. of Canada, Ottawa 2005

Ceres. *Herbal Teas for Health and Healing.* Healing Arts Press, Rochester, Vermont, 1984.

Chan, K, and Cheung L. *Interactions between Chinese Herbal Medicinal Products and Orthodox Drugs.* Harwood Academic Publishers, Canada, 2000.

Chandler, F. *Herbs-Everyday Reference for Health Professionals,* Can. Pharm Assoc. 2000

Chang & But. *Pharmacology &Applications of Chinese Materia Medica,* World Scientific, 86

Chang Chao-liang et al, *Vegetables as Medicine,* Pelanduk Pub, Malaysia, 1999.

Chappell, P. Emotional Healing with Homeopathy. North Atlantic Books. Berkeley, 2003.

Charissa's Cauldron. www.charissacauldron.com

Chase, Pamela & Pawlik, J. *Newcastle Trees for Healing*, Newcastle Pub. Van Nuys,1991

Chatroux, Sylvia. *Botanica Poetica*. Poetica Press 2004 1-877-POETICA.

_____*Materica Poetica*. Poetica Press 1998.

Chen, John K & Chen, Tina T. Chinese Medical Herbology & Pharmacology. Art of Medicine Press, City of Industry, CA 2004.

Chevalllier, Andrew. *The Encyclopedia of Medicinal Plants*. Reader's Digest, 1996.

Chishti, Hakim. *The Traditional Healer*, Healing Arts Press, Vermont,1988.

Christchurch Flower Essences. www.christchurchfloweressences.com

Clark, Ella E. *Indian Legends of Canada*. McClelland & Stewart. Toronto, 1960.

Coats, Peter. *Flowers in History*. Weidenfeld and Nicolson, London. 1970.

Coffey, Timothy. *The History and Folklore of North American Wildflowers,* Houghton-Mifflin, 1993.

Cohen, Kenneth. *Honoring the Medicine*. Random House, Toronto. 2003.

Conrad, Chris, *Hemp for Health,* Healing Arts Press, Rochester, Vermont, 1997.

Cook, Wm.H. *The Physio-Medical Dispensatory*. 1869. Reprinted by Eclectic Medical Publications, Portland, Oregon, 1985.

_____A compendium of the new Materia medica together with additional descriptions of some old remedies. Wm. Cook Publisher, Chicago, 1896.

Cooper, J.C. *Dictionary of Symbolic & Mythological Animals,* Thorsons, London, 1992.

Cormack, R.G.H. *Wild Flowers of Alberta*. Hurtig Publishers, 1977

Coupland, Francois. *The Encyclopedia of Edible Plants of N. America*. Keats Pub. 1998.

Cousin, Pierre J. *Eat Well, Be Well*. Thorsons, London. 2001.

Cowan, Eliot. *Plant Spirit Medicine*. Swan Raven & Co. Box 726 Newberg, Oregon, 1995.

Cowan, Thomas. The Fourfold Path to Healing. New Trends Pub. Washington DC 2007.

Crane, Eva. *Honey- A Comprhensive Survey* , Heinemann Pub. London 1975.

Craydon D. & Bellows W. Floral Acupuncture. The Crossing Press Berkeley CA 2005.

Creekmore, H. *Daffodils are Dangerous*. Walker and Co. New York. 1966.

Crow, Tis Mal. *Native Plants, Native Healing*. Native Voices Book Pub. Box 99 Summertown, Tennessee, 2001 1-888-260-8458.

Crowell, Robert L. *The Lore & Legends of Flowers*. Thomas Crowell, New York, 1982.

Crowfoot & Baldensperger. *From Cedar to Hyssop*. Sheldon Press, London, 1932.

Cruden, Loren. Medicine Grove. Destiny Books. Inner Traditions Vermont. 1997.

Cummings, S. and Ullman, Dana. *Everyone's Guide to Homeopathic Medicines,* St. Martins

Cupp, Melanie. *Toxicology and Clinical Pharmacology of Herbal Products*. Humana P. 1999

Curtin, LSM. *Healing Herbs of the Upper Rio Grande*. SouthWest Museum, Los Angeles 1965

Cutler & Cutler Eds. Biologically Active Natural Products: Agrochemicals, CRC Press 1999.

Dai Yin-fang&Liu Cheng-jun. *Fruit As Medicine*. Rams Skull Press, Kuranda, Aust. 1987

Dalton, David. Stars of the Meadow. Lindisfarne Books. Great Barrington, Mass. 2006.

D'Amelio Sr. Frank. *Botanicals A Phytocosmetic Desk Reference* CRC Press, Boca Raton, 99

Darby,Wm et al. *Food: The Gift of Osiris,* Vol 1. Academic Press, San Francisco, 1977

Darwin, Tess. The Scots Herbal, the Plant Lore of Scotland. Birlinn Ltd, Edinburgh 2008

Davidow, Joie. *Infusions of Healing, A Treasury of Mexican-American Herbal Remedies,* Fireside Books, New York, 1999.

Davis,W. *El Gringo, New Mexico and Her People*. Harpers, New York, 1857.

Demargaux, N. *Phytotherapy*. Herbal Health Publishers Ltd. 1989

De Bairacli Levy, Juliette. *Herbal Handbook for Farm and Stable*, Faber and Faber 1952

Deer Lame, J & Erdoes, R. *Lame Deer Seeker of Visions.* Washington Sq Press, 1976.

Deer, Thea Summer. Wisdom of the Plant Devas. Bear&Company Vermont 2011.

Delta Gardens Flower Essences. www.deltagardens.com

De Smet et al. *Adverse Effects of Herbal Drugs.* Springer-Verlag, Berlin. 1997.

Der Marderosian, Ara & Liberti L. *Natural Product Medicine,* George Stickley Co, Philadel.

DeRios, Marlene D. *Hallucinogens: Cross Cultural Perspectives.* U. New Mexico Press, 1984

DeSmet, P. et al. *Adverse Effects of Herbal Drugs. vol 2* Springer-Verlag

Devi, Lila. The Essential Flower Essence Handbook. Crystal Clarity Pub. Nevada City 2007.

Dewey, Laurel. *Plant Power- revised.* Safe Goods/New Century Pub, Markham Ont, 2001.

Dewick, Paul M. *Medicinal Natural Products.*3rd Ed John Wiley and Sons, West Sussex, 2009.

Diederichsen, Axel. *Coriander.* Int. Plant Genetic Resources Institute. Rome, Italy. 1996.

Dixon, Bernard.*Power Unseen, How Microbes Rule the World.* W.H. Freeman, Oxford, 1994

Dow, Elaine. *Simples and Worts.* Historical Presentations, Topsfield, MA. 1982.

Duke, James. *Handbook of Medicinal Herbs.* CRC Press, Boca Raton, Florida, 1985

_____*Handbook of Edible Weeds.* CRC Press. 1992

_____*The Green Pharmacy,* Rodale Press, Emmaus, Pennsylvania, 1997.

_____*The Green Pharmacy Herbal Handbook,* Rodale Press, 2000.

_____*Anti-aging Prescriptions.* Rodale Press. 2001.

Dumas, Anne. Book of Plants and Symbols. English Ed. Octopus Pub. London 2004.

Dymock,Wm. *Pharmacographia Indica, Vol 2*, Kegan Paul, Trench, Trubner and Co. 1891

Earle, Liz. *Vital Oils,* Ebury Press, London, 1991.

Eason, Cassandra. Fabulous Creatures, Mythical Monsters… Greenwood Press, CT. 2008.

Eastman, John. *The Book of Swamp and Bog...* Stackpole Books, Mechanicsburg, Penn, 1995

Ebadi, M. *Pharmacodynamic Basis of Herbal Medicine,* CRC Press, Boca Raton. 2002.

Eckey, E.W. *Vegetable Fats and Oils,* Rheingold Publishing Co, New York, 1954.

Eclare, Melanie. *Flower Spirit Cards.* Quadrille Publishing, London, England, 2004.

Edwards, Lawrence. *The Vortex of Life.* Floris Books. Edinburgh 2nd Ed. 2006.

Eisner T et al. *Secret Weapons.* Belknap Press, Harvard U Press. Cambridge & London 2005.

Ellingwood F. *American Materia Medica,* Eclectic Med. Pub. Portand, Oregon, reprint, 1983

Elliot, Douglas B. *Roots* . Chatham Press, Old Greenwich Conneticut.

Ellis, Hattie. *Sweetness & Light.* Hodder and Stoughton, London, 2004.

Erdoes & Ortiz. *American Indian Myths and Legends,* Pantethon Books, New York, 1984.

Erichsen-Brown,Charlotte. *Use of Plants for the Past 500 Years,* Breezy Creeks Press, 1979

_____*Medicinal and Other Uses of North American Plants,* General Pub, 1979.

Erickson, David, Wai Kit Nip *Food uses of whole oil and protein seeds,* Amer. Oil Chemists Society, 1989.

Eskin, N. A. Michael, Tamir, S. *Dictionary of Nutraceuticals and Functional Foods.* CRC Press, 2006.

Etkin, Nina. Edible Medicines, An Ethnopharmacology of Food. U Arizona Press. 2006.

Evans, W.C. *Trease and Evans' Pharmacognosy.* WB Saunders Co. Toronto, 2000.

Fang Jing Pei, Dr. *Natural Remedies from the Chinese Cupboard.* Weatherhill, 1998.

Farmer-Knowles,Helen. *The Healing Garden.* Sterling Publishing, New York, 1998.

Fielder, Mildred. *Plant Medicne and Folklore,* Winchester Press, New York, 1975.

Felter, Harvery and Lloyd, John. *King's American Dispensatory* . 1898. Reprinted by Eclectic Medical
        Publications, Portland Oregon, 1983.

Ferguson, Gary. *Spirits of the Wild.* Clarkson Potter/Random New York, 1996.

Fernie, W.T. Dr. *Old Fashioned Herbal Remedies.* Coles Pub. Toronto, 1980. Reprint.

Fingerman M. et al editors. *Bioremediation of Aquatic and Terresrial Ecosytems.* Sci Pub. Enfield NH 2005.

Fischer-Rizzi, S. *Complete Aromatherapy Handbook,* Sterling Pub. New York. 1990.

_____*The Complete Incense Book,* Sterling Pub. New York. 1998.

_____*Medicine of the Earth,* Rudra Press, Portland, Oregon, 1996

Florey, H.W. et al. Antibiotics vol 1. Oxford University Press. London 1949.

Ford, Gillian. *Plant Names Explained.* Friends of the Devonian Botanic Garden, #16, 1984

Foster, Steven. *Herbal Renaissance,* Gibbs Smith Pub. Salt Lake City

_____& Yue Chongxi. *Herbal Emissaries,* Healing Arts Press, Vermont, 1992

_____& Johnson R. *Desk Reference to Nature's Medicine.* Nat Geographic. Washington, D.C.

Fox, H. M. Gardening with Herbs. Macmillan Pub. New York 1933.

Freeman, D. & Mongeau D. Nettles and More…Vol One. Self published 2nd printing 2009.

Freeman, Lyn. *Mosby's Complementary & Alternative Medicine.*3rd Ed. Mosby Elsevier 2009

Friedman, Sara Ann, *Celebrating the Wild Mushroom,* Dodd, Mead & Co. New York, 1986

Friend, Tim. The Third Domain: the Untold Story of Archaea. Joseph Henry Press. 2007.

Fugh-Berman, Adriane. *The 5-minute Herb &Dietary Supplement Consult.* Lippincott Williams &Wilkins, Philadelphia 2003.

Gaertner, Erika. *Reap without Sowing.* General Store Publishing, Burnstown, Ont. 1995

Galun, Margalith. *Handbook of Lichenology,* CRC Press, 1988

Garran, Thomas. *Western herbs according to Traditional Chinese Medicine.* Healing Arts Press. 2008.

Garrett, J.T. *The Cherokee Herbal.* Bear&Company, Rochester, Vermont. 2003.

Genders, Roy. *Floral Scents of the World* . St. Martin's Press, London, 1977

Geuter, *Herbs in Nutrition.* Bio-Dynamic Agricultural Assoc. London. 1978.

Gildemeister, E. *The Volatile Oils.* John Wiley and Sons, New York. 1916

Gifford, Jane. The Wisdom of Trees. Sterling Pub. New York 2000.

Gill S. & Sullivan I. *Dictionary of Native American Mythology.* Oxford U Press 1992.

Gilmore, M.R. Uses of Plants by Indians of the Missouri river region. 33rd Annual Report Bureau American Ethnology, 1911-12, Washington D.C. 1919.

Gladstar R & Hirsch P. *Planting the Future.* Healing Arts Press, Rochester, Vt. 2000.

Gladstar, Rosemary. *Family Herbal.* Storey Books, North Adams, Mass. 2001.

Glasby, J.S. *Dictionary of Plants Containing Secondary Metabolites,* Taylor & Francis, London 1991.

Godfrey, A & Saunders P. Principles and Practices of Naturopathic Botanical Medicine, Vol 1, CCNM Press Toronto ON 2010.

Goodrick-Clarke, Clare. Alchemical Medicine for the 21st Century. Healing Arts Press. 2010.

Gordon, David G. *The Compleat Cockroach.* Ten Speed Press, Berkeley, CA. 1996.

Gordon, Lesley. The Mystery and Magic of Trees & Flowers. Grange Books. London 1993.

Gottesfeld, Leslie M. Johnson. *Plants, Land and People, A Study of Wet'suwet'en Ethnobotany.*U of A, 1993.

Grae, Ida. *Nature's Colors, Dyes From Plants.* Macmillan Pub. New York, 1974.

Graham, Frances K. *Plant lore of an Alaskan Island.* Alaska Northwest Pub. 1985

Grandparents of the Forest flower essences. www.grandparentsoftheforest.com

Grange, Michael etal, *Handbook of Plants with Pest Control Properties,* J. Wiley& Son 1988

Gray, Bev. The Boreal Herbal. Wild Food & Medicine Plants of the North. Aroma Borealis Press 2011

Green, James. *The Male Herbal* . Crossing Press, Freedom, California, 1991.

_____*The Herbal Medicine-Maker's Handbook.* Crossing Press, Freedom CA 2000

Green, Jonathan. *Consuming Passions.* Sphere Books, London, 1985.

Grey Wolf. *Earth Signs,* Raincoast Books, Vancouver, B.C. 1998.

Grieve, M. *A Modern Herbal.* Jonathan Cape. 1931

Griffiths, Deirdre. *Elk Island National Park.* U. of Alberta Press, 1979.

Grigson, Geoffrey. *A Herbal of All Sorts*. Phoenix House, London

Grimaud, Baptiste,Paul. *TAROT DES FLEURS*, France Cartes, France 1989

Grimshaw, John. *The Gardener's Atlas*. Firefly Books, Willowdale, Ont. 2002.

Grohmann,Gerbert. *The Plant Vol 2,* Bio-Dynamic Farming & Gardening Assoc. 1989.

Gruenwald et al, Ed. PDR for Herbal Medicines. 4th Ed. Thomson Pub. 2007.

Guillet, Alma. *Make Friends of Trees and Shrubs*. Doubleday & Co. New York, 1962.

Gumbel, Dietrich. *Principles of Holistic Skin Therapy with Herb Essences*. Haug Pub. Heidelberg 1986.

Gurudas. *The Spiritual Properties of Herbs* , Cassandra Press, 1988

_____*Flower Essences and Vibrational Healing,* Cassandra Press, 1983

Hageneder, Fred. The Spirit of Trees. Continuum. NY and London. 2005.

Hale, Mason. *The Biology of Lichens*. Edward Arnold Pub. London, 1967.

Hall, Dorothy. *Creating Your Herbal Profile* , Keats, 1988

Hallworth, B & Chinnappa CC. *Plants of the Kananaskis Country* U of A Press 1997.

Hanchuk, Rena. *The Word and Wax*. Can Inst of Ukrainian Studies Press, Edmonton, 1999.

Hanson, J, & Morrison D. *Of Kinkajous, Capybaras, Horned Beetles...*Harper Collins, NY '91

Harbourne & Baxter. *The Handbook of Natural Flavonoids Vol 1&2*. John Wiley & Sons, 1999

_____*Phytochemical Dictionary*. Taylor & Francis 1993.

Harrington, Geri. *Growing Your Own Chinese Vegetables,* MacMillan, N.Y. 1978.

Harrington, H.D. *Edible Native Plants of the Rocky Mtns*. U. of New Mexico Press, 1967.

Harris, Ben C. *Eat the Weeds,* Keats Pub. New Cannan, Conneticut 1973.

_____*Make Use of Your Garden Plants*. General Pub. New York. 1978.

Harris, Marjorie. *Botanica North America*. Harper Collins, New York, 2003.

Harrison, Nora. *Flower Remedy Rhymes* , self published, England, 1990.

Hart, Jeff. *Montana Native Plants and Early Peoples,* Montana Historical Society Press. '92

_____The Ethnobotany of the Northern Cheyenne Indians of Montana. Journal of Ethnopharmacology 1981 4.

Hartung, Tammi. *Growing 101 Herbs That Heal*. Storey Books, Pownal, Vt. 2000.

Hartwell, Jonathan, *Plants Used Against Cancer*. Quarterman Pub. 1982

Hartzell, Jr. H. *The Yew Tree A Thousand Whispers*. Hulogosi, Box 1188, Eugene, OR 1991.

Harvey, C & Cochrane A. *The Healing Spirit of Plants*. Godsfield Press, Sterling Pr N.Y. 1999

Harvey Clare. The New Encyclopedia of Flower Remedies. Watkins Pub. London 2007.

Hatfield, Gabrielle. *Encyclopedia of Folk Medicine*. ABC CLIO Santa Barbara. 2004.

Haughton, Claire. *Green Immigrants*. Harcourt Brace Jovanovich. New York and London.

Hawksworth, Frank & Wiens, D. Dwarf Mistletoes, Ag Handbook 709, USDA, Wash, DC, '96

Health Canada, Native Foods and Nutrition. Medical Services Branch, 1995.

Heatherington, M. and Steck,W. *Natural Chemicals from Northern Prairie Plants,* Ag West Biotech Publishers, Saskatoon, Canada. 1997.

Heilmeyer, Marina. The Language of Flowers-Symbols & Myths. Prestel Pub. Munich 2001.

Heinerman, John. *Encyclopedia of Nuts, Berries and Seeds,* Parker Publishing, 1995.

_____*Encyclopedia of Healing Herbs & Spices*. Parker Pub. N.Y. 1996.

Heinrich, Bernd. *Winter World The Ingenuity of animal survival*. HarperCollins. NY 2003.

Heinrich, Clark. *Magic Mushrooms in Religion and Alchemy*. Park St. Press, VT. 2002.

Heiser, Charles B. Jr. *Of Plants and People*. U. of Oklahoma Press, 1985.

Hellson, John C, *Ethnobotany of the Blackfoot Indians* No. 19, National Museums of Canada, Ottawa 1974.

Henderson, Robert K. *The Neighborhood Forager*. Key Porter Books, Toronto, 2000.

Hendrickson, Robert. *Encycl of Word and Phrase Origins*. Facts on File Inc. NewYork, 1997.

Hendry, G. *Natural Food Colorants* , Blackie and Son, Glasgow Scotland, 1992.

Henry, J. David. *Canada's Boreal Forest.* Smithsonian Institute. 2002.

Hilarion. *Wildflowers, Their Occult Gifts.* Marcus Books, Queensville, Ont. 1982.

Hobbs, Christopher. *Usnea : The Herbal Antibiotic.* Botanica Press. 1986.

_____*Medicinal Mushrooms*, Botanica Press, Santa Cruz, 1995.

Hoffman, David. *The Holistic Herbal.* Findhorn Press, 1983.

_____*Welsh Herbal Medicine.* Abercastle Publications, Dyfed, 1978.

_____*Medical Herbalism.* Healing Arts Press, Rochester, VT, 2003.

Hole, Lois. *Favorite Trees and Shrubs.* Lone Pine Pub. Edmonton Alta. 1997.

_____*Perennial Favorites.* Lone Pine Pub. 1995.

Holm, LeRoy G. *World Weeds,* John Wiley and Sons, 1997.

Holmes, Peter. *The Energetics of Western Herbs, Vol 1 and 2,* Artemis Press, 1989.

_____*Jade Remedies, Vol 1 and 2,* Snow Lotus Press, Boulder 1996.

Hopman, Ellen. *A Druid's Herbal,* Destiny Books, Rochester, Vermont. 1995.

Howarth, D& Kahlee Keane. *Wild Medicines of the Prairies* Self Published, 1995.

_____*Native Medecines* Self Published , 1995

Hozeski, Bruce. *Hildegard's Healing Plants.* Beacon Press. Boston, Mass. 2001.

Hsu, Hong-Yen. *Oriental Materia Medica,* Keats Publishing,Connecticut, 1986.

Huang, Kee Chang. *The Pharmacolocy of Chinese Herbs.* 2nd Edition, CRC Press, 1999.

Hu-Nan. *A Barefoot Doctor's Manual.* Running Press, Philadelphia, 1977.

Hudson, James B. *Antiviral Compounds from Plants,* CRC Press, Florida, 1990

Hudson, Rick. *A Field Guide to Gold, Gemstone and Mineral Sites.* Orca Pub, Victoria, 1999

Hurley, Judith. *The Good Herb* Wm. Morrow and Co. New York, 1995.

Hutchens, Alma. *Indian Herbology of North America.* Merco. 1969

Ingram, Cass. *Supermarket Remedies.* Knowledge House, Buffalo Grove, Ill. 1998.

Injoynow essences.

Inkpen W & Van Eyk, R. *Guide to the Common Native Trees and Shrubs of Alberta,* Government of Alberta, Environmental Protection, 1995.

James & Keeler, *Poisonous Plants- 3rd Int. Symposium,* Iowa State U. Press, 1992.

Jason, Dan & Nancy. *Some Useful Wild Plants,* Talon Books, Vancouver, 1972.

Jiao Shu-De. *Ten Lectures on the Use of Medicinals.* Paradigm Pub. Brookline, Mass. 2003.

Johnson, Kershaw, MacKinnon & Pojar *Plants of the Western Boreal Forest and Aspen Parkland,* Lone Pine Press, Edmonton, Alberta 1995.

Johnson, L. *Tending the Earth A Gardener's Manifesto.* Penguin Books, Toronto, 2002.

Johnson, Leslie. Journal of Ethnobotany and Ethnomedicine. 2006 2:29.

_____*Health, Wholeness & the Land: Gitksan Traditional Plant Use and Healing.* U of Alberta 1997.

Jones, Alison. *Larousse Dictionary of World Folklore.* Larousse, New York, 1995.

Jones, Pamela. *Just Weed, History, Myths and Uses.* Prentice Hall Press, Toronto, 1991.

Kamm, Minnie W. *Old Time Herbs for Northern Gardens* Little Brown & Co. 1938.

Kane, Charles W. Herbal Medicine of the American Southwest. Lincoln Town Press. 2007.

_____Herbal Medicine: trends and traditions. Lincoln Town Press 2009.

Kapoor, L.D. *CRC Handbook of Ayurvedic Medicinal Plants,* CRC Press, Boca Raton, 1990.

Kari, Priscilla. *Tanaina Plantlore.* National Park Service, Alaska Region 1987.

Kaur, Sat Dharam. *The Complete Natural Medicine Guide to Breast Cancer.* Robert Rose Inc Toronto, 2003.

Kavash E, Barrie & Barr K, *American Indian Healing Arts.* Bantam Books, Toronto 1999.

_____*The Medicine Wheel Garden.* Bantam Books, N.Y. 2002.

Kay, Margarita Artschwager. *Healing with Plants in the American and Mexican West,* The University of Arizona Press, Tucson. 1996

Kays, S & Nottingham S. Biology and Chemistry of Jerusalem Artichoke. CRC Press 2008.

Keane, Kahlee & Howarth,D. *The Standing People.* Saskatoon, Saskatchewan. 2003.

Kee Chang Huang, *The Pharmacology of Chinese Herbs,* 2nd Edition, CRC Press, 1999.

Kemp, Cynthia. *Cactus and Company.* Desert Alchemy, Tucson, Arizona, 1993.

Kenner D &Requena Y. *Botanical Medicine:* .Paradigm Pub. Brookline, Mass, 1996.

Kerik, Joan. *Living with the Land:Use of Plants by the Native People of Alberta,* Alberta Culture, Circulating Exhibits Program, National Museums of Canada Fund, 1981.

Kershaw, Linda. Edible & Medicinal Plants of the Rockies, Lone Pine, Edmonton 2000.

_____*Alberta Wayside Wildflowers.* Lone Pine, Edmonton, 2003.

_____*Saskatchewan Wayside Wildflowers.* Lone Pine, Edmonton, 2003.

_____*Manitoba Wayside Wildflowers.* Lone Pine, Edmonton, 2003.

Kershaw, L. et al. *Rare Vascular Plants of Alberta.* U. of Alberta Press, Edmonton, 2001.

Kershaw, MacKinnon & Pojar. *Plants of the Rocky Mountains.* Lone Pine, Edmonton 1998.

Keys, John. D. *Chinese Herbs,* Charles E. Tuttle Co. 1976.

Kimmerer,Robin. *Gathering Moss.* Oregon State University Press, Corvallis, 2003.

Kindscher, Kelly. *Medicnal Wild Plants of the Prairies.* Univ. Press of Kansas. 1987.

King, Francis X. *Rudolf Steiner and Holistic Medicine.* Rider & Co. England, 1986.

Klein, Carol. Plant Personalities. Timber Press, Portland, Oregon. 2005.

Klein, Richard. *The Green World.* 2nd edition. Harper Collins, 1987.

Kloss, Jethro. *Back to Eden.* Woodbridge Press Pub.Co. Santa Barbara, Ca. 1975.

Knab, Sophie H. *Polish Herbs, Flowers and Folk Medicine.* Hippocrene Books, N.Y. 1999.

Knowles, Hugh. *Woody Ornamentals for the Prairies.* U. of Alberta , 1995.

Knudtson,P & Suzuki D. Wisdom of the Elders. Greystone Books. Vancouver BC 2006.

Kraft, K & Hobbs C. *Pocket Guide to Herbal Medicine.* Thieme, N.Y. 2004.

Kranich, Ernst M. Planetary Influences Upon Plants. Bio-Dynamic Lit. Wyoming RI 1984.

Krymow, V. Healing Plants of the Bible. Wild Goose Pub. Glasgow, UK 2002.

Kuhnlein, Harriet and Turner, Nancy. *Traditional Plant Foods of Canadian Indigenous Peoples.* Gordon and Breach Science Publishers. 1991.

Kuijt, Job. *The Biology of Parasitic Flowering Plants,* U. of California Press, 1969

Kunkele, U. & Lohmeyer, T. *Herbs for Healthy Living.* Parragon Pub. Bath UK 2007.

Lacey, Laurie. *Micmac Medicines Remedies and Recollections.* Nimbus Pub. Halifax, 1993.

Lahring, Heinjo. *Water and Wetland Plants of the Prairie Provinces,* Can Plains Research Center, U. of Regina, 2003

Lambert, Grant. *Falling Leaf Essences.* Healing Arts Press, Rochester Vermont, 2002.

Lamont, SM. *The Fisherman Lake Slave and their environment: a story of floral and faunal resources.* Master's thesis. U. of Saskatchewan, Saskatoon, 1977.

Langenheim, Jean. *Medicinal Plant Resins.* Timber Press Portland Oregon 2003.

Larsen,Henning. *An Old Icelandic Medical Miscellany,* Norske Akademi, Oslo, Norway '31

Lavabre, Marcel. *Aromatherapy Workbook.* Healing Arts Press, Vermont. 1990.

Lawless, Julia, *The Encyclopedia of Essential Oils* , Element Books, 1992.

LeClaire,N &Cardinal,G. *Alberta Elders' Cree Dictionary,* U of Alberta Press, 1998.

Leduc, M.A. *The Explorers Guide to Boreal Forest Plants,* Hwy Book Shop, Cobalt, Ont. 1997

Leighton, Anna L. *Wild Plant Use by the Woods Cree (NIHITHAWAK) of East-Central Saskatchewan* . Paper no. 101, National Museums of Canada, Ottawa, 1985

Lepore, Donald. *The Ultimate Healing System.* Woodland Books, Provo, Utah, 1988.

Le Strange, Richard, *A History of Herbal Plants.* Arco Pub. New York. 1977.

Leung, Albert. *Chinese Herbal Remedies.* Universe Books, New York, 1984.

Leung & Foster, *Encyclopedia of Common Natural Ingredients,* J. Wiley&Sons, N.Y. 1996.

Levey,M. *The Medical Formulary or Aqrabadhin of Al-Kindi* U of Wisconsin Press, 1966

Leyel, C.F. *Elixirs of Life,* Faber and Faber, London.1948

Li, Thomas. *Medicinal Plants, Culture, Utilization & Phytopharmacology.* Technomic Publishing, Lancaster, Pennsylvania, 2000.

Li, Thomas. *Chinese and related North American Herbs.* CRC Press, Boca Raton, 2002.

Libster, Martha. *Delmar's Integrative Herb Guide for Nurses.* Delmar, 2002.

Lininger et al. *The Natural Pharmacy.* Healthnotes, Prima Pub. Rocklin Ca, 1999.

L'Orange Darlena, *Herbal Healing Secrets of the Orient.* Prentice Hall, New Jersey, 1998.

Lock, Carolyn. *Country Colours.* Nova Scotia Museum. 1981

Lovejoy, Sharon. *Sunflower Houses.* Workman Pub Co. New York 2001.

Lu, Henry. *Using Foods to Stay Young,* Sterling Press, New York, 1996.

_____*Chinese Natural Cures.* Black Dog & Leventhal Pub. New York, 1994

Luetjohann, Sylvia. *The Healing Power of Black Cumin.* Lotus Light, Twin Lakes, WI, 1998

Lyle, Katie Letcher. *The Wild Berry Book,* NorthWord Press, Minocqua, WI, 1994.

Mabey, Richard. *Plantcraft.* Universe Books. 1978.

MacKinnon, Pojar, Coupe. *Plants of Northern British Columbia.* Lone Pine Press, 1992.

Mailhebiau, Philippe. *Portraits in Oils.* C.W. Daniel Company, Essex, England, 1995.

Malmud, René. *The Amazon Problem,* trans by M. Stein, Spring Pub. Dallas TX, 1980.

Maloof, Joan. *Teaching the Trees, Lessons from the Forest.* U Georgia Pr, Athena GA. 2005.

Manandhar, N.P. *Plants and People of Nepal.* Timber Press, Portland, Oregon, 2002.

Maple, Eric. *The Secret Lore of Plants and Flowers.* Robert Hale Ltd. London 1980.

March, Kathryn & Andrew. *The Wild Plant Companion.* Meridian Hill Pub. 1986.

Marles, Robin. *The Ethnobotany of the Chipewyan of Northern Saskatchewan,* 1984. Thesis.

_____et al. *Aboriginal Plant Use in Canada's Northwest Boreal Forest.* UBC Press, Vancouver, and Natural Resources Canada, 2000

McBride, L.R. *Practical Folk Medicine of Hawaii.* Petroglyph Press, Hilo,Hawaii, 1975.

McCune B. & Geiser L. *Macrolichens of the Pacific Northwest.* Oregon State U. Press, 1997

McFarland, Phoenix. *The Complete Book of Magical Names.* Llewellyn Pub. St Paul 1996

McGrath, Judy. *Dyes from Lichens and Plants.* Van Nostrand Rheinhold, 1977.

McGuffin, Nancy. *Spectrum: dye plants of Ontario.* Burr House Spinner, Richmond Hill '86

Mc Intyre, Anne. *The Complete Woman's Herbal,* Henry Holt, New York, 1995.

Mears, R & Hillman,G. Wild Food. Hodder and Stoughton

MELODY. *Love is in the Earth, A Kaleidoscope of Crystals.* Earth Love Pub. Col. 1995.

Mercatante, A. S. The Facts on File Encyclopedia of World Mythology. New York 1988

Merriam, C. Hart. *Dawn of the World, Weird Tales of Mewan Indians.* Arthur H. Clark, Cleveland, 1910

Meyer, George et al. *Folk Medicine and Herbal Healing,* Charles Thomas, Springfield, 1981

Meyerowitz,Steve. *Sprout It!* The Sprout House, Box 1100,Great Barrington, MA, 1993.

Meyers, Edward C. *Basic Bush Survival,* Hancock House, Surrey, B.C. 1997.

Miller, L &Murray,W. *Herbal Medicinals A Clinician's Guide.* Hawthorn Press, N.Y. 1998.

Miller, Sandra. Editor Echinacea- Medicinal and Aromatic Plants. CRC Press, 2004.

Mills S. & Bone,K. *Principles and Practice of Phytotherapy.* Churchill Livingstone, 2000.

_____*The Essential Guide to Herbal Safety.* Churchill Livingstone, 2005.

Mills, Simon. *Out of the Earth.* Viking Penquin Books, Toronto. 1991.

Millsbaugh, Charles. *American Medicinal Plants,* Dover Pub. New York, 1974

Milne, Courtney. *Visions of the Goddess,* Penguin Studio, Toronto, 1998

Minnis & Elisens. *Biodiversity and Native America.* U. Oklahoma Press, 2000.

Mitchel, Jr. Wm. *Plant Medicine in Practice.* Churchill Livingstone, St. Louis, 2003.

Moerman, Daniel, *Medicinal Plants of Native America.* U of Michigan No. 19, 1986

Mohammed, G. *Catnip & Kerosene Grass* Candlenut Books, Sault Ste. Marie, Ont, 2002.

Montgomery, Pam. *Plant Spirit Healing.* Bear and Company, Rochester, VT 2008.

Moore, Michael. *Los Remedios.* Red Crane Books, 1990

_____*Medicinal Plants of the Desert and Canyon West.* Museum of New Mexico Press 1989

_____*Medicinal Plants of the Mountain West,* Museum of New Mexico Press '79

_____Med Plants of the Mountain West. Revised, expanded. 2003

_____*Medicinal Plants of the Pacific West,* Red Crane Books, 1993

More, Daphne. *The Bee Book,* Universe Books, New York, 1976.

Morelli, I. et al. *Selected Medicinal Plants.* University of Pisa. FAO 53/1

Morton, Julia. *Major Medicinal Plants* . Charles Thomas, Springfield, Illinois 1977

_____*Atlas of Medicinal Plants of Middle America, Bahamas to Yucatan.* 1981

Moss, E.H. *Flora of Alberta.* University of Toronto Press. 1983

Mother, The. *Flowers and their Messages.* Sri Aurobindo Ashram Trust, India 1979.

Mourning Dove. Coyote Stories. Caxton Press Caldwell Idaho. 1933.

Mowrey, Daniel. *The Scientific Validation of Herbal Medicine.* Cormorant Books, 1986.

Mucz, Michael. *Baba's Kitchen Medicines.* U of Alberta Press, Edmonton, 2012.

Mulders, Evelyn. *Western Herbs for Eastern Meridian & 5 Element Theory. Self publ. 2006.*

Mulligan, G editor *The biology of Canadian Weeds,* 1-32 Pub. 1693 Ag Canada 1979

_____33-61 Pub. 1765 Ag Canada 1984

Murphy, Cristine Editor, *Practical Home Care Medicine,* Lantern Books, New York, 2001

Murray, Michael. *The Pill Book Guide to Natural Medicines.* Bantam Books, April, 2002.

_____& Pizzorno, J. The condensed Encycl of Healing Foods. Pocket Books NY 2005.

Naegele, Thomas A. *Edible and Medicinal Plants of the Great Lakes Region,* Wilderness Adventure Books, Davisburg, Michigan. 1996.

Naiman, Ingrid. *Cancer Salves, A Botanical Approach to Treatment.* N. Atlantic Books, 99.

Nesse R & Williams G. *Why We Get Sick.* Vintage Books/Random House, New York, 1996.

Neuwinger H.D. *African Traditional Medicine.* Medpharm Sci. Pub. Stuttgart 2000.

_____African Ethnobotany, Poisons and Drugs. Chapman & Hall, London 1996.

Newcombe C.F. unpub notes on Haida plants. Dept of Anthro. Am Mus Nat Hist. NY 1897

_____unpublished papers. Prov Archives B.C. Victoria. 1898-1913.

Nicander. *The Poems and Poetical Fragments.* Cambridge U. Press, New York, 1953.

Norman,Howard. *Northern Tales.* Pantheon Books, New York, 1990.

Northcote, Rosalind. *The Book of Herbs.* John Lane: The Bodley Head, London, 1912.

Null, Gary. *The Clinician's Handbook of Natural Healing.* Kensington Books, N.Y. 1997.

Olive, Barbara. *The Flower Healer.* Cico Books, London and New York. 2007.

Ollsin, Don. *Herbal Healing Journey-Playful Workbook.* Aquiline Comm, Victoria,BC 1998.

Ootoova I. et al. *Interviewing Inuit Elders, Perspectives on Traditional Health.* Vol 5, Nunavut Arctic College, Box 600, Iqaluit, Nunavut X0Z 0H0.

Page, George. *Inside the Animal Mind.* Doubleday, New York, 1999.

Pallasdowney, Rhonda. *The Complete Book of Flower Essences.* New World Library, 2002.

Pappalardo, Joe. Sunflowers (the secret history). The Overlook Press. Woodstock NY 2008.

Parish, Coupé & Lloyd. *Plants of S. Interior British Columbia*. Lone Pine Edmonton 1996

Park, Willard Z. *Ethnographic Notes on the Norhern Paiute of Western Nevada, 1933-40* compiled by Catherine Fowler, U. of Utah, Salt Lake City, 1989.

Parvati, J. *Hygieia, A Woman's Herbal*. Freestone Collective. 1978

Paturi, Felix *Nature, Mother of Invention*. Harper and Row Pub. New York. 1976.

Peirce, Andrea. *Practical Guide to Natural Medicines*. Stonesong Press. 1999.

Pelikan, W. Healing Plants. Mercury Press, Spring Valley NY 1997.

Pellowski, Anne. *Hidden Stories in Plants*. MacMillan Pub. New York. 1990.

Penoel, Daniel & Franchomme, P. *L'Aromatherapie Exactement* , Roger Jollois, France, 1990

Peneol, Daniel. *Medecine Aromatique, Medecine Planetaire*. Roger Jollois France 1991.

_____& Peneol, Rose-Marie. *Natural Home Health Care Using Essential Oils*. Osmobiose Pub. 1998.

People of 'Ksan, The. *Gathering What the Great Nature Provided*. Douglas & Mc Intyre. Vancouver, B.C. 1980.

Peters, Josephine & Ortiz B. After the First Full Moon in April. Left Coast Press. Walnut Creek CA, 2010.

Pettitt, Sabina. Energy Medicine, Healing from the Kingdoms of Nature, Pacific Essences, Box 8317, Victoria, B.C. V8W 3R9 Canada, 1999

Phaneuf, Holly. Herbs Demystified. Marlowe and Company, New York. 2005

Pielou, E.C. *The Naturalist's Guide to the Arctic*. U. of Chicago Press. 1994.

Pieroni, A & Price L. Eating and Healing, Trad Food as Medicine. Haworth Press. N.Y. 2006.

Pfeiffer E. *The Earth's Face and Human Destiny*, Rodale Press, Emmaus, Pa. 1947.

Plotkin, Mark. *Medicine Quest*. Viking Penguin Books, New York, 2000.

Pojar, J & MacKinnon, A. *Plants of Coastal British Columbia* Lone Pine Edmonton 1994.

Pollock, L. With Faith and Physic: the life of a tudor gentlewoman. Collins & Brown,1993.

Polya, Gideon. *Biochemical Targets of Plant Bioactive Comp*. CRC Press, Boca Raton 2003

Pond, Barbara, *A Sampler of Wayside Herbs*, Chatham Press, Riverside, Conn.

Pressor, Arthur, *Pharmacist's Guide to Medicinal Herbs*, Smart Pub. Petaluma, CA,2000

Price, Len & Shirley. *Understanding Hydrolats*. Churchill Livingstone, Toronto, 2004.

_____Aromatherapy for Health Professionals. Churchill Livingstone 1995.

Purvis, William. *Lichens*. Smithsonian Institution Press. Washington D.C. 2000

Quin, Frederick F. *The Flora Homoeopathica*. B. Jain Pub. New Delhi, India. 1997.

Radin, Paul. *The Winnebago Tribe,* Bur of Am Ethnology, Smithsonian Inst. 37th. 1923.

Rätsch, C. *Plants of Love, The History of Aphrodisiacs*. Ten Speed Press, Berkeley,1997.

_____The Dictionary of Sacred & Magical Plants. ABC-CLIO St Barbara 1992.

_____The Encyclopedia of Psychoactive Plants. Park St Press. 2005.

Raven Essences. www.ravenessences.com

Ravenworks flower essences. www.ravenworksministries.weebly.com

Reaume, Tom. 620 Wild Plants of North America. Nature Manitoba. Canadian Plains Research Center, U of Regina, U of Toronto Press. 2009.

Reckeweg, Hans-Heinrich, *Materia Medica, Vol 1. Aurelia-Verlag GmbH, Baden Baden* 1996.

Reich, Lee. *Uncommon Fruits Worthy of Attention,* Addison-Wesley Pub. 1991.

Reid, Daniel, *A handbook of Chinese Healing Herbs,* Shambala, Boston, 1995

Rhode, David. Native Plants of Southern Nevada. U of Utah Press. 2002.

Richards B & Kanecko A. *Japanese Plants- Know Them &Use Them*. Shufunotomo, Tokyo 1995

Richardson, David. *The Vanishing Lichens*. David and Charles, Vancouver, BC, 1975

Riddle, John M. *Eve's Herbs*. Harvard U Press. Cambridge Mass. 1997.

_____Goddesses, Elixirs and Witches. Palgrave MacMillan. England 2010.

Rister, Robert. *Healing Without Medication.* Basic Health Pub. N. Bergen, N.J. 2003.

Roberts, Jonathan. *The Origins of Fruit and Vegetables.* Universe Pub. New York. 2001.

Robicsek, F. *The Smoking God: Tobacco....*Norman: U. of Oklahoma Press, 1978.

Robinson, Peggy. *Profiles of Northwest Plants.* Far West Book Service. Portland, OR 1979

Rogers, Dilwyn. *Edible, Medicinal, Useful & Poisonous Wild Plants of the Northern Great Plains —South Dakota Region.* Buechel Memorial Lakota Museum, St. Francis,SD, 1980.

Rogers, Pattiann. *Firekeeper:New & Selected Poems.* Milkweed Editions, 1994.

Rogers, Robert Dale. *Sundew Moonwort Vols-1-7, self-published.* Edmonton 1995-present.

_____Rogers' Herbal Manual. Karamat Wilderness Ways, Edmonton, 2000.

_____& Capital Health, Herbal Drug Interactions. Mediscript Comm. 2003.

_____The Fungal Pharmacy, The Complete Guide to Medicinal Mushrooms and Lichens of North America, North Atlantic Books 2011.

Rombi, Max. *Phytotherapy.* Herbal Health Publishers. U.K. 1990.

Rosengarten,Jr. F. *The Book of Edible Nuts.* Walker and Co. New York. 1984.

Ross, Gary. *Nature's Guide to Healing.* Freedom Press, Topanga, Ca. 2000.

Ross, Ivan. *Medicinal Plants of the World.* Vol 1 Humana Press, Totowa, New Jersey. 1999.

_____ Vol 2 Humana Press, Totowa, N. J. 2002.

Rotella, Rev. Alexis. *The Essence of Flowers,* Jade Mountain Press, N.J. 1991.

Royer F. & Dickinson R. *Plants of Alberta.* Lone Pine Pub. Edmonton, AB. 2007.

Rudginsky, Marlene *The Flower Speaks.* U.S. Games Systems, Stamford, Conn. 1999.

Rupp, Rebecca. *Red Oaks and Black Birches* , Storey Comm. Garden Way Publishing. 1990

Russell, Sharman Apt. *Anatomy of a Rose.* Perseus Pub. Cambridge, Mass. 2001.

_____An Obsession with Butterflies. Perseus Publishing 2003.

Ryan, J et al, *Traditional Dene Medicine.* Lac La Martre NWT, 1993.

Ryden, Hope. *Wildflowers around the year.* Clarion Books, New York. 2001.

Ryrie, Charlie. Garden Folklore That Works. Reader's Digest. Pleasantville, NY 2001.

Sagadic O. & Ozcan M. *Food Control* 2003 14.

Salmon, Wm. *Botanologia: The English Herbal.* London: I. Dawkes, 1710.

Sandberg & Corrigan. *Natural Remedies, their origins and uses.* Taylor & Francis 2001.

Sanders, Jack. *The Secrets of Wildflowers.* The Lyons Press, Guilford, CT, 2003.

Sapolsky, Robert. *The Trouble with Testosterone.* Scribner, New York. 1997.

Sauer, Johann Christopher, Compendious Herbal-see Weaver below.

Savage, Candace. Bees, Nature's Little Wonders. Greystone Books. Vancouver 2008.

Schalkwijk-Barendsen, Helene. *Mushrooms of Western Canada* . Lone Pine Pub. 1991.

Schar, Douglas. *The Backyard Medicine Chest.* Elliott&Clark Pub. Washington, DC. 1995.

Scheffer, Mechthild, *Bach Flower Therapy, Theory and Practice,* Healing Arts Press, 1988

Schenk, George. *Moss Gardening.* Timber Press, Portland Oregon. 1997.

Schnaubelt, Kurt. *Medical Aromatherapy.* Frog Ltd. Berkeley CA. 1999.

Schneider, Anny. *Wild Medicinal Plants.* Key Porter Books, Toronto. 2002.

Schnell, Donald. *Carnivorous Plants.* 2nd Ed. Timber Press, Portland, Oregon, 2002.

Schofield, Janice. *Discovering Wild Plants.* Alaska Northwest Books. 1989.

_____*Nettles.* Keats Publishing, New Canaan, Conneticut, 1998.

Schulman, Robert. *Solve It With Supplements.* Rodale Press. New York. 2007.

Shapiro, R & Rapkins J. Awakening to the Plant Kingdom, Cassandra Press 1991.

Shauenberg, Paul and Paris. *Guide to Medicinal Plants.* Keats Publishing, 1977.

Shook, Edward Dr. *Advanced Treatise on Herbology* . Reprint Health Research.

Shosteck,Robert. *Flowers and Plants.* Quadrangle/The New York Times Book Co. 1974.

Siegfried, EV. Masters Thesis, Ethnobotany of the Northern Cree of Wabasca/Desmarais. U of Calgary, Alberta. 1994.

Silverman, Maida. *A City Herbal.* David R. Godine , 1990.

Silvertown, Jonathan. An Orchard Invisible. U of Chicago Press. 2009.

Simonot, Danielle. *Bio-Manufacturing in Saskatchewan-* Assessment of the Manufacturing Potential of Select Saskatchewan Plants, Sask. Nutraceutical Network, Saskatoon, 2000

Simpson, Brenan, M. *Flowers At My Feet,* Hancock House, Surrey, B.C. 1996.

Sionneau, P. *An Introduction to the Use of Processed Chinese Medicinals.* Blue Poppy Press, Second Printing 2003, Translated by Bob Flaws.

Smagghe, Guy Ed. Ecdysone: Structures and Functions. Springer Sci 2009.

Small, E & Catling, P. *Canadian Medicinal Crops,* NRC Research Press, Ottawa 1999.

Small, Ernest. *Culinary Herbs, Second Ed.* NRC Research Press, Ottawa, 2006.

_____*Medicinal Herbs,* NRC Research Press, Ottawa, 2000.

_____Top 100 Food Plants. NRC Press, Ottawa. 2009.

Smith, Andrew. *Strangers in the Garden, the Secret Lives of Our Favorite Flowers.*McClelland & Stewart 2004.

Smith, Annie Lorrain. *Lichens,* Cambridge at the University Press, 1921.

Smith, Harlan, *Ethnobotany of the Gitksan Indians of B.C.* Edited by B. Compton, B. Rigsby, and M.L. Tarpent, Mercury Series, Can Ethno Service, Paper 132, Can Mus of Civil. 1997.

Smith, Huron H. Manataka American Indian Council. www.manataka.org.

Snell, Alma Hogan. A Taste of Heritage. Crow Indian Recipes and Herbal Medicines. University of Nebraska Press 2006.

Soule, Deb. *The Roots of Healing, A Woman's Book of Herbs.* Citadel Press, 1995.

Spencer, Kate. *The Magic of Green Buckwheat* ,Richard Clay, England, 1987.

Spinella, Marcello. *The Psychopharmacology of Herbal Medicine.* MIT Press, 2001.

Steedman, E.V. *The Ethnobotany of the Thompson Indians of British Columbia.* 1930.

Stein, Sara. *My Weeds, A Gardener's Botany.* Harper and Row, 1988.

Stern, Gai. *Australian Weeds.* Harper and Row, Australia 1986

Stern Wm. *Stern's Dictionary of Plant Names for Gardeners.* Cassell Pub, London, 1972

Stewart, Hilary. *CEDAR.* Douglas & Mc Intyre. Vancouver/Toronto, 1984.

Storl, Wolf D. Healing Lyme Disease Naturally. NorthAtlantic Books, Berkeley, CA 2010.

Strehlow,W & Hertzka,G. *Hildegard of Bingen's Medicine* Bear & Co. Santa Fe 1988

Stuart, David. *Dangerous Garden.* Harvard University Press, Cambridge, Mass. 2004

Sturdivant L.&Blakley,T. *Medicinal Herbs in the Garden, Field and Marketplace* Bootstrap Guide, San Juan Naturals, Friday Harbor,WA, 1999.

Sumner, Judith. *The Natural History of Medicinal Plants.* Timber Press, Oregon, 2000.

Sun Bear & Wabun, *The Medicine Wheel* Prentice Hall, NJ 1980.

Swanton, J.R. *Haida Texts and Myths.* Bureau Am Ethnol, Bull #29. Smithsonian Inst. Washington, D.C. 1905.

_____*Bureau of Am Ethno 26th Ann Report.* Smithsonian Inst. Washington, 1908.

Szczeklik, Andrzej. Kore: On Sickness, the Sick and the Search for the Soul of Medicine. Counterpoint Berkeley 2012.

Tainter, D& Grenis A, *Spices and Seasonings* , VCH Pubishers, New York, 1993.

Talalaj,S.& Czechowicz,A S. *Herbal Remedies,* Hill of Content Press, Melbourne, 1989

Taylor, Wm &Farnsworth,N. The Vinca Alkaloids, Marcel Dekker, New York, 1973.

Teeguarden, Ron. *The Ancient Wisdom of the Chinese Tonic Herbs.* Warner Bros. 1998.

Telesco, Patricia. *The Victorian Flower Oracle,* Llewellyn Pub. St. Paul 1994

Temple, Robert. *The Genius of China*. Simon and Schuster. New York. 1986.

Thompson, Gerry, *Astral Sex to Zen Teabags*. Findhorn Press, 1994.

Thoreau, Henry David. *Wild Fruits*. W. W. Norton & Co. New York, 2000.

Throop, Priscilla. *Hildegard von Bingen's Physica*. Healing Arts Press, Vt. 1998.

Tick, Edward. *The Practice of Dream Healing*. Quest Books Wheaton, Illinois, 2001.

Tierra, Michael. *The Way of Herbs- revised Pocket Rooks*, New York, 1998.

Tigner, Daniel. *Canadian Forest Tree Essences,* self published,1998. ISBN 0968365809

Tilford, Gregory. *Edible and Medicinal Plants of the West*. Mountain Press, Missoula 1997.

Timbrook, Jan. Chumash Ethnobotany. St. Barbara Mus, Heyday Books, Berkeley Ca 2007.

Traill, E.C. *Studies of Plant Life in Canada*. A. S. Woodburn, Ottawa, 1885.

Traill, C. P. *The Backwoods of Canada*. McClelland and Stewart. Toronto. 1846.

Tobyn, G., Denham, A., Whitelegg, M. The Western Herbal Tradition. 2000 years of medicinal herbal knowledge. Churchill Livingstone Toronto 2011.

Toop, Edgar W & Williams, Sara. *Perennials for the Prairies*. U of A&Saskatchewan. 1991.

Treben, Maria. *Health Through God's Pharmacy*. Wilhelm Ennsthaler. 1982.

Tresidder, Jack. Symbols and Their Meaning. Friedman/Fairfax Pub. 2007.

Tucker A. & DeBaggio,T. *The Big Book of Herbs*. Interweave Press. Loveland CO. 2000.

_____The Encylcopedia of Herbs. Timber Press, Portland. 2009.

Turkington, Carol. *The Home Health Guide to Poisons and Antidotes,* Facts on File 1994

Turner, Nancy J. *Food Plants of Interior First Peoples*. UBC Press, Vancouver, 1997.

_____*Food Plants of Coastal First Peoples*. UBC Press, Vancouver, 1995.

_____*Plant Technology of First Peoples in B.C.* UBC Press, Vancouver, 1998.

_____et al. *Thompson Ethnobotany*. Memoir #3, Royal B.C. Museum, 1996.

_____*Plants of Haida Gwaii*. Sononis Press, Winlaw, B.C. 2004.

_____The Earth's Blanket. Douglas & Mc Intyre. Vancouver. 2005.

Turner, N & von Aderkas, P. Common Poisonous Plants and Mushrooms. Timber Press 2009

Turner, W.B. *Fungal Metabolites,* Academic Press, London and New York, 1971.

Twitchell, Paul. *Herbs The Magic Healers*. Eckankar, Box 3100 Menlo Park, CA, 1986.

Vermeulen, Nico. *Encyclopedia of Herbs*. Whitecap Books, Vancouver B.C. 1998.

Viereck, Eleanor, G. *Alaska's Wilderness Medicines*. Alaska Northwest Pub. 1987

Vitt, Marsh and Bovey, *Mosses, Lichens, and Ferns,* Lone Pine Press, 1988.

Vogel, A. *Swiss Nature Doctor*. A. Vogel, Switzerland. 1952

_____*Nature-Your Guide to Healthy Living*. Verlag A. Vogel, Teufen, Switzerland 1986.

Vogel, Virgil. *American Indian Medicine,* U. of Oklahoma Press, Norman, 1970

Vortex Essences (Mt. Shasta Essences) www.vortexessences.com

Walker, Barbara. *The Woman's Dictionary of Symbols&Sacred Objects*. Csstle Books, 1988.

Walker, Marilyn. Wild Plants of Eastern Canada. Nimbus Pub. Halifax NS. 2008.

Ward, Bobby J. The Plant Hunter's Garden. Timber Press, Portland. 2004.

Ward-Harris, Joan.*More Than Meets the Eye, The Life and Lore of Western Wildflowers* Oxford University Press, Toronto, 1983

Watanabe & Shibuya. *Pharmacological Research on Traditional Herbal Medicines*. Harwood Academic Publishers, 1999.

Watt, John, and Breyer-Brandwijk, Maria *The Medicinal and Poisonous Plants of Southern and Eastern Africa* . E and S. Livingstone. Edinburgh and London. 1962.

Watts, Donald. Elsevier's Dictionary of Plant Lore. Elsevier. 2007.

Waugh, F.W. *Iroquois Foods and Food Preparation* #12 Anthropological Series, Ottawa. 1916. Reprinted by
    Iroqrafts, RR #2, Ohsweken, Ontario N0A 1M0, 1991.

Weaver, Wm. *100 Vegetables & Where They Came From.* Workman Pub. New York, 2000.

_____*Sauer's Herbal Cures America's First Book of Botanic Healing 1762-1778,* Routledge, New York, 2001.

Weed, Susan. *Menopausal Years, The Wise Woman Way.* Ash Tree Pub. Woodstock NY, 1992

Weigle, Marta. *Spiders and Spinsters.* U. of New Mexico Press, Albuquerque, 1982.

Weiner, M. *The People's Herbal, A family guide.* Putnam Publishing, New York, 1984.

Weiss, Rudolf. *Herbal Medicine.* Beaconsfield Publishers, 1988.

_____*Herbal Medicine* 2nd Edition. Thieme, Stuttgart, New York, 2000.

Wells, Diana.*100 Flowers and How They Got Their Names,* Algonquin Books, Chapel Hill,97

Westcott, Frank. *The Beaver Nature's Master Builder.* Hounslow Press, Willowdale, ON '89.

Westrich, LoLo, *California Herbal Remedies,* Gulf Pub Co. Houston, TX, 1989.

Wetzel, Suzanne et al. Bioproducts from Canada's Forests. Springer Netherlands 2006.

WHO monographs on selected medicinal plants, vol 1, 1999; vol 2, 2002.

White, Ian. *Australian Bush Flower Essences.* Bantam Books, 1991

White, Florence. *Flowers as Food* . Jonathan Cape. 1934

Whitmont, Edward. *Psyche and Substance.* North Atlantic Books. 1980

Wilkinson, Kathleen. *Trees and Shrubs of Alberta.* Lone Pine Books, Edmonton 1990.

_____*Wildflowers of Alberta.* U of A/Lone Pine Books, Edmonton 1999.

Williams, Jude. *Nature's Gentle Cures.* Sterling Publishing. New York. 1997.

Williamson, Darcy. 130 Medicinal Plant Monographs of the NW. self pub. E-book. 2011.

Williamson, E. *Major Herbs of Ayurveda.* Churchill Livingstone, Elsevier Science, 2002.

FLOWER ESSENCE RESOURCES

Aditi Himalaya Flower Essences, 15,Jaybharat Society, 3rd Road, Khar (W), Bombay 400 052, India.

Alaskan Flower Essence Project, P.O. Box. 1369, Homer, Alaska USA 99603-1369. www.alaskanessences.com.

Australian Bush Flower Essences. Australia. www.ausflowers.com.au.

Bach- Healing Herbs English Flower Essences- in Canada by Self Heal Distributing, Box 95008, Whyte Postal Outlet, Edmonton, AB T6E 0E5, 1800-593-5956 or www.selfhealdistributing.com Also www.healingherbs.co.uk or www.fesflowers.com

Bailey Flower Essences, 8 Neslon Road, Ilkley, West Yorkshire England, LS298HN. www.flowervr.com

Bloesem Remedies. Netherlands. www.bloesem-remedies.com

BrynaHerb Essences. www.brynaherbessences.uk

Canadian Forest Essences, PO Box 29128,1996 W. Broadway, Vancouver, BC V6J 1Z0

Canadian Forest Tree Essences. Ottawa. www.essences.ca. 613-725-9764.

Choming Flower Essences. www.mkprojects.com

Clear Path Essences. www.clearpathessences.com

Dancing Light Orchid Essences. Fairbanks, Alaska. www.orchidessences.com

Desert Alchemy, PO Box 44189, Tucson, Arizona, USA 85733. www.desert-alchemy.com.

Deva Flower Essences BP3 38880, Autrans, France. www.lab-deva.com

Eastern Flower Herbal Essences. julied@hfx.eastlink.ca.

Falling Leaf Essences. Box 78, Kallista, Victoria 3791, Australia. www.advancedalchemy.com.au.

Findhorn Flower Essences, Morayshire, Scotland IV36 0TY. www.findhornessences.com

Florais des Minas, Rua Albita, 194-Sala 408, Cruziero, CEP 30310-160,BH, MG, BRAZIL

FlorAlive˚, Brent Davis. Contact info@floralive.com

FES Flower Essence Society, PO Box 1769, Nevada City, California, USA, 95959. www.fesflowers.com Canadian Distributor- Self Heal Distributing, Box 95008, Whyte Postal Outlet, Edmonton, AB T6E 0E5 – www.selfhealdistributing.com

Green Hope Farm Flower Essences, PO Box 125, Meriden, New Hampshire USA 03770

Green Man Tree Essences. www.greenmantrees.demon.co.uk.

Habundia Flower Essences. c/o Peter Aziz. PO Box 90, Totnes, Devon, England TQ11 0YG.

Harebell Remedies. Scotland. ellie@harebellremedies.co.uk.

Hawaiian Gaia Flower Essences. www.gaiaessences.com

High Sierra Flower Essences. PO. Box 4275 Truclee, CA 96160. holly.hsb@highoctavehealing.com

Horus Flower Essences- horus@floweressences.de.

Hummingbird Remedies, PO Box 50161, Eugene, Oregon, USA 97405

Icelandic Flower Essences. www.kristbjorb.is.

Jade Mountain Flower Essences, Box 125, Mountain Lakes, New Jersey USA 07046-0125

Korte Phi. www.PHIessences.com

Light Heart Essences. England. www.lightheartessences.co.uk.

Light Mountain Flower Essences, Michael A. Vertolli, 1-800-667-HERB.

Living Essences of Australia, Box 355, Scarborough, 6019, Perth, Australia. www.livingessences.com.au

Living Flower Essences, www.livingfloweressences.com . Rhonda Pallasdowney.

Master's Flower Essences, 14618 Tyler Foote Rd Nevada City, California, USA, 95959. www.masteressences.com

Miriana fortem Flower Essences. www.mirianaflowers.com and info@miraflowers.com.

NaturaSacredplay, PO Box 32, Buckhorn, New Mexico, 88025, (505-535-2255).

New Millenium Flower Essences of New Zealand. info@nmessences.com.

New Zealand New Perception Flower Essences, PO Box 60-127,Titirangi, Auckland 7, NZ

Pacific Essences, Box 8317, Victoria, B.C. V8W 3R9. www.pacificessences.com.

Pegasus Products, PO Box 228, Boulder, Colorado, USA 80306-0228. 1-800- 527-6104.

Perelandra, Box 3603, Warrenton, VA. 22186. www.perelandra-ltd.com

Petite Fleur Essence, 8524 Whispering Creek Trail, Fort Worth, Texas, USA 76134. www.aromahealthtexas.com

Prairie Deva Flower Essences, Box 95008, Whyte Postal Outlet, Edmonton, AB T6E 0E5 1-(780) 433-7882. www.selfhealdistributing.com

Ravenworks- joni@ravenworksministries.org

Running Fox Farm PO Box 381,Worthington, Maryland USA 01098

Star Peruvian Flower Essences. Santa Barbara. www.starfloweressences.com

Stars of the Meadow, David Dalton, Lindisfarne Books, Mass. 2006.

Sun Essences. Norfolk, England. www.sunessence.co.uk

Sweetwater Sanctuary Essences. www.plantspirithealing.com

Tree Frog Farm Flower Essences. www.treefrogfarm.com

Whole Energy Essences, PO Box 285, Concord, Mass. 01742

Wild Rose Essences. www.wildrose.com

Woodland Essence, PO Box 206, Cold Brook, New York, USA 13324.

www.ingramcontent.com/pod-product-compliance
Lightning Source LLC
Chambersburg PA
CBHW081108170526
45165CB00008B/2371